# Adaptive Mechanisms in Gaze Control

## Facts and Theories

# Reviews of Oculomotor Research

*Series Editors*

D.A. Robinson     H. Collewijn

*Baltimore*     *Rotterdam*

*Advisory Editors*

R. Baker, A. Berthoz, J.A. Büttner-Ennever, B. Cohen, A.F. Fuchs, V. Henn,
E.L. Keller, G. Melvill Jones, F.A. Miles, W. Precht, A. Skavenski,
D.L. Sparks and D.S. Zee

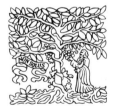

## ELSEVIER

**AMSTERDAM · NEW YORK · OXFORD**

Reviews of Oculomotor Research
Volume 1

# Adaptive Mechanisms in Gaze Control

## Facts and Theories

*Edited by*

A. Berthoz   G. Melvill Jones

*Laboratoire de Physiologie*   *Aerospace Medical Research Unit*
*Neurosensorielle du CNRS*   *McGill University*
*Paris*   *Montreal*
*France*   *Canada*

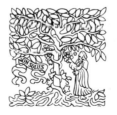

**1985**

## ELSEVIER

**AMSTERDAM · NEW YORK · OXFORD**

ISBN 0–444–80483–8
ISSN 0168–8375

*Published by:*
Elsevier Science Publishers B.V. (Biomedical Division)
P.O. Box 211
1000 AE Amsterdam
The Netherlands

*Sole distributors for the USA and Canada:*
Elsevier Science Publishing Company, Inc.
52 Vanderbilt Avenue
New York, NY 10017
USA

**Library of Congress Cataloging in Publication Data**

Main entry under title:

Adaptive mechanisms in gaze control.

    (Reviews of oculomotor research, ISSN 0168–8375;
v. 1)
    Bibliography: p.
    Includes index.
    1. Gaze—Regulation. 2. Eye—Movements—Regulation.
3. Eye—Accommodation and refraction. I. Berthoz, A.
II. Melvill Jones, Geoffrey. III. Series. [DNLM:
1. Accommodation, Ocular. 2. Adaptation, Ocular.
3. Eye Movements. 4. Fixation, Ocular.
W1 RE253JNM v.1 / WW 400 A221]
QP477.5.A33 1985    612′.846    85–4329
ISBN 0–444–80483–8 (U.S.)

**Printed in the Netherlands**

# Preface

# A review of an unanswered question?

A. Berthoz[a] & G. Melvill Jones[b]

[a] Laboratoire de Physiologie Neurosensorielle du CNRS, F-75270 Paris, Cédex 06, France and [b] Aerospace Medical Research Unit, Department of Physiology, McGill University, Montréal, Canada H3G 1Y6

It is both a privilege and a responsibility to open this new series of Reviews on Oculomotor Research with a book on Adaptive Mechanisms since the topic, in all its facets, represents one of the most fascinating, yet least understood, areas of brain research today. During the past decade or so an intensive burst of research effort has uncovered a broad range of behaviourally induced adaptive responses to sensory rearrangement in the *external* visual environment. Again, there is growing, although as yet limited, evidence of a vigorous potential for central plastic reactions to both central and peripheral neural lesions *within* the vestibulo-oculomotor system. Yet whether or not such lesion-induced plastic reactions in the CNS (e.g., sprouting; reactive synaptogenesis) represent mechanisms which participate in behavioural adaptation still remains an unsettled question; as indeed does the rôle played by underlying neuro-pharmacological processes. As a result, this volume emerges as *a book on an unanswered question*.

Nevertheless, we feel that present knowledge in the field has reached something of a 'critical mass', which is pregnant with possibilities for future developments. Consequently, we have asked a few of the many workers in this area to review each a particular aspect of the field, as viewed within one of three complementary wings of adaptation research, represented respectively by Behavioural, Neuronal and Theoretical studies. Contributors have been encouraged to generate lively reviews of

'facts and theories' with the object of making this book a working tool, rather than a pretentious synthesis of as yet unclear mechanisms. The outcome is a diversity of chapters, some being relatively didactic reviews of a specific question area, others emerging as rather individualistic 'credos', or even short summaries of recent experiments when we thought they were milestones for the understanding of the main question.

Before introducing the streamline of these various chapters it is appropriate to indicate absent topics. The reader will not find here recent data concerning axonal plasticity after peripheral motor lesions, such as has been studied by Baker et al. (1981b). Indeed, contrary to the fields of vision or olfaction, the topic of neuronal regrowth mechanisms represents something of a lacuna in the study of adaptive mechanisms in vestibulo-oculomotor pathways. Another area which will only be treated in a few of its extensive ramifications is the behavioural response to peripheral vestibular lesions, known as 'vestibular compensation'. A number of reviews of this subject are available elsewhere (e.g., Kornhuber, 1974; Cohen, 1981; Precht, 1979; Hecaen & Jeannerod, 1979) and we have preferred to focus on the neuronal and neuropharmacological correlates of functional recovery (see Chapters 17 & 18). Also, the subject of central neurophysiological correlates of adaptation to altered visual-vestibular interactions, as inferred from unit neural recordings, has been treated rather selectively, owing to the excellent recent reviews of Miles & Lisberger (1981b) and Ito (1982a) on this topic. Finally, it is unfortunate that, owing to repeated flight delays, we have not been able to include a review of currently emerging results from human experiments on adaptation to microgravity, conducted in the European Space Agency Spacelab, carried on the recent Columbia Shuttle mission of December, 1983. Preliminary results concerning gaze control have, however, been published (Von Baumgarten et al., 1984; Young et al., 1984; see also chapters 10 & 12).

The contents of the book follow a rationale which starts with an holistic approach. One of the most intriguing aspects of the adaptive phenomenon is that rather than being a mere curiosity of brain function, we believe it constitutes a fundamental property of the nervous system, responsible for active matching both between related subsystems within the CNS and between them and their daily encounter with the external physical world. In a comprehensive sense we envisage this general process operating over the three-fold perspective of phylogenetic evolution, ontogenetic development and moment-to-moment events in the everyday life of an individual organism. All these 'dimensions' are currently under investigation and one purpose of the book is to begin rationalizing the relations they bear to one another.

In another introductory chapter, Simpson & Graf examine phylogenetic and theoretical evidence for the evolution of a preferred set of internal coordinates for the inertia-sensing vestibular end-organs. From this stand point they go on to demonstrate that these particular coordinates appear to have called forth matching sets of 'internal' coordinates in both the relevant visual optokinetic system and the oculomotor efferent channels, as ultimately determined by the planes of action of the extraocular muscles. The facts and ideas which emerge serve to emphasize the fundamental need for proper matching between allied sensory-motor systems generally.

This brings us to the main content of our book, which focusses on a variety of adaptive mechanisms which evidently serve this rôle within the overall system responsible for the control of gaze. In the section on Behavioural studies we begin by reviewing those adaptive changes in the vestibulo-ocular reflex (VOR) which were first shown to be evoked by systematic rearrangement of the external visual environment. This is followed by an extension of visually induced adaptive phenomena to the combined interactions of vestibulo-ocular, optokinetic and pursuit mechanisms. Next are detailed the various adaptive consequences of modifying vestibular cues. Particularly important here is the likely difference between effects due to peripheral receptor changes (physical obstruction of fluid circulation in the canal for instance) and the central consequences of peripheral whole nerve section. Both kinds of manipulation produce vigorous adaptive responses, but do the mechanisms concerned represent fundamentally different kinds of central processes?

The last part of this section extends beyond the oculomotor system per se, to a consideration of integration with other allied systems. First, a perusal of clinical implications takes us through a variety of system interactions made apparent by the ubiquitous reach of pathological interference. The next chapter is devoted to head-eye coordination, which stands here as an example of how complex rearrangements can be produced by a graded action of subsystem manipulation. Finally, we offer a short account of a recent study demonstrating that alteration of mental set alone (i.e., in the absence of vision) proves sufficient to produce lasting alteration of the inherent goal-directed VOR. The additional fact that correlated perceptual changes emerge, raises intriguing philosophical questions concerning the rôle of adaptive mechanisms in establishing valid perceptual interpretation of events in the physical world around us.

The next main section on Neuronal Mechanisms opens with an appraisal of the current standing and significance of those findings and hypotheses which have emerged from the extensive studies of M. Ito and his colleagues (Ito, 1984). In turn, the controversial issue of cerebellar participation in adaptive processes is further examined from the view point of R. Llinás and his colleagues. Subsequent chapters in this section address questions of comparative functions in cerebellar cortex and vestibular nuclei and those plastic mechanisms, both neuronal and neuropharmacological, which accompany vestibular compensation after peripheral lesions. It will be found that the contents of this section are largely confined to studies at the level of brain stem and cerebellum. However, bearing in mind the evident participation of higher, including cognitive, levels in adaptive responses described in the latter chapters of the Behavioural section, there would seem to be a pressing need to extend future neuronal studies beyond the brain stem level.

The last section on Systematic Interpretations presents a number of formal hypotheses of possible adaptive mechanisms. Here we have not tried to be exhaustive, but rather to give some of our colleagues room to summarize the current state of their thinking on the matter. This is not a section on 'models' per se; the reader will find formal models throughout the book. Rather, it is a section concentrating on what we consider at this time in history to be the most promising theoretical advances in the field. These latter contributions have been chosen to help us move on from the essential, but relatively simplistic, description of experimentally observed phenomena, to a functionally meaningful interpretation of the system working as an integrated whole towards identified physiological goals.

No doubt these working statements of theoretical hypotheses will eventually suffer the fate of most useful 'models': they are made to be falsified in favour of better hypotheses. This may well also be the fate of the present volume, since the essential core of adaptive *Mechanisms* still remains to be discovered. We shall be happy if our book contributes in any way to the generation of new approaches and further understanding.

# Acknowledgements

We would like to thank the following organizations for their support in the accomplishment of this book:

Centre National de la Recherche Scientifique, France
McGill University, Montreal, Canada
Programmes d'Echange France-Quebec
Medical Research Council of Canada
Club Vision E.D.F., France
Centre National d'Etudes Spatiales, France.

The Editorial Secretary was M. Reda-Berthoz. Her contribution together with those of E. Wong, M. Franchetcau, H. Mayer, as well as the help of colleagues from the board of Editors and from our laboratories for reviewing the manuscripts is gratefully acknowledged.

# List of Authors

W. ABELN
*Fachbereich 3 (Biologie/Chemie) der Universität Bremen, Universität Bremen, NW2, Leobener Strasse, 2800 Bremen, F.R.G.*

A. BERTHOZ
*Laboratoire de Physiologie Neurosensorielle, CNRS, 15, rue de l'Ecole de Médecine, 75006 Paris, France*

B. COHEN
*The Mount Sinai Medical Center, One Gustave L. Levy Place, New York, NY 10029, U.S.A*

H. COLLEWIJN
*Department of Physiology, Erasmus University Rotterdam, P.O. Box 1738, Rotterdam, The Netherlands*

M. CYNADER
*Departments of Psychology and Physiology, Dalhousie University, Halifax, Nova Scotia, Canada B3H 4J1*

N. DIERINGER
*Institut für Hirnforschung der Universität Zürich, August Forelstrasse 1, Postfach, 8029 Zürich, Switzerland*

H. FLOHR
*Fachbereich 3 (Biologie/Chemie) der Universität Bremen, Universität Bremen, NW2, Leobener Strasse, 2800 Bremen, F.R.G.*

H. L. GALIANA
*Aerospace Medical Research Unit, McGill University, McIntyre Building, 3655 Drummond Street, Montréal, Québec, Canada H3G 1Y6*

W. GRAF
*Rockfeller University, 1230 York Avenue, New York, NY 10021-6399, U.S.A*

## V. HENN

*Kantonsspital Zürich, Neurol. Universitätsklinik U. Poliklinik, Rämistrasse 100, 8006 Zürich, Suisse*

## M. ITO

*Department of Physiology, Faculty of Medicine, University of Tokyo, Hongo, Bunkyo-Ku, Tokyo, Japan*

## M. JEANNEROD

*INSERM U. 94, Laboratoire de Neuropsychologie Experimentale, 16, Avenue du Doyen Lépine, 69672 Bron, France*

## S. G. LISBERGER

*Department of Physiology 762 - S, University of California, San Francisco, CA 94143, U.S.A*

## R. LLINÁS

*Department of Physiology and Biophysics, New York University Medical Center, 550 First Avenue, New York, NY 10016, U.S.A.*

## U. LÜNEBURG

*Fachbereich 3 (Biologie/Chemie) der Universität Bremen, Universität Bremen, NW2, Leobener Strasse, 2800 Bremen, F.R.G.*

## G. MELVILL JONES

*Aerospace Medical Research Unit, McGill University, McIntyre Building, 3655 Drummond Street, Montréal, Québec, Canada H3G 1Y6*

## F. A. MILES

*Laboratory of Sensorimotor Research, National Eye Institute, N.I.H., Building 10, Room 6C420, Bethesda, MD 20205, U.S.A*

## L. M. OPTICAN

*Laboratory of Sensorimotor Research, National Eye Institute, N.I.H., Building 10, Room 6C420, Bethesda, MD 20205, U.S.A*

## G. D. PAIGE

*Department of Ophthalmology, U – 490, School of Medicine, University of California, San Francisco, CA 94143, U.S.A*

## A. PELLIONISZ

*Department of Physiology and Biophysics, New York University Medical Center, 550 First Avenue, New York, NY 10016, U.S.A*

## W. PRECHT

*Institut fur Hirnforschung der Universität Zürich, August Forelstrasse 1, Postfach, 8029 Zürich, Switzerland*

T. RAPHAN
*Department of Computer and Information Science, Brooklyn College of CUNY, Bedford Avenue & Avenue H, Brooklyn, NY 11210, U.S.A*

D. A. ROBINSON
*Departments of Ophthalmology and Biomedical Engineering, The Johns Hopkins University, 355 Woods/Wilmer, 601 N. Broadway, Baltimore, MD 21205, U.S.A*

R. SCHMID
*Instituto di Elettronica dell Universita di Pavia, Strada Nuova 106/c, 27100 Pavia, Italia*

J. I. SIMPSON
*Department of Physiology and Biophysics, New York University Medical Center, 550 First Avenue, New York, NY 10016, U.S.A*

W. WAESPE
*Kantonsspital Zürich, Neurol. Universitätsklinik U. Poliklinik, Rämistrasse 100, 8006 Zürich, Switzerland*

L. R. YOUNG
*Man-Vehicle Laboratory, Department of Aeronautics and Astronautics, Room 37-219, M.I.T., Cambridge, MA 02139, U.S.A*

D. S. ZEE
*Department of Neurology, The Johns Hopkins University, School of Medicine, Blalock Room 1422, 601 N. Broadway, Baltimore, MD 21205, U.S.A*

# Contents

# Introductory Chapter

**Chapter 1.** The selection of reference frames by nature and its investigators      3
by *J. I. Simpson and W. Graf*

# Part I. Goal-Directed Adaptive Changes: Behavioural Studies

•

## IA. Effects of visual modification on oculomotor control

**Chapter 4.** Adaptive properties of the saccadic system ............................... 71
       by *L. M. Optican*

**Chapter 5.** Adaptive regulation in the vergence and accommodation control
         systems ........................................................................................... 81
       by *F. A. Miles*

**Chapter 6.** Effects of visual deprivation on properties and modifiability of
         compensatory eye movement systems ....................................... 95
       by *M. Cynader*

·

## IB. Effects of vestibular modification on oculomotor control

·

**Chapter 10.** Adaptation to modified otolith input ........................................ 155
          by *L. R. Young*

## IC. Multimodal nature of the adaptive responses

**Chapter 11.** Studies of adaptation in human oculomotor disorders ........................ 165
          by *D. S. Zee and L. M. Optican*

# Part II, Internal Processes Underlying Adaptation

•

## IIA. Neuronal mechanisms

## Chapter 17. Neuronal events paralleling functional recovery (compensation) following peripheral vestibular lesions ..................................... 251
by *W. Precht and N. Dieringer*

## Chapter 18. Neurotransmitter and neuromodulator systems involved in vestibular compensation ................................................. 269
by *H. Flohr, W. Abeln and U. Lüneburg*

## IIB. Systematic interpretation of neuronal mechanisms

# List of Abbreviations

CCR,          cervico-collicular reflex
CCW,          counter clockwise
CF,           climbing fibre
COR,          cervico-ocular reflex
CV,           circularvection
CW,           clockwise
EPSP,         excitatory post synaptic potential
HC,           horizontal canal
IO,           inferior olive
MF,           mossy fibre
OKAN,         optokinetic afternystagmus
OKR,          optokinetic reflex
OVAR,         off-vertical axis rotation
PRN,          post-rotatory nystagmus
RSD,          right side down
SCEP,         slow cumulative eye position
SP,           smooth pursuit
SPEV,         slow phase eye velocity (also SP Vel)
SS,           simple spike
VCR,          vestibulo-collicular reflex
VN,           vestibular nuclei (L, lateral; D, descending; M, medial; S, superior) VN is also used for vestibular nystagmus and this is defined in the respective Chapters
VOR,          vestibulo-ocular reflex (H, horizontal; S, sagittal)
VVI,          visual-vestibular interaction

# Introductory Chapter

Adaptive mechanisms in gaze control
Facts and theories
*Eds. Berthoz & Melvill Jones*
© 1985 Elsevier Science Publishers BV (Biomedical Division)

# Chapter 1

# The selection of reference frames by nature and its investigators

## J. I. Simpson[a] & W. Graf

[a] *Department of Physiology and Biophysics, New York University Medical Center,
and The Rockefeller University, New York, U.S.A.*

## 1. Approaches to selecting reference frames

### 1.1. Reference frames and sensorimotor integration

The allure of eye movements, for investigators of sensorimotor integration, comes initially from their seeming mechanical simplicity and the conciseness with which their several tasks can be described. These features of the outward manifestations of eye movements are taken as auspicious for arriving at an understanding of the inward nervous manifestations of eye movements. Even if this extrapolation is correct, we must be mindful of the likelihood that the way in which we have framed our external descriptions of eye movements differs from the way in which they appear framed in the brain. Although a particular reference frame may be quite appropriate for describing externally observed eye movements, it may be ill-suited for promoting understanding of the underlying central processes of sensorimotor integration.

Even without stating what is meant by sensorimotor integration, we can appreciate, by considering the following three points, that the idea of reference frames is central to constructing a definition of sensorimotor integration. First, our descriptions of motor behavior require the formulations of mechanics, which use the idea of a frame of reference at one or another level of abstraction.

Second, reference frames underlie the making of measurements, which is itself the sensory process. Third, sensorimotor integration, at least in its simpler forms, can be thought of as a transformation, and the term 'transformation' calls forth the idea of reference frames.

The generation of eye movements compensatory to head movements serves as an example of sensorimotor integration useful for discussing issues of reference frames and transformations in specific terms. The desired outcome of the sensorimotor transformation of compensatory eye movements is believed to be known and can be simply stated — the entire retinal image should remain stationary on the retina during certain types and conditions of head movements so as to prevent the degradation of visual acuity that would result from retinal image movement. The tolerance for retinal image movement likely varies across species, depends on the task, and is not well known in most cases (e.g., Mackworth & Kaplan, 1962; Kelly, 1979; Steinman et al., 1982; Collewijn, this volume), so the goal of 'stationarity' should be qualified by the modifier 'functional'.

### 1.2. Mechanics and muscles

Reference frames and mechanics are directly introduced when the task to be accomplished by compensatory eye movements is defined in geometrical terms — when the head moves in space, the eye is to move relative to the head so that the configuration of the eye in space is preserved. If the eye is treated as a rigid body, its unconstrained change in configuration can be specified using six variables, three to account for translation of a point fixed in the eye and three to account for rotation about that point. The description of rigid body motion as a translation plus a rotation can take on many forms, depending on the particular reference frames used. The most concise general description is Chasles' central axis theorem, which states that at any instant of time the motion of a rigid body can be represented as a rotation about an axis combined with a translation along that axis (Routh, 1960). If the head undergoes only translation, then preservation of the eye's configuration in space requires that it translates relative to the head by the same amount that the head moves in space, but in the opposite direction. In most animals, the mechanical coupling between the head and the eye permits only a very small amount of relative translation. However, if the head can translate relative to the rest of the animal, then intermittent preservation of global image stability can be achieved by keeping the head stationary in space during translation of the body, as is done by some birds. (The relations between head and body are of great relevance in a general consideration of the task of retinal image stabilization, but we will not consider them in this paper.) Although it has been known for decades that the human eye indeed translates, as well as rotates, relative to the orbit (Berlin, 1871; Weiss, 1875; see also Helmholtz, 1910), mechanical analyses of eye movements neglect this small translation and proceed as if the eye only rotates about a (notional) center of rotation fixed in both the eye and the orbit. With this simplifying constraint, only three independent variables are necessary and sufficient to give the configuration of the eye in the head, in contrast to the six independent variables that would otherwise be required. When the only significant possible movement of the eye in the head is rotation, the objective of keeping the eye stationary with respect to the visual world can be realized only for the rotatory component of head movement. Furthermore, this objective can be strictly met only for an infinitely distant visual world because the

axes of rotation of the head and eye are not collinear. That is, even though the eye and head rotate at the same angular speed but in opposite directions, the eye translates into a new position in space. By rotating the eye at a different angular speed from that of the head the image of a small near object can be kept stationary on the retina.

The analysis of the mechanical behavior of rigid body movement is traditionally divided into two parts — kinematics and dynamics. (The dynamics part is sometimes called kinetics, and then dynamics encompasses both kinematics and kinetics, and is contrasted to statics.) Kinematics is the study of the nature and characteristics of motion (displacements, velocities and accelerations) of particles and rigid bodies without consideration of the underlying forces and torques. Kinematics is an aspect of geometry, and in a sense it is preparatory to the use of dynamics, in which the relations between the forces and the motion are considered and expressed. Here we shall be concerned only with kinematics. The formalisms of kinematics require the idea of a reference frame but can be expressed in general terms without invoking any particular reference frame until one is needed to analyze a particular problem. In treating a specific mechanical behavior, the analyst often finds that one particular reference frame proves favorable over others, not only because the kinematic formulations are simpler, but also because the movement processes become easier to understand. The particular mechanical arrangement under study often provides guidance in selecting what particular reference frame will be advantageous. Reference frames suggested by the organization of the physical system can be called natural (or intrinsic) reference frames. Natural reference frames for motor behavior of animals are apparent from the arrangement of the muscles themselves. These natural or intrinsic motor reference frames differ from the commonly used extrinsic rectangular Cartesian reference frame because the arrangement of muscles acting at a joint typically establishes a reference frame that is not orthogonal. Furthermore, when each muscle is considered as a dimension then the dimensionality of the reference frame is typically greater than the number of degrees of freedom of the joint. Such a mechanical arrangement is said to be indeterminate (over-determined; overcomplete) because the available equations determine not just one solution, but an infinity of solutions. When the number of equations is less than the number of variables (i.e., dimensions) then a unique solution exists only if other conditions are fulfilled.

Even though the eye is a limb of only one joint, it serves as a general mechanical example, for in contrast to most joints, the eye can be moved with three degrees of rotational freedom. Each of the six eye muscles can be considered kinematically as capable of rotating the eye about an axis passing through the notional center of rotation. For any orientation of the eye in the orbit the axis associated with each muscle is perpendicular to the plane defined by the following three points: the effective point of insertion (where the muscle leaves the surface of the globe), the point of muscle origin and the notional center of rotation. This approach dates from the last century (Volkmann, 1869) and has evolved through the work of Krewson (1950), Boeder (1962) and Robinson (1975b). Taken collectively, the six muscle axes of rotation serve as a natural reference frame for the execution of eye movements. As mentioned above, this reference frame has two characteristics that are out of the ordinary. First, the axes of rotation are not orthogonal, and second, the number of dimensions (6) exceeds the number of degrees of freedom (3) of the physical rotatory movement. At each instant during an eye movement the eye can be considered as rotating about a particular axis of rotation with a particular instantaneous angular velocity. Since angular velocity, in contrast to finite angular displacement, can be represented as a vector, it can be treated as compounded according to the parallelogram rule from components directed along the six eye muscle axes. In the terminology of mechanics, the problem of determining the components, knowing their resultant, is referred to as the inverse kinematic problem. In the direct kinematic problem the components are known and the task is to compound them into their resultant. For compensatory eye movements, it is the inverse kinematic problem that we must address because the desired resultant angular velocity is known and the components are sought. Without additional constraints the solution is non-unique because there are more components (6) than degrees of freedom (3). How the central nervous system arrives at a particular solution from among the set of non-unique solutions is an intriguing aspect of motor coordination. The approach of tensorial analysis (covariant-contravariant transformation based on intrinsic coordinate systems) suggests one way of selecting a particular solution (Pellionisz & Llinás, 1980, 1982a; Pellionisz, 1983b; this volume). Another approach to a particular solution is to reduce the dimensionality of the muscle reference frame by averaging the classical agonist-antagonist muscles in pairs to create three imaginary muscle rotation axes (Robinson, 1982; Ezure & Graf, 1984a,b). The accuracy of this approximation is dependent upon the presence of a reciprocal excitatory-inhibitory innervation pattern and the degree of deviation from collinearity of the two muscle rotation axes.

### 1.3. Sensory reference frames and environmental invariants

Let us now turn to the sensory reference frame associated with the vestibular semicircular canals. The structural relations among the six semicircular canals (three on each side) reveal an intrinsic sensory reference frame made up of axes orthogonal to the planes of the semicircular canals (Figs. 1; 2A,E). Although a given semicircular canal usually does not lie strictly in a single plane, a best-fit plane may be calculated (see Blanks et al., 1972) and an axis orthogonal to this plane can be taken as an axis of the vestibular sensory reference frame. Such axes will be called 'principal axes'. The neural response of each canal is scaled in proportion to the cosine of the angle between its principal axis and the head angular acceleration vector. These projection-type vectorial components differ from the parallelogram-type components and may serve different biological functions (Pellionisz & Llinás, 1980). Three linearly independent principal axes must be established by the semicircular canals so that the three dimensional angular acceleration can be adequately measured. Theoretically, the principal axes need not be orthogonal, but practical considerations of signal detection point to the benefits of having the three principal axes mutually orthogonal (Robinson,

6

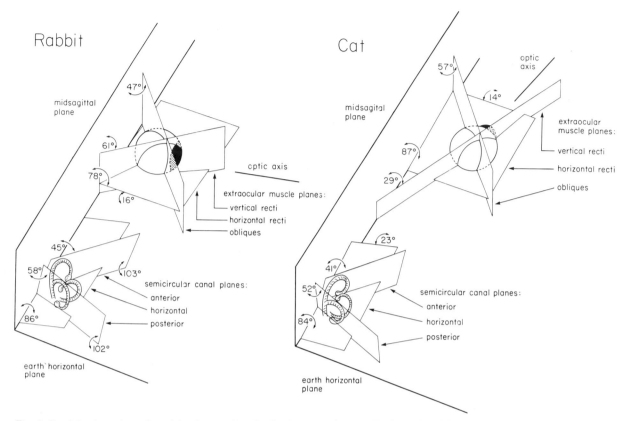

*Fig. 1.* Spatial orientation of semicircular canal and paired extraocular muscle planes in rabbit and cat. In the rabbit, the frontal plane is defined to be perpendicular to the horizontal canal planes, which brings both horizontal canals close to the earth horizontal plane. All angles for the geometry of the sensory and motor periphery in the rabbit are calculated for this particular head position. For the cat, all angles are given for the head in the stereotaxic position. The angles for the eye muscle orientation in both species were calculated from muscle action vectors, determined by the center of rotation and each muscle's origin and insertion points (from Ezure & Graf, 1984a).

1982; this volume). By invoking the primacy of bilateral symmetry and the desirability of a push-pull operation between parallel canal pairs, it follows that the orthogonality condition is met only for two arrangements of the six canals in the skull. In one, the vertical canals are at 45° to the mid-sagittal plane (Fig. 2A,E); the other possibility will be discussed later. Comparison of the semicircular canal geometry of various vertebrates shows a clear tendency towards orthogonality, but examples of marked non-orthogonality can be readily found (e.g., guinea-pig and man) (Blanks et al., 1975a; Curthoys et al., 1975). The implications of reference frame goniometrics for our understanding of sensorimotor integration and compensatory eye movements are topics of active theoretical and experimental study (Pellionisz & Llinás, 1980; Robinson, 1982, this volume; J.

Baker et al., 1982; R. Baker et al., 1982; Simpson, 1983; Graf & Ezure, 1983; Ezure & Graf, 1984a,b; Pellionisz, this volume).

Presumably one of the earliest sensory capabilities of animals in the primordial oceans was that of determining their spatial relation to the earth. Perhaps initially the only measure required was simply that of orientation with regard to a single direction — namely that of gravity. Setting apart the possibility of detecting magnetic fields and the ability to use patterned light (stars), the other available reference for orientation was provided by sunlight striking the ocean surface. This indicator of direction is in fact used and can be seen as the dorsal light reflex of fish (v. Holst, 1935; Graf & Meyer, 1978, 1983). This postural control reflex causes fish to orient their dorsal surface towards a light source. Fish illuminated from the side will tilt

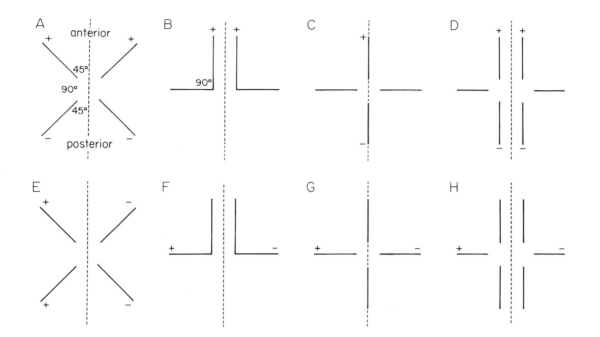

*Fig. 2.* Possible arrangements of vertical semicircular canals, as projected onto a horizontal plane. The midsagittal plane is indicated by the broken lines. Orthogonality among the individual canals will provide the best signal-to-noise ratio. In addition, the canals are depicted as a push-pull system (+ = excitation; − = inhibition). A schematic diagram of the vertical semicircular canal configuration in vertebrates and its operation during head movements is given in (A) for a pitch-down movement (about the bitemporal axis), and in (E) for a left-side-down roll movement (about the naso-occipital axis). The semicircular canals depicted in (B) and (F) are orthogonal, but push-pull operation is possible only for roll movements (F). Starting from the arrangement depicted in (A), rotation of the semicircular canals by 45° about the vertical axis would maintain both orthogonality and push-pull operation, but two canals would be located in the midsagittal plane (C and G). However, such an arrangement has not been found. If the number of vertical canals is greater than four, then additional possibilities arise, as illustrated in (D) for pitch-up and (H) for right-side-roll. The squid possesses six vertical semicircular canals, which are oriented approximately in the transverse and parasagittal body planes. The spatial arrangement of the squid semicircular canals preserves orthogonality, bilateral symmetry and push-pull operation for both pitch (D) and roll (H) movements.

toward the light source until the effect initiated by the light is counterbalanced by that from the vestibular system. In some sense, the direction of greater light intensity indicates the direction opposite to that of gravitational attraction. Gravity, however, provides the only reliable reference available both day and night. Detection of relative internal displacements brought about by an animal's changing orientation with respect to the gravitational field could have been the beginning of the type of global spatial analysis that is inertia-dependent. The direction of gravitational attraction between a body and the earth provides one dimension of a basis for spatial analysis, but as physical directions are, in general, represented by three-dimensions, two other dimensions or directions must also be selected. The three directions need not be orthogonal, but they must be linearly independent. In bilaterally symmetric animals one of the two additionally needed directions could be orthogonal to both gravity and the midsagittal plane, which is usually positioned by the animal so as to contain the direction of gravity. The third direction then would be one that was in the midsagittal plane. These directions might be presumed to be preferred axes of an intrinsic reference frame for global spatial analysis, but it is argued below that the principal axes of the semicircular canals constitute the fundamental intrinsic reference frame for global spatial analysis.

Mechanisms other than inertia-dependent ones are available for measuring orientation and movement; the more global of these would involve movement detection within the earth's magnetic field, as in sharks (Kalmijn, 1974), detection of relative motion by vision, and electrolocation (Scheich & Bullock, 1974; Heiligenberg, 1977). In vertebrates, use of visual and vestibular mechanisms to establish spatial references is virtually universal, whereas use of magnetic field detection and electrolocation is not. Chemical and tactile mechanisms can be used to gain information about orientation and movement, but they seem to be involved more with detecting local, varying properties of the environment, rather than with global, constant properties. Vestibular and visual measures of orientation and movement share the property of relying on an environmental invariant. For the vestibular system the invariant is the direction of gravity; for the visual system it is the global stationarity of the external world.

## 2. Lessons from lateral-eyed and frontal-eyed animals

Head rotation in animals with different interocular angles seemingly requires different compensatory eye movements. For instance, when the head rotates about the naso-occipital axis, the resulting compensatory eye movements will be vertical in rabbit, but torsional in man. In fact, whether or not there is a difference in the description depends upon the reference frame selected by the observer. If the reference frame is tied to the optic axis in primary position, then the above description results, but if the reference frame is tied to the head, then there is no difference.

To compare and contrast compensatory eye movements produced in lateral-eyed and frontal-eyed animals by identical head movements, we have to consider several parameters: the orientation in the head of both the semicircular canals and the extraocular muscles, the neuronally imposed organization of visual space, and the neuronal network connecting the labyrinths with the eye muscles.

### 2.1. The orientation of the semicircular canals in the head

The orientation of the semicircular canals in the head remains qualitatively constant with respect to the midsagittal plane in all vertebrates examined. The variations are far less than those found in the orientation of the optic axis (Retzius, 1881, 1884; Gray, 1908; Rothfeld, 1913; de Burlet & Koster, 1916; Vilstrup, 1950; Baird, 1974; Blanks et al., 1972, 1975a; Curthoys et al., 1975, 1977; Blanks & Precht, 1976; Graf & Simpson, 1981; Simpson & Graf, 1981; Ezure & Graf, 1984a). All vertebrate species exhibit a characteristic 'diagonal' orientation of the vertical semicircular canals in the head, with the anterior canal on one side and the posterior canal on the opposite side being close to coplanar (Figs. 1, 2A,E). These features are apparent in fossil fish where only the vertical canals are present (Stensiö, 1927) and can also be distinguished to some extent in lampreys (de Burlet & Versteegh, 1930; Löwenstein et al., 1968). Even in animals with 'bent' labyrinths (e.g., birds) the same basic structural plan is readily visible (Retzius, 1881, 1884; Gray, 1908; Werner, 1933, 1960; Baird, 1974), and it is also found in sharks and rays where the anterior and posterior semicircular canals are not connected by the common crus as in other vertebrates. The common crus in sharks and rays is formed between the anterior and the horizontal semicircular canals (Retzius, 1881; Daniel, 1928; Werner, 1930). The presence of only two semicircular canals in fossil fish as well as in remnants of the Late Silurian and Devonian Agnatha (extant cyclostomes) seem to reflect the ontogenetic order of appearance of the canals, as the anterior canal and the posterior canal are formed before the horizontal canal (Streeter, 1906/1907; Bast et al., 1947).

The labyrinthine organization of the cyclostomes (Agnatha) has several peculiarities that may bear on the natural evolution of reference frames. Living representatives of the cyclostomes are hagfish (*Myxine*) and lampreys (*Lampetra, Petromyzon*). The hagfish possess only one semicircular canal on each side, but each of them contains two ampullae (Retzius, 1881). The canal itself is oriented in space as follows: it encloses an angle of 30° (open to the front) with the midsagittal plane, and it is tilted 60° off vertical. The hair cells of the cristae are unidirectionally polarized.

The hagfish labyrinth has been reported to monitor well movements about the vertical axis; movements about the pitch axis are less well monitored, while those about the roll axis are not monitored (Löwenstein & Thornhill, 1970). In contrast, the lamprey labyrinth with its two pairs of anterior and posterior ampullae, which are homologous to the anterior and posterior semicircular canal ampullae in gnathostomes, is able to detect reliably all body rotations (Löwenstein et al., 1968). The cristae ampullares in the lamprey are composed of three 'arms', which are directed in different, roughly perpendicular planes (Löwenstein et al., 1968). Compensatory eye movements following labyrinthine stimulation in the lamprey can be induced in any direction, despite the absence of horizontal semicircular canals (Rovainen, 1976).

A great variety of statoreceptors is found in invertebrates (see Bullock & Horridge, 1965). A full presentation of invertebrate angular acceleration and gravity detection systems is not within the scope of this paper. However, to give an idea about some of the structures used by invertebrates for three-dimensional angular acceleration analysis, three examples are briefly introduced.

The statocysts of the fast moving squid and cuttlefish include grooves which, in a similar way as vertebrate semicircular canals, direct endolymph flow towards a sensory crista with a cupula (Stephens & Young, 1978). These invertebrate semicircular canals, like vertebrate semicircular canals, are oriented in space in a roughly orthogonal three-dimensional planar arrangement (Young, 1960; Budelmann, 1977; Stephens & Young, 1978). Four subdivisions of the sensory crista on each side of the animal are distinguished; they are oriented approximately in the main planes of the body, in contrast to the vertebrate arrangement. There is one longitudinal subdivision (longitudinal crista), which responds to movements around the longitudinal body axis (excitation occurs when the ipsilateral side rolls upward), and a vertical subdivision (vertical crista), which responds to movements about the yaw axis (excited during contraversion). Two roughly parallel cristae are found in the transverse body plane (anterior and posterior transverse crista), of which the posterior transverse crista deviates to some degree from the true transverse body plane. The anterior transverse crista is excited during pitch-up movements, and the posterior transverse crista during pitch-down movements. The latter crista is also assumed to detect fast foward and backward

linear accelerations as occur during jet propulsion of the animal (Stephens & Young, 1982).

The operation of the squid statocysts in detecting movements in space remains to be determined quantitatively. However, we shall discuss briefly how this bilaterally symmetric system could monitor three-dimensional angular acceleration in conformity with the idealized vertebrate conditions of push-pull operation and orthogonality. Orthogonality of the semicircular canals would provide an optimal signal-to-noise ratio (Robinson, 1982; this volume), but in order to achieve paired orthogonality, the vertical semicircular canals need not necessarily be arranged in the familiar diagonal fashion (Figs. 1, 2A,E). One alternative arrangement is pairs in parasagittal and coronal planes (Fig. 2B,F) but this arrangement does not fulfil the condition that the paired canals are to operate in a push-pull fashion (Robinson, 1982). Another vertical canal configuration meeting the conditions of orthogonality and push-pull operation is that shown in Fig 2C,G, where two of the four vertical canals lie in the midsagittal plane (see also Robinson, this volume). Thus, two antagonistic canals would be located in the coronal plane and respond best to roll movements of the head (Fig. 2G). The other two canals would be in the midsagittal plane (one behind the other), responding best to pitch movements of the head (Fig. 2C). To our knowledge such a configuration has not been described for vertebrates or invertebrates, but the squid statocyst system seems to be a variant of this arrangement. The left and right longitudinal cristae respond in a push-pull manner to movements of the body around the longitudinal (roll) axis; the vertical cristae (corresponding to the horizontal canals of vertebrates) respond in a push-pull manner to movement about the yaw axis. The disposition of the transverse cristae in squid (Fig. 2D,H) shares features of the configurations shown in Fig. 2B,C. The introduction of a second pair of transverse cristae permits push-pull pairing and bilateral symmetry, with the anterior transverse cristae excited by pitch-up and the posterior transverse cristae excited by pitch-down.

In the octopus the sensory crista on each side consists of nine subsections, and is divided in three main planes which are approximately orthogonal to each other (Young, 1960). The spatial arrangement of the sensory crista suggests an angular acceleration detection system similar to that of vertebrates (Budelmann & Wolff, 1973; Budelmann, 1977).

The third type of 'semicircular canal' system discussed here in the context of invertebrates is found in crabs, which possess one horizontal and one vertical toroidal structure on each side. Depending on the species, these 'toroids' can be either open or can form a closed canal system (Sandeman & Okajima, 1972; Sandeman, 1983; Fraser, 1981). In the freely moving crab the horizontal canals are held in the earth horizontal plane, and since the horizontal and vertical canals are close to orthogonal, the vertical canals are nearly vertical. Each vertical canal lies at an angle of 45° to the midsagittal plane in a configuration comparable to that of the anterior semicircular canal in vertebrates. Although there is only one vertical canal on each side, each one responds preferentially to movements about orthogonal axes and thus the canals of crabs are collectively capable of accurately transducing three-dimensional angular accelerations (Fraser & Sandeman, 1975).

In their 'natural' posture most animals orient their head so that the horizontal semicircular canals are nearly in the earth horizontal plane (Lebedkin, 1924; de Beer, 1947). Man and some other primates depart from this behavior (de Beer, 1947), and an extreme deviation is found in flatfish (Jacob, 1928; Schöne, 1964; Platt, 1973a). Since flatfish undergo a 90° tilt to one side or the other during metamorphosis, while the labyrinths remain in their original position in the head, the horizontal canals in the adult flatfish are no longer oriented horizontally but are vertical with respect to earth horizontal (Jacob, 1928).

## 2.2. The orientation in the head of the extraocular muscles and their kinematic characteristics

Throughout the vertebrate subphylum the extraocular muscle apparatus is configured in a characteristic way (see Edgeworth, 1935; Prince, 1956, among many others). There are always six external eye muscles which execute rotation of the globe: superior rectus and inferior rectus, superior oblique and inferior oblique, and medial rectus and lateral rectus (in this context retractor bulbi or laevator palpebrae superioris muscles are not considered). The geometry of the muscles suggests pairing into three agonist-antagonist pairs (e.g., superior rectus and inferior rectus) although the degree of deviation from coplanarity varies among the different species. If the agonist-antagonist muscles are paired, a common plane of action can be defined (Robinson, 1982; Ezure & Graf, 1984a,b).

With regard to the spatial relationship of extraocular muscles and semicircular canals we observe that the axes of rotation of extraocular muscles in frontal-eyed animals as compared to lateral-eyed animals change with respect to the optic axis so that the rotation axis of each muscle remains most nearly parallel to the principal axis of that semicircular canal from which it receives its primary excitatory input (Rothfeld, 1913, 1914; Ohm, 1919; Graf & Simpson, 1981; Simpson & Graf, 1981; Ezure & Graf, 1984a; Figs. 1,4). These primary excitatory relations are referred to as the principal three-neuron-arc connections of the vestibulo-ocular reflex (Szentágothai, 1943, 1950; see also below). Moreover, there is also a difference in the location of the insertion points of the extraocular muscles between lateral-eyed and frontal-eyed animals (Wessely, 1916; Graf & Simpson, 1981; Simpson & Graf, 1981), which results in different extraocular muscle kinematics when referenced to the eye (Ohm, 1919; Graf & Simpson, 1981; Simpson & Graf, 1981). For example, in the neighborhood of the primary position, contraction of the superior oblique muscle causes intorsion, depression and abduction of the eye in man (Alpern, 1969; Moses, 1970), whereas in the rabbit, the same muscle causes intorsion, elevation and adduction (Ohm, 1919; Graf & Simpson, 1981; Simpson & Graf, 1981). We have concluded (see below) that these differences in kinematic characteristics are in accord with the requirements of compensatory eye movements in animals with different interocular angles. Although the above description was fundamental, it did not reflect the full complexity of the canal-eye muscle coordinate relations. The semicircular canal planes and the extraocular muscle planes are only approximately, but not perfectly, parallel, thus revealing an incongruence between the vestibular and the extraocular muscle reference frames. Furthermore, the change of muscle action (with respect to the eye) with change in the eye bulb orientation in the orbit has to be considered for a given species. For example, the superior rectus of man can act as a pure rotator or as a pure elevator depending on whether the eye is in one or the other of its eccentric horizontal positions with respect to the head (see Alpern, 1969). Such changes of muscle action seem to be responsible for the production of appropriate compensatory eye movements even if the eyeball is in an eccentric position in the orbit during a given vestibular stimulus (see also Szentágothai, 1943). This is possible because the orientation of muscle axes with respect to the head seems to change little with changing eye position in the head (see Robinson, this volume).

A pronounced incongruence between vestibular and oculomotor reference frames is present in flatfish (Jacob, 1928; Schöne, 1964), where the typical structural relation between eye muscles and canals has undergone a 90° relative displacement. The consequences for the vestibulo-ocular reflex (VOR) connectivity in the flatfish are dramatic and will be given in detail below.

In comparison to vertebrates, a much more complicated and heterogenous extraocular muscle arrangement is present in invertebrates. For example, in the octopus seven eye muscles are found in each eye (Budelmann & Young, 1982), although their gross anatomy bears a clear resemblance to that of lateral-eyed vertebrates. *Sepia* possess fourteen eye muscles, one of which has a tendon running across the midline to insert on the other eye, suitable for producing vergence eye movements (J. Z. Young, personal communication; see also Packard, 1972). In the crab, 26 muscles are involved in moving the eye assembly (Burrows & Horridge, 1968).

### 2.3. The organization of visual space in relation to optokinetic eye movements and convergent visual-vestibular signals

The importance of vision in equilibrium control was pointed out first by Mach (1875). This contribution of vision is particularly important during slow movements (low frequencies at physiologically normal amplitudes) and during constant

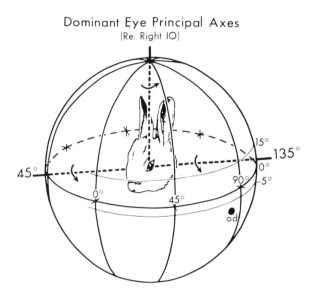

Dominant Eye Principal Axes
(Re: Right IO)

*Fig. 3.* Spatial organization of the three principal axes of rotation for visual modulation of right dorsal cap neurons during monocular stimulation. Two of the principal axes (the vertical axis and the 135° axis) are associated with the contralateral eye; the third axis (45°) is associated with the ipsilateral eye. The arrow about each axis indicates the direction of eye rotation, relative to a stationary visual world, that would result in an increase of activity of each class of dorsal cap neurons (od, optic disc; IO, inferior olive) (from Simpson, Graf & Leonard, 1981a).

velocity rotation when the signal from the vestibular afferents becomes inadequate (Fernandez & Goldberg, 1971; Precht et al., 1971; Wilson & Melvill Jones, 1979; Barmack, 1981). Visually derived information about the relative movement between an animal and its environment reaches the vestibular nuclear complex, as reported for a number of species (Dichgans et al., 1973b; Henn et al., 1974; Allum et al., 1976; Allum & Graf, 1977; Keller & Precht, 1979b). In these studies only horizontally moving stimuli were used. An appreciation of three-dimensional, visually based global spatial analysis became available from investigations in rabbit of the accessory optic system, which processes visual signals about self motion (Simpson et al., 1979). These visual signals are transmitted either directly or indirectly to a variety of vestibular and oculomotor related regions, including the inferior olive and the cerebellar flocculus (Maekawa & Simpson, 1973; Alley et al., 1975; Brecha et al., 1980; Takeda & Maekawa, 1976; Maekawa & Takeda, 1979; Blanks et al., 1982). The visually modulated neurons in the dorsal cap of the inferior olive can be divided into three main categories according to the spatial orientation of the axis of visual world rotation that yields the best modulation from the dominant eye (Simpson et al., 1981a). The three categories were named Vertical Axis, Anterior (45°) Axis, and Posterior (135°) Axis cells (Fig. 3). The Vertical Axis cells exhibit their best responses when the visual world rotates around an axis oriented vertically with respect to the rabbit positioned with its head and eyes in the freeze position. Anterior (45°) Axis cells are best modulated when the visual world is rotated around an approximately horizontal axis oriented about 45° posterior to the nose; Posterior (135°) Axis cells are best modulated when the visual world rotates about an approximately horizontal axis at about 135° posterior to the nose. One of the features that distinguishes these two latter types from each other is that they receive their dominant input from opposite eyes. The preferred rotation axes for these three cell types are oriented in a fashion strikingly similar to that of the principal axes of the vestibular canals (compare Figs. 1 and 3), noting, however, that the rotation axes of the eye muscles are not far divergent from the canal axes. Further measurements of the canal and muscle geometry may help in deciding whether the climbing fiber visual input to the flocculus is referenced to the canals or the muscles (Graf & Ezure, 1983; Simpson, 1983; Ezure & Graf, 1984a).

An exact analysis of the eye muscle groups activated by floccular stimulation is not available (but see, e.g., Dufossé et al., 1977). We can assume, however, that since floccular Purkinje cells are exerting inhibitory effects on secondary vestibular neurons (Baker et al., 1972; Highstein, 1973b; Ito et al., 1977), that the innervation pattern determined by the axonal arborization of the secondary vestibular neurons is predominant (see below). For example, a Purkinje cell projecting onto an ipsilateral (inhibitory) anterior canal vestibular nucleus neuron would bring about a disinhibition of at least the inferior rectus muscle of the ipsilateral side and the superior oblique muscle of the contralateral side.

### 2.4. The neuronal networks connecting the labyrinths with the eye muscles

Studies on the connections between the semicircu-lar canals and the extraocular muscles in different species began with Högyes in 1880–1884 and include Szentágothai's (1943, 1950) now classical description of the three-neuron-arc. More recently, a variety of techniques, including electromyograms, intracellular recordings and single cell staining methods, have been used to reveal vestibulo-ocular relations (Fluur, 1959; Cohen & Suzuki, 1963; Cohen et al., 1964; Suzuki et al., 1964; Highstein, 1971, 1973a,b; Ito et al., 1973a,b, 1976a,b; Kim, 1974; Baker & Highstein, 1978; Uchino et al., 1978, 1980a,b; Ishizuka et al., 1980; McCrea et al., 1980, 1981; Furuya & Markham, 1981; Graf et al., 1981, 1983). All of these studies confirmed the basic structural pattern of the three-neuron-arc, with so-called principal excitatory connections from particular semicircular canals to particular eye muscles, i.e., from the anterior semicircular canal to the ipsilateral superior rectus and the contralateral inferior oblique muscles; from the posterior canal to the ipsilateral superior oblique and the contralateral inferior rectus muscles, and from the horizontal canal to the ipsilateral medial rectus and the contralateral lateral rectus. The principal inhibitory connections link the respective main antagonists of these muscles to the same semicircular canals. Only these canal-muscle relationships are the principal VOR connections, as defined by Szentágothai (1943, 1950).

More recent experiments have demonstrated that in the case of the vertical canals secondary vestibular neurons branch to contact their two respective principal extraocular motoneuron pools (Uchino et al., 1980a, 1982; Uchino & Suzuki, 1983; Graf et al., 1981, 1983; McCrea et al., 1982). This arrangement emphasizes that the coupling between a particular vertical canal and the most nearly aligned eye muscles is securely established. Besides these principal connections there are other canal-eye muscle relationships. Regardless of the number of synapses involved, these other connections are termed accessory (secondary) connections (Szentágothai, 1943, 1950; Graf et al., 1983; Ezure & Graf, 1984b), although, in fact, for some of these accessory connections a three-neuron-arc pattern has been established (Uchino et al., 1980b; Graf et al., 1981, 1983). One such accessory connection underlies the activation of the *ipsilateral* inferior rectus muscle from the

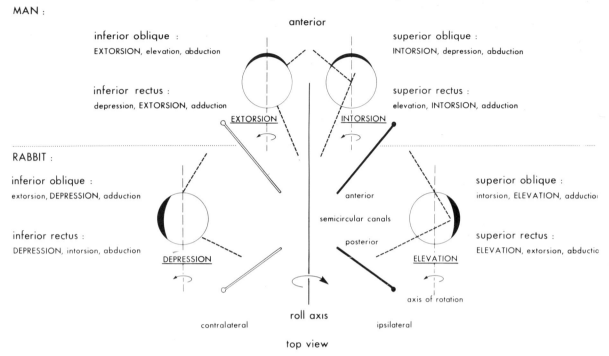

Fig. 4. Combined muscular actions appropriate for compensatory eye movements for head tilt (right-side down) about the roll axis. During this head tilt, the anterior and posterior canals on the right (ipsilateral) side are excited (indicated by the solid canal symbols). In both species, increase in firing frequency of the ipsilateral anterior ampullary nerve activates the ipsilateral superior rectus and the contralateral inferior oblique; excitation of the ipsilateral posterior ampullary nerve effects contraction of the ipsilateral superior oblique and the contralateral inferior rectus. Thin dashed lines indicate the axes of rotation for the compensatory ocular movements. The major participating muscles are indicated next to the eye upon which they act (muscles are symbolized by the thick dashed lines). Although the compensatory eye movements are different for man and rabbit, they are effected primarily by the same muscles connected to the same semicircular canals. This is possible because of the species differences in synergistic and antagonistic kinematic characteristics of the extroocular muscles. Synergistic components are given in capital letters, while components that are in the appropriate direction to cancel each other are given in small letters (from Graf & Simpson, 1981; Simpson & Graf, 1981).

posterior canal in the cat (Cohen et al., 1964); the three-neuron-arc nature of this connectivity has been demonstrated both electrophysiologically (Uchino et al., 1980b) and morphologically (Graf et al., 1983).

The possible functional role of the accessory connections has been discussed in the context of stabilizing the rotation point of the eye during eye movements (Lorente de Nó, 1932), or of compensating for the misalignment between the vestibular and the extraocular muscle planes (Simpson & Graf, 1981; Graf et al., 1983). This adjustment can be viewed as a coordinate transformation from sensory (vestibular) to motor (eye muscle) reference frames, as was first formalized by Pellionisz

and Llinás (1980). Further theoretical treatment of the spatial coordination of the VOR supports the latter role of the accessory connections (Robinson, 1982; Ezure & Graf, 1984b; Pellionisz, this volume).

### 2.5. Compensatory eye movements — a synthesis

The data presented above demonstrate that in both the sensory and motor periphery, as well as within the central nervous system, there are geometrically closely related intrinsic reference frames whose basic three-dimensional organization is given by the principal axes of the vestibular semicircular canals (Fig. 1) (see also Cohen et al.,

1965; Schaefer et al., 1975; Simpson et al., 1979, 1981a). These intrinsic reference frames contrast with the extrinsic rectangular Cartesian reference frame that is commonly applied to describe events in external space, using orthogonal x,y,z axes in the midsagittal and bitemporal planes. Thus, it is likely that the commonly used extrinsic Cartesian coordinate system has no intrinsic relevance for the central nervous system, at least in relation to compensatory eye movements. When eye movements are constrained to only two degrees of freedom, as when Listing's law applies to voluntary eye movements, then other intrinsic reference frames may be revealed. But even then, their axes may not necessarily be horizontal and vertical (see Westheimer & Blair, 1972).

The information provided above can be combined to contribute to the better understanding of visuo-vestibulo-ocular reflexes. In particular, the functional concept of the vertical vestibular systems needs to be viewed in quite a different way from the horizontal system because the signals from the bilateral vertical canals are combined in different synergistic patterns depending on the particular head movement. For example, during nose-down head movement around the bitemporal axis both anterior canals provide excitatory afferent activity (Fig. 2A), but during a head movement around the naso-occipital axis the ipsilateral (with respect to head-down tilt) anterior and posterior semicircular canals provide afferent excitatory neuronal activity (Fig. 2E). The subsequent compensatory eye movements emerge from the structure of the vestibular and eye muscle reference frames. These reference frames are conveniently applied to describe how the observed eye movement results from the collective actions of the individual eye muscles (Meyer zum Gottesberge & Maurer, 1949; Hassler & Hess, 1954; Schaefer et al., 1975). For example, during a head movement around the naso-occipital axis (Fig. 4) humans show an intorsion of the ipsilateral eye (with respect to side down tilt) and an extorsion of the contralateral eye. Rabbits, on the other hand, show a vertical upward movement of the ipsilateral eye and a vertical downward movement of the contralateral eye. In both species, side down tilt excites both ipsilateral vertical semicircular canal nerves, resulting in a co-contraction of the ipsi-

lateral superior rectus and superior oblique and the contralateral inferior rectus and inferior oblique (principal vestibulo-ocular reflex connections). In man, the intorsion components of the actions of the superior rectus and the superior oblique are synergistic, while the other kinematic components are antagonistic. For the rabbit, a similar scenario can be gone through to illustrate the phenomenologically different compensatory eye movements resulting from the synergistic elevation component of the extraocular muscles for the ipsilateral eye and synergistic depression component for the contralateral eye. In both species the collective actions are appropriate for producing the different compensatory ocular movements. Thus, the primary connections of the three-neuron-arcs of the vestibulo-ocular reflexes are preserved by the changes in muscular organization.

Compensatory eye and head movements are also present in invertebrates (Schöne, 1954; Dijkgraaf, 1959, 1961, 1963) and ocular nystagmus can be elicited by vestibular, optokinetic and combined visual-vestibular stimulation (Burrows & Horridge, 1968; Horridge & Burrows, 1968; Barnes & Horridge, 1969; Collewijn, 1970b; Messenger, 1970; Sandemann & Okajima, 1972, 1973a,b). Even pursuit movements have been reported (Tompsett, 1939). However, the invertebrate statocyst-ocular reflex has not yet been analyzed in such detail as the vertebrate VOR and anatomical data are less explicit (see, e.g., Sandeman & Okajima, 1973b; Budelmann & Young, 1982).

### 2.6. Vestibulo-oculomotor coordination in flatfish

Flatfish are one of the few bilaterally asymmetric animals and constitute a natural paradigm to study adaptive changes of the vestibulo-ocular reflex. During metamorphosis all species of flatfish undergo a 90° change in orientation between their vestibular and ocular reference frames (Jacob, 1928; Schöne, 1964; Platt, 1973a). This rearrangement occurs because the body tilts 90° to one side and the eye that would have faced the sea bottom migrates around the dorsal aspect of the fish (Williams, 1902; Norman, 1934; Policanski, 1982). A more proper description of this phenomenon is

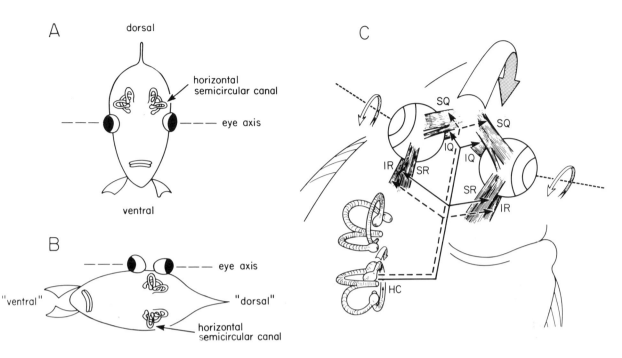

Fig. 5. Spatial relationship of labyrinths and eye axes before metamorphosis (A) and in an adult flatfish (B). The horizontal (lateral) semicircular canals become oriented vertically, while the eyes retain their orientation with respect to the environment. Thus, a 90° relative displacement of semicircular canal and eye axes occurs.

Extraocular muscle co-contractions required for the production of compensatory eye movements during a pitch-down movement of the head are illustrated in (C). Backward rotations of the eyes (small arrows around the optic axes, which are symbolized by broken lines) would be produced by contractions of the superior rectus (SR) and inferior oblique (IQ) muscles. The downward head movement (large arrow) eliciting these compensatory eye movements would activate the vertically oriented horizontal (lateral) semicircular canals (HC). The direction of canal displacement is shown by the small arrow above the left (lower) horizontal canal. Ampullopetal endolymph current is illustrated by the arrow inside the canal. The solid and broken arrows connecting labyrinth and eye muscles suggest the prospective excitatory and inhibitory connections required for an appropriately functioning vestibulo-ocular reflex. The horizontal canal pathways have to undergo a rearrangement leading to new extraocular motoneuron termination sites on both sides of the brain. IR, inferior rectus; SQ, superior oblique (from Graf & Baker, 1983).

that the eyes remain stationary in space while the rest of the fish rotates about them (Fig. 5A,B). As a result the optic axes maintain their orientation with respect to earth horizontal but the horizontal semicircular canals become vertically oriented. Since the flatfish propels itself with the same body referenced swimming movement as a normal fish (Olla et al., 1972), the horizontal canals are still exposed to angular acceleration identical to those present prior to metamorphosis, even though they have rotated 90° with respect to the earth. The appropriate compensatory eye movements during swimming are now simultaneous rotations of both eyes forward or backward (Platt, 1976) in contrast to the situation in upright fish where one eye moves forward while the other

moves backward (Harris, 1965; Easter et al., 1975). Since no qualitative differences between flatfish and other fish were found at the level of the oculomotor system (Graf, 1981), a reorganization of vestibulo-ocular pathways had to be hypothesized (see also Platt, 1973b, 1976). Indeed, a dramatic reorganization of second order horizontal canal neurons was revealed (Graf & Baker, 1983), while vertical canal neurons remained unchanged (the three-neuron-arc connectivity of the flatfish vertical vestibular systems is substantially sufficient for the production of compensatory eye movements for rotations about the longitudinal axis of the animal). Two distinct types of second-order vestibular neurons were observed morphologically in the horizontal canal system (see Fig.

24 of Ch. 2). For both types the axons crossed the midline and ascended in the medial longitudinal fasciculus. In the first type major termination sites were in the inferior oblique and superior rectus subdivisions of the oculomotor nucleus; axonal branches recrossed the midline at the level of the oculomotor nucleus and terminated in identical locations on the contralateral side. For the second type, the major termination sites were in the trochlear nucleus and in the inferior rectus subdivision of the oculomotor nucleus; axonal branches also recrossed the midline and termined in identical motoneuron pools on the contralateral side. For both types, contralateral and ipsilateral termination sites were equally numerous. These termination sites were exactly those expected on the basis of geometrical consideration to be used during compensatory eye movements (Fig. 5C). For example, a head-down movement in the flatfish would excite the side-down horizontal canal, producing contractions of both superior recti and inferior obliques, as well as relaxation of their antagonists, the inferior recti and superior obliques. Therefore, it was proposed that the cell type first described above provides the excitatory pathways to the agonist muscle groups and that the second cell type provides the inhibitory connections to the antagonists (Graf & Baker, 1983).

The flatfish clearly demonstrates central rewiring of the vestibulo-ocular reflex pathways at a level of the secondary vestibular neurons subsequent to a change in the geometrical relations between the semicircular canals and the eye muscles. While one cannot be certain that the adaptive change prompted by the flatfish metamorphosis is equivalent to adaptive plasticity occurring in response to an experimental perturbation, changes observed in some properties of vestibular neurons during adaptive plasticity (Lisberger & Miles, 1980; Keller & Precht, 1979a), in conjunction with the findings in the flatfish, may point to a functional role for secondary vestibular neurons in adaptation. Although the appropriate compensatory eye movements in most species occur, in large part, as a consequence of preserving the geometric relationships between the semicircular canal and extraocular muscle reference frames, the flatfish are an interesting exception.

## 3. Conclusions

The scheme of spatial coordination of compensatory eye movements utilizing intrinsic reference frames of vestibular canal and extraocular muscle axes contrasts with that based on the extrinsic rectangular Cartesian frame composed of vertical, torsional and horizontal axes. The intrinsic reference frames discussed above suggest that in connection with compensatory eye movements no special homage be given to vertical and torsional axes and the attendant notion of vertical and torsional coordination centers. The importance of the spatial arrangement of the vestibular canal reference frame and its primary reflex connectivity for the functioning of basic brain stem circuits is underlined by the findings that eye muscle kinematics change among species to preserve a common primary central connectivity and that other sensory systems also use this reference frame. Therefore, we, together with other investigators (Cohen et al., 1965; Schaefer et al., 1975; Simpson et al., 1979, 1981a), hypothesize that the basic architecture established by the principal axes of the semicircular canals is a common vertebrate 'Bauplan' for the sensorimotor integration underlying compensatory eye movements. Other intrinsic reference frames likely prevail in other contexts and the search for reference frames selected by nature should provide revealing perspectives for understanding the brain.

### Acknowledgements

The authors' research was supported in part by USPHS Grants NS-13742 and EY-04613, the Irma T. Hirschl Trust, the Grass Foundation and the Deutsche Forschungsgemeinschaft (Gr-688/1).

# Part I

# Goal Directed Adaptive Changes:
# Behavioural Studies

# Section 1A

## Effects of visual modification on oculomotor control

Adaptive mechanisms in gaze control
Facts and theories
*Eds. Berthoz & Melvill Jones*
© 1985 Elsevier Science Publishers BV (Biomedical Division)

# Chapter 2

# Adaptive modulation of VOR parameters by vision

## G. Melvill Jones

*Aerospace Medical Research Unit, Dept. of Physiology, McGill University, Montréal, Québec, Canada H3G 1Y6*

## 1. Introduction

The previous chapter examines some fundamental anatomical and physiological properties within the system for gaze control, suggesting that strong evolutionary pressures have predicated an intimate level of functional accord between visual and vestibular inputs into this system. As we shall see below and in later chapters, the concept of a 'symbiotic' relation between these and allied inputs extends further to their dynamic integration, expressed at both the behavioural and central neurophysiological levels. In the present chapter we concentrate specifically on one aspect of the problem, namely the effect of persistent dysmetria between visual and vestibular sensory stimuli, *caused* by artificial alteration of the visual input during natural vestibular stimulation, and *manifest* as retained changes in the dark-tested vestibulo-ocular reflex.

The author's interest in the matter was first kindled in the late 1950s by the simple observation that clear vision of a stationary target is possible at frequencies of angular head oscillation well above the normal limit for visual following of a target which oscillates relative to the stationary head. Thus, whereas the human visual tracking system shows a sharp cut-off at frequencies above about 1 Hz (e.g., Melvill Jones & Drazin, 1961; Young, 1962; Stark et al., 1962; Dallos & Jones, 1963), clear vision was obviously possible at frequencies of head oscillation well above this value, as has since been demonstrated quantitatively by a num-

ber of authors (Benson & Barnes, 1978; Tomlinson et al., 1980; Steinman & Collewijn, 1980). Hence non-visual influences introduced by head rotation must be responsible for the improved upper frequency response of visual fixation introduced by head movement. These and other findings pointed to the vestibulo-ocular reflex (VOR) as one of the likely sources of added oculomotor drive in these circumstances. However, if this reflex were solely responsible for good ocular stabilization at frequencies too high for effective visuo-oculomotor control, it would have to operate consistently at close to unity gain (eye vel./ head vel. = 1), and notably in the absence of useful visual feedback. How, then, could the internal neural parameters (e.g., neural gain and pathway time constants) controlling this sensory-motor system continue to be appropriately adjusted in the face of the many changing conditions of everyday life; for example, alterations of size during growth, loss of neural tissue due to age, normal diurnal and hormonal cycles, exposure to the abnormal movement environments of flight or space, and even the magnifying and diminishing optics of clinical prescription spectacles. That such internal parameters do come under some kind of powerful behaviourally activated adaptive control seemed likely from the then recent psychological experiments of Kohler (1956; 1962) and his colleagues, who found that when wearing inverting Dove prism spectacles their subjects could eventually (4–8 weeks) engage in quasi normal sporting activities (see also related psychological studies of Stratton, 1897; and Taylor, 1962). On the assumption that the specrum of head movement frequencies would then have extended beyond the normal limits of the purely visuo-motor system, it was no great step to guess that in Kohler's subjects either the frequency limit of visual tracking had been adaptively extended, or the inherent characteristics of the VOR had been drastically altered; even reversed. Additional potential factors, such as modified influence of neck afferents (e.g., Dichgans et al., 1973a) and the introduction of new central programs will be treated later (Chapter 12).

## 2. Human Studies

### 2.1. Reversed visual-vestibular dysmetria

#### 2.1.1. Short-term exposure

These expectations led to a series of experiments on human subjects to explore the consequence to the dark-tested VOR of maintained exposure to the reversed visual experience during head movement in the light (Gonshor & Melvill Jones, 1969, 1971, 1973, 1976a,b, 1980; Melvill Jones & Gonshor, 1975, 1982; Melvill Jones, 1977; Melvill Jones & Mandl, 1979, 1981, 1983). An initial study of short-term effects yielded encouraging results, summarized in Fig. 1. A group of seven subjects engaged in two sets of experiments. The first series examined only the potential habituating effect on the VOR of the intended rotational stimulus profile. For this the basic stimulus was a horizontal sinusoidal oscillation of 60° amp. and 1/6 Hz, chosen to lie within the natural range of velocity transduction by canal hydrodynamics (Jones & Spells, 1963; Jones & Milsum, 1965; reviewed in Melvill Jones, 1974a). Usually this was continued over 20 cycles to yield a 2 min test module, conducted in the dark with the subject performing mental arithmetic to stabilize a non-related mental state. The 2 min module was then repeated ten times, with 3 min rest intervals between modules. Finally, the whole sequence was repeated on three consecutive days, with normal activity between days. During all these runs VOR gain was measured as the ratio of peak compensatory eye velocity to peak head (i.e., table) velocity, the cumulative results being shown

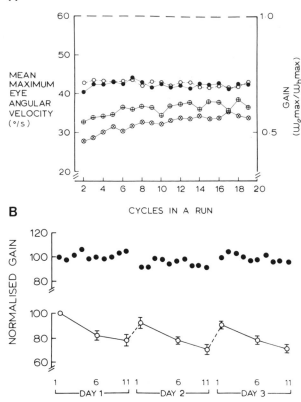

Fig. 1. Short-term changes of dark-tested VOR gain measured over the three time scales of (i) the 2 min period of a 20 cycle test run, (ii) the 50 min period of the daily experiment, and (iii) the 3 days of a complete experiment. (A) Cycle by cycle estimates within test runs Nos. 1 (●, control), 6 (⊕, after four 2 min periods of reversed vision) and 11 (⊗, after a further 8 min of reversed vision). Open circles show corresponding control data obtained from the same subjects 6 months earlier. Note (i) the successive attenuation of gain after each 8 min exposure to rotation with vision reversal, and (ii) the relatively rapid recovery of gain *within* each dark-tested period of 20 cycles (n = 21 for each point, i.e., three estimates from each of seven subjects). (B) Normalized gain during the initial control experiment (upper points, demonstrating no vestibular habituation) and with reversed vision during runs 2–5 and 7–10 (lower curves, demonstrating successive gain attenuation within the daily test sequence and some retention of this effect between days; n = 7 subjects for each point). (Composite data from Gonshor & Melvill Jones, 1976a and Melvill Jones, 1977.)

in the top data points of the upper and lower sections of Fig. 1. No change was seen over any of the three times scales of (i) a 20 cycle run (top curves of Fig. 1A), (ii) the 10 runs of each day (top data points of Fig. 1B), and (iii) the 3 day sequence (also the top data points of Fig. 1B).

These results permitted a second series of similar experiments on the same seven subjects to examine specifically the effect of reversed vision. This was achieved by exposing them to vision of the external world as seen through a plane mirror attached to the turntable. They were required to look at the (moving) mirror-reversed scene during (i) the 2nd to 5th runs and (ii) the 7th to 10th runs on each of three consecutive days. VOR gain was measured in the dark as before during the first, sixth and last (eleventh) runs, as depicted by the points on the lowest curve of Fig. 1B. Three notable features emerged. *First,* in contrast to the initial set of control results, the reversed vision experience consistently produced suppression of the dark tested VOR gain. In Fig. 1A this is seen as the successive lowering of curves produced by the first (i.e., runs 2–5) and second (i.e., runs 7–10) periods of reversed vision, each period comprising a mere 8 min (i.e., four sessions of 2 min each) total duration of visual-vestibular dysmetria. *Second,* as seen in the lower two curves of Fig. 1A, there was a relatively rapid recovery of gain *during* the 2 min testing periods in the dark. As we shall see below, this latter feature becomes much less marked with longer periods of active adaptation; the permanency of change appears to depend on the duration of adaptive stimulation. *Third,* there was a tendency for some day to day retention of the attenuative effect, even though subjects engaged in normal vision and movement during most of the intervening (dashed lines) periods of wakefulness.

## 2.1.2. Long-term effects

These results indicated without doubt that the dark-tested adult VOR is not a stereotyped reflex having fixed input-output characteristics. On the contrary, even short periods of encounter with altered peripheral stimuli can change central parameters controlling the reflex. How far could this kind of alteration be 'pushed'? Were Kohler's subjects modified, perhaps even to the point of reflex reversal? To examine these questions a series of long-term studies was embarked upon, using Dove prism goggles, rather than a mirror, to produce horizontal image inversion and yet permit freedom of movement for the subject. The first pair of these goggles was generously donated for the purpose by Ivo Kohler. Fig. 2 shows the time

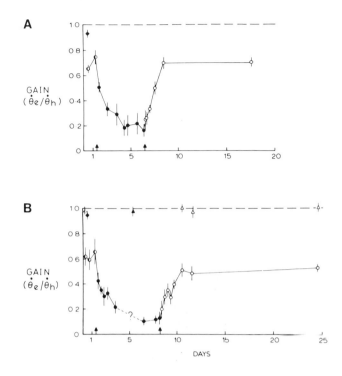

Fig. 2. Gain changes from two subjects exposed to about one week of continuous reversed vision. All points give mean VOR gain ($\dot{\theta}e/\dot{\theta}h$ = eye vel./head vel.) obtained from 20 cycle test runs in the dark. Half filled points, controls; filled points, during the period of reversed vision; open points, after return to normal vision. Diamonds show control results with normal vision. Triangles in B give dark-tested vertical (sagittal) VOR gain, which did not change. Vertical arrows show beginning and end of the period of reversed vision. (Reproduced from Gonshor & Melvill Jones 1976b.)

course of gain changes, measured as before, in two medium term subjects each of whom wore the reversing prisms continuously for periods of about one week. Very similar patterns of response were obtained from both subjects, demonstrating (i) progressive VOR attenuation from day to day over a quasi-exponential time course, which plateaued out at gain values between 0.1 and 0.2 over a period of 5–7 days; (ii) the acquired attenuation was retained over night; (iii) progressive, but not immediate, recovery occurred on return to normal vision; and (iv) recovery (or near recovery) of original control conditions was achieved within a week or two.

Some of the final dark-tested records from the 7 day subject (see question mark in B) hinted at more radical changes, amounting to commence-

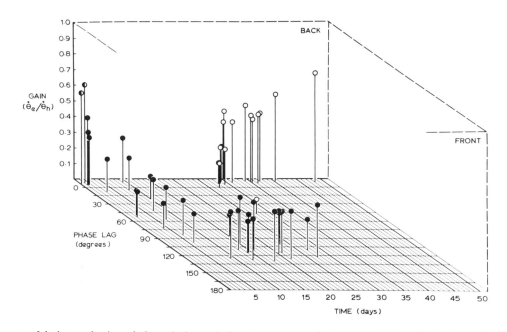

*Fig. 3.* Changes of dark-tested gain and phase during and after about one month of reversed vision. Symbols as in Fig. 2. Note than 180° phase would represent VOR reversal. (Reproduced from Gonshor & Melvill Jones, 1976b.)

ment of large but variable changes of phase, albeit at very low gain. Accordingly a longer duration of exposure, amounting to 27 days of continuous prism vision, was undertaken, with the overall outcome illustrated in Fig. 3. All points on this three dimensional display represent the dark-tested VOR. The height of each 'stalk' gives gain (ordinate) as before, whilst the abscissa gives time in days. The third, or z coordinate, depicts the phase of eye velocity, relative to that of the idealized normal compensatory response. Half filled circles show control values, filled circles those obtained during the period of reversed vision and open circles the time course of recovery after return to normal vision. If values obtained during the first 7 days are projected onto the gain-time plane (back 'wall' of the figure) the time course of adaptive attenuation is seen to lie close to those of Fig. 2. However, a notable additional feature seen here, is a progressive migration of phase in a lagging direction toward that of reversal (180°), plateauing out at between 120° and 130° phase lag, as tested at 1/6 Hz and 60° amp. in darkness. Note also the partial recovery of gain after the quasi reversed state had become stabilized.

Evidently the changes incurred are *adaptive,* in the sense that instead of 'mere' habituative atten-

uation, they trend progressively in a complex fashion towards the functional goal of automatic retinal image stabilization during head movement with reversed vision. The strictly adaptive nature of the process is further highlighted by the fact that changes were restricted to the plane in which they would be functionally useful. Thus, as shown by the triangular points at top of Fig. 2B and also in the long-term subject (not shown), no changes were seen in the sagittal vertical plane (SVOR), in which the Dove prisms produced no optical reversal of vision. The adaptive characteristic was later reinforced by findings described below which demonstrate upwards gain increment when this is called for by magnifying optics (Miles & Fuller, 1974; Gauthier & Robinson, 1975). The changes were considered *plastic* (Barlow & Gaze, 1977) in the sense that there was extensive and retained remodelling of the reflex in a functionally useful manner, with the added feature that complete recovery to normal conditions could be brought about, but only when this was called for by return to normal vision. However, the return sequence was not simply an inverted replica of the original adaptation. Instead of the slow original emergence of phase changes, there was very rapid restoration of phase to near normal within 1–2 h after remov-

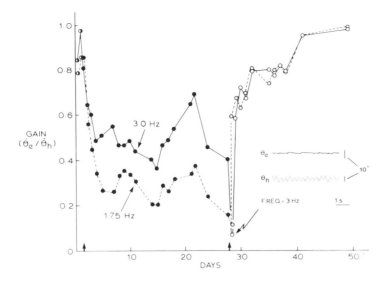

*Fig. 4.* Gain changes measured at 3.0 and 1.75 Hz during active 'sinusoidal' head oscillation (about a vertical axis) and temporarily non-reversed vision for all tests. Same subject and symbols as in Fig. 3. Inset shows the virtual absence of response at 3 hz half an hour after permanent removal of reversing optics. Vertical arrows as in Fig. 2. (Reproduced from Melvill Jones & Gonshor, 1982.)

ing the prisms. Nevertheless, thereafter the recovery of gain did follow roughly the same 2–3 week time course as that of its original modification. Apparently the gain and phase characteristics reflect more than one process in the adaptive mechanism, a matter considered in more detail later.

### 2.1.3. *Frequency-dependent characteristics*

The results of Fig. 3 were obtained at low frequency oscillation (1/6 Hz) in the dark. Fig. 4 shows additional results obtained with the (same) subject actively oscillating his head in the light, with the reversing prisms removed just for this test (i.e., with temporarily 'normal' vision). Only ocular gain is shown here, frequency dependence of phase being characterized separately in Fig. 5. As in Figs. 2 and 3 there were large and rapid initial changes of ocular gain (despite the presence of normal vision), plateauing out at values dependent on the frequency of oscillation. Note particularly the larger degree of attenuation at the lower frequency, which is contrary to expectation based on the frequency response of normal visual tracking. Note also the transient very low values of gain obtained shortly (half an hour) after final prism removal; and compare this with the corresponding

very low gain obtained at the same time during low frequency oscillation in the dark (first open circle in Fig. 3). This almost imperceptibly weak response is exemplified in the inset figure. It is also seen in long-term experiments on cats, as discussed later in connection with Fig. 15. Lastly, note the recovery curves of Fig. 4. As in Fig. 3 gain recovery was quasi-exponential, occupying a total of 2—3 weeks, but notably *with no further frequency dependence between the two curves.*

That novel frequency-dependent characteristics are present in the well-adapted state is clear from Fig. 5, in which sections A and B show gain and phase obtained over a decade of frequencies from 0.5 to 5.0 Hz. Here again head oscillation was active, with eyes open and reversing prisms temporarily removed for the test only, primarily to avoid confusion due to anticompensatory eye movements which can occur in these circumstances in the dark (Melvill Jones, 1964; Barnes 1979a). Open circles in Fig. 5a show (expected) control results, with gain close to unity and phase (not shown) close to that of perfect compensation. The filled circles in Fig. 5a and b show gain and phase over the same frequency range, pooled from four different days in the 2nd two weeks of the adapted period. Bearing in mind that at the low

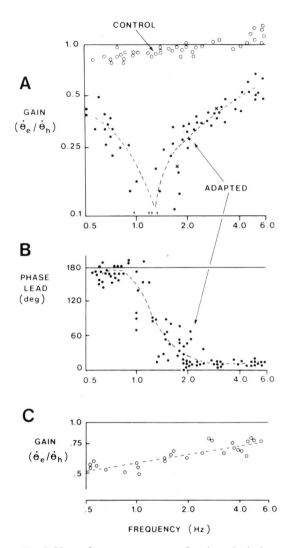

Fig. 5. Upper frequency response of ocular gain during control (upper open circles in A) and fully adapted (filled circles in A and B) states and 36 h after return to normal vision (C). In the fully adapted state note (i) the reversed phase at 0.5 Hz (despite temporarily non-reversed vision during the tests), (ii) the plunging gain and return to normal phase between 1 and 2 Hz, (iii) the monotonic increment of gain with frequency above 2 Hz, and (iv) the relatively simple attenuation of gain seen in C shortly after permanent removal of reversing optics. (Composite figure from data of Melvill Jones & Gonshor, 1982.)

end of the frequency range (0.5 Hz) visual tracking per se (i.e., with head still) could normally cope readily with the imposed task, and also the fact that for this test the reversing prisms were temporarily removed, it is remarkable to see that actual eye movement was reversed, thereby substantially worsening retinal image slip and hence also per-

ceptual visual blur (Barnes & Smith, 1981). Next, note the dramatic transitions of gain and phase between about 1 and 2 Hz. During this transition gain fell to values almost indistinguishable from zero, whilst phase underwent almost complete return to normal, albeit in a somewhat erratic manner. The feature referred to in the recovery phase of Fig. 4, namely loss of frequency lability on return to normal vision, is reaffirmed in the results of Fig. 5c. Here we see the corresponding gain plot obtained 36 h after permanent return to normal vision. At this stage the phase (not shown) was consistently near normal, whilst the gain, although depressed, showed a similar monotonic dependence on frequency to that of the control values at top of Fig. 5a.

### 2.1.4. 'Simple' and 'complex' components

What kind of clues do these findings offer for elucidation of the adaptive mechanism? The matter is discussed in detail elsewhere (Melvill Jones & Gonshor, 1982) and later in this chapter in connection with related results from animals. Briefly, it seems that at least two quite different adaptive processes must be at play when reflex reversal is called for by overt reversal of vision: one responsible for the relatively simple monotonic changes of gain, the other for more complex changes of phase (and dependent additional alteration of gain). Notable characteristics of the 'simple' gain changes are their gradual build up and gradual decay (time constants of days, see Figs. 2 and 3), and the monotonic dependence of gain upon frequency during most of the readaptation to normal vision (Figs. 4 & 5c). Notable features of the more 'complex' phase characteristics are (i) the long duration required for acquisition of phase 'reversal' (see Fig. 3; also Fig. 15), (ii) the very rapid loss of phase reversal on return to normal vision, and (iii) the apparent filtering out of phase reversal in the fully adapted subject at frequencies above about 1.0–2.0 Hz (Fig. 5a and b). It seems that whilst gain change obeys almost machine like rules (Miles & Eighmy, 1980), phase is highly frequency labile and, whilst taking weeks to acquire, can be 'forgotten' in a matter of hours when called upon to do so (but notably not overnight in darkness). One suggestion is that whilst the monotonic gain changes

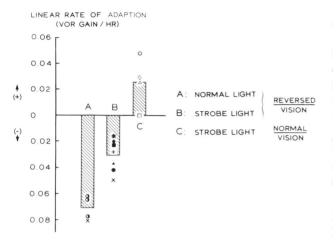

LINEAR RATE OF ADAPTION
(VOR GAIN / HR)

A: NORMAL LIGHT } REVERSED VISION
B: STROBE LIGHT } REVERSED VISION
C: STROBE LIGHT   NORMAL VISION

*Fig. 6.* Rates of change of dark-tested VOR gain (per hour) estimated over 6 h periods of (A) reversed vision in normal light, (B) reversed vision in 4 Hz strobe light, and (C) normal vision in strobe light. Each symbol represents a given subject and shaded columns give overall mean values. (Data adapted from Melvill Jones & Mandl, 1979.)

adaptive response (Ito, 1970; Gonshor & Melvill Jones, 1976b; Robinson, 1976; Chapter 14). An indirect way to test the hypothesis in a behavioural context would be to replace smooth retinal image slippage by intermittently stabilized retinal images, using stroboscopic illumination of short flash duration. Following this approach, human subjects were exposed to 6–7 h of active movement with horizontally reversing Dove prism vision in stroboscopic light of 4 Hz flash frequency and around 5 µs flash duration (Melvill Jones & Mandl, 1979). VOR gain was measured in the usual way by passive sinusoidal rotation in the dark whilst performing mental arithmetic to maintain mental alertness. Fig. 6 shows that despite complete elimination of smooth slippage, sizeable rates of adaptive attenuation still occurred (column B), amounting to roughly half that to be expected in similar circumstances in normal light (column A). The effect could not have been due to strobe illumination per se, since as shown in column C, control runs with normal vision in strobe light surprisingly tended to produce an opposite effect, namely augmentation of gain, perhaps called for by a need to bring the inherent VOR gain closer to unity due to the stroboscopically degraded visuomotor input. Clearly, continuous slippage of the image over the retina is not a necessary condition for production of adaptive change.

Possibly the discontinuous image displacement ($\Delta\Theta_e$) with respect to time ($\Delta\Theta_e/\Delta t$) could activate neural movement detectors in a manner similar to, but less effective than, continuous displacement ($d\Theta_e/dt$). The suggestion is in line with the similarity between neural responses in superior colliculus to discontinuous and continuous retinal image movement stimuli (Outerbridge et al., 1977), and with the recent human experiments of Barnes & Edge (1983). Alternatively, given a reversed final oculomotor drive "the possibility arises that an efferent copy of this drive (which is opposite to the vestibular one) might be responsible for changing the VOR" (Gonshor & Melvill Jones, 1976a). A similar principle has recently been incorporated into a new hypothesis of adaptive plasticity in this system (Miles & Lisberger, 1981b). This raises the question of whether in the human strobe experiments there was in fact effective modification of oculomotor outflow by the

might depend upon 'simple' plastic changes of synaptic efficacy in recognised VOR pathways (Wilson & Melvill Jones, 1979; see also Chapter 14), the added phase phenomena might derive from the more elaborate addition of a predictively generated periodic function (perhaps akin to that of Collewijn & Grootendorst, 1979 or Eckmiller & Mackeben, 1978), based on the predictable nature of the notably unchanging primary afferent vestibular input (Miles & Braitman, 1980). Such a function would take time to 'learn' but could be readily 'switched off' when no longer appropriate. That predictability may be involved is suggested by the fact that the presumed 'complex' component of response (calculated by vectorial subtraction of the 'simple' component from the fully adapted state) demonstrates frequency dependent characteristics similar to those associated with visual tracking of a predictably moving target (Melvill Jones & Gonshor, 1982).

### 2.1.5. Experiments in stroboscopic light

All the adaptive oculomotor phenomena mentioned so far trend in a direction suitable for reducing image slippage on the retina during head movement. Hence a reasonable guess would be that it is this slippage which constitutes the peripheral error message responsible for activating the

28

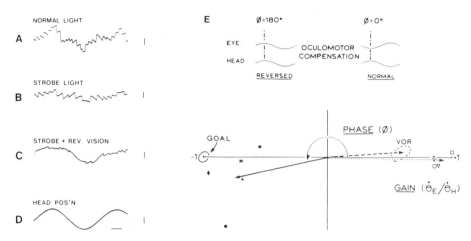

*Fig. 7.* Visual reversal of oculomotor output in a 'naive' subject during vestibular stimulation in 4 Hz strobe light. (A) Normal compensatory nystagmus during sinusoidal head rotation (D) in normal light. (B) Same, but in 4 Hz strobe light. (C) Reversed vision in strobe light produces reversed smooth eye movement, in opposition to the prevailing vestibular stimulation. (D) Polar plots of (i) dark-tested VOR (dashed vector), (ii) ocular response with non-reversed vision in strobe light (dotted vector extending to +1 goal), and (iii) mean vector of approximately reversed eye movement (such as in C) produced by reversed vision in strobe light (solid line vector directed towards −1 goal). Plotted points obtained from individual subjects. Inset diagram defines 0° and 180° phase. (Composite figure from data of Mandl & Melvill Jones, 1979.)

reversing prisms during head rotation in the strobe light environment?

To examine this question, eye movements of a subject wearing reversing prisms were recorded during sinusoidal rotation of the whole body in strobe light (Mandl & Melvill Jones, 1979). Fig. 7 illustrates a set of records from one subject, exposed to (A) normal vision in normal light, (B) normal (i.e., non-reversed) vision in strobe light, and (C) reversed vision in strobe light. It was remarkable to find that even though strobe flashes occurred at only 4 Hz with no more than 0.002% of time in the light, there was almost perfect reversal of smooth eye movement with, incidentally, appropriately placed (i.e., reversed), although unusually small, intervening saccades. Fig. 7E shows the general outcome of this study obtained from subjects whose adaptive results are shown in Fig. 6. Note that this study was undertaken at least one week before obtaining the results of Fig. 6. In the polar plot of this figure the length of the radius vector gives the numerical value of mean ocular gain, whilst the phase angle gives the difference between that of actual slow phase eye velocity and ideal normal compensation, the latter being defined as having a gain of +1 and zero phase. Conversely, with vision reversal the ideal response would reach the −1 goal with 180° phase (see inset diagram). The dashed vector gives mean VOR

with mental arithmetic in darkness. The dotted one shows the corresponding vector obtained with non-reversed vision in the strobe light. The main feature here is the third, solid line vector, pointing generally towards the −1 goal, and representing the (vectorial) mean outcome from records such as that in Fig. 7C. Individual means are shown as the five filled points distributed around the arrow-head of the mean vector. This approximately 'reversed' mean vector has a length (gain) of 0.77 and phase angle of +192° (or −168°). Clearly the reversed stroboscopic vision did produce marked and continuous modification of actual oculomotor outflow relative to the incoming vestibular drive. Hence, it is indeed possible that, according to the Miles/Lisberger hypothesis (1981a), it was this form of oculomotor-vestibular dysmetria which activated the adaptive response, rather than the presence of retinal image slip per se.

It is important to note that this visual production of an oculomotor signal which is opposite to that of the prevailing vestibular drive, took place before there were any parametric changes in the dark tested VOR. Thus, it transpired that the effect is almost instantaneous even in a subject who has never been exposed to the reversed vision condition. For example, when using a reduced flash frequency of 2 Hz, only the minimum necessary visual information (i.e., two strobe flashes in an otherwise dark room) was found to generate appropriate smooth eye movement, even when such movement was in a direction opposed to that of the prevailing vestibular drive. This raises the intriguing question of the extent to which generation of a 'mental' intent to achieve an identifiable goal might participate in producing this kind of response, particularly in view of the demonstrated effectiveness of purely mental effort, both in 'naive' subjects (Barr et al., 1976) and in the production of an adaptive change in the VOR (Melvill Jones et al., 1984). These latter questions are examined at greater length in Chapter 13.

### 2.1.6. Adaptation sickness

In normal light, active movement during prism-reversed vision quickly (5–15 min) generates a strong and lasting sense of malaise and nausea (Gonshor & Melvill Jones, 1980; Oman et al., 1980) akin to, perhaps the same as, the well known phenomenon of motion sickness (c.g. Money, 1970; Reason & Brand, 1975; Reason, 1978; Oman, 1982a,b; Igarashi et al., 1983). Similarly, as noted above, after equally short exposures to vision reversal in normal light, the already altered VOR leads to perceptual movement of the seen world during high frequency (3 Hz) oscillation of the head with prisms temporarily removed.

Neither of these two phenomena were evident in the strobe experiments (Melvill Jones & Mandl, 1981); which raises significant questions about the otherwise apparent similarity of results in strobe and normal light. That the lack of 'motion' sickness was due to selective resistance in the chosen subjects would be a statistical anomaly, especially since one of them had previously been troubled with severe and long lasting nausea during reversed vision experiments with normal light. Indeed, that subject admitted to having been apprehensive of anticipated nausea in strobe experiments, and yet experienced none. Again, another subject of the strobe experiments later quickly made himself nauseated simply by walking around for 20 min with the reversing prisms on in normal light. The lack of prism-free perceptual oscillopsia at 3 Hz head movement corresponded with complete absence of measured gain attenuation at this frequency (see Table 1 of Melvill Jones & Mandl, 1981).

Does this failure to generate the usual adaptive correlate of nausea represent an important finding? Or was it simply due to the reduced rate at which measured adaptive changes occurred in strobe light? Possibly it could be associated with the above-mentioned absence of measured gain change at higher frequencies, although there seems no obvious rationale for this. Alternatively, speculating rather wildly, could it be that presumed synchronous bursts of retinal afferent activity generated by the intermittent strobe flashes might in some way disorganize the (still mysterious, e.g., Miller & Wilson, 1983) link between neural phenomena responsible for adaptive and maladaptive components of the whole adaptation syndrome?

Be that as it may, the lack of VOR change at high frequency in the strobe experiments is of interest in its own right, especially in view of contemporary controversies concerning the dependence of adapted VOR dynamics upon conditioning stimulus frequency. (See section below on frequency dependence; also Chapters 21 & 22). Why should there have been selective low frequency (i.e., VOR attenuation at 1/6 Hz but none at 3 Hz) adaptation when the conditioning stimuli were provided by the broad spectrum of natural movement? Certainly, there was no such selective frequency dependence in the early phases of corresponding experiments conducted with reversed vision in normal light. One possibility is that with strobe illumination the high frequency components of head movement would generate widely separated, and relatively few, individual image placements on the retina per stimulus cycle, thus resulting in spatio-temporal patterns of image dispersion relatively devoid of meaningful velocity information. If this were so, then one might guess that the adaptive system had in fact been selectively stimulated by the low frequency components of natural movement, which in turn might account for the selective implementation of adaptive change at these frequencies. Does the coincident absence of nausea and of high frequency adaptation in the strobe experiments point to a link between nausea and high frequency stimuli? Clearly, the matter calls for further study, especially in view of the severe penalties currently experienced by astronauts during the early days of adaptation to zero gravity in orbital flight (e.g., Benson, 1977; Graybiel et al., 1974; Matsney et al., 1983; Money & Oman, 1983; Oman, 1982b).

### 2.1.7. Directional specificity of VOR adaptation

We have seen that reversal of vision in a horizontal plane produces adaptive changes in the horizontal VOR (HVOR). It was also noted (see Fig. 2B, upper triangles) that in the orthogonal sagittal plane, in which the horizontally arranged Dove prism produced no optical inversion, no such change occurred in the VOR tested in that plane (SVOR). This rather striking example of adaptive specificity seems physiologically plausible on the grounds that essentially separate sensory-motor pathways subserve the horizontal and vertical vestibulo-ocular reflex systems (Wilson & Melvill Jones, 1979). However, the same cannot be said for the orthogonal sagittal and frontal planes within the 'vertical' system, since each of these employs both sets of diagonally oriented vertical canal-muscle pairs, as illustrated in Fig. 8B, which is reproduced from Simpson & Graf (1981). Bearing in mind that the Dove prism does produce image movement reversal in the frontal plane (i.e., a plane perpendicular to the optical axis of the prism), an interesting question arises: does differential adaptation occur between SVOR and torsional VOR (TVOR) despite the fact that the same four sensors (anterior and posterior vertical canals) and same four effector muscles (superior and inferior recti and obliques) participate in the production of response in both these planes?

Investigating this phenomenon, Berthoz et al. (1981a) first determined that long-term exposure to horizontally investing Dove prisms does indeed produce attenuation in the normal TVOR (Fig. 8A), as well as in HVOR. Using a sensitive test of perceptual blur during head oscillation (Melvill Jones & Drazin, 1961; Melvill Jones & Gonshor, 1982), and bearing in mind the fact that no change in measured SVOR was ever found in previous and similar long-term experiments (Gonshor & Melvill Jones, 1976b), it was concluded that in the absence of any change in SVOR, TVOR could indeed be attenuated proportionally with HVOR (Fig. 8C). The finding would seem to exclude the use of synapses in the direct pathways of the vertical canal-muscle reflexes as targets for adaptive

'teaching' influences. Rather, it tends to implicate other neuronal pools in which the sensory-motor information becomes transformed into sagittal and frontal planes. Indeed, this could provide an indirect rationale for convergence of orthogonal canal afferent information, which although not frequent at the monosynaptic input level (e.g., Markham & Curthoys, 1972; Wilson & Felpel, 1972) appears to be much more common in the awake, unanaesthetized animal exposed to natural stimulation (Curthoys & Markham, 1971; Baker et al., 1983). The nature of the necessary central transform, and the required adaptive changes in central matrices at that level is explored in later chapters (Chapter 19 & 20).

### 2.1.8. Implications for postural control

In view of the significance of vision in the control of posture (e.g., Nashner & Berthoz, 1978; Nashner et al., 1982) and the normal reliance on VOR for the stabilization of vision, it becomes interesting to enquire how adaptive reorganization of VOR affects the visual control of posture. To this end, Gonshor & Melvill Jones (1980) studied balance control in subjects adapting to vision reversal in horizontal and frontal planes, as judged by their ability to walk along a thin rail with eyes open after the well tried method of Fregly & Graybiel (1970). It was not surprising to observe severe postural disturbance when first donning the reversing optics, as illustrated in Fig. 9. The figure demonstrates three notable features of postural disorganization in a long-term vision-reversed subject. First, after an initial almost catastrophic destabilization (subjects positively threw themselves against padded safely bars), marked improvement developed towards the original capability with normal vision. The time course of this recovery was notably similar to that of adaptive HVOR changes in the same subject (Fig. 3).

Theoretically this could have been the result of an acquired ability to disregard adverse visual inputs in favour of direct vestibulo-spinal signals, which might be thought to have remained unchanged. That this was not so is indicated by two significant findings. On the one hand, return to normal vision (second arrow on the abscissa) immediately produced a recurrence of the violent loss of balance seen when first donning the prism

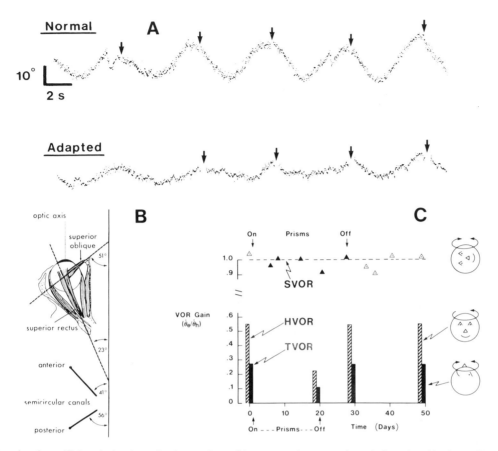

*Fig. 8.* Directional specificity of adaptive gain changes in a subject exposed to approximately 3 weeks of horizontally reversing Dove prism vision. Oriented in this way the prisms also produced optical reversal of vision in the frontal plane, but NOT in the sagittal vertical pane. (A) Normal and adapted torsional eye movements recorded under infra red illumination without vision (TVOR); note the marked adaptive attenuation of TVOR after approximately three weeks of Dove prism vision. (B) Roughly parallel orientation of vertical canal planes and those in which the vertically acting eye muscles operate in man. (C) Adaptive attenuation (and recovery) of HVOR and TVOR in response to horizontally reversing Dove prisms, which also reversed image movement in the frontal plane, but not the sagittal plane. Note the absence of change in the vertical sagittal VOR (SVOR) (triangles) recorded in the subject of Figs. 2 and 3. (A & C, data from Berthoz et al., 1981; B, reproduced from Simpson & Graf, 1981.)

goggles (first abscissal arrow). This could not have occurred if visual signals had been disregarded. Indeed the recurrence of a state of active destabilization on return to normal vision may well reflect the presence of a successfully reversed visuo-spinal reflex, perhaps worsened by a now adversely adapted TVOR (see previous Section and Fig. 8A). Changed perceptual interpretation of the visual scene noted in the next section on 'perceptual correlates', probably further contributed to the problem, since the subject described the visual world as apparently rotating in the frontal plane in the *same direction* as he was falling, which is opposite to normal experience.

On the other hand, the premise that the vesti-bulo-spinal system for balance control should not be altered by optical modification of vision seems untenable in the light of experimental results. Thus, there was marked (80%) deterioration in the *dark-tested* balance, suggesting that either vestibulo-spinal, or somatic limb reflexes (or both) had become in some way altered as part of the overall adaptive phenomenon. Perhaps this might be attributable to the fact that the final motor outflow to postural muscles would likely be the consequence of superimposed influences from multiple sources. If the visuo-spinal component of those influences had become adaptively altered, then accordingly so presumably should those from non-visual sources.

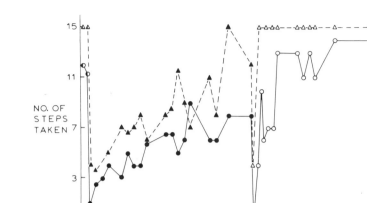

*Fig. 9.* Postural disorganisation and its recovery, produced by prolonged Dove prism vision. With eyes open the subject attempts to walk heel-to-toe along a thin rail. Half filled, filled and open symbols as in Figs. 2, 3 and 4. Continuous and dashed lines give data from narrow (0.75 in) and wide (2.25 in) rails respectively. Note (i) the sharp reduction of postural achievement on first donning the prism goggles (first abscissal arrow), (ii) the smooth pattern of progressive recovery during adaptation to reversed vision, (iii) the return of severe postural instability on return to normal vision (second arrow), and (iv) the prolonged period of recovery after prism removal, as reflected by performance on the narrow rail. (Reproduced from Gonshor & Melvill Jones, 1980.)

### 2.1.9. Perceptual correlates

The effects of vision reversal are not confined to purely reflex mechanisms. As mentioned earlier, after a mere 10–15 min of reversed vision, return to normal vision is associated with perceptual movement of the seen world on moving the head (Gonshor & Melvill Jones, 1980). More dramatically, Oman et al. (1980) have clearly demonstrated an associated reversal of the relation between seen movement of the external world and self-motion perception. In fact they showed that this radical alteration of visually perceived self-motion can be brought about within a few hours of commencing Dove prism vision. Normally the leftward rotating head is associated with relative right-going movement of the seen stationary world, and this visual stimulus then contributes to the perceptual sensation of self-rotation to the left. The phenomenon, known as circularvection, can conveniently be realized as a compelling sensation of body turning (say left), when the *stationary* subject looks at an artificially rotating (right-going) full field visual scene. The striking experience of circularvection (CV) has been known for many years (Mach, 1886), but has recently been inten-

sively studied in the modern context of visual-vestibular interactions on the ground (Dichgans & Brandt, 1972; reviewed 1978) and in flight and space (Chapter 10). Typically, in the laboratory a subject is seated on a fixed chair at the centre of an optokinetic 'drum' in the form of a concentric vertical (i.e., horizontally rotating) cylinder. The drum is then set in constant velocity (e.g., right-going) motion in darkness. On turning on the light one first sees the proper drum motion, knowing oneself to be still. Then some 5–20 s later the whole body is positively felt to start rotating relative to space in the opposite direction (left) and with increasing speed. Eventually most subjects report an apparently stationary drum, whilst the body continues seemingly to rotate relative to space at 'full' speed (to the left). The sensation tends to be correlated with on-going nystagmus, which in animals is in turn correlated with appropriate neural signals in the vestibular nuclei (see Chapter 16).

In Oman et al.'s first series of five subjects, all showed normal CV before donning the prisms. However, after 3–4 h of active reversed vision experience, "with a latency of between 10–42 s, all

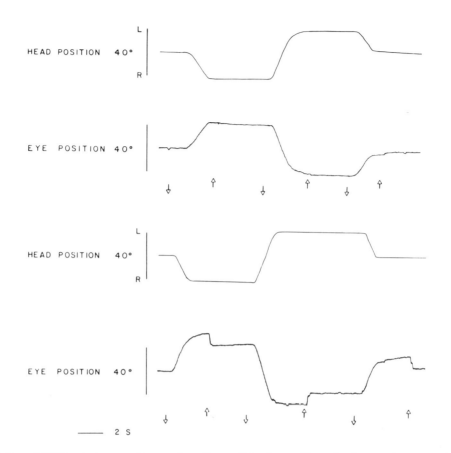

HEAD POSITION 40°

EYE POSITION 40°

HEAD POSITION 40°

EYE POSITION 40°

2 S

*Fig. 10.* Augmentation of VOR gain in man after wearing ×2 magnifying lenses. Top pair of traces show normal changes of eye position induced by stepwise head rotations in the dark (down and up arrows show moments of switching lights off and on, respectively). Lower pair shows the consistent overshoot of compensatory eye movement due to an augmented VOR after wearing ×2 lenses. With lenses removed for this test, the overshoot is corrected by a suitable short-latency saccade onto target after switching on the lights. Perceptually the (stationary) target appears to have moved (relative to space) in the direction of the saccade. (Reproduced from Gauthier & Robinson, 1975.)

five subjects reported an unequivocal sensation of motion in the *same direction* as the seen stripe (drum) motion" (i.e., to the *right* in our example). With this relatively short duration of reversed vision experience the phenomenon of reversed circularvection (RVC) appears to be somewhat labile, as observed in a second series of subjects. However, consistent within those experiencing RVC was the interesting feature that its presence was strictly confined to optokinetic stimulation within the limited visual field of previous Dove prism experience. Invariably, extension to wide field vision caused reversion to the normal direction of CV. The authors concluded from this that "visual information from the exposed central visual field is transmitted centrally along pathways

separate from those carrying information from the peripheral visual field". As we shall see below this is not an isolated example of correlated adaptive changes in related perceptual and reflex phenomena. The finding raises important questions concerning the commonality (or separateness) of the underlying plastic processes responsible for reflex and perceptual changes, and concerning the means by which perceptual veracity is both achieved and maintained in normal life (Melvill Jones, 1983a).

## 2.2. Non-reversed visual vestibular dysmetria

### 2.2.1. Experiments with magnifying lenses
The truly adaptive nature of the VOR's response to modified visual stimuli is high-lighted by

the fact that magnifying optics call for, and achieve, augmentation of gain, a phenomenon which could not possibly be accounted for by habituation (see Chapter 7). Following the premise that underwater divers should augment their VOR due to magnification of the scene viewed through a diving mask (Gauthier, 1974), Gauthier & Robinson (1975) studied the human VOR during and after several days of wearing ×2 magnifying spectacles. As did Miles & Fuller (1974; see below) in monkey, they observed systematic augmentation of the dark-tested gain and its progressive reversal to normal values after return to normal vision. Large gain magnification factors were achieved, up to around 1.7. Moreover, despite large differences in absolute values, these general patterns of change were present in each of three different mental sets, in which the subject, whilst in the dark, (i) tried to 'look' at the stationary outside world, (ii) performed 'non-committal' mental arithmetic, or (iii) tried to 'look' at a head-fixed target, after the methods of Barr et al. (1976).

Although their main results were obtained using conventional sinusoidal stimuli, they also employed an alternate method in an attempt to estimate perceptual correlates, as illustrated in Fig. 10. With head fixed to the turntable, subjects were asked to fixate a small earth-fixed target. Then, in complete darkness, but with the subject attempting continued fixation on the target, the turntable was rapidly rotated through 20–40° to a new stationary location, after which the stationary fixation point was again made visible. In control conditions (top pair of records) the VOR, operating at close to unity gain, ensured good spatial stabilization of gaze, and notably with the associated percept of the target having remained still in space. In contrast to this, after adaptation to the magnifying spectacles (lower set of records) the augmented VOR gain drove the compensatory eye movement through a larger angle than that of the head, so that the line of gaze moved away from the target in a direction opposite to that of the head movement, incurring a large corrective saccade in the same direction as the head movement. Thus, after a right-going head rotation, the gaze became shifted to left of the target. On re-illumination (upward arrow) the target was therefore seen to be

located to the right of the direction of regard, and this was associated with the percept that it (i.e., the target) appeared to have moved to the right; which is reminiscent of the altered sensation of circular-vection described in Section 2.1.9. This important demonstration of a tight correlation between perception of movement and gain of the VOR led the authors to conclude that adaptive recalibration had occurred at the vestibular input. Since no such changes have been found in the monkey primary vestibular neural signal (Miles & Braitman, 1980), this recalibration presumably reflects a central adaptive phenomenon which may provide a common basis for the changes observed in reflex and perceptual mechanisms (see also Chapter 13).

### 2.2.2. Adaptation to clinical prescription spectacles

Thus far we have described adaptive phenomena in response to abnormally large visual-vestibular discrepancies. Presumably, neither overt reversal of vision, nor two-fold changes of optical magnification have ever been experienced during the course of evolution. It is indeed remarkable to find such vigorous and extensive reactions to these grossly abnormal conditions; reflecting perhaps an evolved potential for contending with major pathological disturbances. Collewijn et al. (1983) have recently studied responses to relatively minor calls for change, such as those incurred by the lenses of normal prescription spectacles. Clinically it is well known that new prescription lenses tend at first to destabilize the seen world during head movement; and indeed the subsequent resolution of this effect has been investigated at a subjective level long ago (Rönne, 1923). Collewijn and colleagues were able to measure oculomotor correlates of the phenomenon by using high precision recording techniques employing the magnetic search coil method originated by Robinson (1963) and modified by Collewijn & Kleinschmidt (1975) and Collewijn (1977a).

Fig. 11 illustrates the time course of adaptive changes brought about in one eye of a myopic subject who normally wore negative corrective lenses, but for this experiment exchanged these for +5D spectacles, calling for an overall VOR gain increase of around 36%. In this particular experiment all conditioning and test stimuli were performed with active head oscillations of 0.66 Hz and

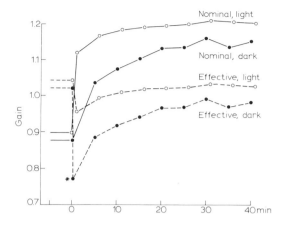

**Fig. 11.** Rapid gain changes induced in a subject converting from his normal negative spectacle lenses to positive ones of ×5D, representing an optical magnification factor of around 1.33. Continuous lines show the actual (nominal) ocular gain in dark and light, measured as eye movement relative to head movement. The corresponding 'effective' curves include the added effect of projecting gaze through the spectacles. For these tests active head oscillations (at 0.66 Hz and 17° amp.) were made continuously during a period of 40 min. The star (see foot of effective-dark curve) gives the theoretical value to which effective VOR gain in the dark was reduced from the pre-existing value by the magnifying lenses. Note the rapid approach of the 'effective, dark' curve from this starred value towards the ideal value of unity. (Reproduced from Collewijn et al., 1983.)

17° amplitude. Four curves are shown, open and filled circles representing conditions in the light and dark respectively; dashed and continuous lines giving, respectively, effective (i.e., including the effect of the worn lenses) and nominal (i.e., using actual eye movement relative to skull) gain values. Consider first the two continuous 'nominal' curves. The normal (control) ocular gain in the light was 0.9, reduced below unity due to the requirements called for by the subject's normal negative lenses. Note that in accord with this, his normal dark-tested VOR produced a similar sub-unity value. Then, on changing to +5D spectacles at time zero, there was immediate gain enhancement in the light, not far removed from that called for by the new lenses. The subsequent approach to this plateau was notably rapid, compared with those found in the larger percentage changes called for and described in earlier sections. Particularly interesting are the almost equally rapid changes in the dark-tested data, demonstrating that with these relatively moderate

demands the requisite adaptive changes can be induced over periods of minutes, rather than hours and days.

Turning to the dashed lines of 'effective' gain, we see similar time courses, with the functionally significant feature that both curves trend towards the required value of unity. In another subject (their Fig. 11) they noted an intriguing phenomenon, reminiscent of that described by Keller (1978) in monkey, whereby the effective light gain amounted virtually to unity immediately after donning the new lenses, implying little or no relative slippage of the retinal image during the active 'conditioning' head movements. Yet a progressive readjustment of dark-tested ocular gain took place in the usual way. The authors drew the interesting conclusion "that stimulation of the peripheral retina is unnecessary for adequate, fast adaptation of the V.O.R.".

These authors also compared the effectiveness of active versus passive head rotations, concluding in all cases that active movements are (slightly) more effective than passive ones, even when the subject tries to 'look' at an earth-fixed target in the dark. More significant in the present context is the striking finding that when different degrees of adaptive change are called for in the two eyes of a given subject, differential adaptation to the unequal demands proved difficult or impossible. Thus, it was concluded that when the conflict was mild, a compromise solution tended to yield residual errors distributed symmetrically between the two eyes. If, on the other hand, the interocular discrepancy was large, then the adaptive process of both eyes appeared to be controlled by the one eye found to yield the most meaningful information, as has been found in the adaptive control of saccadic gain (Chapter 4). Interestingly, the fundamental aspect of this resistance to differential changes in the two eyes has recently been called in question by studies of Snow & Vilis (1983), who were able to produce independent gain adjustments for each of the two eyes by imposing simultaneous conflicting visual error signals. The latter finding is particularly significant since it tends to violate Hering's (1868) law of equal innervation.

### 2.2.3. Rapid effects of transient VOR suppression
Another form of rapid adaptive change in the

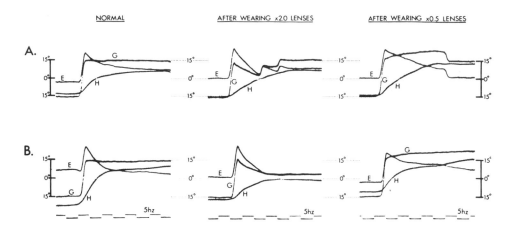

*Fig. 12.* Effects of magnifying and diminishing lenses on ocular compensation induced by active head movement in the trained monkey. (A) Target light on throughout (note that these tests were performed without lenses in place). (B) Total darkness during the head and eye movements. H, E and G: head re world; eye re head; gaze (H + E) re world. Note (i) the normal (left side of figure) cancellation of head movement by VOR, to produce stationary post-saccadic gaze, (ii) the over and under compensation produced after adaptation (several days) to magnifying and diminishing lenses, respectively, and (iii) the effects were relatively independent of whether the target light was visible or not. (Reproduced from Miles & Fuller, 1974.)

dark-tested VOR has recently been demonstrated following very short durations of visual suppression of the reflex (Segal, 1985). Human subjects were vestibularly stimulated by rotational oscillation on a conventional turntable in darkness, except for a small head-fixed point source of red light which could be switched on and off intermittently. Stimulus conditions were chosen so that when the light was on, almost perfect visual suppression of the VOR was possible. Therefore, not only was the reflex suppressed, but also presumably 'velocity storage' (Cohen et al., 1977; see Chapter 8) build up was prevented by elimination of dynamic motor output. Typically the light would be repetitively turned on for 9 s and off (total darkness with eyes open) for 2 s over a total period of 2 min. The 2 s periods in the dark thus permitted measurement of eye movements in the presence of a standard periodic vestibular stimulus, but notably after repetitive short periods of visual VOR suppression. By choosing an appropriate relation between sampling intervals and periodic time of the vestibular stimulus, sampling bins could be distributed evenly over the sinusoidal stimulus cycle, thereby allowing a description of 'post-suppression VOR' dynamics.

Assuming that any residual influence of pursuit would be lost after the first 200 ms in each dark period, one might expect a normal VOR to be present in the latter half of those periods. In fact it turned out that the measured gain in this time slot consistently remained some 60% below that to be expected during an equivalent vestibular stimulus in permanent darkness. Recall that the experimental design aimed at exclusion of effects due to both short latency pursuit mechanisms and accumulation of 'velocity storage'. What else could be responsible for this large percentage suppression in the dark? Certainly it does not represent a long-term adaptive phenomenon since, (i) there was no cumulative effect over the 2 min test period (or from one test period to another), and (ii) there was always full recovery to normal VOR gain within 30 s of continuous oscillation in complete darkness. Possibly the effect might be attributable to retention of a mental set associated with intended fixation on the head-fixed target (Barr et al., 1976), although this seems unlikely since subjects were required to concentrate on an *earth*-fixed location when in the dark. Alternatively it may represent a truly adaptive phenomenon acting over an even shorter time scale than that described in the previous section; in which case perhaps there may eventually prove to be a continuum extending from very rapid to very prolonged mechanisms in the overall adaptive process.

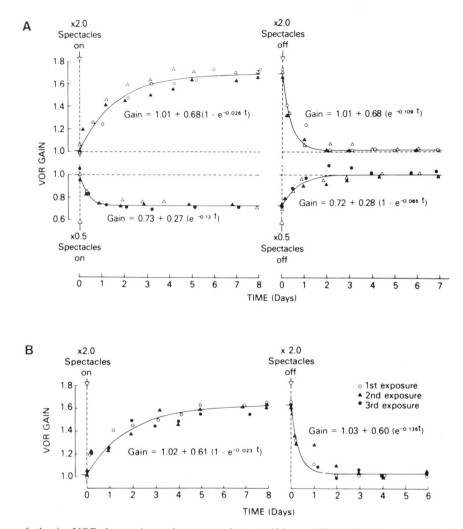

*Fig. 13.* Time course of adaptive VOR changes in monkeys exposed to magnifying and diminishing lenses. (A) Consistency of effects between different animals. (B) Consistency of repetitive exposure to the same adaptive (and readaptive) stimuli in one animal. Note that in the equations time is given in hours. For example the time constant of gain augmentation with ×2 spectacles was 1/0.026 = 38 h. (Reproduced from Miles & Eighmy, 1980.)

## 3. Studies on intact animals

### 3.1. Simple lenses

Miles & Fuller (1974), noting the excessive demands of the vision-reversed paradigm described in earlier sections, argued that simple magnifying or reducing lenses would better reflect any naturally evolved adaptive capability. Furthermore, as mentioned earlier, by calling alternately for augmentation or reduction of gain in the same animal, this approach should distinguish more clearly between simple habituative attenuation and a truly adaptive goal-seeking phenomenon. In Miles' initial study three monkeys were equipped with either ×2 magnifying or ×0.5 diminishing spectacles for durations of 3–21 days. During periods of optically modified vision, while the animals were free to move the head, they were not free to make natural body movements since they were constrained in a primate chair to avoid locomotor and postural coordination problems and to prevent manual interference with the lens fixtures.

After wearing ×0.5 diminishing lenses all animals reduced their dark-tested VOR gains in about 3 days from control values in the range of

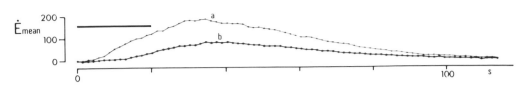

*Fig. 14.* Slow phase eye velocity induced by caloric stimuli (solid bar) (a) after adaptation to ×2 magnifying spectacles, and (b) in the normal animal. The mean post caloric a/b ratio was 2.15, which is to be compared with a corresponding VOR gain ratio of 2.03 obtained by passive oscillatory rotation in the dark. (Reproduced from Miles & Eighmy, 1980.)

0.9–1.0, to new minimum values in the range 0.6–0.7 (i.e., to within 20–40% of the ideal value, 0.5). Similarly in about 3 days the ×2.0 magnifying lenses produced gain augmentation to around 1.7 and 1.8 (i.e., within 10–15% of the ideal value, 2.0). An important additional finding was the significance of dynamic interaction of visual and vestibular signals in producing change. Thus, whereas monkeys who were returned to the free movement environment of their colony readapted to normal vision in 2–3 days, one animal whose fully adapted gain was 1.6 still retained an augmented gain of 1.3 after some 14 days of head immobilization in the light. Similar findings have been reported for free moving cats in the dark (Robinson, 1976), with the difference that here it was the visual, rather than vestibular, interactive component which was excluded. Paige (1983a and b), using alternately (i) darkness with free movement, and (ii) head immobilization in the light, confirmed the general phenomenon in canal-plugged monkey (see Chapter 9).

Fig. 12 demonstrates how the adapted gain changes extend to active as well as passive movements. The records are from a trained (Wurtz, 1969) monkey making sudden voluntary gaze shifts (with head free and without lenses on) between two dimly lit targets separated by 30°. Normally (left hand records) even with the target extinguished by initiation of the ocular saccade (row B), an accurate gaze shift was well stabilized due to near unity gain in the compensatory VOR during the ensuing head movement (Morasso et al., 1973). In contrast, after adaptation, despite retention of a generally appropriate ocular saccade, the subsequent direction of gaze was systematically forced away from the target location by an altered VOR. Of additional interest is the fact that retention of an illuminated target (row A) made little difference; which is reminiscent of the adap-

ted VOR's dominance over vision during active head oscillation in man (left side of Fig. 5A and B).

A later and more extensive behavioural study (Miles & Eighmy, 1980) generally confirmed these findings and emphasized the almost 'machine-like' nature of the adaptive process. Thus, the four curves in Fig. 13A show the time courses of adaptive and recovery changes induced in three separate animals (separate symbols) by magnifying and diminishing lenses (upper and lower curves, respectively). Note first that there were no great differences between animals in any of the curves, suggesting the action of a fundamental neurophysiological process rather than an idiosyncratic psychological learning phenomenon peculiar to each animal. Second, except for some of the earliest data points, each of the patterns of change generally follows a single exponential curve. Thus, the rate of change is closely related to the prevailing difference between present gain and that of the final 'goal' (i.e., plateau of achievement); which difference therefore represents a plausible index of 'adaptive drive'. Third, the rate of gain suppression was much faster (five-fold) than that of its augmentation, suggesting that gain reduction may be a less demanding process than its enhancement, a feature also noted in cat (Demer & Robinson, 1982; unpublished observations of the author). Fourth, although the rate of recovery from amplified gain was *faster* (four-fold) than its induction, the recovery from diminished gain was somewhat *slower* (two-fold), than its induction, demonstrating that return to the normal condition is not necessarily a faster process than adaptation to the abnormal one. Rather, both these latter observations tend to endorse the view that gain enhancement is generally slower than its reduction, independently of initial conditions.

Another 'machine-like' aspect of the adaptive process is shown in Fig. 13B where three succes-

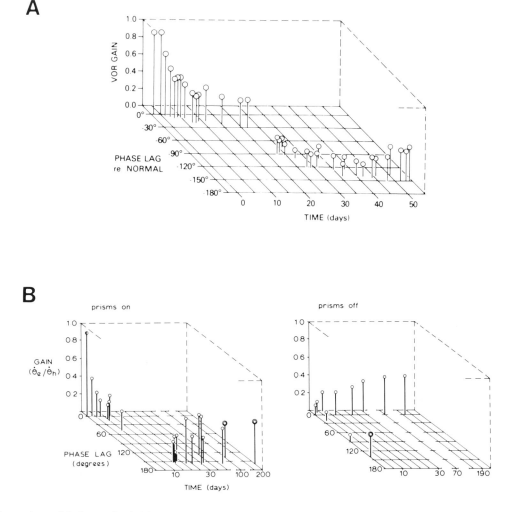

*Fig. 15.* Comparison of dark-tested gain/phase changes induced in (A) monkey (tested at 0.2 Hz and 25°/s amp.) and (B) cat (tested 0.125 Hz and 4°/s amp.) during (and after) long-term exposure to vision-reversing optics. Compare these 3-D plots with the human data of Fig 3. Note (i) the sharp transition of phase produced by introduction of forcing stimuli in monkey after 21 days, (ii) the close approach to reflex reversal (180° phase) in both animals, (iii) the relative stability of the adapted response after 2–4 weeks, despite very long-term exposure in cat (note the abscissal time gaps), and (iv) the two stage process of recovery (cat) on return to normal vision, similar to that for man in Fig. 3. (Reproduced from (A) Miles & Eighmy, 1980 and (B) Melvill Jones & Davies, 1976.)

sive cycles of adaptation to, and recovery from, ×2 lenses in the same animal are shown superimposed on one another. The three successive data sets are indistinguishable from one another, demonstrating unequivocally that over this sequence there was no evidence of 'acquired' enhancement of the adaptive capability.

Also in line with the 'machine-like' behaviour of the process are the responses to unilateral caloric stimuli, exemplified in Fig. 14. The two plots of induced eye velocity ($\dot{E}$) show the pooled means from three separate trials on the same animal, (a) after wearing ×2 spectacles and (b) in the normal condition. After completion of caloric irrigation (thick bar) there was a highly consistent ratio of adapted to normal gain, amounting to 2.15; which compares favourably with a corresponding VOR gain ratio of 2.03 based on conventional passive oscillatory tests in the dark.

All these factors led the authors to conclude that with non-reversing optics (including a visual field which does not move with the head) they were

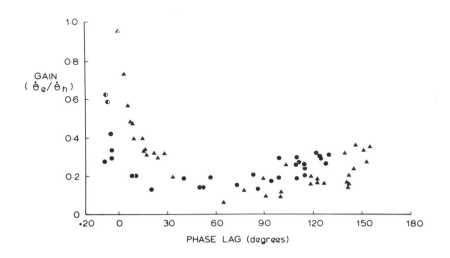

*Fig. 16.* VOR gain vs. phase replotted from the human data of Fig. 3 (circular points) and monkey data of Fig. 15A (triangular points), to illustrate the similarity of apparently 'fixed' relations between these two variables during the adaptive process. Each point represents the mean gain/phase value obtained from an individual test run at a given time during the adaptive process. Note the remarkably consistent pattern of gain phase relations both within and between species, suggesting a tight inter-dependence between these two variables. (Data from Gonshor and Melvill Jones, 1976b and Miles & Eighmy, 1980.)

observing the response of a single state system, characterized by a gain which is invariant at any given time. This conclusion implies that the established ability of man to superimpose influential strategic changes of the intended goal (Barr et al., 1976; Baloh et al., 1984; Melvill Jones et al., 1984; also Chapters 12 & 13), were unlikely to have been at play in these experiments on monkey. The implication is particularly significant for interpretation of their extensive correlated neurophysiological findings (Miles & Braitman, 1980; Miles et al., 1980a,b; Lisberger & Miles, 1980; reviewed by Miles & Lisberger, 1981a,b).

### 3.2. Reversing optics

However, this concept of a single state system cannot be extended to long-term results from animals exposed to the vision-reversed paradigm described in earlier sections of this chapter on human experiments. The general nature of this conclusion is made clear by comparing results in Fig. 15 obtained from (A) monkey and (B) cat, with corresponding results from man in Fig. 3. The data in Fig. 15A represent a two stage development of the monkey's adaptive response to vision reversal. For the first 3 weeks the animal's visual-vestibular conflict was restricted to that provoked

by head movement alone, through being constrained in the primate chair. As in man there was rapid VOR gain attenuation but, unlike the actively locomoting human, only minor changes of phase developed, although those which did occur were indeed in the same lagging direction. The animal was then force-oscillated in the light with prisms on whilst still in its chair, on a daily basis. Thereafter, gain-phase changes were remarkably similar to those of the freely locomoting human subject. Indeed, the apparently stereotyped gain-phase relations in the two species is highlighted in Fig. 16 by the superposition of human (filled circles; replotted from Fig. 3) and monkey (triangles; replotted from Fig. 15A) data points projected onto the gain-phase plane. The two data sets emulate one another to a remarkable degree, especially bearing in mind that the normal human control data are shifted downwards and to the left relative to those of the normal monkey. This degree of stereotype argues against these admittedly rather bizarre gain-phase characteristics being some kind of ephemeral phenomenon dependent on whimsical fluctuations of 'concentration' or 'effort'. Indeed, this conclusion is strengthened by the very close similarity of cycle by cycle gain-phase relations found even in separate individual test runs exhibiting large gain-phase fluctua-

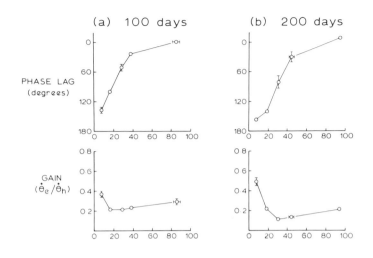

(a) 100 days  (b) 200 days

PHASE LAG (degrees)

GAIN ($\dot{\theta}_e/\dot{\theta}_h$)

STIMULUS pp AMPLITUDE (°/s)

*Fig. 17.* Amplitude dependent of the (dark tested) adapted response in cat, after (a) 100 and (b) 200 days of Dove prism vision. Note (i) reflex reversal was confined to low amplitude stimuli, (ii) gain attenuation was retained even at high stimulus amplitudes, and (iii) both gain and phase curves were considerably modified between 100 and 200 days. In the normal control animal the gain was stable at around 0.8 over the whole of this range. (From Melvill Jones & Davies, 1976.)

tions within the run (compare this Fig. 16 with the cycle by cycle data from three separate tests run at early, middle and late stages of adaptation, shown in Fig. 15A of Gonshor & Melvill Jones, 1976b).

An important additional feature of the vision-reversed adapted state, which contrasts markedly with that of the non-reversed condition produced by lenses, is its frequency and amplitude lability. Thus, whereas magnifying and diminishing lenses produced gain changes with relatively unchanged VOR dynamics (Miles & Eighmy, 1980), the reversal paradigm has already been seen to produce what might be termed an 'exotic' upper frequency response in man (Fig. 5), a feature also closely replicated over the tested range in monkey (i.e., up to 1.0 Hz; Fig. 9E of Miles & Eighmy, 1980). Moreover, as detailed in a later section (see Fig. 20), there was marked frequency lability of the dark-tested VOR in the reversed-vision adapted cat. Again, the long-term adapted cat demonstrated a heavy amplitude dependence of its response at a given frequency (see below and Fig. 17), indicating the introduction of marked non-linearities which defy simulation by contemporary linear models.

It seems that, whereas the simple changes of gain produced by non-reversing stimuli would be consistent with relatively simple changes of synap-

tic efficacy in known neural pathways, this is unlikely to be so for the reversal phenomenon. Rather, the demand for reversal appears to call up a more complex mechanism which, nevertheless, seems remarkably consistent within the different species so far examined. It could be argued that the reversal phenomenon represents no more than an artifact, introduced by the quite unnaturally extenuating circumstances of 'asking' for reflex reversal. On the other hand the clear facts that (i) the phenomenon does occur, and (ii) when present it obeys highly stereotyped, if complex, rules, point to an important versatility in the nervous system which does exist. As mentioned earlier it has been argued on an analytical basis that the 'complex' element may represent a learned predictive capability (Melvill Jones & Gonshor, 1982), perhaps analogous to that evidenced elsewhere (Collewijn & Grootendorst, 1979; Eckmiller & Mackeben, 1978). Whatever the mechanism, it requires no great stretch of the imagination to envisage a functionally useful role in the radical central neural reorganizations often called for by internal neural (or even external) pathology; or perhaps today in the quite unrevolutionary problem of adaptation to maintained zero gravity in space flight (Melvill Jones, 1974b; Ch. 10).

The three dimensional plot of Fig. 15B demon-

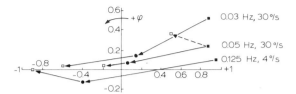

Fig. 18. Comparison of polar plots obtained from cats producing 'reversed' and non-reversed dark-tested responses. +1 and −1 represent the respective goals for vision stabilization with normal and reversed vision. Phase advancement (φ) of VOR relative to ideal normal is represented anticlockwise from the +1 abscissa. Filled squares show normal dark-tested VOR; filled circles show fully adapted dark-tested responses; open squares show responses in the presence of reversed vision, that in the upper right quadrant (dashed lined vector) being before adaptation, those on the left being after long-term adaptation. Results at 0.03 Hz, 30°/s amp. and 0.125 Hz, 4°/s amp. from Davies (1979); those at 0.05 Hz, 30°/s amp. from Robinson (1976). Note (i) the expected phase advancement of normal VOR with decreasing frequency (filled squares), (ii) the apparent continuum of adapted responses (filled circles) across the ordinate from non-reversed to 'reversed' conditons, and (iii) the very considerable advantageous effect of adaptation on the reversed vision performance (compare the open square in top right quadrant with the corresponding one in the adapted state). Arrowed lines show the vectors (i.e., gain = length, phase = direction) of change between connected points; e.g., as tested at 0.125 Hz, 4°/s the adaptation produced a change of dark-tested gain equivalent to 1.36 and a phase change of +189° (or −171°).

strates that the vision reversed paradigm can be made to produce gain and phase changes in the dark-tested VOR of cat (Melvill Jones & Davies, 1976) which strongly resemble those in man (Fig. 3) and monkey (Fig. 15A). Note incidentally that, at least under the test conditions employed here (see below), the major effects were produced within 3–4 weeks, both during adaptation to reversed vision and readaptation to normal vision. Even very long exposure (note the large abscissal time gaps in Fig. 15B) failed to produce more than minor improvement beyond this period, as tested at this frequency and amplitude. Note also the different time courses of phase changes during original adaptation and recovery, which are very similar to those commented on in connection with the human data of Fig. 3.

However, an important point to note is that whereas the human and monkey data of Figs. 3 and 15A were obtained with velocity amplitudes of 60°/s (1/6 Hz) and 25°/s (1/5 Hz), respectively, those of Fig. 15B for cat were tested at 4°/s amp. (1/8 Hz).

The cat's adapted response proved highly non-linear in the sense that it was very dependent on stimulus amplitude, as revealed in Fig. 17. Note particularly the very large changes of both phase and gain with stimulus amplitude over the tested range. Possibly similar non-linearity would be manifest in man and monkey if examined over a higher amplitude range, although this has not yet been examined in the present context. Here we do incidentally see a significant consequence of very long adaptive periods, by comparing the two data sets obtained at (a) 100 days (left side of figure) and (b) 200 days. Eventually (dark-tested) VOR reversal occurred with a gain of 0.5, although this high level of reversed gain was restricted to the very low stimulus amplitude of 4–5°/s, perhaps associated with the noted slow head movements made by these prism-reversed animals during their ambulatory excursions around the laboratory (Melvill Jones & Davies, 1976).

Incidentally, this high degree of amplitude lability nicely accounts for the fact that a parallel study of Robinson (1976), although revealing large gain changes, did not yield the large changes of phase seen in Figs. 15B and 17. Nevertheless, the two experimental series did in fact yield thoroughly comparable response characteristics under similar test conditions, as illustrated in the polar plots of Fig. 18 (compare with Fig. 6 of Robinson, 1976). Here the layout is similar to that of Fig. 7E, so that +1.0 and −1.0 on the abscissa represent the oculomotor goals for normal and reversed vision, respectively. Symbols are chosen similar to those in Robinson's figure, with solid squares and solid circles showing normal and adapted dark-tested VORs respectively and the open squares showing performance with prisms on in the light. First note Robinson's results, obtained at 0.05 Hz and 30°/s amp. (middle line of arrows in Fig. 18). Adaptation brings the dark-tested response from close to +1 to close to zero (intersection of coordinates), with the addition of reversed vision taking the response across the ordinate towards the new goal of −1. Note that the approximate 180° phase of the latter point represents approximate reflex reversal. Davies' (1979) data obtained at 0.03 Hz and 30°/s amp. (top line of arrows) follow a somewhat phase advanced version of Robinson's 0.05 data (as is to be expected at the lower frequency, see

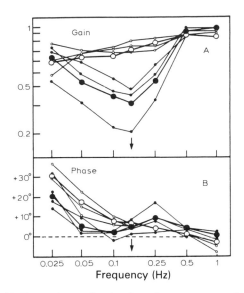

*Fig. 19.* Dependence of cat's adapted response upon the sinusoidal frequency of adaptive conditioning. Open and closed symbols show normal and adapted VOR. The arrows show the conditioning frequency. Each individual graph represents the mean of two experiments with an individual cat. The heavy line gives mean data from six experiments on three cats. Note (i) that this frequency-specific effect was produced by confining the conditioning stimulus to a single sinusoidal frequency with no free movement in the light, and (ii) the phase effects either side of the arrow, which conform with those predicted by the multiple pathway model proposed by Miles et al. in Chapter 21. (Reproduced from Godaux et al., 1983b.)

Wilson & Melvill Jones, 1979, Chapters 3 and 8), with generally similar trends. For comparison, an example of Davies' results obtained at the very low amplitude of 4°/s (1/8 Hz) (compare with Fig. 15B) is also shown (bottom line of arrows in Fig. 18). The normal dark-tested VOR was closer to zero phase (again, as is to be expected at this higher frequency), but the adapted one has already crossed the ordinate at close to 180° phase shift, so that approximate reversal is evident even in the dark. The functional adequacy of this degree of modification at this stimulus amplitude is evident from the close approach of the light-tested response to the new (i.e., reversed) goal of −1. Note particularly that seen in this format, the transition from the non-reversed adapted response at 30°/s to the reversed one at 4°/s (lower two filled circles) appears in reality to represent a graded, amplitude dependent, phenomenon rather than a fundamental difference. Note also the functional advantage of the adaptive phenomenon, by comparing

the reversed vision achievement of a naive cat (open square in top right quadrant at tip of the dashed line vector), with the adapted performance of the same cat (open square at left of the ordinate, close to −0.2 on the abscissa).

### 3.3. Dependence on conditioning stimulus frequency

Several investigators have addressed the interesting question of frequency specificity in the adaptive response. The matter is treated at length in another chapter (Chapter 21). Briefly, although some studies suggested but a weak effect (Robinson, 1976) or none at all (Davies, 1979; Ito et al., 1979a), others have identified a distinct, although variable, measure of dependence upon the frequency of conditioning stimuli (Collewijn & Grootendorst, 1979; Schairer & Bennett, 1981; Wallman et al., 1982; Lisberger et al., 1983). Possibly the variability of reported effects in the literature arises from the variety of different kinds of environmental experience encountered during or between conditioning stimuli. Thus, at one extreme, although Melvill Jones & Davies (1976) exposed both control and reversed-vision cats to very long periods of daily 2–3 h sinusoidal 'forcing' stimuli at 1/8 Hz, neither control nor adapted animals produced any sign of selective effect at this frequency in the dark-tested VOR's frequency response. However, between conditioning stimuli, these animals were treated as pets and although permanently equipped with reversing optics, were allowed free run of the lit laboratory environment. Consequently they were presumably exposed to a broad frequency range of reversed visual-vestibular interactions between forcing sessions.

At the other extreme, Godaux et al. (1983b) used a paradigm in which the only exposure to visual-vestibular interaction was at a given single frequency, all the intervening periods being spent in the dark. In these circumstances there was progressive development of clearly defined notching in the VOR frequency response at the conditioning frequency, as shown in Fig. 19. Presumably, therefore, the development of frequency specificity represents a basic property of the adaptive process, although it seems that, given adequate exposure to the broad frequency range of natural

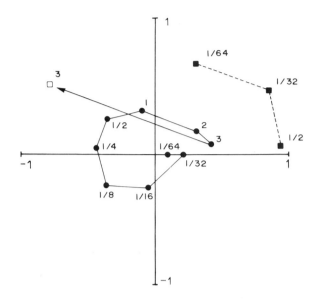

Fig. 20. Anomalous effects of vision on adapted responses illustrated in polar plot form. Data from long-term vision-reversed cat (Davies, 1979). Filled squares show normal phase dependence of dark-tested VOR upon test frequency (compare with filled squares of Fig. 18). Filled circles show the peculiar dynamics (gain/phase characteristics) of the adapted (dark-tested) response. The open square shows the effect of reversed vision in the adapted animal, tested at 3.0 Hz. The arrowed line shows the vector of visual influence at this frequency, which in normal circumstances is too high to produce a significant visuomotor effect per se. Numbers and fractions associated with plotted points refer to test stimulus frequency in Hz. (Modified from Davies, 1979.)

head movement, this property can readily be masked. Alternatively, as noted in connection with the strobe light experiments of Section 2.1.5., the adaptive attenuation may have been restricted to that frequency range in which the spatio-temporal dispersion of separately flashed images is compatible with the generation of meaningful retinal afferent information. The question of frequency selectivity in the adaptive process is of considerable contemporary interest and has indeed led to the development of a new proposal for the central mechanisms concerned (Lisberger et al., 1983; see also Chapter 21).

Another aspect of frequency-dependent changes is introduced by the vision-reversed paradigm. We have already seen that complex patterns of frequency response were produced by the prism-adapted human in the upper range of 0.5–5.0 Hz

(Fig 5). Fig. 20 illustrates in polar plot form the peculiar but definitive effects reported by Davies (1979) in the same animal as that of Fig. 15B after 250 days of permanent Dove prism vision. As in Fig. 18 filled squares (joined by dashed lines) give control values of gain (distance from origin) and phase (phase angle positive in anticlockwise direction), illustrating the normal pattern of amplitude and phase dependence in the dark-tested VOR (e.g., Robinson, 1976). In marked contrast, filled circles show the corresponding and additional points obtained in the dark-tested but fully adapted animal. Clearly the adaptive process produced large frequency-dependent changes, with only the 1/2 to 1/8 Hz range demonstrating approximate reversal; perhaps reflecting the major power spectral content of free head movement during the free locomotor activity of this animal.

### 3.4. Experiments in strobe light

The stroboscopic experiments on humans described in Section 2.1.5. were followed up with a related set of investigations in alert cats. Rather surprisingly, the outcome was that, at least with 8 Hz strobe light, the normal animal adapted similarly to the vision-reversed conflict, independently of whether illumination was normal or stroboscopic (Mandl et al., 1981), thus confirming the earlier conclusion that continuous image slip is not necessary for activation of the adaptive process. An extension of these experiments to animals reared exclusively in 8 Hz strobe light demonstrated that these also responded with a generally normal adaptive time course (see Fig. 3, Chapter 6), although their dark-tested VOR did tend to lie in the lower range of normal values (mean value of 0.72). The significance of this retained adaptive capability rests on the knowledge that cats reared exclusively in strobe light are deficient in the directional and orientation sensitivity of movement-detecting neural units in visual cortex (Cynader & Chernenko, 1976; Olson & Pettigrew, 1974; Pasternak et al., 1981; Pearson et al., 1983) and the functionally related superior colliculus (Flandrin et al., 1976; Kennedy et al., 1980). Hence the apparent lack of interference with the adaptive process found in these experiments with strobe-reared animals tends to exclude these com-

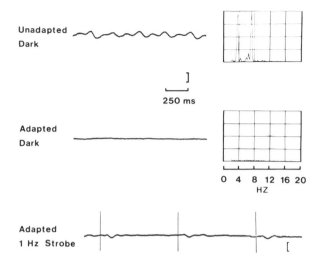

Unadapted
Dark

250 ms

Adapted
Dark

0  4  8  12  16  20
HZ

Adapted
1 Hz  Strobe

*Fig. 21.* Pendular nystagmus in a cat reared from birth in 8 Hz stroboscopic light (see also Chapter 6, Fig. 6) and its disappearance after adaptive attenuation of VOR. The top power spectrum at right shows concentration of spontaneous oscillations in the dark at the strobe rearing frequency of 8 Hz and its subharmonic of 4 Hz. The middle trace shows that these oscillations disappeared after 50–60% adaptive attenuation of VOR. The bottom trace shows retention of a latent tendency to activate the oscillatory system with intermittent single flashes (eye cal., 1°). (Reproduced from Melvill Jones et al., 1981.)

ponents of the visual system as important participants in the adaptive process. A similar conclusion could be drawn from the earlier experiments of Ito et al. (1974a) on rabbits, in which ablation of visual cortex did not materially alter their short-term adaptive capability. Feran & Douglas (unpublished) have recently drawn a similar conclusion from visually decorticated cat. The results of these studies emphasize the likely involvement of non-cortical visual pathways notably in the accessory optic system (see Chapter 1), in which the neural signal retains its directional characteristic in the strobe reared animal (Chapter 6).

Important to note is the fact that, although strobe rearing at 8 Hz does not apparently interfere seriously with either the normal development of VOR, or its adaptive modifiability, this conclusion does not apparently hold for all rearing frequencies. Thus, Kennedy et al. (1982) found an abnormally low VOR gain of around 0.45 in cats reared in 2 Hz strobe light. Moreover this value of gain was not adaptively raised towards the ideal value of unity, even after long periods (up to 5 months) of free movement in the light. It would be

interesting to know whether these animals would be equally resistant to adaptive attenuation of gain (e.g., as in Fig. 3 of Chapter 6), especially in view of the apparently greater ease of gain attenuation than augmentation noted above in connection with Fig. 13. Possibly the different effects of rearing at 8 and 2 Hz might represent part of a continuum from light to dark rearing, since complete denial of any visual contact during development has indeed been shown to produce abnormally low VOR gain, as well as impaired adaptability, at least in the direction of gain augmentation (Collewijn, 1976, rabbit; Harris & Cyander, 1981a, cat; see also Chapter 6). In this connection it is interesting to note that the newly hatched chick excluded from light also shows abnormally low VOR gain, although in this case there does appear to be a vigorous potential for visually induced adaptive changes in the reflex, both in the upward and downward directions and even to the point of reflex reversal (Wallman et al., 1982; Chapter 6).

An interesting additional feature of the strobe-reared animal, which also may have more general implications, is the appearance of oscillatory eye movements having their fundamental frequency close to that of the strobe light in which they grew up (Melvill Jones et al., 1981; see also Chapter 6). The phenomenon is of interest in its own right (Cynader & Chernenko, 1976; Conway et al., 1981). But in the present chapter its main significance lies in the fact that these self-sustaining oscillations were suppressed (yet latent) after marked adaptive attenuation of the strobe-reared animal's VOR gain. Fig. 21 shows first a sample of the oscillatory activity of a strobe-reared cat in the dark, together with its power spectrum. Two clear peaks occur, one close to the 8 Hz rearing frequency and one at half that value. However, both these peaks disappeared in the adapted state when VOR gain was reduced from 0.82 to 0.33, although, as seen in the bottom trace, a damped oscillation of roughly 8 Hz could be triggered by single intermittent flashes at one second intervals. It seems likely that central neural parameters controlling VOR gain are involved in the dynamics underlying this oscillatory condition, emphasizing the close interdependence of allied systems; a matter which will be developed in later chapters (3, 12, 22).

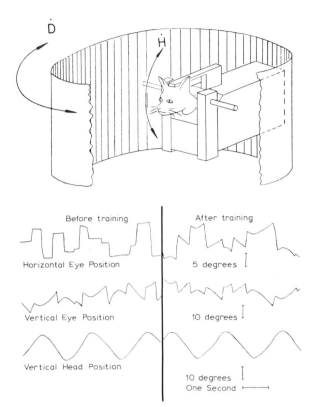

*Fig. 22.* Adaptive cross-coupling of horizontal and vertical components of VOR. The alert cat is oscillated in the sagittal vertical plane, with a strictly correlated horizontal oscillation of an optokinetic drum. The traces before and after several hours of exposure to this condition show the adaptive introduction of significant horizontal nystagmus by purely vertical oscillation of the animal in the dark. (Reproduced from Schultheis & Robinson, 1981.)

### 3.5. Directional plasticity

In Section 2.1.7 it was emphasized that there is high directional specificity in the human adaptive process: vision reversal in horizontal and frontal planes, but not the sagittal plane, produced proportionate adaptive changes in HVOR and TVOR, but none in SVOR (Fig. 8). Schultheis & Robinson (1981) adopted another approach to the general question of directional plasticity, using cats exposed to the experimental paradigm sketched in Fig. 22. The method builds on earlier psychophysical studies (Hay, 1968; Wallach et al., 1969) which demonstrated interesting perceptual rearrangements introduced by changing the usual relation between directions of visually and vestibularly sensed head rotation. In the figure, rotation

of the cat in its vertical sagittal plane induced strictly correlated horizontal rotation of the seen world (an optokinetic drum). Thus, when sagittal vestibular stimulation occurred, the functional need was to generate horizontal eye movement to follow the relative movement of the drum.

As seen in the records of Fig. 22, before training vertical head movement in the dark produced purely vertical (SVOR) compensatory eye movements, as is to be expected. However, after about 5 h training (right side of figure) the same head movement in the dark consistently produced a horizontal component (HVOR) of compensatory eye movement, with an HVOR/SVOR ratio of around 0.25. This interesting finding leads to important inferences about responsible central mechanisms, a matter examined in detail by Robinson in Chapter 20 and, in connection with a related topic, by Pellionisz in Chapter 19.

Another directional effect has been reported by Harris & Cynader (1981b), whereby a unidirectional bias can be built into the dark-tested cat VOR by combination of a sinusoidal vestibular stimulus with the unidirectional rotation of a surrounding optokinetic drum. The effect is relatively rapid in onset, being well marked after a mere 2 h exposure. Particularly notable is the fact that the observed changes of velocity bias were not associated with any change of VOR gain as such, which consistently remained at the pre-experiment value. In addition there are interesting developmental implications bearing on the similarities and differences of gain and bias control mechanisms, and their susceptibility for independent adaptive modulation, as discussed in Chapter 6.

### 3.6. Anomalous visual effects

A significant question arises as to whether the adaptive process extends to alteration of the effect of vision on oculomotor control. Several aspects of this question are currently under investigation. For example, Melvill Jones & Gonshor (1982) showed no alteration of visual tracking per se (i.e., with head still and target moving) in any of their long-term human subjects (see their Fig. 1). However, in Chapter 3 it will be seen that a number of authors have demonstrated modification of the wide field optokinetic reflex (OKR) which is

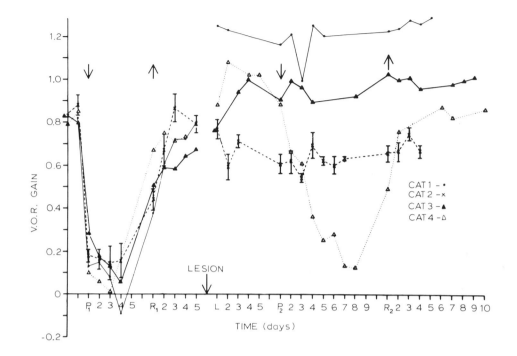

*Fig. 23.* Effect of lesioning the dorsal cap of inferior olive (IO) on the adaptive response of cat. On the left hand side four cats responded as expected to maintained vision reversal and subsequent return to normal vision. The right hand side shows the response of the same animals to the same adaptive stimuli after dorsal cap lesion. Three of the four showed no further adaptive response. Arrows at top indicate direction of expected adaptive change. P, prisms applied; R, return to normal vision; L, lesion of IO. (Reproduced from Haddad et al., 1980.)

closely associated with adaptive modification of the VOR: and recent evidence suggests that enhanced visual control of the VOR in the light may represent another component of the adaptive process (Douglas et al., 1982). The 3 Hz data from cat in Fig. 20 illustrate one aspect of this latter feature. Note especially the large amplitude of the vector joining the adapted data points in dark and (reversed vision) light. At this frequency visual stimulation alone normally has little effect, since it is above the upper cut off for normal visual following; yet here we see a large vector of visually induced change. Possibly a goal-directed change of mental set akin to that discussed above for humans (Barr et al., 1976) could be at play, although the contemporary data of Douglas et al. (1982) suggests there may be a superadded adaptive enhancement of the visual control of central mechanisms responsible for the VOR, as was also suggested by the findings of Keller in monkey (1978) and the human studies of Gonshor & Melvill Jones, 1980 (see their Fig. 8).

## 4. Ablation studies

This chapter is primarily concerned with behavioural phenomena in the intact animal, the question of central mechanisms being reserved for Part II of this book. However, Part II is mainly devoted to neurophysiological and analytical studies. Consequently, it is appropriate here to review briefly behavioural studies conducted in conjunction with selective ablation of central structures. The matter has been recently reviewed by Ito (1982a,b, 1984).

Early approaches were based on the contemporary development of Ito's hypothesis of cerebellar participation in the organization of motor control generally (Ito, 1970, 1972; see Chapter 14). The parallel development of this hypothesis and the behavioural experiments demonstrating adaptive plasticity specifically in the VOR (Gonshor & Melvill Jones, 1969, 1971) pointed to the cerebellum as a target for ablative interference with VOR adaptation.

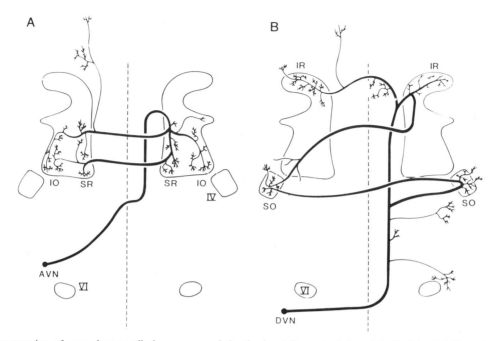

*Fig. 24.* Reconstruction of secondary vestibular neurons of the 'horizontal' canal of the adult flatfish. (A) Type 1 prospective excitatory neuron. (B) Type 2, prospective inhibitory neuron. Compare these pathways with those idealised in the right hand section of Fig. 5 in Chapter 1. AVN, DVN, anterior and descending vestibular nuclei, respectively. IV and VI, trochlear and abducens nuclei, respectively. IR, SR, IO, SO, inferior and superior rectus, and inferior and superior oblique muscles, respectively. Other abbreviations as in Fig. 24. (Reproduced from Graf & Baker, 1983.)

The first essentially simultaneous studies of Ito (Ito et al., 1974a,b) on rabbit, and Robinson (1975, 1976) on cat, produced similar results. Thus, in both laboratories, cerebellectomy, and in particular flocculectomy, prevented the ability of modified visual-vestibular interactions to produce lasting adaptive changes in the dark-tested VOR. Hassul et al. (1976) made similar observations in the chinchilla, whilst Takemori & Cohen (1974) and Daniels et al. (1978), working in a related but somewhat different context, observed impairment of rapid readjustments of VOR by vision in monkey and chinchilla, respectively. More recently, Lisberger et al. (1984) have confirmed the inability of monkey to produce any adaptive changes of VOR gain after complete flocculectomy.

Ito's hypothesis, based on the Marr (1969) Albus (1971) concept of climbing fibre (CF) control of Purkinje cell inputs in cerebellar cortex, pointed further to the significance of the inferior olive (IO) as the source of CF neurons projecting to floccular cortex (Desclin & Escubi, 1974; Alley et al., 1975). Ito & Miyashita (1975) there-fore placed lesions in the dorsal cap of IO and found that this too abolished behavioural adaptive plasticity in the rabbit's reflex. Later, Haddad et al. (1980) made a similar observation in cat, as illustrated in Fig. 23. At the left hand side are curves demonstrating the normal adaptive attenuation and recovery of reversed vision in unlesioned cats, whilst the remaining curves show the predominant lack of adaptive response in the same cats after selective bilateral dorsal cap lesions.

At this stage the search for the 'teaching line' of Ito's hypothesis seemed well under way, particularly in view of the earlier demonstration of suitable visual signals in this CF pathway (Simpson & Alley, 1974). However, serious complicating issues arose. First, ablation of flocculus tends to produce retrograde degeneration of dorsal cap neurons, prejudicing discrimination between lesions in the two sites (Barmack & Simpson, 1980; Ito et al., 1980). Second, it was found by Dufossé et al. (1978b) and Ito el al. (1979b) that destruction of olivary neurons can have remote consequences due to reduction of the effectiveness of Purkinje cell projections on their target neurons, although Montarolo et al. (1981) could not confirm this.

Attempting to circumvent this latter problem, Demer & Robinson (1982) argued that blockade of electrical activity in CF, without obstructing axonal transport, should resolve the issue. Accordingly they used local microinjection of anaesthetics at the CF decussation to produce reversible local arrest of CF neural signals projecting to the cerebellum. This invariably produced reversible *augmentation* of VOR, independently of whether the animals were normal, or preadapted to reversing prisms or magnifying lenses. From these results they concluded that "when climbing fibres are silenced but not killed, a learned behaviour (altered VOR gain) is readily abolished. This would suggest that the modifiable synapses storing learned behaviour are not in the cerebellum, since these would not be expected to change rapidly in the absence of climbing fibre activity".

The matter is however by no means settled at the time of writing. As the above authors cautiously point out, the loss of CF input could lead to Purkinje cell 'saturation' by augmented simple spike input, which in turn could invalidate their main conclusion. Perhaps more telling are the recent neurophysiological findings of Ito et al. (1982c; and Chapter 14) which demonstrate a marked potential for selective alteration of parallel fibre influence on Purkinje cell responses induced by coincident stimulation in the two systems (i.e., vestibular input via mossy fibers and IO input via climbing fibers).

Llinás et al. (1975) introduced a further complication by demonstrating that chemical destruction of CF projections invariably abolished or prevented, vestibular *postural* compensation after unilateral 8th nerve section; whilst cerebellar decortication did not. Important to note is the fact that their demand for adaptive change called specifically for readjustment of bilateral vestibular imbalance, rather than VOR gain per se which has been the main topic of this chapter (see Chapters 9, 17, 18, 22). And indeed, subsequent experiments of Haddad et al. (1977) suggest that different mechanisms may be involved in remodelling gain and bias (but see also Chapter 22).

Nevertheless, the view of Llinás and Walton (1979b; see also Chapter 15) that adaptive plasticity

may be represented by a distributed system rather than a particular component of the CNS is not to be taken lightly. As we will see unfolding in subsequent chapters of this book, a wide range of different autoadaptive mechanisms (Melvill Jones, 1983b) has already emerged within the neural systems for control of gaze. Moreover other systems, notably vestibulo-spinal reflex (Watt and Tomi, 1983) and even the short latency spinal reflex (Wolpaw et al., 1983a,b) have recently 'joined the club'. Evidently the time is ripe for new approaches to the elucidation of common processes involved. Falling into this category is a recent proposal of Ito (1984; see also Chapter 14) that cerebro-cerebellar connections generally may prove susceptible targets for adaptive modulation according to prevailing behavioural needs. No doubt parallel studies at the molecular level should in due course uncover common cellular and/or humoral neuromodulatory mechanisms.

## 5. Concluding remarks

In this chapter we have seen beyond doubt that visual alteration of behavioural context can be made to produce radical rearrangement of sensory-motor relations in the VOR. However, as noted in the Introduction to this book, and elaborated later in Part II, the underlying central mechanisms remain uncertain. In particular, can the *behaviourally* induced adaptive drive call forth reactive *central* plastic responses of the kind known to result from neural lesions (reviewed by Tsukahara, 1981)? We will find evidence of altered synaptic efficacy in the vestibular cerebellar cortex (Chapter 14) and of reactive synaptogenesis in central vestibular commissures during compensation for peripheral neural lesions (Chapter 17). These and other findings (e.g., Tsukahara & Fujito, 1976) do suggest that parameters such as neural gain can be altered in established central pathways by remote influences. However, this is not to say that 'rewiring' has occurred, in the sense of building new pathways which did not exist before.

At this point we may turn back to the remarkable flatfish for provocative implications. In Chapter 1, Simpson & Graf described a (so-far) unique form of adaptation in the VOR of this animal, associated with its metamorphosis from the normal swimming orientation shown in (their) Fig. 5A to the adult condition of (their) Fig. 5b (Graf & Baker, 1983). Recall that, as the body changes attitude by rotation through 90° about its long axis, so the 'under' eye (but *not* the vestibular system) also migrates to the new position shown in (their) Fig. 5B. As a result a new geometric relation is established between the sensor (vestibular end organ) and effector (ocular) mechanisms, such that the optic axes and the 'horizontal' (i.e., lateral) canals become (abnormally) perpendicular to one another. And yet, the above authors have established that the muscular insertions of the extraocular muscles do not change relative to the optic axis; they remain generally oriented as in any normal fish, or for example the rabbit. Hence, since the adult flatfish continues to exhibit a functionally appropriate VOR, it was argued that abnormal neuronal pathways must surely be developed to properly link up this anatomically modified sensory-motor reflex system. For example the disynaptic reciprocally acting pathways originating from the lateral canals should now project to the vertically acting eye muscles, as depicted on the right hand side of their figure.

Using HRP tracing this was indeed found to be so in the adult animal, as exemplified in Fig. 24 (from Graf & Baker, 1983), which reconstructs secondary vestibular neurons of the lateral ('horizontal'; but now vertically oriented) canals. The left side (A) shows a prospective Type 1 excitatory neuron projecting as it should to motoneuron pools innervating superior rectus (SR) and inferior oblique (IO) muscles. The right side (B) shows a

Type 2 prospective inhibitory neuron, also projecting as it should to motoneuron pools innervating inferior rectus (IR) and superior oblique (SO). Note particularly the (appropriate) cross linkages to corresponding bilateral sites in both instances. None of these connections appear to have been reported for second order vestibular neurons related to the 'horizontal' canal in other animals. Thus, Graf & Baker (1983) concluded that "the extensive axonal aborizations of flatfish horizontal canal neurons onto the oculomotor and trochlear nuclei seems to be a novel development initiated by the necessity to adjust eye movements to a new environmental situation".

Of course one can only speculate on the part played by vision in this adaptive reorganization of internal neuronal connections. It would indeed be interesting to know whether these idiosyncratic pathways would fail to emerge in the dark-reared flatfish. If so, this would provide strong presumptive evidence for behavioural determination of target sites for specific *new* neuronal projections, in this case ultimately controlled through behaviourally induced visual afferent stimuli. If the veracity of this presumption were proven it would surely open a new perspective on potential mechanisms at play in the visual control of VOR modifiability. Alternatively, of course the novel neural connections which are anatomically defined here, could be the outcome of morphogenetic control. The topic is pregnant with fruitful potential: but at this time in history the matter remains one of the many unanswered questions in this field.

Adaptive mechanisms in gaze control
Facts and theories
*Eds. Berthoz & Melvill Jones*
© 1985 Elsevier Science Publishers BV (Biomedical Division)

# Chapter 3

# Integration of adaptive changes of the optokinetic reflex, pursuit and the vestibulo-ocular reflex

H. Collewijn

*Department of Physiology I, Faculty of Medicine, Erasmus University, Rotterdam, The Netherlands*

## 1. The limited tolerance for retinal image slip

The relation between the amount of retinal image motion and the quality of vision is not known with great precision and has been investigated mainly for human subjects. Recent measurements have been reviewed by Steinman et al. (1982). When a subject's head is stabilized on a biteboard the standard deviation of horizontal eye angular position is about 3 min of arc (3′) on a single meridian and retinal image speeds are on the order of 15′/s. When the head is unsupported and the subject stands or sits still, the standard deviation of eye position rises to about 15′ and retinal image speeds increase to about 27′/s. When, in addition, natural head movements are encouraged, the standard deviation of eye position during a fixation task is augmented to about 30′ with retinal image speeds of about 97′/s. As retinal image speeds as high as 100′/s do not adversely affect vision of detail (Westheimer and KcKee, 1975; Murphy, 1978), and the diameter of the iso-acuity area is as large as 50′ (Millodot, 1972), the precision of gaze during bodily movement is sufficient in terms of position as well as speed to permit clear vision. On the other hand, retinal image velocities are high enough to prevent visual fading even when head movements are kept to a minimum (Skavenski et al., 1979). However, we are ignorant of the limits for perceptual fading or blurring in animals with a different retinal organization such as the cat and rabbit.

Limitation of retinal slip velocities is achieved by the generation of continuous, smooth eye movements through the optokinetic reflex (OKR), the vestibulo-ocular reflex (VOR) and the smooth pursuit (SP) system. However, the process of automatic stabilization is not simple. First, the origin of retinal image motion is both in the subject (eye, head and body motion) and in the external world (object motion). Second, the degrees of freedom are numerous since the locations of the eyes as well as of a target can change by rotations around three orthogonal axes and translations in three dimensions. Compensatory eye movements in mammals on the other hand consist only of rotations of the eye in the orbit. This calls for a complex guidance system and even this can provide only partial stability (Carpenter, 1977). Translation of the eye relative to the world is caused by linear head movements and locomotion. Such a motion cannot be truly neutralized by rotation of the eye, which can give an approximate compensation only for one plane of depth, and a strict one only for a single point in object space. Therefore, in species with foveal vision, stabilization is likely to be optimized for the central visual axis. Although a truly effective mechanical solution for the compensation of translation has been developed by several birds (pigeon, chicken, duck) in the form of a linear head nystagmus made during walking, this path has not been followed by mammals with lateral eyes such as the rabbit. Possibly the mass of the head and the compactness of the neck do not allow a similar solution. Another complication in the use of rotations is that several axes of rotation do not coincide. Particularly those of the eye and head can be rather far apart. As a consequence, the gain of the VOR has to be adjusted for distance (Blakemore & Donaghy, 1980; Collewijn et al., 1982b). The OKR, SP and VOR subsystems have to cooperate precisely to achieve their mutual goal of image stability. When the result is not satisfactory, adaptive changes occur in one or more of the subsystems to improve stability.

In most experiments on adaptation, the emphasis has been on parametric changes in the VOR caused by simultaneous vestibular and (modified) visual input, i.e., dissociation between head and eye movements (Chapter 2). Less attention has been given to long-term changes in OKR and smooth pursuit induced by prolonged motion stimuli. Improved visual tracking might also enhance retinal stability of targets during movements of the object or head. As VOR, OKR and smooth pursuit have certain neuronal circuits in common, (part of) an adaptation may be shared by several of them. Before examining some of the evidence of the integration of adaptive changes in the several subsystems it is necessary to briefly review their properties in several species.

## 2. Stabilizing subsystems

### 2.1. The optokinetic system of the rabbit

The rabbit is the best studied example of non-foveate species. Its visual field is virtually panoramic, although not homogeneous, as a visual streak and a sector of potentially binocular vision are present. Preferential looking behaviour is only expressed in the production of large saccades combined with head movements (Collewijn, 1977a). Visual acuity is about 20′. No independent eye movements are generated and no smooth pursuit of small moving targets can be elicited. When the head of the alert animal is immobilized, eye movements are virtually suppressed. All that remains is

a rather coarse tremor and a drift not faster than about 0.1°/s, occasionally interrupted by a saccade which usually returns the eye towards the mid-position (see Collewijn, 1981a).

The stability of the eye is due to an active process and is lost in darkness, which may result in a ten-fold increase of drift velocities. When the light is turned on again the eye will come to rest without returning to the position taken prior to the period of darkness. The system at work here is the OKR. In the absence of head movements it is the only system capable of preventing (or at least reducing) slow drift of the eye in the orbit. Also, drift caused by very slow head movements, which are not an effective stimulus for the labyrinth, is only compensated by the OKR. In the rabbit, OKR has the following response characteristics when exposed to a suddenly imposed constant velocity optokinetic stimulation in the horizontal plane. A 'direct' and 'indirect' system can be distinguished similarly as in the monkey (Chapter 16) but the contribution by the direct system is small. After a latency of about 100 ms, a 'direct' response with slow-phase eye velocities up to about 2°/s is rapidly generated (Fig. 1A). Higher eye velocities (in response to rotations faster than a few degrees per second) are developed only gradually (Figs. 1B and 2A) with an average acceleration of no more than about 1°/s² (Collewijn, 1969). Once slow-phase eye velocities have surpassed the 'direct' range of a few degrees per second, sudden darkness will result in optokinetic afternystagmus (OKAN). The slow phase velocity of OKAN decays linearly with time in the rabbit (Collewijn et al., 1980a), which is in contrast to the traditional description of this decay as exponential in primates and cat. The steady-state velocity gain (after build-up) for constant stimulus velocities is shown in Fig. 3. Gain is not better than about 0.8 for stimulus velocities up to 12°/s. For higher velocities gain decreases progressively, with a steep decline for velocities higher than 60°/s. The gain values shown for the rabbit in Fig. 3 (means of four animals) are somewhat higher than the ones previously published (Collewijn, 1969, 1981a, b). This is in part due to improvement of the stimulus. A drum lined with a random dot pattern (elements about 1°) is more effective than a stripe pattern. In contrast, we recently found that a projected stripe

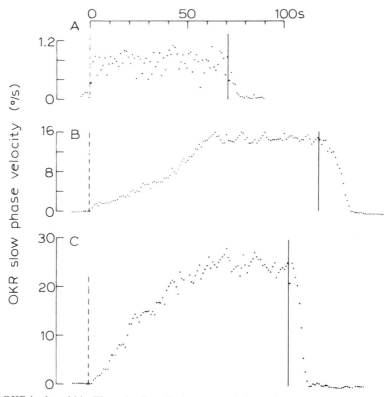

*Fig. 1.* Characteristics of OKR in the rabbit. The animal was in the center of a large drum which rotated around a vertical axis. Slow phase eye velocity is shown as a function of time. Beginning (light on) and end of stimulation (light off) are marked by broken and solid lines, respectively. A, immediate response to low velocity stimulus (1.2°/s). B, slow build-up during stimulation with 30°/s. C, slow build-up during open-loop stimulation with 1.2°/s. (from Collewijn, 1981b).

pattern, filling the entire visual field, is a very ineffective optokinetic stimulus for the rabbit. The gradual building up of slow-phase velocity can take place only incompletely when a periodic (e.g., sinusoidal) stimulus motion with frequent changes in direction is administered (Fig. 4A). It is also abolished after bilateral labyrinthectomy (Collewijn, 1976). In these circumstances mainly the 'direct' (short-time constant) response is seen, with a cut-off at lower stimulus velocities than with constant velocity stimulation. For the rabbit, this cutoff velocity (Fig. 4A) is about 5°/s, independent of frequency and amplitude of the stimulus. The OKR system is most simply described as a closed-loop velocity feedback system with the retinal slip velocity as input to the feedback pathway, encoded by retinal direction-selective ganglion cells (Oyster et al., 1972) and subsequently converging in the pretectal nucleus of the optic tract (NOT; Collewijn, 1975b). The neural velocity signal is a non-linear function of retinal image velocity with relative insensitivity for higher velocities. However, this is not the main cause of the inferior response to high stimulus velocities. This is shown in studies in which the visual oculomotor feedback loop is opened mechanically or optically so that the retina receives a constant motion stimulus, uninfluenced by the elicited eye movements. Open-loop stimulation of the rabbit's retina with low velocities (Collewijn, 1969; Dubois & Collewijn, 1979a) elicits an OKR with eye velocities much higher than the stimulus velocity (open-loop gain up to about 100), but also this velocity is built up gradually (Fig. 1C). Thus, in closed as well as open loop conditions, visual motion signals can elicit a direct motor response not faster than a few degrees per second in the rabbit; higher visually elicited eye velocities are only developed after long periods of continued stimulation. This behaviour has been simulated in a model by a direct pathway (with low gain) and an indirect pathway containing an integrator (with long time constant) in parallel

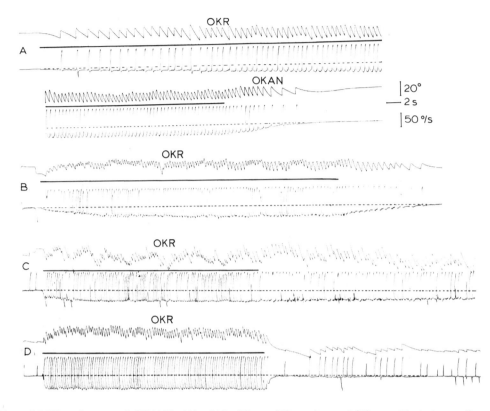

*Fig. 2.* Build up of OKR and course of OKAN in (A) rabbit, (B) cat, (C) monkey and (D) man. Typical recordings obtained with the scleral coil method while the animal or subject was positioned in the center of a similar real drum, lined with a random dot pattern (elements about 1°) which rotated around a vertical axis at a constant velocity of 60°/s clockwise. The horizontal bars mark the period in which the light was on. Upper traces, eye position; lower traces, eye velocity. Continuous recordings. For the monkey, only the initial period of OKAN is shown.

between the sensory input and the slow phase generator (Collewijn, 1972).

In view of the many speculations on the role of the central and peripheral retina in the generation of OKR it is important to note that the rabbit's visual field is not spatially equipotent in mediating the OKR, but that on the contrary this potential is concentrated in and congruent with the visual streak. The periphery beyond the streak is incapable of inducing OKR, and the optokinetic sensitivity runs parallel with the density distribution of retinal ganglion cells (Dubois & Collewijn, 1979a).

### 2.2. Integration between VOR and OKR in the rabbit

The dynamic range of the VOR is more or less complementary to that of OKR, specifically when

the canal-ocular response is tested with horizontal rotation in darkness. The responses of the rabbit to sinusoidal oscillations can be approximately predicted on the basis of the traditional model of the cupula-endolymph motion as an overdamped second-order system with a long time constant in the order of 3 s (Baarsma & Collewijn, 1974). The best performance is found for stimulus frequencies above 0.3 Hz with a gain of about 0.8. The VOR responses to oscillation are fast, both in the sense of latency (about 10 ms) and of rapid development of high eye velocities, which occasionally reach 400°/s in spontaneous head shaking behaviour (Collewijn, 1977a).

In normal head rotations in all species the integral of accelerations in opposite directions over time periods of a few seconds is always virtually zero and the VOR shows no aftereffects. Only unidirectional velocity steps (acceleration impul-

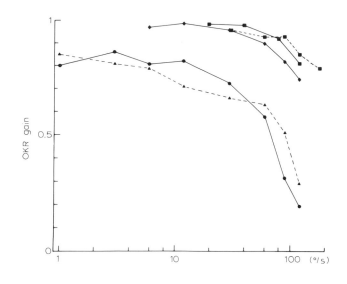

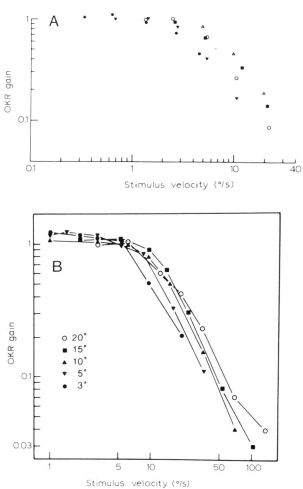

Fig. 3. Steady-state gain of OKR for rabbit, cat, monkey and man as a function of stimulus velocity. Measurements were obtained with the scleral coil method inside a real drum rotating around a vertical axis. (●) rabbits ($n=4$); (▲) cat ($n=2$); (◆) man ($n=1$); (■) monkey; interrupted lines: from Lisberger et al., 1981; solid lines, after Paige, 1983a.

Fig. 4. Optokinetic gain as a function of stimulus velocity for sinusoidal oscillation of a drum surrounding the animal around the vertical axis. These periodic stimuli predominantly excite the direct OKR. A, rabbit (from Collewijn, 1981a); B, cat (from Godaux et al., 1983a).

ses) in darkness elicit a long-lasting per- or post-rotatory nystagmus (PRN).

The time course of PRN in the rabbit is much longer than that of the cupula and similar to that of OKAN, even to the extent that after rotation in the light OKAN and PRN cancel each other perfectly, so that no afternystagmus occurs (Ter Braak, 1936; Collewijn, 1981a). This suggests that PRN and OKAN are mainly controlled by similar central storage mechanisms for visual and vestibular motion information, and that cupular dynamics are of secondary importance. In the rabbit the decay of PRN (as well as OKAN) is linear, although in man it is exponential (Collewijn et al., 1980a; Baloh et al., 1983).

Under normal conditions, the direct OKR and VOR will act in concert with, as a result, relatively good stability throughout the naturally occurring range of head and ocular drift velocities. The actual level of stability during spontaneous behaviour in the rabbit is reasonably good, although not perfect and somewhat dependent on the type of behaviour. It is best in the frontal plane, somewhat less good in the horizontal plane, and rather poor in the sagittal plane (Fig. 5) (Van der Steen &

Collewijn, 1984). There are indications that periods of very good stability occur during periods of apparently increased visual activity with increased saccadic frequencies (see Collewijn, 1981a, Figs. 20, 21). However, the typical stability in the moving rabbit is probably lower with horizontal retinal slip velocities up to about 5°/s occurring most of the time (Van der Steen & Collewijn, 1984). In a way these estimates of stability are academic, because they are based on the ratio between eye and head rotations, which is a true measure of stability only for visual targets at infinite distance in the absence of translations. In

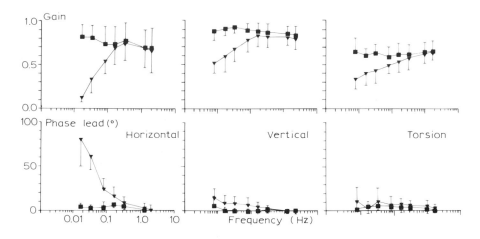

Fig. 5. Gain of the VOR (oscillation of the animal in the dark) and combined VOR and OKR (oscillation in the light) of the rabbit, oscillated in three different planes. (■) light (OKR + VOR); (▼) dark (VOR) (from Van der Steen & Collewijn, 1984).

reality the rotational axes of eyes and head are spatially separated, visual objects of interest are close or distant and locomotion involves a great deal of linear displacement. True stabilization of the retinal image by ocular rotation alone is clearly impossible. The normal level of performance of the rabbit's compensatory systems may strike some compromise which optimizes the average amount of retinal image motion. Possibly, the rabbit with its rather primitive retina and low visual acuity is also relatively tolerant to retinal image slip.

### 2.3. Optokinetic and vestibular reflexes in the cat

In the cat, the eyes have moved to a frontal position. A central area has developed in the retina, but the overall distribution of ganglion cells has also retained features of a visual streak and a true fovea has not formed (Stone, 1978). In this respect the cat occupies an intermediate position between the rabbit and primates. The cat makes independent eye movements in the head and its saccadic gaze displacements are smaller than in the rabbit (Collewijn, 1977b). However, its oculomotor responses to moving objects are rather similar to those of the rabbit. As shown by Evinger and Fuchs (1978) horizontal smooth pursuit of small moving targets is very poor, with maximal eye velocities of only 0.6°/s. Addition of a background moving together with the target augmented this

maximal pursuit velocity to 8.5°/s. To reach higher tracking velocities, prolonged stimulation in an optokinetic drum is necessary (Honrubia et al., 1967; Collins et al., 1970). Evinger and Fuchs mention a maximal OKR velocity of 28°/s, reached after 15–20 s. They noticed that the recruitment of the slower, indirect pathways was very dependent on a sufficient level of attention. Keller and Precht (1979) show eye velocities of about 45°/s during optokinetic stimulation of 60°/s. Haddad et al. (1980), using a scleral coil and a real rotating striped drum mention a steady-state gain of about 0.82 at 20°/s and about 0.65 at 40°/s. In addition, they specify an initial pursuit velocity of 2.4°/s (reached within 0.2 s) and a time constant for the build-up of the indirect response of 2.7 s. Figs. 2 and 3 show some recent results obtained in my laboratory with cats stimulated in an optokinetic drum lined with a random dot pattern (the same one as used for the rabbits). Slow phase velocities as high as 57°/s were observed. As Fig. 3 shows, the steady-state gain-stimulus velocity relationship is not significantly different from that for the rabbit if both species are investigated under optimal circumstances. Less favorable stimulus conditions may have led to Donaghy's (1980) estimate of 4–8°/s as the cut-off stimulus velocity for the OKR of the cat; this is probably about an order of magnitude too low. The real break in the gain curve seems to occur for stimulus velocities around 60°/s.

It is worth emphasizing that maximal opto-kinetic performance is only obtained under optimal circumstances. The animals have to be alert, but also the stimulus configuration has to be optimal. A real rotating drum is more effective than a projected pattern, and a random dot pattern is probably a better stimulus than a regular grating. Fig. 2B suggests that the major difference between rabbit and cat is the magnitude of the acceleration of the gradual, indirect component of the OKR. While in the rabbit this is about $1°/s^2$, in the cat a value of $5°/s^2$ is typical, at least in the first few seconds of stimulation (acceleration decreases at later stages). Thus, the charging of the velocity storage integrator is faster in the cat than in the rabbit. A true direct pursuit pathway as found in primates seems to be poorly developed in the cat, as suggested by the poor pursuit of small targets (Evinger & Fuchs, 1978), and the small immediate component in the build-up of velocity and its decrease; OKAN in darkness has practically the same initial velocity as the steady-state OKR (Fig. 2) without a significant sudden drop in velocity.

The responses to periodic motion of the surroundings is best described as a function of the maximal stimulus velocities, independent of the amplitude and frequency of the stimulus (Fig. 4B) (Godaux et al., 1983a), as was also found for the rabbit. However, the cut-off velocity is higher (about $10°/s$) than in the rabbit.

The frequency response of the VOR of the cat has been measured with electro-oculography by Landers & Taylor (1975), Donaghy (1978) and Godaux et al. (1983a), and with the scleral coil technique by Robinson (1976). All authors agree that the response is flat in the range 0.1–7 Hz, with a phase lead not exceeding 10°. The gain found with the scleral coil method is about 0.9. A second order system characterized by two time constants of 21 s each fitted Robinson's data best, while a single cupular time constant of 4 s described the data poorly, in contrast to the findings for the rabbit. This difference may reflect the faster charging of the velocity integrator, which will improve the responses to low frequencies.

The synergic action of horizontal OKR and VOR during head oscillation in illuminated, stationary surroundings results in a flat gain close to unity and a negligible phase error for amplitudes of 3–20° and frequences of 0.025–1Hz (Godaux et al., 1983a).

## 2.4. Optokinetic reflex and smooth pursuit in primates and humans

The development of foveal vision in primates induces a marked heterogeneity in the distribution of visual acuity. Optimal use of the foveal high quality sector of the visual field (about 1° in diameter) requires excellent oculomotor control. In addition to stability, which is no less important than in the rabbit, positional accuracy is of supreme importance. Thus, whereas a tight coupling between eye and head movements serves the limited needs of the afoveate rabbit well enough, the foveated primate requires independent fine control of eye movements relative to the skull in addition to automatically coupled eye and head movements (see Berthoz, Chapter 12). It may be no coincidence that this achievement is paralleled by the capacity for detailed motor control of the distal extremities.

Although the functional demands on the primate's oculomotor system are high, in one sense they are simplified by foveal vision: the direction of looking is no longer ambiguous. The critical requirement for detailed vision is that the line of sight (the projection of the fovea in space, shortly defined as gaze) intersects with the target. Mechanically, this goal can always be achieved by rotations, whatever the complexity of the head or target motion. Of course this will require deviations from a simple one-to-one relation between eye and head rotations, and also the inclusion of vergence movements to retain binocular fixation. The selective control of foveal vision will involve complex and often uncorrelated motion of the peripheral retinal images due to the non-coincidence of rotational axes of eye and head, linear displacements with parallax motion, and also motions of the target relative to the background. The required control of gaze direction in the primate is achieved by a combination of saccades (which correct position) and smooth movements (which control velocity as well as position). The saccadic component will not be discussed in detail in this review. Smooth oculomotor control has been well investigated in monkey and man.

### 2.4.1. The monkey

In the monkey, optokinetic responses to whole-field rotation can be divided into immediate, short-time-constant and delayed, long-time-constant components (Cohen et al., 1977, Lisberger et al., 1981) (Chapter 16). This division is qualitatively similar to that described above for the rabbit, but the quantitative relations are quite different. The initial component shows accelerations of several hundred degrees per $s^2$ and although this maximum is maintained only for a couple of hundred ms, slow phase velocities close to $100°/s$ are reached within a second (Lisberger et al., 1981). Higher velocities are built up gradually through a long-time-constant system. When darkness is introduced after complete development of OKR, there is a sudden drop in slow phase eye velocity, corresponding to the immediate ending of the short-time-constant component, whereas the long-time-constant component lingers on as OKAN with a gradual decay. OKAN is abolished by bilateral destruction of the labyrinth (Cohen et al., 1973). In order to estimate the relative strengths of the two mechanisms, Lisberger et al. (1981) employed the initial acceleration of the eye in the first 0.1 s of stimulation and the initial velocity of OKAN.

An example of the very rapid development of the OKR in a monkey, exposed suddenly to rotation at 60°/s in the same drum as used for the rabbit and cat is shown in Fig. 2C. The steady state OKR gain for the monkey is shown in Fig. 3, based on the data published by Paige (1983a) for squirrel monkeys and those of Lisberger et al. (1981) for the rhesus monkey. All those data are in good agreement and show a substantially higher OKR gain in the monkey than in the rabbit and cat throughout the velocity range, but particularly above 60°/s. All these data were obtained with real rotating drums and electromagnetic search coils. We found that the use of a projected stripe pattern resulted in markedly lower OKR gains in the monkey, especially above 30°/s.

Unlike the rabbit, the monkey is able to track small moving objects with the central retina. This is the smooth pursuit system. There is of course no reason why this system would not also be activated by whole field stimulation and indeed many arguments have been advanced to support the notion that the direct component of the monkey's OKR is nothing else than smooth pursuit (Lisberger et al., 1981). Both have short latencies and fast dynamics. Although smooth pursuit can generate some afternystagmus (Muratore & Zee, 1979), Lisberger et al. (1981) emphasize that this effect is relatively small.

The direct component of OKR as well as smooth pursuit is severely depressed after bilateral ablation of the cerebellar flocculus (Zee et al., 1981; Waespe et al., 1983). The optokinetic responses and visuo-vestibular interactions in the monkey after flocculectomy show all the characteristics of the indirect system controlled by velocity storage which is typical for the normal cat and rabbit. Actually, the acceleration of the OKR response was reduced to $3–5°/s^2$ (Waespe et al., 1983) which is the normal value for the cat.

### 2.4.2. Man

In man, oculomotor responses to moving visual patterns are not very different from those in the monkey. Results for a human subject, recorded in the same drum used for the species discussed above, are shown in Figs. 2D, and 3. Surprisingly, we find that even in highly cooperative and motivated human subjects the OKR induced by a real drum lined with a random dot pattern is substantially better than that elicited by a stripe pattern projected on a hemicylindrical screen, as used for instance by Van Die and Collewijn (1982). A main difference with the monkey appears to be a still greater dominance of the direct, short-time-constant response. An immediate OKR response with high velocities is normally seen in man (Cohen et al., 1981). This response is replaced by a gradual build-up described in patients with maldeveloped foveas (Baloh et al, 1980), lesions of the vestibulocerebellum (Yee et al., 1979) and hereditary cerebellar ataxia (Zee et al., 1976a). Vestibulocerebellar lesions in man also lead to decreased ipsilateral slow phases of OKR and smooth pursuit movements (Dichgans et al., 1978). Also, during open-loop stimulation with a low, but non-corregible retinal slip velocity high eye velocities are built up within a few seconds (Dubois & Collewijn, 1979b). OKAN is present in normal humans but less vigorous, shorter and more variable than in the monkey, rabbit or cat (Collins, 1970; Brandt et al., 1974; Zee et al., 1976b; Koenig & Dichgans, 1981). Human OKAN saturates at about 20°/s (Cohen et al., 1981).

Bilateral dysfunction of the labyrinths abolishes or strongly attenuates OKAN in man (Zee et al., 1976b; Zasorin et al., 1983) and also produces some defect in the optokinetic tracking of higher drum velocities. The abolishing of OKAN after destruction of the peripheral vestibular organs seems to be a universal phenomenon in mammals. It is due to the loss of the primary afferent fibers with their tonic resting discharge, because simple plugging of the canals, which leaves the resting discharge unaffected, does not interfere with OKAN in the rabbit (Barmack & Erickson, 1981) and in the monkey (Cohen et al., 1982) (see also Chapter 9). The phenomenon may be primarily caused by the silencing of vestibular nuclear activity (see Chapter 17, this volume) due to the loss of the tonic afferent input, but more research on this defect and the lack of recovery seems needed.

The classification of oculomotor responses to moving targets into a direct OKR, identical to SP, and an indirect OKR seems to be a valid and useful concept which can be applied to all mammals. The neurophysiological backgrounds of this division are discussed in Chapter 16. One should be cautious in associating these two forms too readily with foveal and peripheral stimulation. Extra-foveal smooth pursuit has been demonstrated in man (Winterson & Steinman, 1978). In monkey and man OKR is heavily dominated by the central retina (Koerner & Schiller, 1972; Cheng & Outerbridge, 1975; Dubois & Collewijn, 1979b; Van Die & Collewijn, 1982). OKAN is not effectively stimulated in the monkey by peripheral field stimulation during foveal suppression of OKR (Lisberger et al., 1981). This implies that in the monkey large field, extrafoveal stimulation is relatively ineffective in producing OKAN, and that the long-time-constant response is only adequately activated by full-field stimulation. In man, however, the existence of peripherally induced OKAN has been emphasized by Brandt et al. (1974). The short-time-constant system can be activated by either

full-field or small stimuli but has no access to the OKAN storage system. An extra factor to be reckoned with is selective attention which can modify the local weight of different parts of the retina in producing oculomotor responses (see Collewijn et al., 1982a). In particular peripheral stimuli require special attention from the subject to be effective (Cheng & Outerbridge, 1975; Dubois & Collewijn, 1979b). However, it seems likely that in general oculomotor and adaptation processes in man are largely controlled by the central retina, which tends to be aligned with the features attracting the momentary attention.

Although OKR in man seems to be heavily dominated by the 'direct' pathways, one should also be cautious in considering the human response to full field stimulation as identical to the voluntary pursuit of a small target. Some recent results on the gain of human smooth pursuit of a discrete target moving at constant velocity (triangular wave) are shown in Fig. 6 (Collewijn & Tamminga, 1984). These gains are much lower than the OKR gain shown in Fig. 3 for man and fall steeper with the increase of stimulus velocity. The smooth pursuit gain is also lower than that of OKR generated by large projected stripe patterns (Van

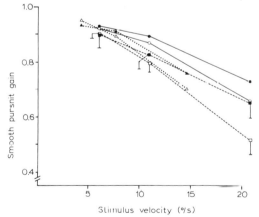

*Fig. 6.* Gain of human smooth pursuit (with saccades deleted) as a function of stimulus velocity. The stimulus was a red laser spot moving at constant velocity in alternating directions (△, ▲) in either one dimension (horizontal or vertical) (—) or in both dimensions simultaneously. In the latter case the target followed a rhomboid (diamond) trajectory. The stimulus amplitude was 7.07 (······) or 10° (—,---) (horizontal (solid symbols) and vertical (open symbols) gains were calculated separately); the frequency was varied from 0.15 to 0.52 Hz. Average results for five subjects (from Collewijn & Tamminga, 1984).

Die and Collewijn, 1982). These findings emphasize that the influence of the physical nature of the stimulus should not be underestimated in quantitative assessments of oculomotor tracking.

### 2.5. The VOR in primates and man

The horizontal VOR in the monkey under normal circumstances, measured in darkness, appears to be very stable and well-calibrated. The gain has been reported as very close to unity (Miles & Eighmy, 1980; Zee et al., 1981) and recently as 0.85 at the average in the squirrel monkey (Paige, 1983a). The phase deviates by not more than a few degrees from a perfect compensation in the frequency range 0.1–1 Hz. For lower frequencies, the properties of the VOR depend on the previous experience of the animal, as will be discussed later. The gain of the human VOR seems considerably more flexible and actually highly contingent on the conditions under which it is measured. Traditionally, the VOR is assessed by passive oscillation of human subjects, alertness of whom is secured by making them do mental arithmetic during the test. Although values vary somewhat, most investigators have found relatively low gains under such circumstances. For frequencies between 0.1 and 1.0 Hz, Benson (1970) found a gain of 0.70; Meiry (1971, his Fig. 4) about 0.43; Gonshor & Melvill Jones (1976a, their Table I) about 0.70; Barr et al. (1976) 0.65–0.83; Barnes & Forbat (1979) 0.54–0.90; Wall et al. (1978) about 0.52. Such values are surprisingly low and would suggest a poor calibration of the human VOR with a continuous need for suppletion by OKR-SP subsystems. However, as Barr et al. (1976) first described, the performance level of the human VOR is strongly influenced by specific instructions to the subject concerning the mental spatial frame of reference. Imagination of a stationary target in space made the gain of the VOR in darkness rise to 0.95; a functionally much more meaningful level. On the other hand VOR gain declined to 0.35 if the subject imagined that a target was fixed to the chair and rotating with him. Such flexibility calls for careful choice of specific control of mental set if one wants to investigate systematic changes such as adaptive phenomena with any precision, but some recent findings suggest that most of the ambiguity is abolished by

studying head movements produced actively by the subject. Takahashi et al. (1980) and Tomlinson et al. (1980) found relatively high values for the VOR gain during active head movements in the dark. Collewijn et al. (1983), using a very precise scleral coil technique found an average effective VOR gain for active head movements in the dark (corrected for spectacles) of 0.96 ± 0.04 (S.D.), which was only 0.05 lower than for similar movements in the light. For passive motion in the dark an average gain of 0.82 ± 0.12 was found in the same subjects, who were instructed to keep looking at the imagined stationary target. Thus, in darkness gain was not only lower but also more variable. It appears that active production of head movements automatically involves the decision to fixate the stationary world with activation of the VOR, in a similar way as achieved by the imagination of a fixed target (see also Chapter 12).

During active movements in the light, human compensatory eye movements have a gain close to unity, but rarely precisely one. Collewijn et al. (1983) found an average gain of 1.01 ± 0.03 (S.D.), with each subject deviating consistently by a few percent from the unity value. The resulting imprecisions in gaze have been mentioned in the introduction and extensively discussed by Steinman and Collewijn (1980), Collewijn et al. (1981a, b) and Steinman et al. (1982) (see also Ch. 12).

The interaction between the VOR, indirect OKR and direct OKR (smooth pursuit) are too complex to be understood quantitatively unless suitable mathematical models are used. To appreciate the evolution and explanatory power of such models the reader should consult Robinson (1977a,b, 1981a), Henn et al. (1980), Buizza and Schmid (1982), Buizza et al. (1980), Berthoz and Droulez (1982) and Waespe et al. (1983a).

### 3. Adaptation and habituation

Changes in properties of oculomotor reflexes after repeated testing have been recognized long ago. Specifically, changes in the time constant of postrotatory vestibular nystagmus due to repeated velocity steps, administered in darkness, have been described as habituation of the VOR (Collins, 1974) (Chapter 7). Habituation in general has the significance of a diminished response to repeated stimuli which prove to be behaviorally irrelevant. Due to its use in association with very diverse changes in biological processes, the term 'adaptation' is rather ambiguous, even in vestibular physiology, where one of its meanings is the diminishing response of vestibular hair cells to prolonged accelerations. In the present context I shall use 'adaptation' to indicate processes which change the parameters of systems in such a way that the eventual performance is better suited to the requirements of the (changed) surroundings.

## 3.1. The time constant of OKR and VOR

In 'naive' monkeys (i.e., monkeys adapted to their customary behaviour) the time constant of the VOR may be as long as 40 s (Skavenski & Robinson, 1973; Blair & Gavin, 1979). This is considerably reduced by repeated stimulation with velocity steps but also by sinusoidal oscillation at frequencies below 0.1 Hz. This process can reduce the time constant of the VOR to about 7 s (Blair & Gavin, 1979; Buettner et al., 1981; Jäger & Henn, 1981a,b). This is not significantly above the accepted time constant of the peripheral sense organ as reflected in the activity profiles of primary canal afferents (Fernandez & Goldberg, 1971; Büttner & Waespe, 1981).

In contrast to the findings in the rabbit, time constants calculated from the responses to sinusoidal motion and to velocity steps in the monkey appear to be identical if measured in the same state of habituation; they also correspond to the time course of unit activity in the vestibular nuclei. As vestibular unit activity also closely parallels OK(A)N activity (up to a saturation velocity of 60°/s) it is tempting to suppose that the same long-time-constant storage system is involved in both OKR and VOR (Raphan et al., 1977; Robinson, 1977a,b; Waespe & Henn, 1977a,b). However, this tight link has been questioned by Skavenski et al. (1981). A program of spins and stops reliably produced in three monkeys a symmetrical reduction in the time constant of PRN from more than 30 s to about one third of the starting value. Although in 78% of these cases this was accompanied by a reduction of the time constant of OKAN from a similar initial value of about 30 s to half of that, the authors interpreted these changes

conservatively in view of statistical unreliability. Later, OKAN was habituated in the same monkeys by repeated exposure to a drum rotating at 80°/s followed by a Ganzfeld, in alternating directions. Twenty exposures of one min duration were sufficient to half OKAN time constants, but these were accompanied by reliable decreases of the PRN time constant in only half of the cases. It is important to note that the symmetrical habituation of OKAN and PRN involved a reduction of the time constant, but not of the initial gain of the response. A similar observation was made by Lisberger et al. (1981). The measurements of Skavenski et al. (1981) should be followed up by more experiments in monkeys and other species to evaluate the amount of linkage between PRN and OKAN time constants more firmly. If the interaction between OKAN and PRN serves to cancel afternystagmus after rotation in the light (Koenig et al., 1978; Raphan et al., 1977, 1979; Igarashi et al., 1978a) a similar time constant of both subsystems would seem intuitively highly desirable. However, Demer and Robinson (1983) have pointed out that a common velocity storage system for OKAN and PRN can not be discarded on the basis of the findings of Skavenski et al. (1981), because the decay of PRN is determined by the interaction of two time constants: the one of the semicircular canals as well as that of the storage system. Theoretical combinations of values of these parameters can be found which fit Skavenski's results.

Sinusoidal oscillation in darkness at very low frequencies (0.01 Hz) induces shortening of the VOR time constant also in man (Jäger & Henn, 1981b), but on the other hand the responses to frequencies above 0.1 Hz remain unaffected by long-term stimulation of the VOR by either low or high frequencies (Jäger & Henn, 1981b; Gonshor & Melvill Jones, 1976a).

## 3.2. The effect of the unidirectional visual stimulation

Whereas symmetrical excitation of the VOR and OKR by low frequencies or symmetrical velocity steps affects only the time constant and not the gain or bias, asymmetrical visual stimulation of sufficient duration induces a systematic bias and

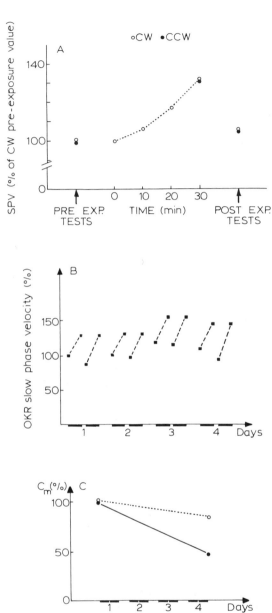

*Fig. 7.* Effects of OKR training (stimulus velocity 30°/s CW) in the cat. A, increase of OKR slow phase velocity (SPV), given as per cent of the starting value, during a training period of 30 min. The increase is bilateral and of short duration. B, increase of OKR velocity during a series of (CCW) OKR trainings, without significant retention. C, values of cumulative slow phase deviation during post-rotatory vestibular nystagmus before and after a CW optokinetic training. There is a significant uni-directional vestibular effect with a greater depression of the side contralateral to the direction of optokinetic training (from Jeannerod et al., 1981).

sometimes changes in gain.

There seems to be agreement that long-term stimulation of OKR does not reduce OKR gain by habituation but, in contrast, increases it. This effect has been described by Miyoshi and Pfaltz (1972) and Miyoshi et al. (1973) for man. It was elicited by small as well as large field stimuli and seemed to persist over long periods. Van Die and Collewijn (unpublished) also informally observed an improvement of human OKR gain in the course of repeated sessions. Kowler et al. (1978) described an increase of smooth pursuit gain during daily practice for a month from 0.82 to 0.99 for a 2.4°/s target velocity and from 0.70 to 0.94 for a 5.4°/s target velocity. In the cat, both Harris and Cynader (1981b) and Clement et al. (1981; also reported by Jeannerod et al., 1981) found an increase of OKR gain during continued opto-kinetic stimulation in the same direction by about 30%. These changes are quite remarkable for a feedback system and would reflect a substantial increase of the open loop gain if the optokinetic loop operates indeed as a velocity feedback system with retinal slip velocity as the input and eye velocity as the output (Fig. 7). However, Clement et al. (1981) observed that this effect had a per-sistence of only a few minutes.

Some apparently conflicting results have been obtained with regard to the after-effects occurring when prolonged OKR is followed by darkness. As mentioned before, OKR is normally followed by OKAN in the same direction, which after a var-iable time is often replaced by secondary after-nystagmus (OKAN II) in the reversed direction, and even further reversals may occur at later stages, as described for the monkey by Büttner et al. (1976). It is interesting to notice that OKAN II is especially prominent after prolonged stimula-tion with elevated velocities. Büttner et al. (1976) used a velocity of 60°/s for periods up to 15 min. Clement et al. (1981) elicited OKR in cats using a drum velocity of 30°/s with a duration of 30 min. when they turned the lights off after this period they observed an OKAN II (opposite to the previous OKR) which lasted from several minutes to more than an hour.

Just the opposite result was obtained by Harris and Cynader (1981b) who stimulated cats with a velocity of 6.3°/s for one hour. Afterwards they

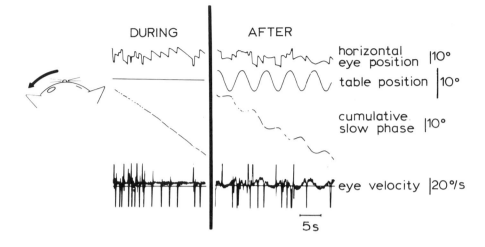

*Fig. 8.* Effects of horizontal OKR training (stimulus velocity 6.3°/s during 1 h) (during, left side) on VOR elicited by sinusoidal oscillation of the cat in darkness (after, right side) (from Harris & Cynader, 1981b).

obtained an OKAN I in the same direction as the previous OKR, lasting about 50 min. I could confirm these effects by stimulating one cat on several days for a period of 30 min. with 6, 30 or 12°/s. After 6°/s the cat showed a very prolonged OKAN I, after 30°/s a very marked OKAN II, whereas after 12°/s practically no afternystagmus was seen. This differential effect of low and high velocities might give us a clue to the adaptive mechanisms activated by prolonged visual slip. The key difference might be the activation of only the short-time-constant (smooth pursuit) system by low stimulus velocities, and activation of the long-time-constant OKR by high stimulus velocities. More investigations in several species are needed in this respect, especially since the same difference is reflected in the transfer of the optokinetic training to the VOR.

Harris and Cynader (1981b), using their stimulus of 6.3°/s noticed that after prolonged OKR the VOR elicited by sinusoidal oscillation was unbalanced by the OKAN I (Fig. 8). As this effect could be accounted for satisfactorily by a linear summation of the OKAN I velocity with the VOR with an unmodified gain throughout the frequency range, it seems that the VOR system was not essentially affected by the procedure. Similar results as after training of OKR alone were obtained by simultaneous OKR training (unidirectional) and VOR stimulation (by oscillation).

Higher OKR stimulus speeds, followed by OKAN II, seem to affect the VOR more profoundly. After optokinetic training at 30°/s, the cumulative slow phase deviation during PRN induced by velocity steps in darkness was reduced by 55% for the nystagmus direction corresponding to the previous OKR training and by 30% in the opposite direction. For sinusoidal stimulation, a reduction in gain for low frequencies (50% at 0.03 Hz and 35% at 0.1 Hz) and increased phase lead were found, but only in the habituated direction. Retention of this visually induced habituation of the VOR was shorter than one day. This lack of retention seems to be the main difference between optokinetic and vestibularly induced habituation (Clement et al., 1981).

Selective habituation of the VOR in one direction by optokinetic training in the corresponding direction has been previously described for man (Young & Henn, 1974; stimulus velocity 60°/s) and monkey (Young & Henn, 1976; stimulus velocity 30°/s). The general results were as described above for the cat, but no changes in OKR during training were observed in the monkey. Gain of PRN (peak slow phase velocity/rotation velocity step) was markedly reduced in the direction of the previous OKR, but on the other hand enhanced in the opposite direction. A spontaneous nystagmus (OKAN II) was seen after optokinetic training, but this was by itself insufficient to account for the changes in the VOR by simple superposition. Also, in the monkey the retention was shorter than one day.

Summarizing the main trends of these optokinetic training experiments, we may conclude that *fast optokinetic stimuli tend to induce after effects in the opposite direction, and reduction of the responses in the same direction.* With unidirectional training, this is expressed as a secondary OKAN and a bias of the VOR. Bidirectional training, as done by Skavenski et al. (1981), reduces the responses in both directions without a unidirectional bias. *Unidirectional optokinetic training at a low velocity on the other hand induces aftereffects in the same direction,* as expressed in a primary OKAN of long persistence and biasing of the VOR to the same side. One might expect then, that bidirectional optokinetic training at low velocities would actually enhance the VOR. This has been shown indeed in a number of cases, as described in the following section.

### 3.3. Training of the VOR by a periodical optokinetic stimulus

An increase in gain of both the OKR and VOR during and after visual stimulation with only a slowly oscillating optokinetic drum has been ob-served both in the rabbit (Collewijn & Kleinschmidt, 1975; Collewijn & Grootendorst, 1979; Honrubia et al., 1982) and the goldfish (Schairer & Bennett, 1978 and in preparation). The frequencies of the stimulus were low (1/8 to 1/6 Hz) with amplitudes of 1–10° so that velocities did not exceed about 10°/s. Although vestibular and visual stimulation were never combined, a marked and similar improvement of OKR as well as VOR gain developed within a few hours in rabbit as well as goldfish (Fig. 9). Unfortunately it has not been possible to replicate this effect in monkey (Miles & Lisberger, 1981a) or man (Steinman & Collewijn, unpublished observations). These negative findings are surprising in the light of the clear effects of unidirectional OKN training in primates. The difference could well be due to the development of a smooth pursuit system; pursuit of a target without head movements is of course not a meaningful reason to change the calibration of the VOR.

### 3.4. Pattern storage

There is some evidence that adaptive processes can be specific for the motion pattern which has been applied. This is obvious for the unidirectional conditioning regimes which induce a bias, and to a certain extent the vestibular habituation to very low frequencies is also specific for that range. However, it seems that time constants are not only indiscriminately shortened, but rather specifically tuned to the trained frequency. It has now been found in the rabbit (Collewijn & Grootendorst, 1979), monkey (Lisberger & Miles, 1981), cat (Godaux et al., 1983b), chicken (Wallman et al., 1982) and goldfish (Schairer & Bennet, in preparation) that adaptive changes of the VOR and OKR are larger for the entrained frequency than for the neighbouring frequencies. Frequency selectivity, which is further discussed in Chapter 21 in terms of a channel-hypothesis, considerably complicates our concepts of adaptation as simple over-all adjustments of gains are not adequate to explain such behaviour.

However, the picture seems to be even more complex because instances have been found in which the entrained motion pattern was spontaneously reproduced as an oculomotor output. This was reported for the rabbit (Collewijn & Grooten-

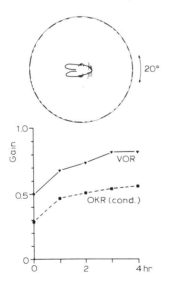

Fig. 9. Gain of VOR and OKR of the rabbit as a function of time, with continuous sinusoidal optokinetic stimulation alone (0.17 Hz, amplitude 20° peak-to-peak). Average values for 6 animals (from Collewijn, 1981).

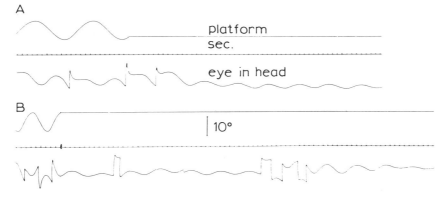

*Fig. 10.* Spontaneous post-oscillatory eye movements as after-effect of conditioning in the rabbit. A, spontaneous oscillation of the eye at 1/6 Hz during and after test of the VOR at 1/12 Hz. The animal had been conditioned for 6 h with visual motion only at 1/6 Hz, 20° p.p. B, similar effect after test of the VOR at 1/6 Hz. The animal had been conditioned for 2 h in a conflict (whole field) situation (from Collewijn & Grootendorst, 1979).

dorst, 1979) as an exceptional phenomenon (Fig. 10), but it was observed in the majority of goldfish (Schairer & Bennett, in preparation). It appeared as a smooth sinusoidal eye movement of approximately the same frequency as the one entrained (1/6 or 1/8 Hz), and both in rabbit and goldfish it was often provoked by oscillation in darkness at a lower frequency. Storage of a motion pattern in connection with phenomena of habituation, motion sickness and after effects of unfamiliar patterns of motion (e.g., of a ship) has been postulated long ago in a general form by Groen (1957). A possibly related phenomenon was reported by Eckmiller & Mackeben (1978) who found that monkeys often continue to pursue a regular target motion for more than a second when the target is suddenly extinguished.

### 3.5. Expression of VOR adaptation in parameters of OKR

In view of the demonstrated tight functional relation between the long-time-constant OK(A)N and VOR subsystems it is opportune to ask whether adaptive changes in the VOR are always shared by the OKR. There are some obvious problems in making this comparison. As the OKR is, in principle, a closed loop system, its performance will not be dramatically changed by mild changes of the open loop gain. To avoid this complication the OKR can be studied with high velocity stimuli, which are matched by the eye only partially and after gradual build-up. Secondly, VOR adaptation is induced by the association of visual slip with head movements; these could of course adapt the OKR system independently of the VOR. Lisberger et al. (1981) adapted monkeys towards a VOR gain of zero or two using fixed field or ×2-telescopic goggles. Such changes had no effect on the short-time-constant (smooth pursuit) component of OKR, measured as the initial acceleration of the eye, i.e., the fast build-up of pursuit velocity. However, the gain of the long-time-constant OKR varied in parallel with VOR gain (Fig. 11A). For example, the initial OKAN velocity ranged from 37 to 120°/s as VOR gain ranged from 0.29 to 1.80. Also, the maximum eye velocity reached during OKR during stimulation with high drum velocities increased together with VOR gain, with some decrease of the time constant of build up. The time constant of OKAN decay decreased in the course of the time over which the experiments extended, but was not sensitive to VOR gain. Recently, a correlation between VOR gain and initial OKAN velocity was found also in humans (Zasorin et al., 1983). Essentially similar results have been obtained by Demer (1981) in the cat, with the difference that in the cat the time constant of OKAN varied from about 2 s at a VOR gain of 0.2, to 10 s at a VOR gain of 1.66 (Fig. 11B). These experiments indicate that, both in a foveate primate and the afoveate cat, the variable gain element of the VOR is shared by the long-time-constant optokinetic system. The

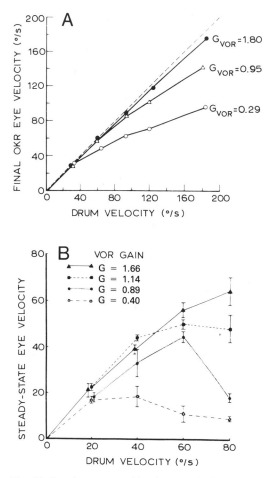

*Fig. 11.* Steady-state optokinetic eye velocity as a function of drum velocity for different adapted values of VOR gain. A, monkey (from Lisberger et al., 1981); B, cat (from Demer, 1981).

smooth pursuit mechanism (which is poorly developed in cats) would gain access to the final oculomotor pathway distal to the variable gain element. Thus, for the monkey it seems that habituating stimuli (Skavenski et al., 1981; Jäger & Henn, 1981a,b) primarily reduce the time constant of the long-time-constant mechanism, without affecting its gain, whereas adaptive changes of VOR gain are reflected primarily in a change of the gain of the long-time-constant OKR.

Although these results are consistent and easily accommodated in models (Lisberger et al., 1981; Demer, 1981) they have one puzzling aspect. The adaptation of the VOR was induced by a period of at least temporarily increased retinal slip. This

would seem to call for an increase in OKR gain, whatever other adaptations may be made. In the rabbit, any condition which augments visual slip raises the OKR gain, even though the VOR gain may decrease simultaneously. The chicken behaves similarly (Wallman et al., 1982). Another difference between the monkey and the rabbit is that in the latter a visually induced increase in OKR and VOR gain at 1/6 Hz was not accompanied by an increased OKR gain for steady velocities, but by a slight decrease (Collewijn & Grootendorst, 1979). As the rabbit's OKR is primarily in the long-time-constant range, there is clearly a conflict with the observations in cat and monkey.

### 3.6. Hypotheses on adaptive mechanisms in visuo-vestibular interaction

Although there is now a lot of evidence on adaptive phenomena in the integrated activity of the visuo-vestibular guidance system of the eye, it is still difficult to formulate a unifying theory which offers an all-encompassing framework and yet has some specific explanatory value.

Stimulation of each subsystem apart may lead to adaptive or habituative changes. Repeated stimulation of the VOR with low frequencies or velocity steps induces, predominantly, shortening of time constants. These changes are at least partially shared with the OKR system, and can be also induced (although apparently less permanently) by similar visual stimuli. The coupling of these changes reflects common elements in both systems and is not dependent on direct interaction between the visual and vestibular sensory input signals. It is a more or less obligate visuo-vestibular integration at the premotor level. Habituation involving the shortening of time constants seems a general phenomenon serving to eliminate prolonged responses to steps or slow oscillations, whatever their origin. Possibly, such a change is useful in the prevention of motion sickness (Jäger & Henn, 1981b). The habituation process may be triggered by the prolonged central neuronal activities (e.g., in the vestibular nuclei) rather than by a specific sensory signal.

The adjustment of directional bias is a somewhat more specific phenomenon. Two mechanisms may be at work here. As we saw, modest retinal slip velocities tend to induce bias changes that reinforce the eye movements elicited by the slip. This slip-induced modification is useful, because it will tend to decrease retinal slip. However, a fast unidirectional nystagmus in real life is a pathological phenomenon which has to be eliminated, independent of slip signals. Unidirectional nystagmus of natural origin is mostly caused by an unbalance in the peripheral or central vestibular apparatus. An extreme example is the response to unilateral labyrinthectomy (Courjon et al., 1977). The ensuing violent nystagmus and central unbalance is probably initially abated by an automatic counter-regulation (see Chapter 18), uncontrolled by retinal slip, which is in a velocity range which is too high to be very useful anyway. This phase is also independent of the cerebellum (Haddad et al., 1977). Once nystagmus velocities have become relatively low, the slip signal is used to adjust the steady eye velocity in the direction of the apparent slip of the world, with as the end point a stable eye in a stable world.

Similarly, optokinetic stimulation of a stationary animal with healthy labyrinths in a rotating drum will, at low velocities, induce a bias controlled by the retinal slip (eye movements, drum movements and slip are all in the same direction). The result will be a moving eye, which is stable with respect to the (moving) world. However, if the OKR velocities are high or continued for a long time, the system will act to repair this unbalance, i.e., create a bias opposite to the ongoing eye movements. The actual expression of these different trends may depend on the intensity and duration of the OKR. After optokinetic stimulation continued for several days at velocities as low as 5°/s in the rabbit, extremely strong secondary afternystagmus (OKAN II) has been observed (Barmack & Nelson, 1982). The nonvisual nystagmus repair mechanisms have been modelled and related to the problem of periodic alternating nystagmus by Leigh et al. (1981).

The most interesting example of integrated visuovestibular adaptivity is the recalibration of the VOR gain. This subject is treated extensively in Chapter 2 but a few points regarding the interaction of the signals will be considered here. As regulation of retinal image slip at a low level is the ultimate purpose of the VOR, there can be little doubt that retinal slip signals are used to control the recalibration process of the VOR when the gain is inappropriate. Retinal slip alone cannot guide the recalibration process; in order to decide whether a decrease or increase in gain is appropriate, slip has to be compared to the direction of the head movements, signalled by the labyrinth. According to Ito's hypothesis (Ito, 1972, 1977, 1982a; Ito et al., 1974b) there is an interaction between visual slip signals and vestibular head velocity signals in a cerebellar side-loop of the vestibulo-ocular reflex arc. This is actually an application of the cerebellar learning theory of Albus (1971) which postulates a lasting decrease in synaptic efficiency of the parallel fiber-Purkinje cell connections induced by simultaneous activation of the climbing fibers terminating on the same Purkinje cells. The long-term adaptation of the VOR by visual signals is accounted for by a change in the balance between the number of Purkinje cells in microzone II of the flocculus which fire in- and out-of-phase with head velocity. Such changes would be induced by visual slip signals carried on the climbing fibers. The modifiable element would thus be the Purkinje cell. Miles & Lisberger (1981b) have extensively argued that this is unlikely to be the case in the monkey, and that the modifiable element is probably located in the brain stem, although the flocculus may be instrumental in providing the signals which induce the plastic changes elsewhere. Although, theoretically, sampling from different floccular microzones in rabbit and monkey could have led to conflicting results (Ito, 1982), for the moment Ito's hypothesis seems to be less satisfactory to account for the findings in the monkey. But even for the rabbit the interaction as postulated by Ito is too limited to explain all known phenomena. Particularly, it cannot explain the optokinetic modification of the VOR observed in the rabbit and goldfish, in which there is no conjunction of visual with vestibular signals. Collewijn and Grootendorst (1979) have proposed as an alternative the interaction between retinal slip signals and a signal representing the ongoing eye movement, equivalent to an efference copy. Slip of the world in the same direction as the ongoing eye movement would indicate a too small eye movement, and thus cause an increase of VOR

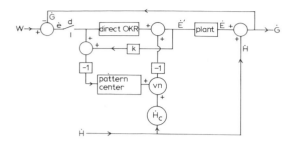

Fig. 12. Diagram of adaptation of the VOR-OKR system hypothesizing a pattern center. For description see text.

and OKR gain; opposite directions of slip and eye movements should induce a reduction of the VOR but still an increase of OKR gain. The attractiveness of this scheme is that it explains all findings in the rabbit, including the purely optokinetic modification of the VOR and the paradoxical increase in VOR gain when the eye moves according to the optokinetic stimulus during a visual inversion paradigm. If the same interaction would operate in the very low frequency range, it would also correct a spontaneous nystagmus of peripheral or central origin. Only nystagmus related to anomalies or unreliabilities in the slip signal itself, as may occur in albinism (Collewijn et al., 1978, 1980b), would remain uncorrected. No specific site for this adaptation was proposed. However, the results in the chicken (Wallman et al., 1982) do not support this theory, as the chicken shows no paradoxical increase of VOR gain during visual inversion. Another problem with the hypothesis is that optokinetic training in the primate does not adapt the VOR gain, although it does affect bias and time constants. As Miles and Lisberger (1981a,b) have pointed out, the use of eye movement as a substitute for head velocity may have been abandoned by animals which have developed a smooth pursuit system which works independently of head movements. However, the activity of the smooth pursuit system during head movements could by itself signal the inappropriateness of the VOR gain, and some central correlate of smooth pursuit could act as a substitute for, or at least complement, slip signals in the interaction with the VOR (Miles & Lisberger, 1981a,b).

Two lines of evidence support the role of smooth pursuit in adaptation. Firstly, fixation of small targets during head oscillation does induce adaptation of the VOR in primates (Miles & Lisberger, 1981a; Collewijn et al., 1983). The role of smooth pursuit is also supported by experiments in man (Collewijn et al., 1983) showing that a mismatch induced by magnifying spectacles can be almost immediately compensated during head oscillations in the light, while adaptation of the VOR measured in darkness follows more slowly. This indicates a gradual substitution of smooth pursuit by the VOR, without much change in actual slip velocities. An interesting point then is that adaptation may be induced via the smooth pursuit system, which may be equivalent to the direct OKR system, but that it is expressed in the dynamics of the indirect VOR-OKR system (Lisberger et al., 1981).

A second argument for the adaptive role of smooth pursuit is the strong association of the flocculus with smooth pursuit as well as adaptation of the VOR in the monkey. Thus, Miles and Lisberger (1981a,b) have proposed that the output signals of the flocculus control smooth pursuit as well as the induction (elsewhere) of a change in VOR gain. Even though the flocculus may not be the site of the variable gain element, its essential role in visuo-vestibular integration seems to be universal as it has been demonstrated in the rabbit, cat, monkey and goldfish (Schairer & Bennett, 1981).

Parametric adjustments of time constants, bias and gain are sufficient to control the VOR to a great extent. The clear examples that have been reported of storage of a pattern seem to indicate that in reality adaptation may be achieved in a more complex way. As postulated in general terms by Collewijn and Grootendorst (1979), consistent patterns of slip (and maybe smooth pursuit) associated with eye (or head) movements might be stored in the nervous system. The stored pattern could later interact with the eye movements when a similar type of motion returns; its retrieval could be based on some principle of resonance. The pattern should always interact with the ongoing eye movement in the correct direction to decrease slip, which means that it has to be read out with correct phase relations. A somewhat similar argument has been adduced by Melvill Jones and

Gonshor (1982) who found a 'complex' element in adaptation of the human VOR which might reflect the central generation of a predicted periodic function.

A possible diagram for the 'pattern center' hypothesis is shown in Fig. 12 (without the pretention of submitting a formal model). It consists of a slightly modified model as developed by Robinson (1977a, 1981a) for the interaction of VOR and OKR. An essential feature of Robinson's model is a positive feedback loop (with gain $k<1$) which adds an eye velocity signal (efference copy) to the visual slip signal.

Such an interaction is essential in Collewijn and Grootendorst's (1979) view on the role of the direction of eye movements and retinal slip in adaptive processes in the rabbit. Although the interaction is symbolized as a simple addition in this diagram, a non-linear interaction might exist in reality. A 'direct' OKR pathway (probably incorporating the visual cortex and the flocculus) has been added to the diagram, without any specification of dynamics. The black box marked 'pattern center' replaces an element $1/(sT_o + 1)$ in Robinson's model. Robinson introduced this lag element as a counterpart of the cupular dynamics, to filter out the higher frequencies from the OKR. Accordingly, $T_o$ was supposed to be equal to $T_c$, the time constant of the canal. Under this condition, the time constant of OKAN as well as PRN was shown to be equal to $T_o/(1 - k)$ (Robinson, 1981a). This means that afternystagmus in this model is caused by a combination of a positive feedback loop and an integrative storage element. The latter is the sole means of velocity conservation in other models (see Waespe et al., 1983). Even without effective positive feedback of eye velocity ($k=0$) Robinson's model will produce OKAN with a time constant $T_o$. The element $1/(sT_o + 1)$ in Robinson's model may be interpreted as an internal model of the canal in negative: it provides the dynamics that the canal lacks so that the OKR and VOR complement each others' frequency response exactly. This seems an ideal situation, which might require adaptive properties in the OKR lag element to be maintained. Actually, possible changes in $T_o$ have been recently discussed in the context of habituation (Demer & Robinson, 1983).

A broader interpretation of the optokinetic lag element would be to view it as a 'pattern center' which would develop an internal model compensating any long-term functional deficit in the VOR-OKR system by changing its frequency response characteristics. Continued stimulation at a specific frequency would lead to tuning of the element to this frequency to produce an optimal response (with minimal visual slip) of the total system. In exceptional cases the element might produce spontaneous oscillations at the trained frequency.

### Acknowledgements

Thanks are due to Miss S. Markestijn and Dr. J. van der Steen for assistance in the preparation of this chapter.

Adaptive mechanisms in gaze control
Facts and theories
*Eds. Berthoz & Melvill Jones*

Chapter 4

# Adaptive properties of the saccadic system

## L. M. Optican

*Laboratory of Sensorimotor Research, National Eye Institute, National Institutes of Health, Bethesda, MD 20205, U.S.A.*

## 1. Introduction

Visual perceptions are formed after acquiring and stabilizing images on the retinal area with the highest visual acuity, the fovea. Preceding chapters have tended to concentrate on those eye movements used to stabilize a given retinal image during head and/or image movements. In foveate animals the voluntary shifts of gaze, made with rapid eye movements called saccades, are of equal functional significance. Normally these saccades are characterized by both a high degree of accuracy (corresponding to the small foveal diameter, e.g., 1–2° in the monkey) and a high angular velocity (100–900°/s in the same species). Another important characteristic, which is particularly relevant to the present chapter, is that saccades end abruptly, i.e., without post-saccadic ocular drift, thereby permitting good visual perception immediately after completion of each saccadic movement. Over the past decade much has been learned about the way the brain generates saccadic eye movements. The present chapter focuses on one aspect of the neural control of saccades: the adaptive ability to maintain saccadic performance (in particular the ability to get the eyes accurately on target and to hold them there without ensuing ocular drift).

The command for a saccade is produced by neurons within the brain stem that are part of the oculomotor control system (Robinson, 1975a; Keller, 1981). When a target is selected as the item of interest, it is the task of this subsystem to generate the neural signal required to take the fovea to the newly selected image and hold it there. As we shall see below, functionally significant aspects of the motor performance produced by this signal are monitored by other parts of the brain. Those other parts can advantageously alter critical parameters within the saccadic motor subsystem, thereby acting as an adaptive control system (Optican & Robinson, 1980).

In natural life these adaptive mechanisms serve to offset degradation of oculomotor performance resulting from interference along the chain of neural conduction, neuromuscular transmission and muscle function, due for example to such factors as aging, injury and disease. Clinical aspects of this matter are reviewed by Zee and Optican in Chapter 11, and by others elsewhere (e.g., Optican, 1982; Stark, 1982). Experimental laboratory studies have shown that at least two mechanisms, one fast and one slow, can alter saccadic movements in response to inappropriate oculomotor performance. The present chapter reviews some of the basic experimental studies which demonstrate the presence of these adaptive mechanisms, and attempts a systematic interpretation of their functional structure and operation.

## 2. Generation of saccades

As shown by Robinson (1964), the description of the mechanical properties of the eyeball, suspensory tissues and extraocular muscles can be simplified by lumping them into viscous and elastic elements, the inertia of the globe being insignificant. To move the eyes rapidly, the muscles must develop a large transient force to overcome the viscous drag of the orbital tissues. To hold the eyes at one point in the orbit, the muscles must develop just enough maintained tension to balance the elastic restoring force of the orbital tissues. Hence a saccade requires a large, brief pulse of torque to move the eye rapidly and a smaller, sustained torque to hold the eye in its new position.

These two components of torque are caused by two corresponding elements in the efferent neural discharge to the extraocular muscles. Thus, the large transient motor output needed to turn the eyes rapidly against viscous drag is generated by a high-frequency burst, or pulse, of phasic neural activity; while the sustained muscle force opposing the elastic tension is generated by a step change in tonic activity (Robinson, 1973). This combined pulse-step pattern of neural activity is now known to be formulated within the brain stem by the motor control subsystem mentioned above, and constitutes the basis of all normal saccade generation (Keller & Robinson, 1972; Luschei & Fuchs, 1972; Keller, 1974).

As implied above, to achieve an ideal saccade the pulse and step of innervation must be adjusted so that the pulse drives the eye to the desired position and the step holds it there. Inappropriate innervations give rise to inaccurate, or dysmetric, eye movements. If both the pulse and step are too small, the eye will not reach the target (hypometria), while if they are too large, the eye will overshoot the target (hypermetria). If the pulse and step are not matched, the eye will move rapidly until the pulse of innervation ends, but then it will drift exponentially to the orbital position determined by the step (glissade). If the step is too large for the pulse, the eye drifts onwards; if too small, it drifts back (see Fig. 2).

## 3. Maintaining saccadic accuracy

The accuracy of saccades appears to be governed by three different mechanisms. One mechanism is under voluntary control and operates over a time scale of seconds, while the other two are involuntary and operate over slower time scales of minutes and days. For reasons given below, only the latter two are considered to function as adaptive mechanisms.

### 3.1. Voluntary goal adjustment

The voluntary control of saccadic accuracy is achieved by changing the selection of the saccade goal. Vossius (1972) studied the ability of subjects to acquire targets that moved when they tried to look at them. By monitoring eye position and adding a fraction of the eye position to the target position signal, the target was made to jump with every saccade in a predictable fashion. After just a few attempts subjects learned to make a single saccade to a location where there was no target, but to which the feedback signal would bring the target. Hallett (1978) has shown that subjects can voluntarily make saccades that are smaller than, larger than, or oppositely directed to target jumps. Such studies indicate a high degree of volitional control over the selection of saccadic goals.

Such a goal changing strategy may be of limited usefulness outside the laboratory. For example, patients with a sixth nerve palsy take several days to improve the accuracy of their saccades, apparently making no use of saccadic goal selection strategies (see below). In the laboratory, goal selection tasks are done with a few points of light that move in a stereotyped fashion. When patients have to cope with saccadic dysmetrias, however, the visual scene is rich with items of interest, and the required goal modification may depend on the position of the eyes in the orbit. Thus, there may not be enough time to make the volitional effort needed to reprogram the goal for every saccade under these conditions. Because of the volitional nature of goal selections, these essentially instantaneous alterations of saccadic gain are excluded from the rest of the discussion of the adaptive properties of saccades.

### 3.2. Normal hypometria

The definition of an adaptive mechanism must be broad enough to deal with more than just simple accuracy, for despite the ability of subjects to rapidly adjust saccadic goals, normal saccades are not always accurate. When the required refixation exceeds 10° of arc in man or monkey, it is usually made with more than one saccade. The first, or primary, saccade almost always falls short of the target, and is quickly followed by a secondary, or corrective, saccade (Becker & Jürgens, 1975; Hallett & Lightstone, 1976). If the target light is turned off just before the primary saccade, an accurate secondary saccade can still be made. Hence, this falling short, or hypometria, does not reflect an inaccuracy of the saccadic system. Instead, saccadic undershoot seems to be preprogrammed (Becker & Fuchs, 1969).

## 3.3. Rapid saccadic adaptation

This normal hypometria has been studied by altering visual feedback conditions. Henson (1978) used an optical system to magnify the effective size of a subject's saccades. This magnification resulted in the usually hypometric saccade falling exactly on the target (orthometria) or even overshooting it (hypermetria). With 10 to 15 min of this altered visual experience the subject's saccades again became usually hypometric. This mechanism seems qualitatively different from the voluntary selection of saccadic goals: it involves a smooth change in saccadic accuracy over a period of time. These experiments indicate that the gain of the saccadic system (size of the primary saccade divided by the size of the initial target eccentricity) is under rapid adaptive control. Furthermore, they demonstrate that the goal of the first saccade is not simply to acquire the target: the primary saccade is intended to fall short.

Most explanations for this undershooting are based on the observation that corrective saccades in the same direction as the primary saccade follow it with a shorter latency than corrective saccades in the opposite direction (Hallett & Lightstone, 1976; Henson, 1978). If the first saccade falls short, the target will still be on the same side of the fovea, and hence its image will project to the side of the brain that generated the primary saccade. If the first saccade overshoots the target, it will then be on the opposite side of the fovea, and its image will project to the other side of the brain. The increase in time required to correct for a hypermetric movement is presumed to have two compo-

nents: one for consolidating information between the hemispheres and one for reprogramming the direction of the corrective saccade.

Two mechanisms have been proposed to account for this form of hypometria. Hallett (1978) proposed a dual saccadic system in which one component is fast, but has a coarse retinal resolution, while the other is slower but more accurate. The primary saccade is made by the faster system. The second, co-activated system gives a better estimate of the target's position. This estimate is combined with eye position information to obtain an anticipated error, which may give rise to a secondary saccade. This dual control would explain the need for corrective saccades, but it would not explain why the primary saccade is usually hypometric. Since the saccadic gain is adaptable, the average of a large number of coarsely programmed saccades should still be orthometric, i.e., exactly on target.

In an attempt to overcome this difficulty, Optican (1982) hypothesized that the undershoot of large saccades is purposeful. Since most saccades are small (e.g., under 15° in amplitude according to Bahill et al., 1975a), an undershoot only on large saccades would provide an occasional perturbation of known size, allowing a 'corrective system' to monitor the accuracy of the saccadic motor system. In order to derive an error signal for saccadic gain control, the target must not move before the result of this perturbation is measured. When the retinal image projects to the opposite hemisphere, the information on target position must be sent back to the original hemisphere to allow for a comparison with the expected error. This must take longer than if the image stayed in the same hemisphere. Since the measurement time will be shorter if the retinal error stays in the same hemisphere, the primary saccade is made hypometric to reduce the probability that the target will move before the actual retinal error can be compared with the expected retinal error. Furthermore, programming a corrective saccade in the same direction as the primary saccade takes less time than programming one in the opposite direction (Hallett & Lightstone, 1976). Hence, the total time to actually reach the target will be less if the perturbed primary saccade falls short, rather than long.

The purpose of the rapid adaptive system that maintains hypometria may be to guarantee that the first saccade falls short. This could be achieved with a relatively simple system, allowing a more complex, but slower, controller to adjust saccadic accuracy by monitoring the effects of amplitude perturbations. The existence of such a gradual controller has been established in both human patients and monkeys.

### 3.4. Gradual saccadic adaptation

The ability of subjects to rapidly restore hypometria in response to altered visual feedback represents a fast form of plasticity, i.e., a gain change that is maintained without conscious effort. The voluntary changes of saccadic goals described earlier represent another fast form of saccadic control. Despite these abilities patients take several days to increase their saccadic system gains to compensate for muscle paralysis (Kommerell et al., 1976; Abel et al., 1978). Presumably patients with peripheral weakness can still alter their saccadic goals voluntarily, but they do not use this ability to compensate for their weakness. Perhaps this is because such compensation requires a large volitional effort for each saccade, especially when oculomotor deficits depend on orbital position. A qualitative difference also exists between the types of saccadic adaptation seen in patients and in the subjects of altered feedback experiments: in altered visual feedback experiments no post-saccadic ocular drift develops. Yet Kommerell et al. (1976) found that patients with a unilateral abducens nerve palsy, when viewing with the normal eye, made saccades with the paretic eye that not only fell short of the target, but also had post-saccadic drift back. Patching the normal eye led to an increase in the size of its saccades, and produced post-saccadic drift in it. These changes were not evident after a short time (15 min), but took several days to develop. Hence patterns of innervation change slowly in patients with abducens nerve palsies.

A gradual form of adaptation for recalibrating the motor system would obviate the need for volitional control over every saccade. The longer time course of a gradual adaptive mechanism would allow it to take into account effects, such as orbital position dependence or post-saccadic drift, which were not evident from the accuracy of a single saccade. These interesting clinical observations have led to controlled experimental studies on laboratory animals. A form of gradual adaptation to peripheral weakness has been studied in monkeys. After weakening the muscles of one eye, patching one eye at a time allows the visual experience of the animal to be controlled. Using this patching paradigm Optican and Robinson (1980) found that adaptive control of saccadic accuracy occurred gradually; compensation for peripheral weakness had a (roughly) exponential time constant of 1.5 days, while return to the original condition occurred more rapidly.

Weakening the muscles of these animals caused a decrease in the ratio of orbital viscosity to elasticity, presumably due to the increased elasticity of scar tissue. Hence, saccades in the weakened eye not only fell short of the target, but were also followed by post-saccadic drift back. When the monkey's normal eye was patched, the saccades of the paretic eye gradually became larger, and its drift was suppressed. The corresponding saccades in the normal eye became too large and had post-saccadic drift onward. This is consistent with Hering's Law, that the same innervation is sent to both eyes. The time course of the amplitude correction and the drift suppression were the same.

These changes in saccadic waveforms can be interpreted in terms of the efferent pulse and step of innervation. When the normal eye is first patched, the brain views the world with an eye that falls short of the target and drifts back. In an effort to improve vision, the pulse is increased until the paretic, viewing eye can reach the target in one saccade. The normal, patched, eye overshoots the target, and thus appears to also receive this larger innervation. The step of innervation is also increased to offset the increase in the orbital elasticity. This suppresses the post-saccadic drift back in the paretic eye. The normal, patched, eye develops a post-saccadic drift onward when it receives the same step.

Optican and Robinson (1980) used this patching paradigm to investigate the dependence of the adaptive control system on the cerebellum. The direct effects of ablating portions of the cerebellum on the saccadic system can be assessed by observing the saccades made by the normal eye. The indirect effect of such ablations on the adaptive mechanism can be assessed by observing the changes in saccades following patching of the normal eye. After the midline portions of the cerebellum (the vermis, paravermis and fastigial nuclei) were ablated in monkeys, the saccades in the normal eye became hypermetric. Patching either eye for several weeks did not cause any change in the saccadic amplitude. However, post-saccadic drift was still suppressed, after several days, in whichever eye was viewing. After total cerebellar ablations, the saccades in the normal eye became hypermetric, and were followed by post-saccadic drift. The direction and amount of the drift depended on orbital position. Neither the hypermetria nor the drift were ever altered by the patching of either eye. These two findings suggest a separate mechanism for drift suppression. Following this lead, it was found that when the floccular lobes of the cerebellum were ablated in monkeys, their saccades did not become hypermetric, but had an enduring post-saccadic drift that could not be modified by optical means (Optican et al., 1980).

Vilis and Hore (1981) found that cooling the midline cerebellar nuclei of monkeys caused dysmetric saccades with post-saccadic drift. When cooling ceased, saccades returned to normal. Vilis et al. (1982) have also found that unilateral cooling of the medial cerebellar nuclei resulted in different degrees of dysmetria in the two eyes. In both the ablation and the cooling experiments the amount of dysmetria and drift depended on orbital position and saccade amplitude, indicating that the cerebellum is involved in matching the pulse to the step as a function of orbital position. Neither study found any change in the dynamic characteristics of saccades (their amplitude-duration and amplitude-peak velocity relationships). An earlier study by Ritchie (1976) did report an altered amplitude-duration relationship in primates with small midline cerebellar ablations, but no explanation exists for this discrepancy.

These experiments indicate that the cerebellum is involved in the adaptive control of both the pulse and step gains of the saccadic system (for recent reviews see Optican, 1982 and Stark, 1982). The pulse gain control seems to depend on midline structures (vermis and fastigial nuclei) while the step gain control seems to depend on lateral structures (flocculus). The cerebellum may also be involved in maintaining conjugacy of the two eyes, and in compensating for position-dependent orbital mechanics. How the cerebellum interacts with the brain stem circuits that generate saccades is not yet known. It will be a great help in studying such interactions if the functional roles of the two regions can be understood in detail. One approach to such a functional description is through modeling.

## 4. Error signals for adaptive control

Quantitative models of physiological processes not only summarize what is known about a system, but allow hypotheses to be tested and new experiments to be designed. Modeling an adaptive control system requires knowledge of two parts of the system. First, the motor subsystem must be understood. This subsystem actually moves the eye, and it will contain parameters, such as gains and time constants, that determine its performance. Second, the adaptive mechanism must be described. This subsystem monitors the performance of the saccadic system. Some measure of performance is combined with other information to derive an error signal. It is the goal of the adaptive mechanism to reduce this error signal by adjusting the parameters of the motor control subsystem, a form of interaction termed parametric feedback.

While quantitative models of the motor control part of the saccadic system have progressed rapidly (Robinson, 1973, 1975a; Zee et al., 1976c), very little is known about the error signals used to achieve adaptive control of saccades. The adaptive control of the pulse gain, which determines saccadic accuracy, is greatly complicated by the need to recognize the target. Since a saccade is made to only one item within a visually rich scene, knowledge that a saccade was inaccurate requires that the same item be identified in different retinal locations before and after the saccade. These different locations must then be compared in some way to determine the error

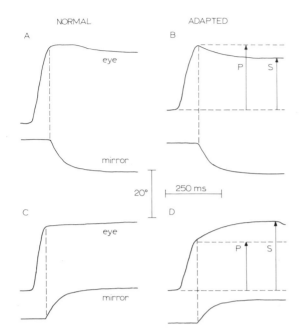

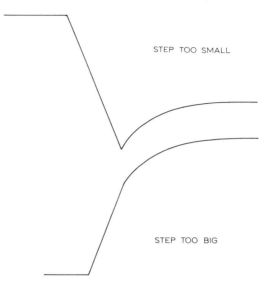

Fig. 2. Schematic representation of a glissade. In the top trace, the step of innervation is too small for the pulse of innervation, causing the eye to drift back. In the bottom trace, the step is too large for the pulse, causing the eye to drift onward. Note that the drift portion of the eye movement is identical in either case, making post-saccadic retinal slip alone insufficient to determine whether the step gain is too large or too small.

*Fig. 1.* Suppression of optically induced retinal slip. The left panels show the movement of the visual field (mirror) triggered by a saccade before the animal has been adapted. The visual field movement in part A causes retinal slip backward, while that in part C causes retinal slip onward. Note the pursuit system response after about 110 ms. The right panels show the same types of movements after several days of experiencing the optically induced slip. There is now a zero-latency ocular drift in the compensatory direction. Part B shows that the gain of the step driven part of the movement (S) has been reduced relative to the gain of the pulse driven part (P). In part D, the gain of the step has been increased.

signal. A preliminary attempt at modeling the adaptive control of saccadic accuracy has been described elsewhere (Optican, 1982). That model depends on a corrective system that generates secondary saccades and derives a post-saccadic amplitude error signal for a cerebellar-dependent adaptive gain controller. The corrective system derives an error signal by comparing the actual retinal error after a saccade with the retinal error expected because of the intentional hypometria of the primary saccade.

Adaptive control of the step gain (to suppress post-saccadic ocular drift) is much easier to model, since drift can be monitored either by extraocular muscle proprioception or by full-field retinal slip. Optican and Miles (1979) reported

studies in primates subjected to saccade-triggered visual slip. In these experiments the visual world was caused to drift after each saccade by a computer controlled optical system involving a mirror galvanometer and a projected visual scene. In one series of experiments the slip was in the same direction as the antecedent saccade (Fig. 1C), while in another series the slip was oppositely directed (Fig. 1A). After several days of such optically-induced slip, the monkey's saccades showed adaptive changes (Fig. 1B,D). These experiments showed that retinal slip is sufficient to elicit adaptive changes in the saccadic system. However, slip alone does not indicate the sign of the necessary gain change. Fig. 2, for example, shows that a saccade to the left when the step is too small for the pulse of innervation, and a saccade to the right when the step is too large, both have identical ocular drifts. Based on the experimental findings given above an attempt has been made to propose a mechanism for adaptive drift suppression in which the relevant error signal is derived by correlating retinal slip im-

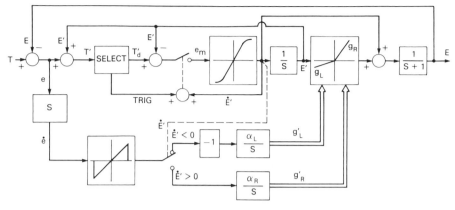

ADAPTIVE CONTROL OF POST-SACCADIC DRIFT

*Fig. 3.* Block diagram of a model for the suppression of post-saccadic drift. The upper pathways represent the saccadic motor control system. The step gain is represented by the box on the right with two line segments whose slopes are variable. The slopes, $g_L$ and $g_R$, represent the gain for leftward and rightward saccades. The bottom pathways represent the adaptive control mechanism for adjusting the step gains. The signal indicating the step gain error is derived by correlating retinal slip with the direction of the antecedent saccade. Single lines represent signal processing paths. Dashed lines indicate switching signals. Double lines represent variable gain controls. See text for explanation of signals.

mediately following a saccade with the direction of that saccade. Fig. 3 shows a model based on this hypothesis.

## 5. An adaptive model of post-saccadic drift suppression

To model drift suppression we start with a model of the normal saccadic system (Robinson, 1975a; Zee et al., 1976c). Fig. 3 shows the neural integrator ($1/S$) and ocular motor plant ($1/S+1$) in Laplace transform notation (Robinson, 1973). There is also a branch for velocity feed-forward compensation of the lag in the plant dynamics.

To make a saccade, a velocity command, or pulse, must be generated and sent both directly and indirectly, through the neural integrator, to the ocular motor neurons; the two pathways contributing the pulse and step signals, respectively (Robinson, 1973). The pulse therefore completely determines the dynamic properties of the saccade. In this model, a pulse generator that is not pre-programmed, and that has as its input the desired target position in spatial, rather than retinal, coordinates is used (Robinson, 1975a). This spatial estimate ($T'$) is obtained by adding the brain's best estimate of where the eye is

(efference copy, $E'$), to the retinal error ($e$). Retinal error ($e$) is determined by the position of the target in space ($T$) relative to the eye position in space ($E$). A selection process determines the desired eye position in spatial coordinates ($T'_d$). A high-gain, nonlinear element generates a large output, or burst, based on an estimate of the motor error ($e_m$) between where the eye is ($E'$) and where it is going ($T'_d$).

Since $e_m$ depends on $E'$, the burst is generated continuously, automatically ending when the motor error ($e_m$) becomes zero. The high gain, non-linear element is based on the 'short lead' burst cells identified by single-unit recordings within the brain stem (Luschei and Fuchs, 1972; Keller, 1974). The burster's high gain makes the saccadic system unstable. Hence to prevent the eyes from oscillating a switch, modeled after the pause cells found in the pons, is included (Keller, 1974). When a trigger is received from some other part of the brain, the switch closes and the burst begins. When $e_m$ reaches zero, the switch opens and the eye is held on target by the neural integrator. Once again, it is important to realize that each part of the model reflects some aspect of the available data. The structure is a hypothesis, but no physiologically unrealistic parts have been added (Zee et al., 1976c).

When assembling these various components, we must include a variable gain element that will allow post-saccadic drift to be adaptively suppressed. Experiments on monkeys (see above) have shown that lesions of the posterior vermis can abolish pulse gain adaptation while sparing step gain adaptation. That being the case, there is one, and only one, place where the variable gain element may be located. Since the step is obtained by integrating the pulse, everything upstream from the neural integrator affects both the pulse and the step. Since the ocular motor neurons carry the combined pulse and step of innervation, everything downstream from this point also affects them both. Hence the variable gain element must be located just after the neural integrator. Since final eye position is based on efference copy ($E'$), the gain element must be outside the efference copy feedback loop. (If it were inside the feedback loop, the steady state eye position would not be affected by the gain, since the burst continues until the desired eye position is reached.) The gain of the step can be altered independently for leftward and rightward saccades, so it is represented in Fig. 3 by two line segments with different slopes: $g_L$ and $g_R$.

The parts of the model described so far represent the structure needed to make the saccade, but not the structure needed to adjust the variable gain element. In order to extend this model, two further components must be added. The first is a parametric gain adjuster. The second is a mechanism for deriving a step gain error signal. The step gain does not jump instantly to new values, but changes gradually over several days. This suggests that the step gain could be set by the output of a neural integrator with a low gain. The step gain would then change gradually, with a time course determined by the gain of the neural integrator. Such slow integration acts as an averager. The retinal slip seen by normal subjects can have any direction, but on the average it should occur equally often in all directions, i.e., the average slip should be zero. A subject with post-saccadic ocular drift, however, would have retinal slip in a direction correlated with the direction of the antecedent eye movement. Hence a retinal slip signal could be used as a step-gain

error signal if it is integrated in a way correlated with saccade direction.

The adaptive controller on the bottom of Fig. 3 monitors retinal slip velocity ($\dot{e}$), with high saccadic speeds clipped out, by feeding them into one of two integrators. Which integrator the slip goes into is determined by a switch set by the direction of the antecedent saccade ($\dot{E}'$ dotted line). The output of the two integrators ($\alpha_L/S$ and $\alpha_R/S$) sets the desired step gains ($g'_L$ and $g'_R$) for the elimination of post-saccadic ocular drift. The gains of the integrators, $\alpha_L$ and $\alpha_R$, determine the time course of the adaptation.

This model is useful in two ways. First, it summarizes what is known about the structure and function of the saccadic system, and second, it allows predictions about the behavior of the system to be made. By extending this model to include other ocular motor subsystems, such as smooth pursuit or the vestibulo-ocular reflex, predictions can be made about the interaction between saccadic and other types of eye movements. Then, by studying the effects of changing the saccadic step gain on other types of eye movements more can be learned about the structure of the ocular motor control system as a whole.

## 6. Conclusion

The saccadic system exhibits both a rapid and a gradual adaptive capability, with the gradual mechanism being known to depend on the cerebellum. Fast adaptation keeps the eyes from overshooting the target, while gradual adaptation appears to compensate for deficits in the motor system that affect saccadic accuracy (even in an orbital-position-dependent way), or that cause post-saccadic ocular drift. These two systems may interact, with the gradual system depending on the faster one for the derivation of its error signal.

The interaction between the visual sensory system and the saccadic motor system is not limited to the selection of visual targets, but also includes complex interactions that are required to maintain saccadic performance. Saccadic amplitude control may depend on the ability to compare the actual retinal error after a saccade (a visual system signal) with the expected retinal error (a motor system signal). Post-saccadic drift suppression may require the correlation of retinal slip (a visual system signal) with the antecedent saccade's direction (a motor system signal). By extending the mathematical models of saccadic motor performance to include adaptation, new roles for visual inputs to the saccadic system are opened to quantitative investigation (an example is given in Ch. 12).

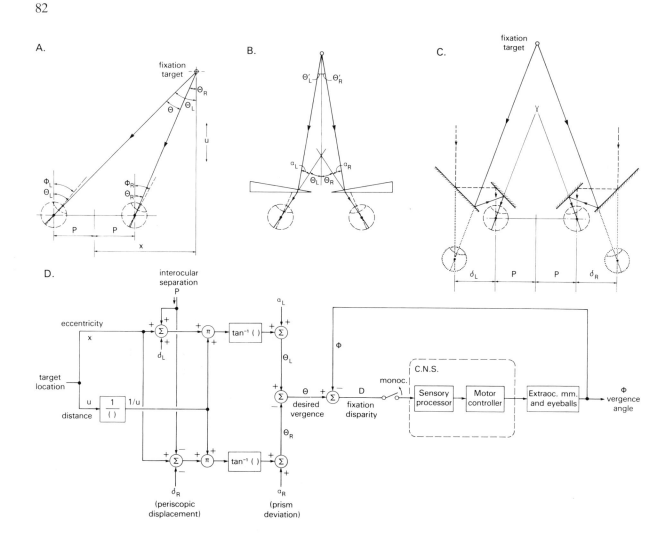

*Fig. 1.* The vergence control system. A. Simple optical geometry indicating the parameters used to define the input ($\theta$) and output ($\phi$). B. Use of base-out wedge prisms to increase the required convergence by a roughly constant amount at all viewing distances ($\alpha_L + \alpha_R$). C. Use of laterally-displacing periscopes to increase the effective interocular separation ($\delta_L + \delta_R$). Note that these optical devices move the subject's effective viewpoint backwards as well as laterally, thereby also increasing the viewing distance, but this effect is negligible, except perhaps for very near viewing. D. Block diagram of the system, including the optical geometry underlying the effects of wedge prisms and periscopes on the visual input (Eqn. 7 in the text).

plete and maintain the appropriate vergence state necessary for perceptual fusion to occur. Since both mechanisms operate on disparity errors, this nomenclature can be misleading. Normally, the vergence output follows the disparity input very closely, with errors — called fixation disparities — of only a few minutes of arc at most (Rashbass & Westheimer, 1961; Riggs & Niehl, 1960).

Recordings in the visual cortex of alert rhesus monkeys have revealed classes of single neurons whose discharges are each selectively sensitive to targets at, nearer than, or beyond the fixation plane, and it has been suggested that such neurons may provide the disparity information mediating vergence eye movements (Poggio & Fischer, 1977). Westheimer & Mitchell (1969) showed that a human subject whose corpus callosum had been surgically sectioned could only make vergence responses to objects that gave rise to images activating regions of both retinae that project (via the geniculostriate system) to the same cerebral hemisphere. Thus, this patient could not converge on objects within the regions bounded by the two lines of sight: when such objects are nearer than the fixation point, they are imaged on the temporal retinae (projecting to ipsilateral cortices), and when they are beyond, they are imaged on the nasal retinae (projecting to contralateral cortices). These observations suggest that the corpus callosum is important for the derivation of appropriate disparity error signals in cases where the two images are initially processed by separate hemispheres.

For a clear understanding of the vergence system and its response to various optical challenges, a precise description of the input to the system, or desired vergence angle, $\theta$, is needed. Referring to Fig. 1A, by simple geometry,

Desired vergence angle ( $\theta$ )

$$= \theta_L - \theta_R \tag{1}$$

$$= [\tan^{-1}\underset{u}{(x+P)}] - [\tan^{-1}\underset{u}{(x-P)}] \tag{2}$$

where $\theta_L$ and $\theta_R$ are the angles of incidence of the light reaching the left and right eyes, respectively, $u$ is the distance to, and $x$ the eccentricity of, the target, and $P$ is half the interocular separation. Note that the vergence error, fixation disparity $D$, defines the extent to which the actual vergence angle $\phi$, falls short of the desired vergence angle $\theta$:

Actual vergence angle ( $\phi$ )

$$= \phi_L - \phi_R; \tag{3}$$

Fixation disparity ( $D$ )

$$= \theta - \phi. \tag{4}$$

Thin wedge prisms are commonly used to challenge the system with a known disparity load (see Fig. 1B). For our purposes it can be assumed that the deviation produced by such prisms is independent of the angle of the incident light. Thus, base-out prisms increase the required convergence by an amount that we can assume is constant for all viewing distances, while base-in prisms have the converse effect. Base-out prisms can be said to have a positive effect on convergence and base-in prisms a negative effect. Referring to Fig. 1B, by simple geometry,

Desired vergence angle ( $\theta$ )

$$= \theta_L - \theta_R,$$

$$= (\theta_L' + \alpha_L) - (\theta_R' + \alpha_R), \tag{5}$$

where $\theta_L'$ and $\theta_R'$ are the angles of incidence of the light at the two prisms, $\theta_L$ and $\theta_R$ are the angles of incidence of the light at the two eyes, and $\alpha_L$ and $\alpha_R$ are the deviations due to the prisms in front of the two eyes.

Horizontally-displacing periscopic spectacles have recently been used to alter the apparent separation of the two eyes and so alter the amount of convergence required to align both eyes on the object of regard (see Fig. 1C). It is important to realise that while the wedge prisms produce a relatively constant change in the desired vergence at all viewing distances, the effect of the periscopes is in inverse relation to the viewing distance. Since laterally-displacing periscopes increase the effective interocular separation they can be said to have a positive effect, while medially displacing periscopes decrease it and can be said to have a negative effect. Referring to Fig. 1C, by simple geometry,

Effective interocular separation

$$= (P + \delta_L) + (P + \delta_R), \tag{6}$$

where $\delta_L$ and $\delta_R$ are the effective lateral displacements of the lines of sight of the left and right eyes, respectively. We can now generate a general description of the input to the vergence control system:

Desired vergence angle ( $\theta$ )

$$= \theta_L - \theta_R,$$

$$= \{[\tan^{-1}\underset{u}{(x + (P + \delta_L))}] + \alpha_L\}$$

$$- \{[\tan^{-1}\underset{u}{(x - (P + \delta_R))}] + \alpha_R\} \tag{7}$$

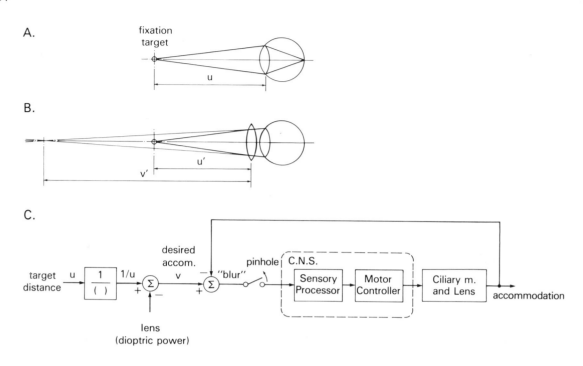

*Fig. 2.* The accommodation control system. A. Minimal representation of the eye indicating that the focusing function of the accommodation system is to bring the retina into optical congruency with the fixation target. B. Convex (positive) spectacle lenses decrease the required accommodation by creating a virtual image of the fixation target that is further away from the eye. C. Block diagram of the system including a much simplified representation of the optical geometry underlying the effects of spectacle lenses on the visual input (Eqn. 9 in the text). Note that V is the desired accommodation in diopters.

A block diagram representation of this visual input to the vergence system is shown in Fig. 1D. The effects of wedge prisms and periscopes are indicated by simple summing junctions with bias inputs. It is a simple matter to eliminate the disparity input merely by covering one eye and, in the block diagram of the system, this has been accomplished with a simple switch positioned in the forward path (labelled 'monoc').

## 3. The accommodation control system

Accommodation operates to eliminate retinal image blur, but blur is a scaler quantity having magnitude without direction. Thus, when blur is the only cue available, the accommodation system must at first 'hunt', just like the projectionist who has only a 50:50 chance of improving the focus of the image on the screen with his first try; it is not until the consequences of this first attempt are known that the direction of the required change in the focusing system can be deduced (Phillips & Stark, 1977; Stark & Takahashi, 1965; Troelstra et al., 1964). Under normal viewing conditions the accommodation system does not 'hunt' and does not initiate alterations in the wrong direction because it has recourse to other distance cues (Campbell & Westheimer, 1960). There are many potentially useful distance cues in the normal viewing situation that the system might utilize: spherical and chromatic aberrations, perspective, size, brightness, relative position, parallax effects associated with eye movements, and so forth (Campbell & Westheimer, 1959; Smithline, 1974). However, the role of these supplementary cues is poorly understood and beyond the scope of the present review; for want of a better collective term, the sensory stimulus to accommodation will be referred to here as blur, but the reader should always bear in mind the several possible supporting cues.

From the optical viewpoint, the function of the accommodation control system is to adjust the eye lens so as to bring the retina and fixation target into congruency (Fig. 2A). Spectacle lenses are commonly used to challenge the system with a known dioptric load. The magnitude of this effect can be estimated using the thin lens equation, which describes the image distance ($v'$) in terms of the object distance ($u'$) and the focal length of the lens ($f$). In gaussian form, this is:

$$\frac{1}{v'} = \frac{1}{f} + \frac{1}{u'} \tag{8}$$

The distances $v'$ and $u'$ are measured from the spectacle lens plane, while the input to the accommodation control system is specified in relation to the nodal point of the eye. However, since the distance separating the spectacle plane and nodal point is very small in relation to the usual target and image viewing distances it will be ignored here. The virtual image created by the spectacle lens provides the drive to accommodation and Eqn 8 can now be rewritten to specify the input to the accommodation control system in reciprocal meter units:

Desired accommodation ($V$, diopters)

$$= U - F, \tag{9}$$

where $U$ is the viewing distance to the object (in diopters) and $F$ is the dioptric power of the lens. Thus, spectacle lenses create a virtual image $F$ diopters away from the object of regard and so merely introduce a fixed dioptric bias into the optical path. Note that positive (convex) lenses decrease the accommodation required to focus the retinal image and negative (concave) lenses increase it. These effects of lenses on the input to the accommodation control system can be represented in the block diagram of the system by a simple summing junction with a bias input whose magnitude is determined by the dioptric power of the lens (see Fig. 2C).

Blur-induced accommodation has a very long latency — about 370 ms (Campbell & Westheimer, 1960) — and objective measures of accommodation usually reveal steady-state errors of half a diopter or more (Alpern & David, 1958; Fincham & Walton, 1957; Heath, 1956a; Morgan, 1944a & b, 1968). This 'lazy lag' led Toates (1972) to argue

for a proportional control system, though much of the error seems to be due to 'dead space', which relates to the system's inability to resolve small focus errors; even during steady fixation, fluctuations of up to 0.4 diopters seem to be normal (Campbell et al., 1959; Denieul, 1982). Presumably this relates in some way to the depth of focus of the system (Campbell, 1957; Green et al., 1980). The latter can be considerably increased experimentally using an artificial pinhole, an approach that is often employed to effectively eliminate the blur drive to accommodation by maintaining a focused image on the retina independent of the dioptric power of the eye lens. In the block diagram of the accommodation control system seen in Fig. 2C, this effect of pinhole apertures has been approximated by a simple switch positioned in the forward path.

## 4. The neural coupling between vergence and accommodation

The two negative feedback systems controlling vergence and accommodation do not operate completely independently of one another. This is perhaps not surprising since both systems are concerned with tracking the same objects, in depth, and so share a common range-finding problem. During monocular viewing, when there are no disparity inputs to the vergence system, blur-induced changes in accommodation also result in parallel changes in vergence, which are similar in form to those that accompany changes in accommodation in normal binocular viewing conditions: the *accommodative vergence* (AV) response (Alpern & Ellen, 1956a, b; Flom, 1960a, b; Kenyon et al., 1978; Maddox, 1886; Mueller, 1826; Semmlow & Venkiteswaran, 1976; Westheimer, 1955a). This response seems to result from cross-coupling between the two negative feedback control systems: It is usual to assume that the blur drive signal emerging from the sensory processor in the accommodation control system not only provides the input to the motor controller driving the ciliary muscles but also provides an input to the motor controller that drives the extraocular muscles mediating vergence eye movements (see Fig. 3). Except towards the extremes of its range, changes in accommodation during monocular

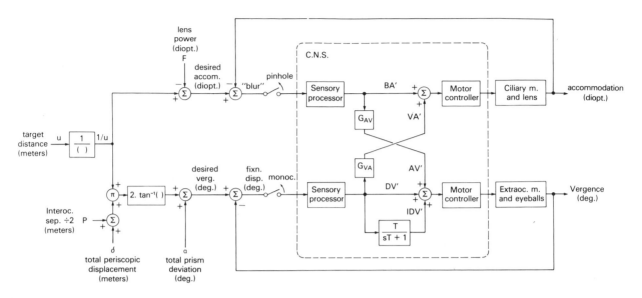

*Fig. 3.* A block diagram of the vergence and accommodation control systems showing the neural cross-links assumed to underlie accommodative vergence and vergence accommodation (after Krishnan et al., 1977). For simplicity, the optical arrangements defining the visual input to the vergence system assume the symmetrical case and have been reduced to their essential canonical form. The forward path in the vergence control system includes a leaky integrator, whose transfer function is shown in Laplace notation, where $s$ is the Laplace complex frequency.

viewing are normally accompanied by linear changes in vergence (Alpern et al., 1959; Flom, 1960a); the slope of this relationship, which indicates the change in vergence per unit change in accommodation, is an index of the strength of the AV response and is referred to in the literature as the AC/A ratio.*

So long as the vergence and accommodation outputs faithfully reflect their respective input drive signals, the value of the AC/A ratio can be totally ascribed to the gain element $G_{AV}$ in the model in Figure 3. However, this assumption would no longer be valid if the peripheral motor apparatus were to become less responsive for some reason. This would happen in the accommodation system, for example, if the ciliary muscle

were to become fatigued, or the lens were to become sclerotic (as in presbyopia), or neuromuscular transmission were to be compromised (as after cycloplegics). All of these conditions might be expected to result in an immediate increase in the measured response AC/A ratio since in each case the subject must employ more than the usual accommodative effort to eliminate blur. If, for example, the accommodative effort must be increased by 25% above its normal level to achieve a satisfactory focus then, in the monocular test situation, the associated change in vergence per unit change in accommodation (i.e., the AC/A ratio) would increase by 25% (c.f., Alpern & Larson, 1960; Breinin & Chin, 1973; Westheimer, 1963). Of course, if the vergence motor apparatus were to be compromised (as in myasthenia gravis, or Guillain-Barré syndrome, or fatigue) an immediate decrease in the measured response AC/A ratio might be expected to result. Thus, before attributing changes in the AC/A ratio to the neural gain element $G_{AV}$, it is necessary to rule out changes in the peripheral motor apparatus.

The accommodation and vergence control systems are also cross-coupled through a second,

---

*Many earlier studies of the AC/A ratio failed to measure the accommodative response directly, often assuming that it followed the accommodation stimulus rather closely; since the accommodation response can deviate considerably from its stimulus, these studies are often difficult to interpret. It is usual to distinguish between the two kinds of measures by referring to them as the stimulus and response AC/A ratios, respectively. To avoid confusion I will only refer to studies using response measures.

quite separate, mechanism. During binocular pinhole viewing, when blur inputs to the accommodation system are negligible, disparity-induced changes in vergence are associated with parallel changes in accommodation, which are similar in form to those that accompany changes in vergence in normal binocular viewing conditions: the *vergence accommodation* (VA) response (Fincham, 1955; Fincham & Walton, 1957; Kent, 1958; Morgan, 1954). It is usual to assume that the disparity error signal emerging from the sensory processor in the vergence control system drives not only the vergence motor controller but also the accommodation motor controller, accounting for the VA response (see Fig. 3). Except towards the extremes of its range, changes in vergence during pinhole viewing are normally accompanied by linear changes in accommodation (Fincham & Walton, 1957); the slope of this relationship, which indicates the change in accommodation per unit change in vergence, is an index of the strength of the VA response and is referred to as the CA/C ratio. This ratio can also be totally ascribed to a single gain element in the model in Fig. 3 — this time, the element $G_{VA}$ — but again it is necessary to point out that this assumes two appropriately responsive motor systems. Any compromise in the operation of the accommodation motor apparatus that renders it less responsive to the VA drive would be expected, initially at least, to decrease the measured CA/C ratio; any compromise in the vergence motor apparatus that necessitates augmented vergence effort to align the eyes would be expected to increase the measured CA/C ratio. Thus, before attributing changes in the CA/C ratio to the neural gain element $G_{VA}$, it is necessary to rule out changes in the peripheral motor apparatus.

## 5. Vergence adaptation to wedge prisms and lenses

### 5.1 Effect on the resting phoria

When an eye is occluded, it adopts a vergence position reflecting (i) any resting bias in the disparity vergence control networks, and (ii) the accommodative state of the other, viewing eye (due to accommodative vergence). In this monocular viewing situation, the extent to which the line of sight of the non-viewing eye deviates from the object of regard of the viewing eye defines the subject's *phoria*. Orthophoria refers to the condition in which the covered eye is accurately aligned with the object of regard; esophoria exists when the eye is over-converged, and exophoria when the eye is under-converged. For distant viewing, most normal subjects are reasonably orthophoric. If during binocular viewing a base-out prism is placed in front of one eye and then a few seconds later that eye is covered, the convergent deviation evident in that eye while the prism was in place is lost within 10–15 seconds as the eye now returns to its usual resting phoria position (Ludvigh et al., 1964). However, if the prism is left in place for several minutes before the eye is occluded, then the convergence induced by the prism persists — as an esophoria — for minutes or even hours (Alpern, 1946; Carter, 1963, 1965; Ellerbrock, 1950; Henson & North, 1980; Kenyon et al., 1978; Morgan, 1947; Ogle & Prangen, 1953; Schor, 1979a; Schubert, 1943). Similarly, prolonged exposure to base-in prisms results in exophoria. A few minutes of normal binocular experience is usually sufficient to re-establish the normal resting phoria.

Schor (1979b, 1980) has argued that such prism adaptation effects can be accounted for by merely incorporating a leaky integrator with a long time constant into the forward path of the vergence control system, which thereby becomes a proportional-plus-integral controller (see Fig. 3). It can be seen that there are now three input signals driving the vergence controller in the model: the direct disparity input (DV'), the accommodative vergence input (AV') and Schor's integrated disparity input (IDV'). With this arrangement, the resting bias in the vergence control networks referred to above is determined by the contribution from the integrator, and it is this contribution that is assumed to alter during prism adaptation, giving rise to the heterophoria evident in monocular test situations.

### 5.2. Effect on steady state errors

When suddenly confronted with a new disparity

load such as a base-out prism, there is an immediate increase in the vergence error drive signal, giving rise to convergence which operates to reduce that error but does not eliminate it entirely. This is to be expected of a proportional control system. However, Carter (1965) and Schor (1979a) have presented evidence which indicates that the unusually large fixation disparity errors initially associated with wedge prism spectacles do not persist, and these authors attribute this improvement to the adaptation mechanism: phoria adaptation is viewed merely as one manifestation of a process that functions primarily to reduce steady-state or long-term vergence errors. The model in Fig. 3 is consistent with this notion. The direct disparity input (DV') that deals with immediate or short-term vergence errors operates as part of a proportional control system that tolerates small steady state errors. However, any persistent residual fixation disparity signal will gradually charge up the integrator, increasing the integrated disparity drive to the vergence controller (IDV') and so gradually reducing the persistent disparity error to its normal low level. Thus, with time, the integrated disparity signal tends to substitute for any persistent disparity errors (Schor, 1979b). This charging process is assumed to take on the order of half a minute to approach asymptote, and if one eye is then covered, the charged state is maintained, giving rise to the observed phoria.

Semmlow and Hung (1979) have recently shown that the augmented fixation disparities initially associated with exposure to prisms are approximately halved during pinhole viewing and hence are due in part to the cross-links between the vergence and accommodation control systems. Careful perusal of the model in Fig. 3 reveals that the cross-links would be expected to exacerbate steady-state disparity errors: any increase in the disparity error results in a corresponding increase in the VA drive to accommodation, leading to a change in accommodation that results in a negative blur drive signal, which tends to offset the increment in the VA drive signal; the reduced blur drive signal will, however, result in a correspondingly reduced AV drive signal, which will operate to cancel some of the effect of the original disparity error signal thereby tending to increase fixation disparity. Clearly, it would be expected from the model that this cross-talk problem would be eliminated by pinhole viewing, since this would obviate the changes in the accommodative vergence drive signal. However, more importantly, it should be realised that insofar as vergence adaptation works to minimize persistent disparity errors, it too would be expected to reduce the potentially disruptive effect of the AV input on steady state binocular fixation.

A further expected consequence of the neural cross-links between the vergence and accommodation control mechanisms is that prolonged exposure to lenses would also influence the resting phoria, e.g., positive lenses that reduce the stimulus to accommodation would be expected to decrease accommodative vergence, resulting in increased reliance on the direct disparity input to sustain convergence, hence leading once more to increased charging of the integrator and esophoria. This has in fact been observed (Ellerbrock, 1950; Schor, 1979b). Note that the placement of the integrator in the model — in front of the summing junction through which the AV' signal accesses the vergence controller — is such that prolonged exposure to lenses would not be expected to influence the resting phoria in monocular viewing conditions when disparity feedback is lacking. This too has been documented (Schor, 1979b).

### 5.3. An example of adaptive offset control

Vergence adaptation to prisms and lenses is manifest as a step-wise shift in the workings of the VA and AV reflexes. For example, prolonged exposure to base-out prism spectacles results in a downward shift in the VA response curve and an upward shift in the AV response curve (see Fig. 4). The reverse effects are seen with base-in prism spectacles, though often less pronounced. Given that the deviation produced by a thin wedge prism is relatively independent of the viewing distance, it is optically appropriate that prism adaptation should result in these step-wise shifts in the VA and AV response curves with little influence on their slopes. However, the changes and interactions underlying these gradual step-wise shifts in VA and AV response curves are quite complex

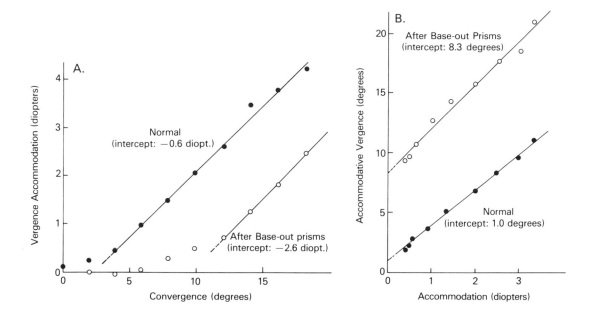

*Fig. 4.* Effect of 30 min of exposure to base-out prisms on the cross-coupling between vergence and accommodation. A. The vergence-induced accommodation response measured during binocular pinhole viewing. B. The accommodative vergence response measured during monocular viewing.

and best explained by recourse to models such as that in Fig. 3.

In the binocular pinhole viewing situation used to evaluate vergence accommodation, the blur-induced drives to accommodation and vergence (BA′ and AV′) will be invariant. However, following adaptation to, say, base-out prisms, when the IDV′ drive has acquired a convergent bias, the DV′ drive associated with any given vergence angle must be less than usual.* Since the VA′ drive to accommodation is assumed to vary along with the DV′ signal, the VA response will also show this bias, i.e., any given vergence state will be associated with *less* accommodation than usual, hence the VA response curve will show a downward shift. A complicating factor here is that the human subject's ability to produce negative accommodation is quite limited, hence for small vergence angles, accommodation simply remains close to zero, and in the case documented in

Fig. 4A, the VA response is only apparent for vergence angles in excess of 6°.

In the monocular situation used to evaluate accommodative vergence, the DV′ drive to the vergence controller is eliminated, and, following adaptation to, say, base-out prisms, the AV′ drive to convergence now merely sums with the newly increased IDV′ convergent drive that constitutes the primary adaptive change. Thus, the amount of convergence associated with any given accommodative state would be expected to increase, thereby shifting the whole AV curve upwards. Base-in prisms would be expected to have the converse effects.

In conclusion, the vergence adaptation mechanism that comes into operation when the system is challenged with wedge prisms or lenses can be viewed as an example of adaptive offset or bias control. Such a mechanism would seem to be important for the establishment and maintenance of a tonic vergence state that allows the system to function with minimal sustained stress on its feedback controller and consequently minimal steady-state vergence errors.

---

*This assumes that the integrator output remains constant throughout the VA calibration, a reasonable expectation provided that the whole procedure takes no more than a few minutes.

## 6. Adaptive regulation in the coupling between vergence and accommodation

### 6.1. Vergence accommodation

The vergence accommodation response seems to play a crucial role in the rapid initiation of changes in accommodation. During monocular viewing, accommodation is very slow to respond to blur and its associated cues, and does so with a latency of about 370 ms. However, when transferring fixation between targets at different distances under normal binocular viewing conditions, the changes in accommodation begin at least 100 ms earlier (Krishnan et al., 1977), largely because of the VA response. Indeed, it seems that blur cues normally perform only a fine-tuning function as the accommodation response nears completion. However, the long latency of the blur-induced effects is not the only reason for this. Blur inputs are only effective within a few degrees of the fovea; if the desired new fixation target is more eccentric than this, then blur cues will not even start to come into effect until the vergence movement and refixation saccade have brought the image of the new target into the immediate vicinity of the fovea (Campbell, 1954; Fincham, 1951; Phillips, 1974; Hennessy & Leibowitz, 1971; Whiteside, 1957). A further problem is that only modest levels of blur seem to be effective as a stimulus to accommodation: blur in excess of 2·D often fails to elicit any accommodation response (Fincham & Walton, 1957; Ogle, 1966; Heath, 1956b). It would, therefore, seem that for much of the time the accommodation system effectively operates open-loop so far as blur is concerned. By contrast, the disparity detection mechanism driving vergence eye movements has a much shorter latency (160 ms), is effective across the entire retina, has a large depth range (Westheimer & Mitchell, 1969) and, most importantly, is not degraded by blurring (Jones & Kerr, 1972). Clearly, in the absence of an adequate blur drive signal to initiate rapid changes, the accommodation system utilizes the superior disparity drive signal, via the VA cross-link.

However, the VA reflex operates open-loop, giving rise to an output, accommodation, that does not directly influence its input, disparity. For maximum effectiveness, the VA reflex should be appropriately calibrated: a given disparity input should generate a commensurate change in accommodation (as well as vergence). In their original study, Fincham and Waltham (1957) showed that the magnitude of the VA response in young adults, as indicated by the CA/C ratio, was close to ideal for maintaining correct focus of the eyes on their object of regard. Recent work suggests that this precision may result from the operation of an adaptive gain control mechanism.

### 6.1.1. Adaptive gain control

In the model in Fig. 3, the pure gain element $G_{VA}$ determines the strength of the neural coupling by which the vergence system influences accommodation. The desired vergence and desired accommodation in normal binocular viewing conditions are linked by simple geometry, and the physical parameter that governs the strength of the relationship is the separation of the two eyes: the greater the separation, the less the required change in accommodation that should accompany a given change in vergence and, hence, the less the required CA/C ratio. If the neural gain element, $G_{VA}$, is subject to adaptive regulation then it should be possible to modify it by changing the apparent separation of the two eyes using horizontally displacing periscopic spectacles (see Fig. 1C). Laterally-displacing periscopes that more than doubled the apparent interocular separation have recently been shown to elicit an adaptive decrease of 50% or more in the CA/C ratio within 30 min (Miles & Judge, 1982) (see Fig. 5A). However, medially displacing (cyclopean) periscopic spectacles that reduced the apparent separation to zero were without significant effect on the VA response. Perhaps the challenge offered by the cyclopean spectacles was too extreme or required more time than the 30 min employed, so that for the present this negative result should be viewed with circumspection.

That the CA/C ratio could be decreased but not increased is especially puzzling since the system showed rapid recovery from the acquired low gain ratio. It is possible that the observed decrease is not due to a genuine adaptive reduction in the gain of the neural linkage, but merely due to fatigue of the accommodative response. Such fatigue might be expected to result from the extreme exertions associated with constantly refocusing and re-aligning the eyes while adapting to the periscopic spectacles. However, this seems to be an unlikely explanation since attempts to induce fatigue effects with controlled 'exercises' were only mildly successful in some subjects. (In these cases it must be conceded that such fatigue effects may account for a small part of the observed decrease in the CA/C ratio and might even have operated to obscure any slight tendency for the ratio to increase with the cyclopean spectacles.)

### 6.1.2. Functional role of the adaptive gain control mechanism

In discussing the functional role of adaptive gain control in other oculomotor subsystems such as the vestibulo-ocular reflex and the saccadic system, it has been usual to invoke the open-loop nature of their operations as the major reason for having some adaptive calibration mechanism to establish the proper gain. It is also generally assumed that there is a continuing need for these adaptive mechanisms throughout life to compensate for the assumed intrinsic long-term instability of neuronal connectivity, as well as to render the system less vulnerable to aging, sickness and trauma. While the present example may share the same needs, its rapid time course would seem to implicate it in more short-term regulation. It is tempting to assume that the asymmetry in the adaptive response is genuine and relates to the fact that the interocular separation increases during normal development, but never decreases. However, the adaptive process is so rapid, with a time constant measured in minutes, that developmental factors extending over years would hardly seem to constitute its primary challenge. In my view, a somewhat more plausible role for this rapid adaptive mechanism would be to combat the tendency for the VA reflex to overdrive accommodation whenever the convergence response is subject to fatigue; such a function would be consonant with both the speed and the apparent asymmetry of the adaptive process. It is generally acknowledged that the nervous system normally deals with disparity errors much more

vigorously than with blur, presumably because diplopia is the more debilitating handicap and disparity the more effective feedback signal. Of all the oculomotor subsystems, those governing binocular alignment are consistently required to perform with the greatest precision. It can be safely assumed that any tendency for the vergence motor mechanism to fatigue would be dealt with promptly and very effectively by disparity feedback, allowing only a very small increase in the fixation disparity; however, the latter could nonetheless have profoundly deleterious effects on accommodation — which is subject to much weaker feedback control — via the VA′ drive signal. A decrease in the gain of the VA response would alleviate this problem. Note that the integrator in the vergence control path could not compensate for the effects of such fatigue since these would be manifest as an apparent change in the gain — rather than the bias — of the vergence response.

### 6.2. Accommodative vergence

The AV response is also generated open-loop and, in the model in Fig. 3, the efficacy of this response is solely determined by the neural gain element $G_{AV}$. An estimate of the value $G_{AV}$ can be obtained from measuring the change in vergence per unit change in accommodation in monocular viewing conditions — the AC/A ratio — provided that, as usual, the two motor systems are appropriately responsive. A number of studies have attempted to modify the AC/A ratio using orthoptics, but reviewers have usually expressed considerable scepticism about their validity and significance (e.g., Alpern, 1969; Ciuffreda & Kenyon, 1983; Westheimer, 1955b). For a variety of reasons, these studies are often difficult to interpret and inconclusive: many assumed and did not measure the accommodative response; others used only patients with known ocular alignment problems and were concerned mainly with enduring changes that might have potential therapeutic value and so would survive subsequent binocular experience; many employed a rather ill-defined optical situation that may or may not have directly challenged the AV response. Whatever the reason, none of these earlier studies reported

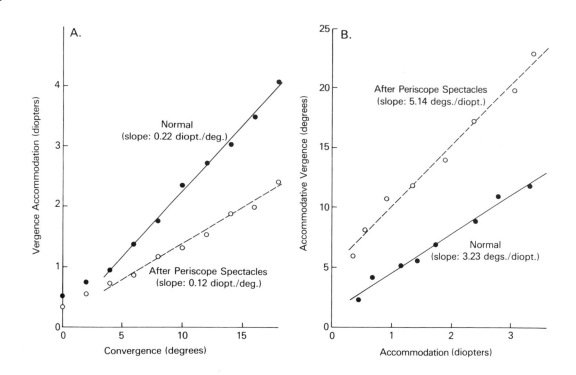

*Fig. 5.* Effect of 30 min of exposure to laterally-displacing periscopic spectacles, which more than double the effective interocular separation, on the cross-coupling between vergence and accommodation. A. The vergence-induced accommodation response measured during binocular pinhole viewing. B. The accommodative vergence response measured during monocular viewing (after Miles & Judge, 1982).

more than minor changes in the AC/A ratio, often of uncertain statistical and functional significance. For a detailed consideration of these earlier studies, the reader is directed to the excellent review by Ciuffreda and Kenyon (1983).

Recently, laterally-displacing periscopic spectacles that more than doubled the apparent separation of the eyes and so presented a direct, vigorous challenge to AV, have been shown to elicit adaptive increases of 50% or more in the response AC/A ratio within 30 min (Miles & Judge, 1982) (see Fig. 5). Once more, however, the cyclopean spectacles were ineffective. As with the previously discussed decrease in the CA/C ratio, the present increase in the AC/A ratio might be due to fatigue of the accommodation response mechanism rather than to a genuine adaptive change in the neural gain element $G_{AV}$. Again, however, the ineffectiveness of cyclopean spectacles and exercise controls would seem to make this an unlikely explanation.

### 6.2.1. Functional significance of the adaptive gain control mechanism

Unfortunately, the functional significance of this adaptive process in the AV mechanism is a matter of some conjecture because the AV reflex itself seems to have only minor functional significance. Blur-induced vergence has a much longer latency (280 ms) than disparity-induced vergence (160 ms) (Krishnan et al., 1977) and also requires stimulation of the central retina (Semmlow & Tinor, 1978) with the attendant disadvantages already alluded to. A careful comparison of the vergence responses generated by simultaneous blur and disparity with those produced by disparity stimulation alone reveals only very minor transient differences during the later stages of the vergence change (Semmlow & Wetzel, 1979). There is no question that AV can be most disruptive, as we shall see when we discuss, for example, accommodative esotropia, and as we saw in considering the cross-talk between vergence and accommodation during prism adaptation when its influence certainly cannot be ignored. However, the AV response in normal subjects would seem to be of very minor functional significance, in marked contrast to the VA response. In this regard, it might be noted that the AC/A ratio is usually much lower than the CA/C ratio and AV responses are always much slower than VA responses. Of course, the functional role invoked for adaptive regulation in the VA reflex — to offset any fatigue of the vergence motor response — can also be argued for the AV reflex even though its contribution might be minor.

If the AV response is normally of minor functional significance as I have suggested, it would seem to indicate that this cross-link is only vestigial in man. In evolutionary terms, we can assume that laterally directed eyes predated frontal, that accommodation predated vergence and that the use of blur and its associated distance cues predated the use of disparity. Thus, as the eyes migrated forwards, it seems possible that the blur signals driving accommodation would at first represent the only central correlates of target distance available to accomplish convergence. Such arguments suggest that accommodative vergence may have been the primordial mechanism for accomplishing convergence. However, once evolved, disparity detectors provided markedly better depth information that allowed the development of a feedback-controlled mechanism for rapidly achieving the precise binocular alignment necessary for good stereoscopic vision, and also provided a useful feedforward boost to accommodation. Blur cues together with the blur-dependent AV mechanism, were then relegated to a minor role.

### 6.3. Related clinical observations

The failure to reduce the AC/A ratio or increase the CA/C ratio with what would seem to be an appropriate optical challenge — cyclopean spectacles — is in accord with several common clinical findings. The first is the esotropia seen in some hyperopic children. This could result from increased AV drive associated with excessive accommodative effort (presumably blur-induced) and/or from voluntary vergence undertaken to augment accommodation through the VA input. In either event it would seem that such patients would stand to benefit from adaptive changes in the cross-coupling networks, or more specifically, from a decrease in the AC/A ratio and/or an increase in the CA/C ratio. Thus, that esotropia sometimes accompanies hyperopia is consistent with the failure of the system to adapt to cyclopean spectacles. That myopes sometimes develop intermittent exotropia may also be in part due to these adaptive insufficiencies. Yet further related clinical findings are the high response AC/A ratio and low CA/C ratio seen in presbyopes (Breinin & Chin, 1973; Fincham & Walton, 1957).

### 7. Gaze specific adaptation in corrected anisometropia

Anisometropes, whose spectacle prescription is slightly different for the two eyes, manage to contend with the differing magnification factors quite successfully. The eye confronted with the more positive lens and hence more magnified image must always make correspondingly larger movements than the other eye to maintain binocular alignment and single vision. The important point so far as we are concerned is that the two eyes experience unequal prismatic deviations during eccentric fixation, e.g., if the right spectacle lens is the more positive one then binocular alignment requires progressively increasing convergence during leftward gaze (quasi-increasing base-out prism effect) and progressively decreasing convergence during rightward gaze (quasi-increasing base-in prism effect). Of course, vertical eccentric deviations will also be greater for the right eye, and it should be noted that vertical binocular alignment is unrelated to the viewing distance. It has been shown that during monocular viewing the phoria in corrected anisometropes varies with gaze position exactly in accordance with the varying prismatic demands of their spectacles (Allen, 1974; Ellerbrock, 1948; Ellerbrock & Fry, 1942). Thus, subjects can selectively adjust their phoria at different orbital positions.

In this regard, Henson & Dharamshi (1982) have recently shown that if gaze is confined to a particular direction during the adaption to wedge prisms, then the changes in phoria are greatest at that position and may, for example, be only half as large, a mere 20° to either side. Furthermore, they showed that normal subjects can successfully adapt their resting phoria to small amount of optically-induced incomitance achieved with a contact lens/spectacle lens combination in front of one eye; this induced a prismatic deviation which increased as the line of sight deviated from the optical center of the spectacle lens. The clear suggestion from this work is that the usual precise binocular synergy characterised by Hering's law is achieved at least in part through the operation of adaptive mechanisms.

Adaptive mechanisms in gaze control
Facts and theories
*Eds. Berthoz & Melvill Jones*
©1985 Elsevier Science Publishers BV (Biomedical Division)

## Chapter 6

# Effects of visual deprivation on properties and modifiability of compensatory eye movement systems

## M. Cynader

*Departments of Psychology and Physiology, Dalhousie University, Halifax, Nova Scotia, Canada B3H 4J1*

## 1. Introduction

It has become clear that most eye movements are not made to look around at a stationary world. Rather, most eye movements, especially slow ones, have as their goal the stabilization of a dynamic visual environment set into motion by the activity of the observer's head and body. Two major compensatory eye movement systems, whose action we measure as the vestibulo-ocular and optokinetic reflexes, share the task of visual stabilization. Other chapters in this volume discuss the characteristics, the underlying neural circuitry, and the modifiability of compensatory eye movement systems. Here we consider the effects of various forms of visual deprivation imposed during the early postnatal life of the organism on the properties and adaptive capacities of compensatory eye movement systems.

We begin by noting that it is most unlikely that the vestibulo-ocular reflex of a normal cat or human would be challenged by a stimulus as unusual as a complete left-right reversal in the field of vision during the course of everyday life (Gonshor & Melvill Jones, 1976a). Yet, evidence presented in this volume and elsewhere makes it clear that the vestibulo-ocular reflex can respond in an adaptive manner to demands of this sort. What rationale can we offer for this amazing plasticity? One possibility is that the capacity to adapt to these extremely unusual visual inputs reflects a more basic ability of the system to compensate for alterations which normally occur during development. The early postnatal period is a period of rapid growth for the eye, and for the oculomotor system as well. Human infants are frequently astigmatic, or show refractive errors during the first few months of life (Mohindra et al., 1978). In addition, the eye muscles themselves are maturing during the early postnatal period. If clear vision is to be maintained during this period of constant adjustment and development of visuomotor systems, then the capacity to modify the VOR in response to persistent retinal slip becomes a valuable, and indeed necessary, characteristic of the oculomotor system.

The need for adaptive capacities during early development has spurred interest in studying vestibular function in very young animals and in animals which have been deprived of visual input during early postnatal development. The vestibulo-ocular reflex operates as an open-loop system and as such is quite vulnerable to errors of calibration. Since no opportunity for calibration exists unless visual input is made available, studies of neonatal subjects and dark-reared animals allow us to determine the vestibular system's inherent biases in the absence of visual input.

The vestibular-ocular reflex is clearly present at birth in chickens (Wallman et al., 1982) and at the time of earliest measurement (10 days postnatal) in kittens (Flandrin et al., 1979). In both

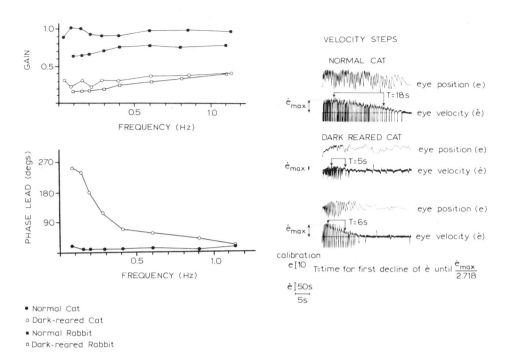

*Fig. 1.* The properties of the horizontal vestibulo-ocular reflex of dark-reared rabbits and cats are compared with those of normally reared animals (figure redrawn from Harris & Cynader (1981a) and Collewijn (1977c). The top left panel compares VOR gain in normal cats and rabbits (filled circles and squares, respectively) and their dark-reared counterparts (open symbols) across a range of sinuosidal frequencies. In both species, VOR gain is reduced by a factor of at least two after dark rearing. The lower left panel shows that, in dark-reared cats, the phase response of the VOR is also markedly anomalous. One observes a large, frequency dependant, phase advance which is not present in normal animals. The right hand panel shows the response of a normal cat (top two traces) and a dark-reared cat (lower four traces) to a step in velocity. The traces begin at the moment of the step. The responses to three steps are shown, each one giving rise to a pair of traces corresponding to eye position (top traces of each pair) and eye velocity (lower trace of each pair). The upper two steps were from 70°/s to zero, and were applied to a normal cat (top pair of traces) and a dark-reared cat (next pair of traces). The results of a further step, of 210°/s to zero, applied to the dark-reared cat are also shown (lower two traces).

species, however, VOR gain is much lower than in adult animals. Mature VOR properties are not observed until about 2 months of age in the cat.

Several workers have studied the consequences of complete visual deprivation, starting near birth, on VOR function and modifiability. The early qualitative investigations of Nasiell (1924) in rabbits, and Mowrer (1936) in pigeons, revealed no impairments in VOR function following a few weeks of dark rearing starting at birth. VOR function as assessed qualitatively with EOG methods also appeared normal in kittens dark reared until 4 months of age (Berthoz et al., 1975a). These workers, however, noted a reduction in the frequency of the quick phases of vestibular nystagmus, suggesting that the gain of the VOR was reduced by a factor of two in dark-

reared kittens. Their conclusions were substantiated in more recent quantitative studies of vestibular function using the scleral search coil technique. These latter studies (Collewijn, 1977c; Harris & Cynader, 1981a) have revealed substantial alterations in VOR properties in both rabbits and cats reared in darkness for prolonged periods of time.

Fig. 1 compares the gain and phase of the VOR as assessed with sinusoidal stimulation, in normal and dark-reared rabbits and cats. In the rabbit, dark rearing reduces the gain of the VOR by a factor of about three throughout the range of frequencies tested. The results in the cat appear very similar, with a clear reduction in gain throughout the frequency spectrum. In addition, the dark-reared cats show substantial anomalies in phase response relationships between vestibular inputs and oculomotor output. The phase anomalies appear as a frequency-dependent phase lead which reaches 180° with sinusoidal stimulation at 0.3 Hz. At this frequency, therefore, the action of the VOR is entirely *anticompensatory* rather than compensatory. The abnormal phase relationship is present only with low amplitude vestibular stimulation (10° peak to peak), and becomes less pronounced with higher amplitude stimuli.

The right hand panel of Fig. 1 illustrates another anomaly of vestibular function which follows dark rearing in the cat. The figure illustrates the response of normal and dark-reared cats to steps of angular velocity, presented in total darkness. The table is rotated at a constant angular velocity of 70°/s for 2 min and then halted abruptly. The normal cat displays a post-rotary nystagmus which persists for some time after such a velocity step (Fig. 1 right, top two traces, corresponding to position and velocity) decaying with a time constant of 18.5 s. The response of the dark-reared cat to the same velocity step is shown in the next two traces in Fig. 1, right. Two features are immediately apparent from a comparison of the normal and dark-reared traces. Firstly the peak 'slow-phase' eye velocity of the dark-reared is much lower than that produced by the normal cat in response to an identical step. Secondly the response declines very much faster.

The decline of eye movement velocity of a normal cat after exposure to a step of velocity is only roughly approximated by an exponential. This is particularly true as the eye velocity approaches zero (Fig. 1, right, top traces). Since the dark-reared cat's response to a velocity step reaches a maximum much closer to zero velocity, the lack of a truly exponential decline may contribute to the observed difference in the duration of post-rotatory nystagmus. The dark-reared cat was therefore subjected to a velocity step of three times that used for the normal cat (i.e., 210°/s). This resulted in a maximum slow-phase eye velocity very close to that of the normal cat's records shown in Figure 1. The records thus obtained from the dark-reared cat are shown as the bottom two traces of Fig. 1. They demonstrate that the rate of decline is independent of the maximum velocity of the slow-phase response over this

range of velocity steps. The time constant in this case was 6 s, a value very close to that achieved with the smaller step in velocity.

It is noteworthy that the time constant of post-rotatory nystagmus in the normal cat (Robinson, 1976) is much longer than that of the semicircular canals (Blanks et al., 1975b). This prolonged time constant apparently reflects the functioning of higher order brain stem circuits, rather than simply mirroring peripheral canal dynamics (Raphan et al., 1977; Robinson, 1977a). In the dark-reared animals, the time constant of the system as a whole is fairly well approximated by the response *of the canals themselves*, suggesting that the higher order circuits (Robinson, 1977a) which prolong vestibular nystagmus are deficient in dark-reared animals.

These findings make it clear that the development of normal vestibular function depends on exposure to visual stimuli in both the cat and the rabbit. It appears, moreover, that there is an, as yet undefined, critical period in the animal's early life during which visual experience is required for the development of normal VOR function. Simply placing a normally-reared adult cat in the dark for up to five months has no effect on either the gain, phase, or time constant of the VOR. (Harris & Cynader, 1981a)

## 2. Does the vestibular system have to learn how to learn?

The results described above make it clear that a variety of VOR properties are altered following prolonged visual deprivation. Since one of the basic properties of the VOR is its modifiability in response to unusual visual demands, it is relevant to ask whether the very capacity for modifiability is degraded if no visual challenges are imposed during development. The evidence indicates that dark rearing has strong effects on VOR plasticity. Fig. 2 shows the results of an effort to modify the VOR of a dark-reared cat. The open circles, taken from Fig. 1, show that VOR gain is low (between 0.3 and 0.5) throughout the range of frequencies tested before the modification attempt. The cat was then rotated in the light for a period of 4 h. Rotation in the light allows both the visual and the vestibular system to participate in the compensation process. Under these cir-

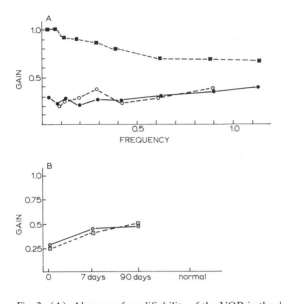

*Fig. 2.* (A). Absence of modifiability of the VOR in the dark-reared cat. The VOR was first measured in darkness (●). Thereafter the animal was subject to forced rotation in the light. This raised the gain of the compensatory responses substantially (■). However no improvement of VOR perform- ance is found when the animal is subsequently tested in the dark (○). (B) This illustrates the permanence of the VOR deficits after dark rearing in the cat (⊙) and rabbit (⊡). When the animals are first brought into the light, VOR gain is near 0.25 in both species. A clear improvement, to values near 0.4, is found in the first week of light exposure, but little further gain improvement is noted over the next 3 months and per- formance never approaches that of the normally reared coun- terparts. Redrawn from Harris & Cynader (1981a,b) and Col- lewijn (1977c)

cumstances, compensation for the table rotation is rather good. As illustrated in Fig. 2, the com- bined visual and vestibular reflexes are able to achieve a gain of close to unity at low frequencies, declining with increasing frequency to 0.7 at 1.0 hz. The phase lead is close to 0° (not shown) throughout the frequency range tested. Yet, when the lights are turned off and the animal's VOR is again tested in darkness, no changes in the gain (or phase) of the VOR are observed. The gain is still as low as it was before the modification attempt. Control data show that a regimen of forced rotation with a mismatch between vestibu- lar output and resulting visual input evokes clear changes in the VOR of normally reared cats (Robinson, 1976; Harris & Cynader, 1981b). The

weak modifiability of VOR gain after dark- rearing contrasts with the situation observed in the neonate. In 1-day-old chickens, Wallman et al. (1982) were able to show a rapid increase in VOR gain (from a similar low baseline) with two hours of 'increased gain' training.

The reduced modifiability of vestibular func- tion after dark rearing can be studied in quite a different way. In a dark-reared animal with a low VOR gain (of less than one), each natural head movement in normal visual surroundings serves as a stimulus for VOR modification. In a normal cat in which VOR gain has been artificially low- ered, (see, for instance, Melvill Jones & Davies, 1976) simply allowing the animal normal vision produces a mismatch between reduced vestibular output and normal visual input. This mismatch results in extremely rapid VOR modification and the gain of the VOR approaches unity over a period of a few days. However, placing a dark- reared cat into a normally lit environment for up to 5 months does not promote substantial recov- ery of VOR gain. The data for recovery of VOR gain with light exposure are compared for dark- reared cats and rabbits in the lower panel of Fig. 2. The rabbit and cat data are similar. As men- tioned, VOR gain is low immediately after dark rearing. Placing the animals into a normally illu- minated environment promotes only a limited re- covery of VOR function. The gain does improve somewhat with light exposure, but the VOR of the dark-reared rabbit or cat remains below nor- mal even after 3 months of light exposure. This finding contrasts with the developmental data for normally reared kittens or chickens in which VOR gain improves steadily in the first few weeks of life (Flandrin et al., 1979b; Wallman et al., 1982).

## 3. Mechanisms underlying the lack of VOR mod- ifiability in dark-reared animals

Several authors in this volume discuss the neural mechanisms which underlie VOR modifiability. While several distinct mechanisms for VOR mod- ifiability have been proposed and remain the sub- ject of active debate, (Ito, 1982a, also Chapters 14, 15; Miles & Lisberger, 1981, also Chapter 21) it seems clear that the mechanism by which VOR gain is altered by visual input depends on the integrity of the cerebellum, particularly the cerebellar flocculus (Ito, 1977; Robinson, 1976). It is possible that the reduced modifiability of the VOR in dark-reared animals may result from a reduced or absent visual input to the cerebellar flocculus in dark-reared animals. If visual input is somehow prevented from reaching the cerebellar neurons involved in the VOR modification process then this could, in itself, explain the reduced modifiability of the VOR in these animals.

It has been found in other contexts that one of the effects of visual deprivation is to reduce the functional effectiveness of some visual pathways. In the deeper layers of the superior colliculus of normal cats, visual input combines with that from other sense modalities resulting in multimodal responses in individual units (Wickelgren & Sterling, 1969; Berman & Cynader, 1972). After dark rearing, visual responses in this part of the superior colliculus are greatly reduced in magnitude. Most units can still be driven by stimulation of other sensory inputs, but responses to visual stimuli are selectively attenuated. It has been suggested that this reduction in efficacy may be brought about by a competitive interaction between visual afferents and those from other sensory modalities (Cynader, 1979; Rauschecker & Harris, 1983). A similar phenomenon may occur with regard to the visual cortex input to the nucleus of the optic tract (NOT) in monocularly-deprived and strabismic cats (Hoffmann, 1979; Cynader & Hoffmann, 1981). The visual cortex output pathway appears to lose its functional effectiveness, with the result that the response properties of NOT neurons in these deprived animals resemble those of decorticate animals (Hoffmann, 1982).

We have no information as yet on the nature and strength of visual inputs to the cerebellum of dark-reared animals. Indeed, the nature and significance of visual inputs to the cerebellar flocculus in normal animals is still uncertain (Maekawa & Simpson, 1972; Maekawa & Takeda, 1976; Simpson et al., 1979; Lisberger & Fuchs, 1978a Takemori & Cohen, 1974). If these inputs are, however, reduced in their efficacy, then it would provide a possible explanation for the relatively low level of VOR modifiability in dark-reared animals. The notion is simply that one effect of visual deprivation would be to prevent visual input from gaining access to the modifiable elements of the VOR pathway and therefore provide the error signal necessary for the modification process to occur.

It is worth noting that most of the effects of visual deprivation are characterized by displaying a clear critical period during which the effects of deprivation are most pronounced. Several months of normal vision, for instance, fails to reverse the consequences of an initial 4 month period of dark rearing on collicular neurons. (Flandrin & Jeannerod, 1977; Cynader, unpublished). Yet, as little as a few days of normal vision allowed during the first 6 weeks of life in an otherwise dark-reared cat largely prevents the deleterious effects of dark rearing on collicular neurons (Cynader, unpublished). It would be most interesting to see whether one could prevent the deficits in VOR gain and dynamics which occur in dark-reared animals by allowing animals periods of visual exposure during the dark-rearing regimen. It is also possible that visual deprivation maintained for shorter periods, or begun only after a period of normal visual exposure early in life would still allow normal VOR function. In each of the rearing conditions described above, it will be important to assess both the basic vestibular functions (VOR gain, phase, frequency response, time constant, etc.) and also the capacity for visual modifiability of these functions. It may be that a regimen of partial visual deprivation will enable us to dissociate modifiability of the VOR from deficits in its routine, day-to-day, functioning.

## 4. The effects of rearing in stroboscopic illumination on VOR properties and modifiability

It is generally accepted that a major goal of the visual and vestibular systems involved in generating compensatory eye movements is to reduce retinal image slip which would otherwise result from head and body movements. While perfect stabilization of the retinal image is not always achieved (Steinman & Collewijn, 1980), the adaptive changes in VOR function described in this volume always have the effect of reducing retinal slip during head movement. In view of the strong effects of dark rearing on both the basic functions and the modifiability of the VOR, compensatory eye movements have been examined in cats reared in an environment in which vision of stationary contours was permitted, but retinal image slip was prevented. This was achieved by rearing kittens in a light enclosure in which the only illumination source was a strobe light (Cynader et al., 1973; Cynader & Chernenko, 1976). The 10 μs flash duration prevents the smooth image slip which normally evokes compensatory eye movements. Before describing the effects of strobe rearing on VOR function, we first consider the effects of the rearing procedure on organization of the visual system.

Rearing animals in stroboscopic illumination throughout the first few months of life results in marked changes in the response properties of neurons in the visual pathways. Since the initial studies in cat visual cortex, the effects of strobe rearing have been examined in several visual structures in rabbits, hamsters and cats (Chalupa & Rhoades, 1978; Flandrin et al., 1976; Pearson & Murphy, 1983). Different investigators have varied the duration of the strobe-rearing period and the interval between strobe flashes. The most consistent effect of this movement deprivation paradigm is to cause a reduction, or loss, of direction selectivity among visual neurons. In the striate cortex of normal cats, for instance, over 80% of the neurons encountered display direction selectivity, producing at least twice as many nerve impulses in response to a bar moving in the presumptive preferred direction as for movement in the opposite (null) direction. After strobe rearing with a 125 ms interflash interval for the first 6 months of life, only 14% of the neurons encountered display this property (Cynader & Chernenko, 1976). This reduction in cortical direction selectivity can be observed in the absence of alterations in other cortical response features, such as orientation selectivity and binocular interaction. In the cat superior colliculus, the incidence of direction selective neurons is reduced from 84 to 12% by rearing in a 4 flashes/s strobe environment (Kennedy et al., 1980). Similar, but in some cases less marked, changes have been observed in the visual cortex and superior colliculus of strobe-reared rabbits and hamsters (Chalupa & Rhodes,

1978; Pearson & Murphy, 1983). As yet, we have no information concerning the effects of strobe rearing on the direction selective responses of neurons in the accessory optic system and the NOT. This lacuna is frustrating because it is now widely accepted that these neurons are a major route by which visual information reaches compensatory eye movement systems (Hoffmann, 1982; Simpson et al., 1979).

In contrast to the substantial effects of dark rearing, cats reared in an 8 Hz strobe environment show little or no reduction in the gain of their VOR, as measured in the dark, relative to normal cats (Melvill Jones et al., 1981). The mean VOR gain for two strobe-reared cats examined by these authors was 0.73, a value only slightly lower than that of normal cats. Strobe-reared cats display a small but consistent advance in phase relative to normal cats studied under the same conditions of sinusoidal oscillation. This phase lead of about 5° is, however, tiny compared to that of over 200° observed in dark-reared cats measured under similar conditions (Harris & Cynader, 1981a). With lower frequencies of strobe rearing (2 Hz), Kennedy et al. (1982) found deficits in VOR gain. VOR gain of their low frequency strobe-reared cats was close to 0.4; a value not far from that of dark-reared animals. In contrast to dark-reared animals however, the low frequency strobe-reared cats showed no anomalies in either the time constant or the phase responses of their VOR.

These studies indicate that measurable changes in VOR properties can be demonstrated in strobe-reared cats. The graded nature of these alterations, depending on the frequency of strobe flashes used during rearing, suggests that these animals may be valuable preparations for future experiments in which deficits of a certain size are desired.

As yet, there have been no studies of VOR modifiability in the low frequency strobe-reared cats described above. However, strobe rearing at 8 Hz, unlike dark rearing, does not markedly affect the adaptability of the VOR. Fig. 3 illustrates the time course of VOR adaptation to vision reversal induced by visual exposure while wearing dove prisms (Melvill Jones & Davies, 1976) in normal and strobe-reared cats. Fig. 3A

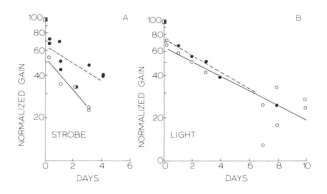

*Fig. 3.* Time course of VOR adaptation to vision reversal. All data points indicate VOR gain (eye velocity/head velocity; ordinate) measured in the dark, and normalized relative to mean control values (□), Linear regression lines have been calculated for control animal C (solid lines, open symbols), and for the two strobe reared animals $S_1$ and $S_2$ (interrupted lines, filled symbols). A, comparison of adaptation, in strobe light, of strobe-reared with normal cats. B, comparison of adaptation, in normal light, of strobe-reared and normal cats. Redrawn from Mandl et al. (1981).

shows the effects of vision reversal induced during a period of stroboscopic illumination, and Fig. 3B the effects of vision reversal in normal illumination. In strobe illumination, it is clear that both the normal and strobe-reared subjects show an initial sharp fall in VOR gain to about 60–70% of initial values with vision reversal. This is followed by a slower decline at an approximate rate of 5–10% per day. The regression line for the slow adaptive process appears to have a somewhat steeper slope in the strobe-reared cat than in the normal animal but this difference does not reach statistical significance. Fig. 3B shows that VOR adaptation follows a very similar course in normal and strobe-reared cats when adaptation occurs in normally lit surroundings. As in Fig. 3A (see also Melvill Jones & Davies, 1976), a fast and slow adaptive process can be observed which appears indistinguishable in the normal and strobe-reared animals.

Strobe rearing at 8 Hz, therefore, in contrast to total visual deprivation, has relatively small effects on VOR properties and adaptability. We may thus conclude that exposure to retinal slip during development and the presence or absence of direction-selective neurons in the superior colliculus and visual cortex of strobe-reared cats

does not play a critical role either in the development of normal VOR properties, or in altering VOR function in response to unusual visual demands.

## 5. Optokinetic nystagmus (OKN)

While the vestibulo-ocular reflex is primarily responsible for generating compensatory eye movements in response to high frequencies of head rotation, the visual system makes its major contribution to compensatory eye movements when low frequencies and velocities of the stimulation are present. We can observe the compensatory behavior of the visual system in isolation by measuring the slow phase of optokinetic nystagmus and comparing the slow phase eye velocity with that of the angular velocity of a textured drum rotating about the animal. Perfect compensation for the drum motion is obtained when the eye velocity matches that of the rotating drum. It should be noted that in contrast to the VOR, the optokinetic system operates as a negative feedback system which normally has a high open-loop gain. The transfer function of the optokinetic system is usually given as:

$$\frac{E}{W} = \frac{G}{1+G}$$

where $G$ is the open-loop gain, $E$ is eye velocity, and $W$ is drum velocity. Under these circumstances even a large loss of neural connections which would, for instance, change $G$ from 20 to 10, would result in only a small change in the closed-loop gain of OKN, from 0.95 to 0.91. Thus, failure to find large deficits in closed loop OKN performance may not rule out the presence of neural anomalies.

Several investigators have studied OKN in visually deprived animals. In qualitative recordings, Mowrer (1936) found a marked depression in OKN capacities in dark-reared pigeons. This recovered after a few days of visual experience. More recent studies using EOG and search coil methods to record eye movements, show that OKN can be elicited immediately after prolonged periods of dark rearing in both cats and rabbits (Vital Durand & Jeannerod, 1974a,b; Harris et

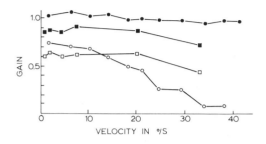

Fig. 4. The 'closed loop' (eye velocity/drum velocity) gain of horizontal optokinetic nystagmus measured in normal and dark-reared cats (●, ○) and rabbits (■, □). Conventions are the same as in Fig. 1. OKN gain values are close to 1 in both rabbits and cats over most of the velocity range tested, but dark-rearing causes a marked diminution of OKN gain especially with higher drum speeds. Redrawn from Harris & Cynader (1981a) and Collewijn (1977c)

al., 1980; Collewijn, 1977c). The gain of OKN is, however, reduced in dark-reared animals. Fig. 4 compares the closed-loop gain of OKN in normal and dark-reared rabbits and cats. The data differ in detail for cats and rabbits, but a clear trend toward reduced OKN gain, especially for high stimulus velocities, is present in both species. This indicates a loss of connections in the optokinetic system of dark-reared animals. The causes and nature of this deficit will be considered in more detail after a description of monocular OKN.

## 6. Monocular OKN

In normal animals OKN can be elicited under conditions of monocular visual stimulation. In many species, however, OKN generated under conditions of monocular viewing displays marked asymmetries when the visual stimulus moves in the two horizontal directions of motion. In studies of lateral-eyed animals, such as rabbits and rats, OKN in response to drum motion directed anteriorly (nasally) is much stronger than responses to posterior (temporal) directed drum motion. This asymmetry is not noted in normal monkeys or humans, and in an extensive survey of 18 mammalian and non-mammalian species, Tauber and Atkin (1968) concluded that the naso-temporal asymmetry in monocular OKN correlated with the presence or absence of the fovea. This correlation is supported by studies of OKN in a rod

monochromat, who lacked a functional fovea, in whom a marked naso-temporal asymmetry in OKN was found. A clear naso-temporal asymmetry in monocular OKN can also be demonstrated in human infants during the first few months of life, while the fovea is still relatively immature (Duke-Elder & Wybar, 1973; Atkinson, 1979).

In the normal cat, a small naso-temporal asymmetry in monocular OKN is present, but it is much less pronounced than in rabbits and rats (Honrubia et al., 1967). In the cat, the naso-temporal asymmetry in OKN appears to be related to the integrity of the visual cortex, rather than the presence or absence of the fovea. Lesions of the cat visual cortex drastically reduce or abolish optokinetic responses to lateral-directed drum motion under conditions of monocular viewing (Wood et al., 1973; Hoffmann, 1982; Strong et al., 1984; Precht, 1981). The lesion has, of course, no effect on the fovea itself, but the effect on OKN is to make the decorticate cat resemble a lateral-eyed animal such as a rat or rabbit in its monocular performance.

Like visual decortication, dark rearing greatly exacerbates the small naso-temporal OKN asymmetry of the normal cat. Fig. 5 compares OKN responses to nasal versus temporal-directed drum motion in normal and dark-reared cats. The left hand side of the figure illustrates responses with nasal-directed drum motion of different speeds while the right hand side describes temporal-directed responses. The figure shows that for dark-reared cats the response to nasal-directed drum motion appears much stronger than normal with low stimulus velocities. Responses decline rapidly with higher drum speeds. The paradoxically large response for low drum speeds in which the eye is actually moving *faster* than the drum (thus, resulting in retinal slip in the temporal direction) is explained by the occurrence of a spontaneous nystagmus, with a nasal-directed slow phase which is observed in dark-reared cats (Harris & Cynader, 1981a). If one eliminates the contribution of this spontaneous nystagmus, then OKN responses, although clearly present, are much weaker than in the normal cat. Nasal directed responses become very weak for drum speeds above 20°/s. For temporal-directed drum

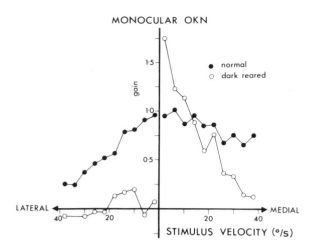

MONOCULAR OKN

gain

• normal
○ dark reared

LATERAL ◄─────

MEDIAL ─────►

STIMULUS VELOCITY (°/s)

*Fig. 5.* The right hand part of the figure illustrates the responses of normal and dark-reared cats to a monocularly-viewed textured drum moving medially (towards the nose) with varied velocity, while the left hand part of the figure illustrates responses to lateral drum motion. In the normal cat, OKN gain is close to 1 for low drum speeds, but drops off with higher speeds. Responses for medial directed drum motion are generally stronger than those for lateral motion especially with high drum speeds. In the dark-reared cat, responses to lateral-directed motion are virtually absent at all drum speeds and the gain is markedly reduced from normal with medial-directed motion above 20°/s. The apparent gain of greater than one results from a spontaneous nystagmus (slow phase medial) found in dark-reared cats. Redrawn from Harris et al. (1980)

motion, dark-reared cats essentially fail to respond effectively regardless of the drum speed. Occasional weak and intermittent slow phases are the only evidence for optokinetic responses.

The optokinetic deficits observed with stimulation of the deprived eye of cats which have been monocularly sutured since birth are even more severe. When the deprived eye is first opened, responses to temporal-directed drum motion are largely absent, as in the dark reared cat. With nasal-directed drum motion, some responses can be obtained, but the gain of the response is much reduced even relative to that of dark-reared cats. (Malach et al., 1981, 1984).

The effects of monocular eyelid suture on OKN elicited via stimulation of the non-deprived eye are somewhat controversial. Van Hof-van Duin (1976) found that monocular eyelid suture caused substantial asymmetries in OKN elicited via the *non-deprived* eye, essentially abolishing

responses to temporal drum motion. Hoffmann (1979) obtained a similar result in some of his monocularly sutured cats, but in others, OKN elicited through the non-deprived eye appeared very similar to that elicited monocularly in normal cats. Several other studies (Malach et al., 1981, 1984; Cynader & Roach, unpublished) found no differences between monocular OKN responses in normal cats and those of the non-deprived eye of monocularly sutured cats. The causes of the divergences in these experimental results remain unclear.

## 7. Mechanisms underlying the monocular asymmetry of OKN

The effects of dark rearing and monocular eyelid suture on OKN behavior may be at least partially explicable in terms of a functional loss of the cortical contribution to the subcortical systems controlling OKN. It is by now well established that the pretectal nucleus of the optic tract is a major subcortical relay station mediating horizontal OKN in rats, rabbits and cats. This conclusion is consistent with the results of lesion (Collewijn, 1975a; Precht, 1981), stimulation (Collewijn, 1975a) and recording studies (Hoffmann & Schoppmann, 1975; Collewijn, 1975b; Hoffmann, 1982) which show that damage to this region severely disrupts OKN and that neurons in this nucleus respond well to stimuli which normally elicit OKN.

In lateral-eyed animals such as rabbits, and also in cats in which the cortex has been removed, NOT neurons are activated by visual stimulation via the contralateral eye only and solely by nasal-directed stimulus motion. This directional bias in the response of monocularly-driven NOT neurons probably accounts for the strong naso-temporal asymmetry in OKN responses observed in normal lateral-eyed animals and in decorticate cats. With the cortex intact, cat NOT cells respond to stimulation via the ipsilateral eye as well. The preferred direction of NOT cells remains the same in visual space and so the directional preference is now in favour of *temporal ward* stimulus motion through the ipsilateral eye. The additional indirect input via the cortex from the ipsilateral eye which emphasises responses to temporal motion probably accounts for the finding that the naso-temporal asymmetry in OKN is less marked in normal cats than in decorticate cats. In addition, NOT cells in unlesioned cats respond to higher stimulus velocities than do NOT cells in decorticate cats. This difference in velocity tuning may be the cause of the reduced high velocity OKN responses in decorticate cats.

The optokinetic capacities of dark-reared cats, may well be explicable by postulating that dark rearing produces a functional decortication with respect to the optokinetic system. Several authors have found that dark rearing produces substantial declines in the responsivity of visual cortex cells (Cynader et al., 1976; Imbert & Buisseret, 1975) as well as causing reductions in the incidence of feature-specific properties, such as direction selectivity. Although there is no direct evidence available on this point, one may speculate that the weakly responding and unspecific cortical cells of dark-reared cats may be unable to exert their influence on subcortical pathways mediating OKN. Results showing that dark rearing appears to prevent the cortex from exercising its normal influence on units in the cat superior colliculus (Wickelgren & Sterling, 1969) are also consistent with this hypothesis.

The effects of monocular eyelid suture may also be interpreted in similar terms. The deprived eye loses its ability to influence cortical cells (Wiesel & Hubel, 1965) and accordingly, loses access to the midbrain via the cortical pathways. A similar loss of cortical influence on midbrain structures may account for the loss of temporal OKN observed in the normal eye of some monocularly-deprived cats.

## 8. Modifiability of the optokinetic system

While most studies of oculomotor plasticity have concentrated on modifiability of the vestibulo-ocular reflex, as tested in total darkness, several recent studies make it clear that normal adult animals (including rabbits, cats and primates) can show marked adaptive changes in optokinetic responses following only a few hours of atypical visual exposure. Several groups of workers (Demer, 1981; Lisberger et al., 1981; Melvill Jones et al.,

1980) (see also Chapters 2, 3, 8) have found that procedures which result in successful VOR adaptation produce correlated changes in OKN performance. Since, as discussed earlier in this chapter, the optokinetic system operates as a closed-loop control system, small changes in system performance may be difficult to measure using conventional closed-loop stimulation techniques. One approach to assessing OKN modifiability has thus been to measure the saturation velocity of closed-loop OKN. Saturation velocity under these conditions is directly related to VOR gain. In cats, for instance, saturation velocity ranged from 10 to 20°/s when horizontal VOR gain had been adaptively reduced to 0.2–0.4. When VOR gain was increased to 1.66, horizontal OKN saturation velocity increased to 65°/s (Demer, 1981). Several other approaches (Collewijn & Grootendorst, 1979; Strong et al., 1984) have demonstrated adaptive changes in OKN after conditions of unusual visual stimulation, or have demonstrated recovery of OKN after cortical lesions which decrease OKN capacities.

The detailed interpretation of these studies is beyond the scope of this chapter, but they made it clear the OKN capacities are subject to adaptive modification in normally reared adult animals just as is the vestibulo-ocular reflex. In this context, it is interesting to consider the developmental effects on OKN modifiability. As yet, only limited data are available on this point. The effects of dark rearing on OKN properties have been described earlier. The gain of OKN is reduced in visually-deprived cats, especially at high drum speeds, and this diminished gain appears to be unmodifiable in animals subjected to prolonged dark rearing (Harris & Cynader, 1981a). In experiments, in which efforts were made to raise the gain of the VOR (see previous section), no alterations in OKN gain were observed, in contrast with modifications obtained in normal cats (Demer 1981). Another way to evaluate the modifiability of OKN capacities in deprived animals is to simply seek changes in OKN gain when dark-reared animals are brought out of the dark and maintained in a normally illuminated environment. This has been done for both cats and rabbits. In neither species were dramatic improvements of the OKN gain observed. The deficits in OKN performance which follow prolonged visual deprivation appear to be permanent in both species.

Thus, in contrast to the modifiability of OKN in normal animals, dark-reared rabbits and cats exhibit little capacity for adaptive modification of OKN. The lack of VOR modifiability in these animals appears to be part of a more global impairment which these visually-deprived animals show in meeting the challenges of a changing visual environment. Evidently, failure to exercise the modifiability mechanisms during early development results in permanent deficiencies in the adaptive process.

## 9. Matching properties of compensatory eye movement systems to special demands of the visual environment

The results discussed earlier make it clear that atypical visual exposure can strongly affect both the normal functioning and capacity for modifiability of compensatory eye movement systems. Most of the special rearing conditions considered thus far result in impaired performance of compensatory eye movement systems and/or of defects in the ability to modify these systems in response to atypical visual exposure. Yet one of the most striking features of the organism's response to unusual visual environments imposed early in development is the tendency for cortical neurons to adapt their properties to match the most probable features of the visual environment. This trend is exemplified by studies of the cortical organization of animals reared in a visual environment consisting primarily of contours of a single orientation (Hirsch & Spinelli, 1970; Blakemore & Cooper, 1970; Cynader & Mitchell, 1977; Stryker & Sherk, 1975). If, for example, kittens' visual experience is effectively restricted to vertical contours, then the vast majority of the striate cortex neurons encountered in the adult cat will respond optimally to vertically oriented stimuli. In horizontally reared kittens, cortical neurons instead prefer horizontal stimuli. A similar tendency for the visual system to alter the characteristics of cortical neurons to match the most probable features of the visual environment appears in investigations of cats reared with stimuli moving primarily in one direction. Under these circumstances, the majority of cortical neurons respond best to the direction of stimulus motion which prevailed during rearing (Cynader et al., 1975; Tretter et al., 1975; Berman & Daw, 1977).

Despite these impressive findings at the level of the visual cortex, only a few studies have sought adaptive changes in compensatory eye movement systems as a result of unusual visual experience during postnatal development. Vital-Durand and Jeannerod (1974a) examined OKN in cats reared in a one-directional environment (rightward). They found that OKN responses were much stronger in response to stimulus motion in this direction than in the opposite direction. This intriguing finding may result from several different mechanisms. The biased OKN could reflect a special adaptation by the directional motion system of these animals, or alternatively it could simply reflect the effects of visual deprivation for the system normally mediating leftward OKN and normal exposure for the system responding to rightward motion. It will be important to see whether the rightward OKN system of these animals is better in its performance than that of normal animals. It would be most interesting also, to see tests of monocular OKN capacities in these unidirectionally reared cats. Since each eye normally responds better to nasal-directed stimuli, it may be that OKN elicited through the right eye would be substantially weaker than that elicited through the left eye. If so, then unidirectional rearing might produce effects similar to that of monocular deprivation for compensatory eye movement systems. In the rabbit, similar efforts to modify neuronal directional preferences in the retina and OKN behavior by means of unidirectional exposure during development have proven unsuccessful (Daw & Wyatt, 1976).

The most comprehensive evidence for long-term adaptive modifications in compensatory eye movement systems after atypical visual exposure in infancy is found in strobe-reared animals (see also Chapter 2). As described earlier, the VOR of strobe-reared cats appears normal, both in its day-to-day functioning and in its capacity for visual modification. Yet striking anomalies are present in both spontaneous eye movements and

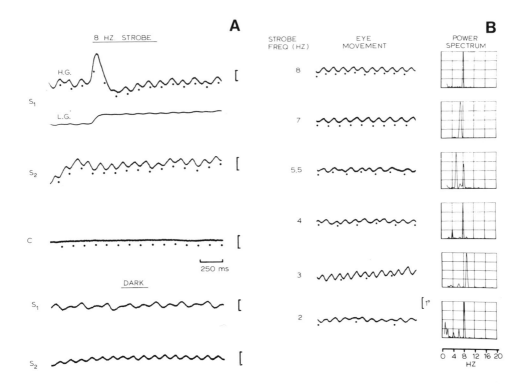

*Fig 6.* (A) Oscillatory horizontal eye movements in strobe-reared and control cats, recorded with head fixed in 8 Hz strobe light and in the dark. All records, except the lower traces for $S_1$ in strobe (L.G., low gain DC, 0.135 times H.G.), were obtained at high gain (H.G., high pass filtered with 0.1 Hz cut-off) to retain trace on recording paper. The control animal showed no eye oscillations, either in strobe light, or in the dark; hence the dark trace for the control cat has been omitted. Dots under H.G. curves indicate the occurrence of strobe flashes. Eye calibrations 1° for H.G. traces, 7.4° for L.G. trace. Time bar 250 ms. All records from right eye; down indicates nasal displacement throughout. Redrawn from Melvill Jones et al. (1981)

(B) Effects of strobe frequency on oscillatory eye movements, obtained from a strobe reared cat before exposure to normal light. Ordinates of power spectrum curves denote relative power density of eye oscillations, expressed in arbitrary units. Power spectra were obtained from original records including, but extending beyond, those shown. Power spectra have been plotted from 2–20 Hz except for the 2 Hz strobe record which extends down to 1 Hz; eye calibration 1°.

in optokinetic reactions of strobe-reared cats. These anomalies appear to represent adaptations by the oculomotor system to the special rearing conditions of these animals (Melvill Jones et al., 1981; Mandl et al., 1981).

## 10. Oscillatory eye movements

Cats reared from birth in stroboscopic illumination at 8 flashes/s develop abnormal spontaneous eye oscillations. These oscillations, as measured in 8 Hz strobe light and in complete darkness are illustrated for two strobe-reared cats and for a control animal in Fig. 6A (left-hand side). The traces illustrate a pendular form of nystagmus with an

amplitude of 0.5–1.0° and a fundamental frequency of 8 Hz. The time of occurrence of the individual strobe flashes is shown by dots in the high gain records of the figure. Note that the oscillatory eye movements are synchronized with the strobe flashes. No comparable pendular nystagmus is observed in normally reared adult cats exposed to strobe illumination. To clarify the significance of this pendular form of nystagmus, cats which had been reared in 8 Hz strobe illumination throughout early development were tested with different frequencies of strobe illumination. The results from one animal are shown in Fig. 6B. The inserts on the right of the figure are power spectra in which the abscissae represent the freqency of eye oscillations and the ordinates are the relative power density of eye oscillation, normalized so that the maximum power density has a value of unity. It is clear that the dominant frequency of eye oscillation varies markedly with the differing strobe light forcing frequencies. Changing the ambient strobe frequency from 8 to 7 Hz reduces the frequency of the oscillation while maintaining the consistency of the phase relationship between the eye oscillations with the individual strobe flashes. Further reductions in strobe frequency to 5.5 and 4 Hz reveal a more complex pattern of eye oscillation. The power spectra show that one component of the oscillations is the same as the imposed 'forcing' frequency of strobe flashes, while another component reverts to the 'natural' frequency of 8 Hz which characterizes the animal's early rearing environment. A similar trend is observed with 2 Hz stimulation, but now subharmonics at 4, 6 and 8 Hz are observed. With 3 Hz strobe flashes, the dominant frequency of nystagmus lies near 9 Hz with smaller peaks at 3 and 6 Hz. The raw traces on Fig.6 show that regardless of the frequency of strobe light employed, the phase relationship between the eyes' oscillation and the occurrence of individual strobe flashes remains rather constant.

These results suggest that an oscillatory process with a dominant frequency close to that of the strobe-rearing frequency has been created in the oculomotor system of strobe-reared cats. It is clearly possibly to modify the frequency of the oscillatory process in adult strobe-reared cats by imposing 'forcing' frequencies of strobe light, but one observes a clear tendency for a return to the oscillation frequency occurring during the rearing history if the 'forcing' frequencies deviate too greatly from that imposed during early development. As already mentioned, no comparable effects are observed in adult cats exposed to strobe light, although normally-reared adult cats have, as yet, been exposed to strobe light for a few days only, rather than for the 6–18 months of exposure employed in the developmental experiments.

The significance of this constant oscillatory motion may appear unclear at first but it should be recalled that the eyes of normal cats (and humans) are in fact undergoing constant motion. Even during fixation, slow drifts and microsaccades are su-

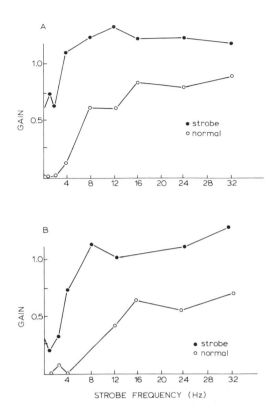

*Fig.* 7. The gain of horizontal optokinetic nystagmus measured under binocular viewing conditions in normal and strobe-reared animals. Responses for a drum speed of 8°/s (A) and for 16°/s (B). The abcissa represents the number of strobe flashes per second. The normal cat (open circles) shows very weak OKN responses with low-frequency strobe flashes. As the flashes become more frequent, OKN gain begins to improve and reaches asymptote near 16 flashes/s. For the strobe-reared cat, OKN performance is much better than that of the normally-reared animal when low frequency strobe flashes are presented and asymptotic performance is reached by about 8 flashes/s. The asymptotic gain is clearly higher in strobe reared cats than in normally-reared animals.

perimposed on a fine (10–30 s arc amplitude) high frequency tremor (Ditchburn & Ginsborg, 1952; Ratliff & Riggs, 1950). These eye movements are essential to normal vision, since most units in the visual system respond best to *changes* in retinal illumination rather than to a given ambient level of input (Hubel & Wiesel, 1962). Visual perception fades after a few seconds if the normal displacements of the eyes are eliminated (Ditchburn & Ginsborg, 1952; Riggs et al., 1953).

After strobe rearing, the drifts and flashes of normal physiological nystagmus are unnecessary for the maintenance of normal vision. The critical requirement for a rapid change in illumination is met by the very intermittency of the light source. Thus, in the presence of the strobe light the requirement is not for continuous destabilization of an ever-present retinal image, but rather for stabilization on the retina of the image of an intermittently illuminated visual world. In the strobe-reared cats this goal appears to have been achieved by synchronizing an ever-present eye oscillation with the ambient strobe flashes. In this context, the continuous eye oscillation appears to represent an adaptive modification to the unusual rearing conditions imposed during postnatal development. It is interesting to note that the eye oscillations disappear within a few weeks of bringing strobe-reared cats into a normally lit visual environment.

Another type of adaptation to the unusual rearing conditions of the strobe-reared cats is observed in the optokinetic system. Fig. 7 illustrates the capacity of normal and strobe-reared cats to perform OKN in the presence of intermittent strobe illumination of different frequencies. The ordinates of the graphs illustrate the gain of OKN in response to the motion of a randomly patterned drum moving at 8 and at 16°/s. The abscissae represent the different frequencies of strobe illumination used during the measurement of OKN. For the normal cat tested with stimulus motion at 8°/s, performance is quite poor at low frequencies of strobe illumination, but improves above 8–12 Hz to approach a gain of about 0.8. For the higher stimulus velocity, even higher frequencies of strobe illumination (16–24 Hz) are required before the gain asymptotes. With intermittent illumination, the performance of strobe-reared cats is markedly superior for both low and high drum speeds. With the slower drum speed, OKN gain reaches asymptote by 8 Hz and even shows a tendency to overshoot with higher frequencies of strobe illumination. With a drum speed of 16°/s, asymptotic gain is also achieved by 8 Hz and maintained for all higher frequencies.

These results thus suggest that some form of adaptive modification has occurred in the optokinetic system of strobe-reared cats, resulting in a marked improvement over normal animals in the ability to perform compensatory eye movements under conditions of intermittent illumination. OKN gain for all stimulus velocities tested is far higher then that of normal cats when the animal is tested with strobe illumination at the rearing frequency of 8 Hz. The relative increase in gain is not sharply turned about 8 Hz. OKN performance is clearly better than normal at 2, 4 and 12 Hz, representing frequencies never experienced during the animal's early life. To perform OKN under conditions of intermittent illumination, the animal must correlate the instantaneous input with that occurring at a later time. For normal cats, the process begins to fail for intervals above 60 ms and performance is extremely poor for intervals of 125–250 ms. These values are close to those obtained in human psychophysical experiments on the perception of apparent motion in random dot kinematograms (Braddick, 1980; Baker & Braddick, 1985). In the strobe-reared cats, performance remains excellent with 125 ms intervals between stimuli and some success is even possible with interflash intervals of up to 500 ms. We have no information on the neural mechanisms underlying this remarkable ability of the strobe-reared cats to adjust the temporal properties of their visuomotor systems, but they may be related in some way to the pendular nystagmus observed in these animals. It will be most interesting to record single unit properties at various levels of the optokinetic pathways in strobe reared animals, searching for the mechanisms underlying adaptation to the unusual rearing conditions.

## 11. Summary, conclusions and lacunae

The capacity for modifiability of compensatory eye movement systems is an important feature of their efficacy. This modifiability may arise from the need to constantly recalibrate these systems during early development as the various parts of the visuomotor apparatus develop in loose concert. The evidence presented here indicates that compensatory eye movement systems must be challenged by persistent error signals during early development if the modifiable subsystems are to develop properly. Dark-reared cats fail to respond adaptively with normal vigor in VOR modification paradigms which are effective in normally reared animals. We still lack information on the neural mechanisms underlying these deficits in visually deprived animals. As well, we need information on the duration and distribution of the dark-rearing period which suffices to interfere with modifiability. In addition, there is a dearth of data available on both the normal postnatal development of VOR properties and on their modifiability. It would be most valuable to learn whether VOR modifiability were especially well developed in young animals who must cope with rapid developmental changes in their visuomotor apparatus. The difficulties in making this determination have been considered by Wallman et al. (1982).

The lack of opportunity for usage causes decreases in the gain of OKN subsystems in dark-reared animals as well. Both cats and rabbits show a pronounced decline in binocularly-elicited OKN. Monocular OKN responses are altered in a selective manner by dark rearing in the cat. The animals lose the ability to generate OKN in response to drum motion directed lateral to the viewing eye. In this sense, dark-reared cats resemble cats who have sustained visual cortex lesions and also resemble normal lateral-eyed animals such as rabbits and rats which show comparable mediolateral asymmetries in OKN. It is noteworthy that human infants also manifest this asymmetry in monocular OKN for the first few months of life (Atkinson, 1979).

Despite these deficits associated with visual deprivation, compensatory eye movement systems can display remarkable adaptation to unusual visual environments imposed on them during early development. Cats reared in an environment in which stimuli move in one direction only eventually develop stronger OKN responses to stimuli moving in that direction. Animals reared in stroboscopic illumination show much stronger OKN responses in stroboscopic illumination than do normal animals tested under the same conditions. Finally these strobe-reared animals develop an unusual pendular form of nystagmus which appears to represent a unique solution to the problem of maintaining visual stability in an intermittently illuminated environment.

# Section IB

## Effects of vestibular modification on oculomotor control

Adaptive mechanisms in gaze control
Facts and theories
*Eds. Berthoz & Melvill Jones*

# Chapter 7

# Vestibular habituation: an adaptive process?

## R. Schmid[a] & M. Jeannerod[b]

*[a]Dipartimento di Informatica e Sistemistica, Universita di Pavia, Italy and*
*[b]Laboratoire de Neuropsychologie Expérimentale, INSERM-U94, Bron, France*

## 1. Introduction

An adaptive system is a hierarchical control system in which at least three levels can be identified: an execution level, a control level and a decision level. An adaptive process is started whenever one of the following situations occurs: a change in the execution level makes it inadequate to perform correctly the function for which it has been designed; the assumptions on which the design was based are no longer valid; the environmental condition is such that the function performed by the execution level becomes useless or even detrimental with respect to the general goal of the system.

Depending on which of these situations takes place, three different classes of adaptive processes can be distinguished. By making reference to the oculomotor control system which has the general goal of ensuring visual fixation and to the vestibulo-ocular reflex which plays within it the role of an execution level with the specific function of visual stabilization during head rotation, the following three adaptive processes can be recognised.

A peripheral or central lesion has modified the gain or the dynamics of VOR and a compensation process is needed to restore VOR function. This adaptive process is described in Chapters 2 & 3.

Unusual visual conditions, such as wearing of prisms or lenses, has changed the relationship required between head and eye movements in order to obtain visual stabilization. A recalibration of VOR gain is therefore needed. This process is described in Chapters 2 & 3.

When the pattern of vestibular stimulation is outside the range considered in the development of the reflex (unphysiological patterns of stimulation) or the environmental conditions (e.g., repeated vestibular stimulation in darkness) the responses evoked may have become meaningless or detrimental. This process, which is normally referred to as vestibular habituation, is described in the present chapter.

## 2. Habituation of vestibulo-ocular responses

Vestibular habituation has been mainly investigated by considering the modifications of vestibulo ocular responses produced by repeated stimulations of the semicircular canals. Habituation produces three major effects, acquisition, retention and transfer (Dodge, 1923).

*Acquisition* is manifested by a progressive decline of VOR response during the period of stimulation.

*Retention* is manifested by the persistence of a modified VOR response after a period of rest.

*Transfer* is manifested by the presence of a modification in responses evoked either by pat-

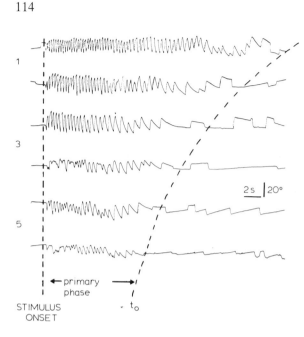

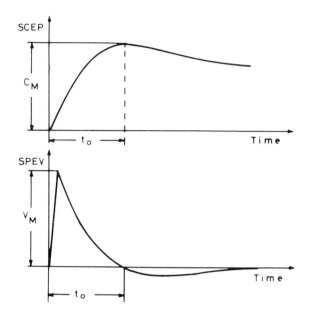

Fig. 1. Horizontal eye movement responses of a cat to repeated CW velocity steps of 160°/s. The first and the last response of the 1st, 3rd and 5th day are represented sequentially.

Fig. 2. Definition of the parameters characterizing the time course of the slow cumulative eye position (SCEP) and of the slow phase eye velocity (SPEV) in response to head angular velocity steps. $C_M$, peak amplitude of SCEP; $V_M$, peak amplitude of SPEV; $t_o$, time of SCEP peak and SPEV zero-crossing.

terns of vestibular stimulation different from that used to provoke habituation or by other sensory stimulations (e.g., optokinetic stimulation). All these three aspects seem to indicate that habituation implies a progressive long-term adjustment of VOR parameters.

Vestibular habituation has been studied in rabbits (Hood & Pfalz, 1954; Kleinschmidt & Collewijn, 1975; Ito et al., 1974a), in cats (Henriksson et al., 1961; Crampton & Schwam, 1961; Crampton, 1964; Collins, 1964a; Jeannerod et al., 1976), in monkeys (Jäger & Henn, 1981a; Collins, 1964b) and in man (Dodge, 1923; Baloh et al., 1982) by using either caloric or rotatory stimulations. It has also been examined in relation to environmental conditions or patterns of stimulation specific to some work or sport practice (e.g., vestibular habituation in pilots, dancers or skaters). An extensive review of the literature has been published by Collins (1974). In the present chapter we shall restrict our description of vestibular habituation to vestibuloocular responses produced by rotatory stimulations of two types, repeated step changes in head angular velocity and prolonged or repeated sinusoidal oscillations.

## 2.1. Habituation to velocity steps

The progressive changes of nystagmic response produced in the cat by repeated velocity steps of 160°/s in the dark are shown in Fig. 1. It can be noted that, as the habituation progresses, the duration of primary nystagmus reduces, the number of beats declines, and their amplitude becomes smaller. A similar description of nystagmus change during habituation has been given by Crampton (1964) and Collins (1964a). These progressive changes can be better appreciated by making reference to some parameters of the diagrams of the slow cumulative eye position (SCEP) and of the slow phase eye velocity (SPEV) obtained from the nystagmic response. A schematic representation of these diagrams is given in Fig 2, where the following parameters are defined: $C_M$, peak amplitude of SCEP; $V_M$, peak value of SPEV; $t_o$, time to SCEP peak or to SPEV zero crossing. The parameter $t_o$ so defined roughly corresponds to the duration of the primary phase of post-rotatory nystagmus.

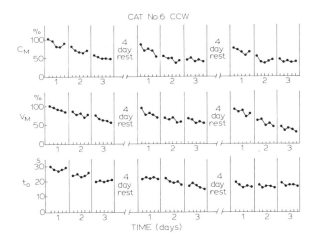

*Fig. 3.* Evolution over time of the parameters $C_M$, $V_M$ and $t_o$ during a long-term bilateral vestibular habituation in the cat. Only values from the CCW responses are represented (from Schmid & Jeannerod, 1979).

The evolution of the parameters $C_M$, $V_M$ and $t_o$ during a process of habituation in the cat is illustrated in Fig. 3. Habituation was provoked by submitting the animal to 10 steps alternatively in the clockwise (CW) and in the counterclockwise (CCW) directions, every day for 3 consecutive days. The animal was then kept at rest for 4 days. This protocol was repeated for 3 consecutive weeks. Acquisition within a session can be appreciated as the difference between the values of each parameter at the beginning and at the end of the session. Acquisition is already present in the first session, and the rate of parameter decline tends to level off in consecutive sessions. Retention from one session to the next (24 h of rest) appears from the difference between the values of each parameter at the beginning of consecutive sessions. Retention increases as habituation proceeds. A retention after 4 days of rest is also present and the acquisition in the successive sessions seems to proceed faster. Combination of acquisition and retention produced a decrease of $C_M$ and $V_M$ to about 30% of their initial values, and a reduction of $t_o$ from about 30 s to about 15 s. A similar pattern of variation of VOR gain and dynamics has been found by Crampton (1964) during habituation to a repeated constant acceleration-constant velocity stimulus. In some cats and with longer sessions of stimulation, habituation

can proceed until a virtually complete extinction of the response.

Acquisition appears to be faster and stronger in animals with a previous experience of habituation protocols (Henricksson et al., 1961; Jeannerod et al., 1976). This fact may be explained by the prolonged retention which is observed following habituation experiments. In one cat submitted to a bilateral habituation protocol (two sessions of ten alternated CW and CCW steps every day for 4 consecutive days), the time course of retention has been studied over up to 46 days. At the end of the last habituation session, the value of $C_M$ was 8.3% of its control value for the step in the CW direction, and 10.7% in the CCW direction. One week later the values of $C_M$ were 37 and 45.2%, respectively. Finally, on the 46th day, these values were 54 and 42%, respectively (G. Clément, unpublished observations).

Habituation to velocity steps has been investigated also in man, but not in the same quantitative way as in cats. The major finding that had been reported was a progressive increase of beat frequency and a decrease of beat amplitude (Collins, 1964a). No systematic investigation of habituation to velocity steps has been done in monkey.

## 2.2. *Habituation to sinusoidal oscillations*

Habituation to sinusoidal oscillations at different frequencies and its transfer to step responses have been shown in monkey (Jäger & Henn, 1981a,b) and in man (Jäger & Henn, 1981b; Baloh et al., 1982).

An example of habituation to sinusoidal oscillations in the monkey is illustrated in Fig. 4A. Habituation was produced by rotating the animal at different frequencies between 0.002 and 0.5 Hz in 17 sessions over a period of 35 days. Each session lasted about 60 min, and each frequency was applied for two or three cycles. For the same frequency of oscillation, there is a progressive decrease of nystagmus frequency and slow phase velocity. The development of habituation has been followed by measuring the gain and the phase shift between head and eye velocity at the different frequencies. The change of the diagrams of VOR frequency response due to habituation is

116

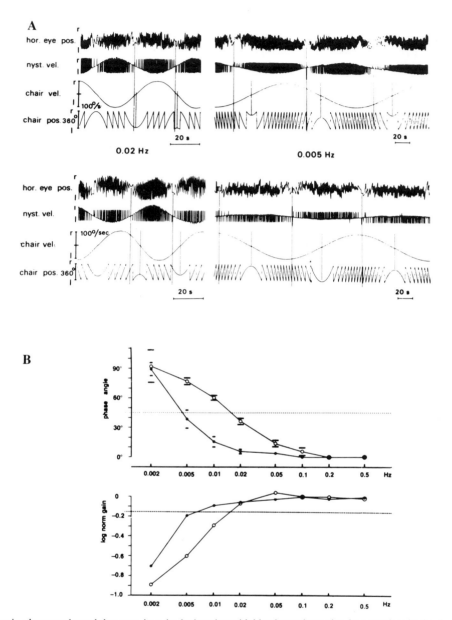

*Fig. 4.* (A) Increase in phase angle and decrease in gain during sinusoidal horizontal rotation in a monkey in the dark. From above, horizontal eye position, horizontal eye velocity, turntable velocity, turntable position. The upper row corresponds to measurements from the naive monkey, the lower row to measurements in the same, habituated, monkey, with the same stimulus frequencies. (B) Frequency response curve from one monkey before and after 17 sessions of sinusoidal rotation. Frequencies of rotation are indicated on the abscissa (from Jäger & Henn, 1981b).

shown in Fig. 4B, which points out that the parametric adjustment occurred in VOR produces greater effects at low frequencies (between 0.005 and 0.05 Hz) than at higher frequencies.

At the beginning and the end of each session, the animal was also submitted to a velocity step in both directions. A transfer of the habituation acquired during sinusoidal rotation was found. Fig. 5 gives a plot of VOR time constant obtained from sinusoidal and from step responses versus

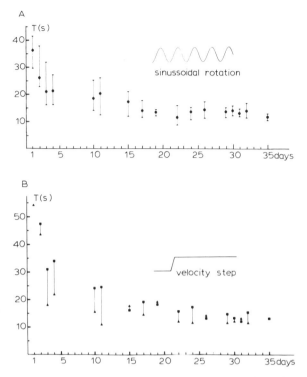

Fig. 5. Shortening of time constants by sinusoidal stimulation with different frequencies in one monkey. Abscissa, number of days; ordinates, value of time constant measured from nystagmus decline of a single velocity step (B) or calculated from frequency response curves (A). Single values and standard deviations (vertical bars) were interpolated from the nearest two frequencies around a phase-lead angle of 45°. In B the time constant was measured as the exponential decay time after velocity steps (100°/s² acceleration, 100°/s, constant velocity rotation). Squares, values before, and triangles values after, sinusoidal stimulation (from Jäger & Henn, 1981a)

the day of stimulation. It is worth noting that the time course of this parameter during habituation nicely corresponds to that of $t_o$ shown in Fig. 3 for the cat.

The occurrence of habituation after exposure to a prolonged oscillation at one frequency was also examined. In accordance with the frequency diagrams in Fig. 4B, no phase change but only a significant gain decrease could be observed at low frequency (0.002 Hz). Nevertheless, the presence of VOR parametric changes due to habituation was also confirmed by measuring the phase shift in the middle range of frequencies (0.005–0.05 Hz) and VOR time constant in step responses before and after the prolonged oscillation at 0.002

Hz. When a middle range frequency (0.01 Hz) was used as the habituating stimulus, the occurrence of habituation was clearly shown by a progressive increase of phase lead and a progressive decrease of gain during the oscillation. Also VOR time constant as measured from step responses before and after the oscillation varied significantly. Finally, when a high frequency (0.15 Hz) habituating stimulus was used, no signs of habituation could be seen to occur during the oscillation nor transfer effects be observed in step responses. This last result is in agreement with previous observations by Gonshor and Melvill Jones (1969) in man (no habituation to rotation at 0.15 Hz with peak velocity of 16°/s applied for 1 h on 3 successive days), by Ito et al. (1974a) in the rabbit (no habituation for a stimulus of 0.1–0.15 Hz with an amplitude of 10° applied for 12 h), and by Kleinschmidt and Collewijn (1975) also in the rabbit (no habituation to rotation at 0.17 Hz with an amplitude of 10° applied for 24 h).

### 2.3. Unilateral vestibular habituation

The possibility of producing a vestibular habituation only to rotations in one direction has been suggested by many authors (Crampton, 1962; Mertens & Collins, 1967) and clearly shown in the cat by Clément et al. (1981). In the experiment by Clément et al. the animal was rotated horizontally with a subthreshold acceleration up to 80°/s always in the same direction. Velocity steps were then produced by sudden stops of the rotation. In each session, eight steps were given, and sessions were repeated twice a day for up to 5 consecutive days.

The development of a unilateral habituation is illustrated in Fig. 6. At the end of the stimulation protocol, the step response in the habituation direction (CW) was reduced to only a few beats occurring during the primary phase of the post-rotatory nystagmus, which lasted less than 10 s. Secondary nystagmus was almost absent. On the contrary, the step response in the other direction was comparable with that recorded at the beginning of the protocol. The time course of the parameters $C_M$ and $t_o$ computed from responses in the habituated direction was very similar to that observed in cats submitted to protocols of bilateral habituation (Fig. 3).

118

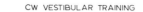

CW VESTIBULAR TRAINING

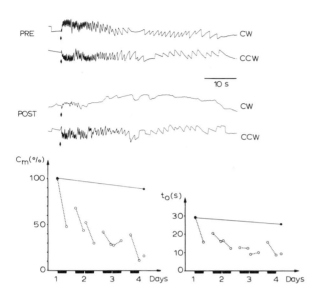

CCW VESTIBULAR TRAINING

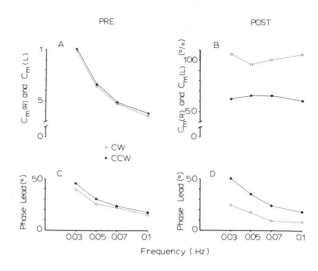

*Fig. 6.* Clockwise (CW) and counterclockwise (CCW) responses to velocity steps before and after unilateral vestibular habituation in the CW direction in the cat. Pre, control values in the naive animal; Post, same animal at the habituated stage. In the lower part of the figure the time course of parameters $C_m$ and $t_o$ in the same animal is represented. $C_m$ is expressed in percent of its initial value, $t_o$ in seconds. For the habituated side, values of $C_m$ and $t_o$ are given for the first and last responses of each session, and for the step response in the post-exposure testing (last value on the abscissae). For the non-habituated side, values of $C_m$ and $t_o$ are given for the step responses in the pre- and post-exposure tests (from Clément et al., 1981).

*Fig. 7.* (A) Amplitude/frequency relationships in the response to sinusoidal oscillations before CCW vestibular habituation. $C_m(R)$ and $C_m(L)$ are given in arbitrary units by assuming the peak-to-peak value during CCW rotation at 0.03 Hz equal to unity. The small differences between $Cm(R)$ and $C_m(L)$ indicate a high degree of symmetry of the responses. (B) Amplitude/frequency relationships in the responses to sinusoidal oscillations after CCW vestibular habituation. The values of $C_m(R)$ and $C_m(L)$ are given in percent of the corresponding pre-habituation values at the same frequency. The amplitude of CCW response is reduced to 60% independently from the frequency. (C and D) Phase frequency relationships in pre- and post-exposure tests, showing an increase of phase lead during rotations toward the 'trained' labyrinth (from Clément et al., 1981).

The unilaterality of the habituation acquired by velocity steps can be transferred to responses evoked by sinusoidal oscillations at different frequencies as shown in Fig. 7. The parameters $C_m(R)$ and $C_m(L)$ plotted in Fig. 7 were defined as the cumulative eye displacement during oscillation to the right and to the left, respectively. The diagrams on the left give the values of these parameters (in arbitrary units) and those of the phase lead prior to the stimulating sessions. The diagrams on the right shows the percent variations of $C_m(R)$ and $C_m(L)$ and the change in phase lead due to habituation. Variations were found only during oscillation in the habituating direction.

The possibility of obtaining unilateral habituation by unidirectional vestibular stimulations excludes a role of unspecific factors, such as changes

in the state of vigilance, in producing the observed modifications of VOR. At the same time it proves that the right and left VOR pathways can be controlled separately in order to obtain a greater system adaptability.

## 2.4. Effects of vestibular habituation on optokinetic responses

It is well established that optokinetic responses are supported by at least two parallel pathways, one reaching VOR at the level of the vestibular nuclei (VN) and the other passing through the flocculus and reaching the brain stem beyond VN (Henn et al., 1974; Cohen et al., 1977; Buizza & Schmid, 1982). It has also been suggested that the first of these two pathways and those responsible for VOR share a common velocity storage mechanism on which both the time constant of vestibulo-ocular responses and that of optokinetic after-nystagmus (OKAN) would depend (Raphan et al., 1977; Robinson, 1977). Thus, it is reasonable to expect that at least some components of optokinetic responses should be modified after a process of vestibular habituation.

The transfer to optokinetic responses of VOR habituation provoked by repeated velocity steps in head angular velocity has been examined by Clément et al. (1981) in the cat and by Skavenski et al. (1981) in the monkey. Steady-state optokinetic nystagmus (OKN) to constant velocity stimulation (from 15/s to 450/s) was tested in the cat before and after a protocol of unilateral vestibular habituation. Clément et al. (1981) could not find appreciable variations neither in OKN morphology nor in its slow phase velocity. The small sensitivity of the closed-loop gain of optokinetic responses to variations of its open loop gain that could have been produced by vestibular habituation has been suggested as an explanation for this lack of an appreciable transfer on OKN.

Optokinetic afternystagmus, which is due to the discharge of the storage mechanism in open loop condition, was tested by Skavenski et al. (1981) in three monkeys before and after repeated (20–40) post-rotatory stimulations (80°/s) in alternated directions. The time constant of post-rotatory nystagmus decreased from an initial value exceeding 30 s to about 10 s or less by the end of the habituating sessions (three sessions separated by 2 or more days). Most (78%) of these decreases were statistically reliable ($P \leqslant 0.01$). Also, the time constant of OKAN decreased by about one-half or more, but 64% of these decreases were not statistically reliable ($P \geqslant 0.05$). In four tests, the OKAN time constant increased after vestibular habituation. As shown in Fig. 8, in two monkeys out of three there is almost no correlation between the variations of OKAN and VOR time constants during habituation. Each data point in the figure refers to the same direction of nystagmus slow phase and to the same stage of vestibular habituation. The data reported by the same authors about VOR and OKAN gains are even less conclusive, probably

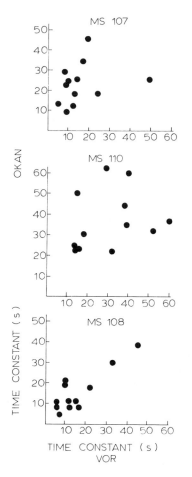

Fig. 8. Relationship between OKAN and VOR time constants measured in three monkeys at different stages of the process of vestibular habituation (from Skavenski et al., 1981).

due to the poor reliability of the method used to measure these gains.

It was nevertheless suggested by the authors that the vestibulo-ocular and optokinetic reflexes do not share a common velocity storage mechanisms. Another possibility is that VOR changes during habituation are not due to parametric variations in a common velocity storage mechanism. A more complete analysis is needed to clarify this point.

## 3. Discussion

Vestibular habituation has sometimes been rejected as an experimental paradigm to investigate VOR plasticity since the progressive modification of the nystagmic response observed during habituation were most likely attributed to unspecific factors rather than to a specific adaptive process. There is now enough evidence to exclude this hypothesis. First of all, during the acquisition of vestibular habituation the gain and the time constant of VOR vary in a regular and strictly correlated way. Their pattern of variation is largely independent from the stimulus used to provoke habituation (e.g., prolonged sinusoidal oscillations at low frequencies or repeated step changes in head angular velocity). This latter result would indicate that a unique strategy is adopted to reach the goal of suppressing a response that became meaningless or detrimental. The second evidence is the possibility of producing unilateral vestibular habituation. Such a specificity can hardly be attributed to unspecific factors. Finally, the presence of retention and the possibility of transfer would indicate that an adaptive process is developing through long-term parametric changes in some neural mechanism, which is also involved in the generation of responses evoked by stimuli different from that used to provoke habituation. Drowsiness and sleep may also temporarily affect VOR parameters. In that case, however, VOR changes appear to be state dependent and to be immediately reversible at the transition between sleep and waking (Flandrin et al., 1979).

VOR habituation should then be considered as an adaptive process, but the neural mechanisms underlying this process are not yet known. The strict correlation between the variations of VOR gain and time constant during habituation suggests that the parameters which are progressively modified to adapt the system influence both the gain and the dynamic characteristics of VOR. Thus, a progressive increase of the gain of the feedforward inhibitory pathway from primary vestibular afferents to VN through the flocculus, which has been suggested as the neural structure supporting a parametric adaptive control of VOR by the cerebellum (Ito, 1972), can be accepted as the basic mechanism for vestibular habituation only if an appropriate dynamics is assumed for that pathway. Otherwise only the gain and not the time constant of VOR would vary during habituation.

What dynamics is needed to explain the experimental results reported in the previous section? An attempt to solve this problem has been made by Jeannerod et al. (1976) as illustrated in Fig. 9. The diagrams of nystagmus slow phase velocity were computed from the first and the subsequent responses to repeated step changes in head angular velocity in the cat. The difference between the diagram obtained from the first response and that computed from the response recorded at a given stage of vestibular habituation was assumed to represent the inhibitory signal sent to VN by the cerebellum at that stage. Then, by comparison with the expected response at the level of primary vestibular neurons, and under the assumption that habituation does not involve that level, it was possible to define (a) what the dynamics of the vestibulo-cerebello-vestibular pathway should be, and (b) how the gain of this pathway should change during habituation. The result was that two parallel dynamic mechanisms should be present, one more sensitive to the low frequency components of the primary vestibular signal (leaky integrator) and the other to the high frequency components (differentiator). Although the frog may not be a good model for testing the mechanisms supporting vestibular habituation, it is nevertheless worth noting that tonic and phasic responses to horizontal constant angular accelerations were actually found by Llinás et al. (1971) in the Purkinje cells of the frog vestibulo-cerebellum. By assuming that the gains of these mechanisms increase linearly with the number of stimulus repetitions, the pattern of variation of VOR parameters within a session of vestibular habituation (acquisition) could be closely predicted (Jeannerod et al., 1976). The pattern of variation of the same parameters throughout subsequent sessions (combination of acquisition and retention) could also be predicted by making the further hypothesis that the values of the adaptable gains at the beginning of one session are proportional to the values reached at the end of the previous session. The factor of proportionality decreases as the time of rest between the two sessions increases. The predicted pattern of variation of the parameter $t_o$ defined in Fig. 1 during five consecutive sessions of repeated post-rotatory stimuli is shown in Fig. 10, and compared to experimental data (from

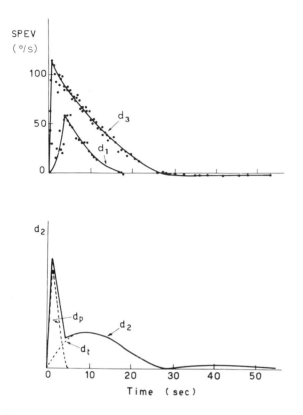

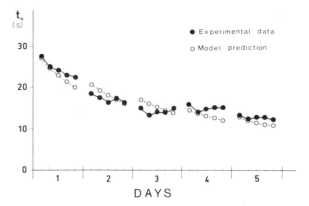

*Fig. 10.* Model prediction and experimental data for the pattern of variation of the parameter $t_o$ defined in Fig. 1 during a process of vestibular habituation to repeated step changes in head angular velocity (from Schmid et al., 1980).

*Fig. 9.* The inhibitory signal ($d_2$) that should be sent to the VN in order to modify the nystagmic response in the way observed at a given stage of vestibular habituation is computed as the difference between the diagrams of nystagmus SPEV in the first response ($d_1$) and in the response ($d_3$) recorded at that stage. This signal can be decomposed into two components, one ($d_p$) generated by a phasic element and the other ($d_t$) by a tonic element (from Jeannerod et al. 1976).

Schmid et al., 1980). It is worth noting that $t_o$ tends asymptotically to a value which corresponds to the expected duration of the primary phase of post-rotatory nystagmus for a VOR time constant equal to the time constant of the semicircular canals.

By using linear system analysis to reformulate the Marr-Albus model of the cerebellum (Marr, 1969; Albus, 1971), Fujita (1982a,b) has recently proposed a model for an adaptive control of VOR by the cerebellum in which a phase lead-lag compensator with learning capability was included in the vestibulo-cerebello-vestibular pathway as previously assumed by Jeannerod et al. (1976).

These theoretical speculations do not exclude

other possibilities of controlling VOR during habituation. Alternatively, it can be assumed that the observed modifications of VOR gain and time constant during habituation are produced by a progressive increase of the leaky factor of the central neural integrator in the vestibulo-ocular pathways. An increase of the leaky factor would actually produce a decrease of gain and a phase lead.

A more general question is whether the same neural mechanism is used for the three types of VOR adaptive processes described in the introduction section. If this is the case, we must assume that the way of using this mechanism changes according to the goal that should be reached through adaptation. For example, VOR adaptation to the wearing of magnifying or reducing lenses (see Chapter 2) requires a gain recalibration with no modification of VOR dynamics. This adaptation occurs with a parallel change of the gain of both VOR and OKAN (Lisberger et al., 1981). Thus, if the neural mechanism for adaptation to lenses is the same as for vestibular habituation, where both gain and dynamics are affected, this mechanism should be used in a quite different way. Lisberger et al. (1981) proposed a model of VOR gain control for adaptation to lenses in which the flocculus is still involved, but the modifiable gain element is placed in the brain stem upstream of the VN.

It is likely that a general and comprehensive

interpretation of the many types of VOR adaptation processes can be reached by looking at the flocculus, not as the relay of a single adaptable or adapting pathway, but as a more complex structure which uses all its sensory and efference copy inputs to decide whether adaptation is needed and what type of adaptation, and implements the correct stategy by using its many outputs appropriately (Ito, 1982a; Courjon et al., 1982).

## Acknowledgements

This work was supported by INSERM (France) and CNR (Italy).

Adaptive mechanisms in gaze control
Facts and theories
*Eds. Berthoz & Melvill Jones*
© 1985 Elsevier Science Publishers BV (Biomedical Division)

# Chapter 8

# Velocity storage and the ocular response to multidimensional vestibular stimuli

## T. Raphan[a] & B. Cohen[b]

[a]*Department of Computer and Information Science, Brooklyn College of CUNY, and* [b]*Department of Neurology, Mount Sinai Medical Center, New York, U.S.A.*

## 1. Introduction

The vestibulo-ocular reflex (VOR) generates compensatory eye movements that stabilize gaze in space. The process is initiated in the peripheral labyrinth where information about head movements and the orientation of the head with regard to gravity is transduced into neural signals in the vestibular nerve. The semicircular canals act as angular accelerometers that respond to angular movements of the head (Steinhausen, 1933; Lowenstein & Sand, 1940; Groen et al., 1952). Over certain frequencies of head movement (0.1–5 Hz) the mechanical characteristics of the canals convert head acceleration into a signal that primarily represents head velocity (Goldberg & Fernandez, 1971). This conversion is due mainly to the interaction of inertia and viscosity of the endolymph and the elasticity of the cupula. The otolith organs act as linear accelerometers. Their mechanical characteristics are such that they respond with rapid dynamics. Consequently, the neural signal they generate gives an accurate representation of head position with regard to gravity over a wide range of frequencies of head movement (Loe et al., 1973; Fernandez & Goldberg, 1976a–c). This information and that from the canals is then conveyed to the central vestibular system, where it undergoes further processing to generate the signal that drives the oculomotor system.

An important part of the processing that takes place in the central vestibular system involves a mechanism for storing activity coming from the visual and vestibular system related to the relative velocity of the head in space. This 'velocity storage mechanism' (Cohen et al., 1977; Raphan et al., 1979) is important for maintaining the firing frequencies of neurons in the vestibular nuclei so that they will be proportional to head velocity during low frequency head movements. It also helps maintain ocular compensatory movements during continued relative rotation of the head and surround. One of the clearest demonstrations of storage of activity in the VOR comes from experiments that show cancellation of post-rotatory nystagmus after rotation in light (Ter Braak, 1936; Mowrer, 1937; Jung, 1948; Raphan et al., 1979). Activity stored during rotation due to the optokinetic stimulation acts to counter and reduce post-rotatory nystagmus at the end of rotation (Fig. 1C). The characteristics of the storage mechanism have been extensively studied for head and environmental movements in the horizontal and vertical planes (Cohen et al., 1977; Raphan et al., 1979; Waespe et al., 1983). Recent evidence suggests that the velocity storage mechanism can also superpose convergent signals about the horizontal component of head rotation from a variety of vestibular receptors, including the otolith organs and the vertical semicircular canals (Raphan et al., 1981, 1983a; Cohen et al.,

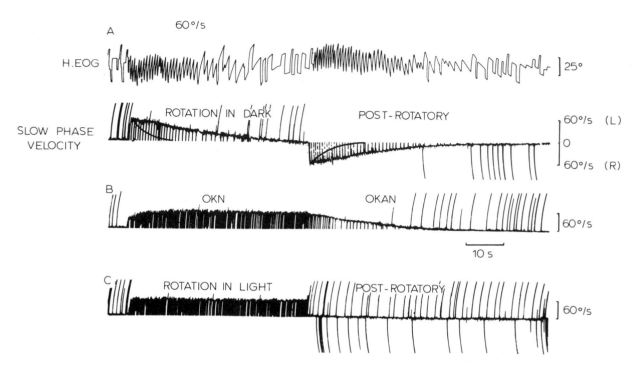

*Fig. 1.* Nystagmus induced in a monkey by a step of platform rotation in dark (A), by a step of surround rotation (B), and by a step of platform rotation in light (C). The top trace in A is the horizontal EOG. The other traces are slow phase velocity. The stimulus velocity was 60°/s in each instance. Note that when rotatory nystagmus and OKN were in the same direction, their after-responses were oppositely directed (A and B). Also note there was only a slight post-rotatory response to the right after rotation in light (C). The solid line in the lower trace in A is the VIII nerve time constant. It shows the time course of eye velocity that would be expected in response to a step of velocity if only activity from the semicircular canals were driving the oculomotor system (from Raphan et al., 1979).

1982, 1983). The purpose of this paper is to review how velocity storage contributes to oculomotor control and to the generation of compensatory eye movements utilizing these various sensory inputs.

Previous work has shown that an intact labyrinth is necessary for the proper functioning of the storage mechanism (Uemura & Cohen, 1973; Cohen et al., 1973; Collewijn, 1976; Zee et al., 1976b). The most likely explanation is that spontaneous activity arising in the periphery plays an important role in maintaining the ability of the CNS to store activity related to slow phase velocity. This paper will also review techniques that cause a modification in labyrinthine input, such as canal plugging and ampullary nerve section and show how these lesions differentially affect the operation of the VOR and visual-vestibular in-

teractions by their effects on velocity storage.

## 2. Storage and its neural representation: basic assumptions and models of visual-vestibular interactions

Insights about the characteristics of velocity storage and how it affects visual-vestibulo-oculomotor control have come from modelling the VOR, optokinetic nystagmus (OKN) and visual-vestibular interactions using control systems theory (Cohen et al., 1977; Raphan et al., 1977, 1979; Robinson, 1977a, 1980; Buizza & Schmid, 1982; Waespe et al., 1983). The models are behaviorally homeomorphic, although they emphasize different aspects of visual-vestibular interaction. There is general agreement that both OKN and vestibular nystagmus are produced by

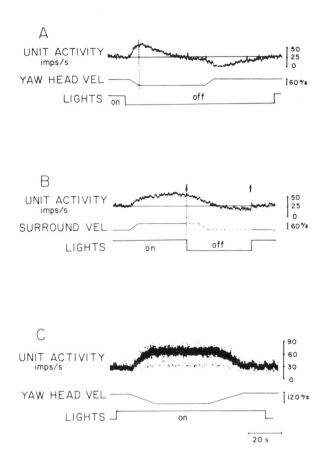

A

UNIT ACTIVITY
imps/s

YAW HEAD VEL

LIGHTS on      off

B

UNIT ACTIVITY
imps/s

SURROUND VEL

LIGHTS      on      off

C

UNIT ACTIVITY
imps/s

YAW HEAD VEL

LIGHTS      on

20 s

*Fig. 2.* Extracellular activity of a neuron in the vestibular nucleus in response to a step in angular velocity of the monkey in darkness (A), to movement of the visual surround (B), and to rotation in light (C). Note the similarity of the frequency curves to the slow phase velocity envelopes shown in Fig. 1. (from Waespe & Henn, 1977a,b).

combined activation of two kinds of processes. During OKN, information is transmitted directly from visual receptors to central neural networks that generate a velocity command signal to the oculomotor system. This type of process follows the input directly. It imposes no additional dynamics, and the output signal is approximately in phase with the input; it has 'memoryless' characteristics (Zadeh & Desoer, 1964). A second type of process is activated by the input and continues to discharge after the input has ceased. Therefore, it introduces its own dynamics in the output and has characteristics that can be viewed as ex-

hibiting a form of 'memory' (Zadeh & Desoer, 1964) or 'storage'. There is considerable evidence that 'memoryless' or 'direct' processes associated with OKN are mediated by different structures and pathways, than are processes associated with OKN and optokinetic afternystagmus (OKAN) that involve 'memory' or 'storage' (Zee et al., 1981; Waespe et al., 1983).

During vestibular nystagmus there is a 'direct' input related to angular head velocity and acceleration coming from the semicircular canals over the vestibular nerve. There is also activation of indirect pathways that add their own dynamics to the response (Raphan et al., 1977; Robinson, 1977a). The summation of both of these processes is seen in the firing frequencies of neurons in the vestibular nuclei (Fig. 2A). These frequencies mirror changes in slow phase eye velocity during vestibular nystagmus (Fig. 1A). Separate vestibular nuclei neurons have not been found that are related only to the direct or to the indirect pathways. Neurons with characteristics of the direct vestibular pathways would have activity that declined with a dominant time constant of the eighth nerve during steps of velocity (Fig. 1A, solid line). Neurons that had characteristics of the indirect pathways would not have a rapid rise in activity at the onset of angular rotation, in contrast to the neuron shown in Fig. 2A. This indicates either that integration responsible for prolonging the time constant of vestibular nuclei neurons is performed elsewhere and the activity is fed back to vestibular nuclei neurons represented in Fig. 2, or that the process of integration responsible for velocity storage is not represented separately in a discrete group of neurons, but is a distributed property of brain stem and cerebellar neurons.

When the visual system activates the storage process, the activation is also reflected in firing patterns of vestibular nuclei neurons (Fig. 2B) (Waespe et al., 1977). Only activity from the indirect pathways is reflected in the firing frequencies of vestibular nuclei neurons during OKN; that is, the contribution of the direct pathways, that causes the rapid rise in slow phase velocity at the onset of OKN (Fig. 1B), does not appear in the firing rates of vestibular nuclei neurons. Unit activity during OKAN (Fig. 2B)

126

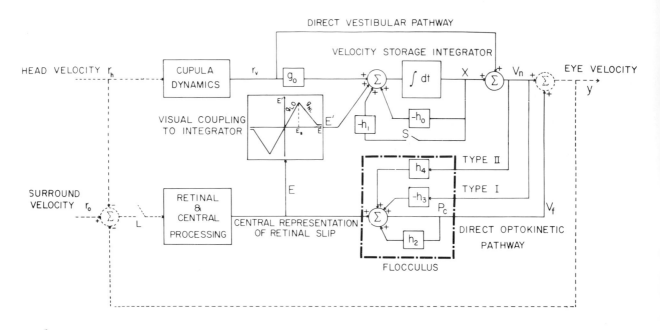

*Fig. 3.* Model of OKN, OKAN, per- and post-rotatory nystagmus and visual-vestibular interactions. Solid lines represent neural signals, dotted lines represent mechanical variables. See text for details (from Waespe et al., 1983).

also reflects activation of indirect pathways. The ability of these units to superpose activity associated with visual and vestibular stimulation during rotation in light (Figs. 1C, 2C) supports the idea that storage for both OKN and vestibular nystagmus is generated by a common mechanism located in the VOR (Raphan et al., 1977, 1979; Robinson, 1977a; Demer and Robinson, 1983).

The mathematical model presented by Waespe et al. (1983) is one of the models that incorporates these concepts (Fig. 3). The model includes the processing up to and including the second order Type I and Type II vestibular nuclei neurons, and shows how they might activate floccular Purkinje cells in the realization of the direct optokinetic pathway. It neglects the positional components introduced by the final neural integrator in the oculomotor system (Skavenski & Robinson, 1973). The model has two inputs: $r_h$ corresponding to head velocity and $r_o$ representing environmental velocity. The former activates the semicircular canals and the latter the visual system. The model representation of the vestibular system responds to the mechanical variable, head velocity $r_h$ and generates an eighth nerve signal represented by $r_v$ that is dependent on the cupula dyna-

mics. Since the signal $r_v$ coming in over the vestibular nerve contributes its activity directly, it has been designated as a 'direct' vestibular pathway. $r_v$ also couples to the storage mechanism which then contributes to the velocity command that reaches the oculomotor system. The storage process has been approximated by a single integrator called the 'velocity storage integrator', and the input-output pathway that contains it has been designated as an 'indirect pathway'. The time course of the storage process is determined by a single parameter which is its time constant ($1/h_o$). The state of the integrator x and the direct pathway summate to form the velocity signal $V_n$ that reflects the activity of 'horizontal' second order neurons in the vestibular nuclei. Because the integrator stores information depending on its time constant, it will continue to have activity even when the eighth nerve activity has diminished to the resting level. This accounts for the longer time constant associated with vestibular nuclei activity and nystagmus as compared to eighth nerve activity (Figs. 1A, 2A).

The model representation of the visual system has retinal slip as its input, formed by subtracting head velocity plus eye velocity from surround

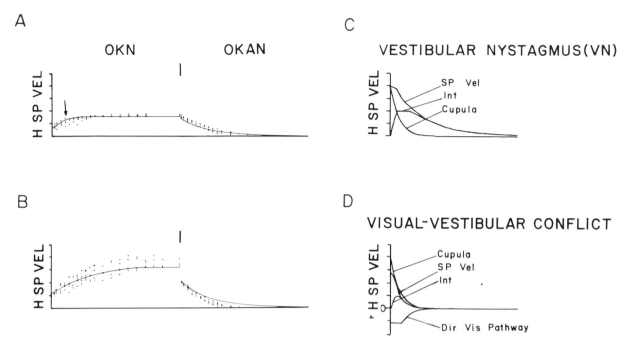

Fig. 4. Comparison of simulation of slow phase velocity of OKN and OKAN (solid lines) at two velocities (60°/s in A and 160°/s in B) with data from a monkey (dots). There was good agreement between the simulated and experimental data. Model simulations of cupula deflection (Cupula), integrator activity (Int) and slow phase velocity (SP Vel) during rotation in darkness (C) and during visual-vestibular conflict (D). Cupula deflection is assumed to reflect activity in the ampullary nerve. Activity in the direct visual pathway (Dir Vis Pathway) is also shown in D. The conflict situation in D is equivalent to that produced by rotating the monkey in light with the OKN drum moving at the same velocity as the rotating platform to produce a subject-stationary surround (from Waespe et al., 1983).

velocity. This signal is transformed into a central representation of retinal slip by visual system processing. The signal E, which is the central representation of retinal slip couples to the velocity storage integrator through a non-linear element ("visual coupling to integrator" of Fig. 3) to generate the velocity command (Waespe et al., 1983). This non-linear element is located in the indirect opto-kinetic pathway. As the integrator becomes charged by a step in velocity, it produces the slow rise in OKN. When the lights are turned off (opening switch L), the integrator is discharged with its time constant ($1/h_o$). Thus, OKAN represents the characteristics of the integrator in the absence of inputs that might contribute their own dynamics (zero input response). It is, in fact, the simplest manifestation of velocity storage.* The suppression switch, S, 'dumps' the integrator rapidly during conflicting visual-vestibular stimuli. It also appears to be responsible for the rapid decline in slow phase velocity when the head is tilted during post-rotatory nystagmus or OKAN (Raphan et al., 1981; Waespe et al., 1985). The structure of the nonlinearity and the 'dump' mechanism can be made to account for many of the nonlinear characteristics of OKN, OKAN and visual-vestibular interactions under normal circumstances and after flocculectomy (Waespe et al., 1983). The central structures involved in the nonlinear coupling are not entirely clear, but it appears to be closely related to the pretectum and visual cortex (Collewijn, 1975; Hoffman, 1981; Hoffman and Schoppmann, 1981; Zee et al., 1982). Recently the dump mechanism, indicated by switch S in Fig. 3, has been shown to be dependent on the nodulus, since it is no longer possible to discharge the integrator rapidly by visual-vestibular conflict or by tilt after nodulec-

*It should be noted that this discussion is confined only to a consideration of primary OKAN, i.e., OKAN in the same direction as the preceding OKN. Secondary OKAN appears to be produced by a separate mechanism (Brandt et al., 1974; Büttner et al., 1976; Zee et al., 1976b).

tomy (Waespe et al., 1985).

The part of the model corresponding to the 'direct' optokinetic pathway is probably mediated by the flocculus, which is represented by the portion of the model enclosed by the heavy dashed lines (Zee et al., 1981; Waespe et al., 1983). The output of the flocculus then combines with activity of Type I and Type II vestibular nuclei neurons, as shown in Fig. 3, to form the velocity command signal, y.

The response predicted by the model to a step in head velocity of 120°/s is shown in Fig. 4C. The model predicts a rapid rise in slow phase eye velocity (SP Vel) due to activation of the semicircular canals and the direct vestibular pathway. There is a plateau in velocity due to a summation of the output of the integrator and the input from the canals (Raphan et al., 1979). This is followed by a brief decline with the cupula time constant due to saturation of the integrator (Int), followed by a slower decline in slow phase velocity as activity is lost from the storage mechanism. For a step in surround velocity during optokinetic stimulation (Fig. 4A,B), the simulation (solid line) shows an initial rapid rise in eye velocity followed by a slow rise to a steady-state level. Due to the structure of the nonlinearity in the indirect pathways, the slow rise has a longer time constant for higher velocities (Fig. 4B), than for lower velocities (Fig. 4A) (See Waespe et al., (1983) for further details). At the end of stimulation, eye velocity drops rapidly and then more slowly with the time constant of the integrator. Experimental data from a monkey is shown by the dots. The model simulations fit the data over a wide range of velocities.

The response of the model to conflicting visual and vestibular inputs is shown in Fig. 4D. The physical representation of the stimulus is a step of head velocity given in a subject-stationary visual surround. Such a stimulus would be produced, for example, by physically coupling the rotating platform and the optokinetic drum and rotating them together. Under such circumstances the vestibular system indicates angular head velocity, but the visual environment remains stationary with regard to the subject, hence the conflict. The step of head velocity that causes the cupula to deflect would drive the eyes with a gain of close to 1 over

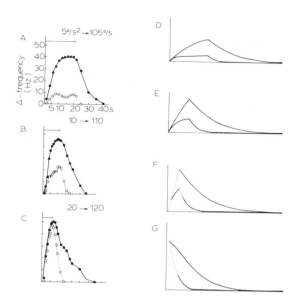

*Fig. 5.* Vestibular nucleus unit activity (A–C) during rotation in dark (dots) and in a subject-stationary visual surround (circles). The monkey was accelerated at 5°/s$^2$ to 105°/s in A, at 10°/s$^2$ to 110°/s in B, and at 20°/s$^2$ to 120°/s in C over the period shown by the solid bar on top of each graph. The time after onset of stimulation is on the abscissa and the change in frequency of firing from the resting level on the ordinate. Note the considerable difference in peak levels of frequency reached during rotation in the two conditions at low accelerations (5°/s$^2$, A). At higher accelerations (20°/s$^2$, C) the peak levels in the conflict situation (circles) approached the level reached in darkness (dots). (From Waespe & Henn, 1978a). D–G, simulations of unit data by the model shown in Fig. 3. The variable $V_n$ is represented. The abscissa and ordinate are the same as in A–C. In each case the lower trace is the value for $V_n$ predicted in the conflict situation, i.e., during rotation in a subject stationary lighted surround. Note the large difference in unit activity during rotation at low accelerations (D, E) and the close approximation of the curves at higher accelerations (G) (from Raphan and Cohen, 1981).

the direct vestibular pathway (cupula). However, in a subject-stationary visual surround, such ocular compensatory movements are opposed by the direct visual pathway (Dir Vis Pathway) which reduces slow phase eye velocity. The integrator is driven by cupula deflection, but this is opposed by the visual coupling to the integrator and by the activation of the suppression switch (S in Fig. 3). This causes the integrator to discharge and decay more rapidly than it would have in darkness (Compare Int in Fig. 4C and D). The model predictions closely approximate eye velocity and unit activity data taken from monkeys given similar conflict stimulation (Waespe & Henn, 1977a; Raphan & Cohen, 1981; Waespe et al., 1983).

Firing rates of Type I and Type II vestibular neurons during rotation in dark were compared to firing rates during rotation in light where there was no relative movement between the monkey and the visual surround (Waespe and Henn, 1978a). The relative subject stationary visual surround was achieved, as described above, by rotating the animal and surrounding OKN drum at the same velocity. Frequencies of firing of vestibular neurons during rotation at low accelerations in darkness were higher (Fig. 5A, dots) than during rotation in a subject stationary visual surround (open circles). As the acceleration increased, however, peak frequencies of unit activity in the relative stationary surround approached those found during rotation in dark (Fig. 5B,C).

If one considers the variable $Vn$, to be the variable related to unit activity, it is possible to simulate the data of Waespe and Henn (1978a) shown in Fig. 5A–C. ($Vn$ represents the summation of direct vestibular input and the signal from the velocity storage integrator.) This simulation is represented in Fig. 5D–G. In each case, the lower trace represents unit activity that would be expected during rotation in light in a subject stationary surround, while the upper trace is the response during rotation in dark. The similarity of the experimental and model predictions suggest the following interpretation: the major visual input to Type I and II vestibular nuclei neurons is through the velocity storage integrator. Because of the lag due to the properties of the integrator, Type I and Type II neurons in the vestibular nuclei are able to respond only to slow changes in the visual input. Since the peripheral vestibular system has a direct pathway into the vestibular nuclei, vestibular excitation can elicit much faster responses in these neurons. In the conflict situation, such as is shown in Fig. 5, the visual system keeps up with the vestibular drive for slow accelerations of $5°/s^2$ and reduces the peak neural activity. As the acceleration increases, however, the vestibular drive on the neurons is too rapid to be affected by the visual system, and the neural activity approaches levels that are found in darkness. Even during high accelerations in a subject stationary visual surround, however, the animal fixates and its eyes move very little (Waespe et al., 1977). This can be explained as being due to the activity of direct visual pathways that cancel activity of vestibular nuclei neurons, thereby reducing eye velocity. Consequently, in this condition eye velocity does not agree with vestibular nuclei activity (Waespe & Henn, 1978a). Similar hypotheses have been proposed to explain the behavior of floccular Purkinje cells during fixation of a point source during head oscillations (Lisberger & Fuchs, 1978a,b; Miles and Fuller, 1975; Miles et al., 1980a,b; Miles and Eighmy, 1980).

Although these simulations conform closely to the general outlines of the ocular responses to visual and vestibular stimuli over a wide range of stimulus conditions, they do not fit the data perfectly. This raises the question of whether a single integrator can accurately represent storage. As the nervous system is complex, a single integrator is undoubtedly not the best representation, and a higher order system giving a sum of exponentials would probably fit the data better. Collewijn et al. (1980a) used a minimum mean square error criteria to show that a linear fit to the data from the rabbit during OKAN was better than a single exponential. There is no particular rationale for fitting OKAN or vestibular nystagmus with a linear function since higher order polynomials would undoubtedly give better fits. On the other hand, approximation of OKAN by a single exponential has an important advantage in that it leads to a model with a simple representation of storage. Derivation of a model based on linear or polynomial fits to the data would be difficult, and as the model resulting from such a fit would be complex, it would not be easy to interpret it in neurophysiological terms. In contrast, approximate closed form solutions can be obtained for parameters of a model in which storage is represented by a single integrator. This facilitates comparisons between normal responses and responses after lesions of the peripheral and central nervous system (Waespe et al., 1983).

In summary, available evidence suggests that there is a velocity storage mechanism in the VOR which is responsible for OKAN and the long time constant of vestibular nystagmus. Models of OKN and the VOR indicate that two processes combine to generate both vestibular and optokinetic nystagmus: one is capable of driving the eyes rapidly; another causes slower changes in eye velocity. In order to adequately evaluate effects of lesions on OKN, the separate contribution of both processes must be considered. Models which represent velocity storage by a single integrator are capable of simulating the dominant characteristics of the VOR and of predicting the major characteristics of visual-vestibular interactions. They provide a theoretical structure for understanding the organization of the VOR. The neural basis for separate portions of the model have been identified. Second order Type I and Type II vestibular neurons contain information related to the velocity storage mechanism in their firing rates as well as the rapid response from the vestibular apparatus. The rapid response from the visual system is mediated through the flocculus. However, where activity from the flocculus interacts with that from Type I and Type II vestibular nuclei neurons is still unknown. Since the major projection from the flocculus is to the vestibular nuclei (Langer et al., 1985), the interaction of the floccular output may be with other classes of neurons in the vestibular nuclei.

## 3. Techniques of selective labyrinthine lesions

Lesion studies have been important in showing the contribution of various sensory inputs to the velocity storage integrator and establishing the origin of activity responsible for the ocular response to various types of complex head movements. Flourens (1842) was one of the first to use labyrinthine lesions to study the function of the vestibular system. When parallel canal pairs were damaged in the pigeon, oscillatory head movements were induced in the plane of the lesioned canals. Goltz (1870), Breuer (1891), Hoegyes (1880), Ewald (1892), Magnus (1924), deKleyn (1914), and Benjamins and Huizinga (1928) among others, used labyrinthine lesions to study the function of the semicircular canals and the otolith organs. An excellent review of the early work is provided by Camis (1930).

Techniques that have been used to study vestibular system function include destruction of the labyrinths on one or both sides, obstruction of endolymph flow in individual semi-circular canals by filling or plugging, section of single or mutliple

nerves from the endorgans, and removal of the otoconia from the otolith organs. Labyrinthectomy has generally been done by surgically destroying and removing the membranous labyrinth and/or sectioning the vestibular nerve before or after Scarpa's ganglia. The goal is to abolish all input to the central vestibular system including the tonic discharge of each of the sensory nerves. This deafferentiation causes a decrease in activity of neurons in the central vestibular system which then gradually recovers (Precht et al., 1966; Ch. 17). The recovery is probably mainly due to central adaptation and not to reestablishing tonic activity in the vestibular nerve (see Schaefer & Meyer (1974), and Precht (1974 and Ch. 17) for reviews). Recently, Jensen (1983) has shown that some spontaneous activity returns in the cut stump of the vestibular nerve if the lesion is made distal to Scarpa's ganglion. There may be functional significance for this low level of spontaneous activity, as there have been reports that postural imbalance recovers more quickly after lesions distal to Scarpa's ganglion (Dohlmann, 1929). Moreover, compensation for postural imbalance after labyrinthectomy made distal to Scarpa's ganglion is made worse after the nerve is relesioned (Jensen, 1983).

Behavioral modifications after unilateral labyrinthectomy are characteristic (Ewald, 1892; Magnus, 1924; Northington & Barrera, 1934; Dow, 1938; Money & Scott, 1962; Uemura & Cohen, 1973; Maioli et al., 1983, see also Ch. 18): there is horizontal rotatory nystagmus with ipsilateral slow phases and contralateral quick phases. The head is tilted to the ipsilateral side, and there is a tendency to circle in that direction. The nystagmus in light quickly disappears, but nystagmus in darkness can persist in darkness for months or years (Stahle, 1958). The gain of the VOR is initially depressed for head movement to the ipsilateral side but soon recovers (Maioli et al., 1983). Permanent postural effects are relatively minor.

After bilateral destruction of the labyrinths there is a more profound behavioral effect. Ocular reflexes dependent on the vestibular labyrinth, including the response to rotation and off-vertical axis rotation are lost, and ocular counter-rolling is abolished (Woellner & Graybiel, 1960) or is seriously impaired (Krejcova et al., 1971). Birds can no longer fly, although they recover the ability to stand or walk (Ewald, 1892). Both animals and humans may have dystaxia. In addition to abolishing the response of each of the labyrinthine receptors, bilateral destruction of the labyrinths also has an important effect on optokinetic nystagmus. After unilateral labyrinthectomy, OKAN becomes shorter to both sides, with ipsilateral OKAN being more affected than contralateral OKAN (Uemura & Cohen, 1973; Cohen et al., 1973). After bilateral labyrinthectomy, OKAN and the slow rise in OKN (shown in Fig. 1B) can no longer be evoked (Uemura & Cohen, 1973; Cohen et al., 1973; Collewijn, 1976; Zee et al., 1976b). The loss of OKAN is permanent and never recovers. The implication of this is either that OKAN is mediated through the efferent vestibular system, possibly causing excitation or inhibition of semicircular canal afferents, or that tonic activity arising in the periphery helps maintain the response. It is unlikely that OKAN is mediated through the afferent vestibular system, since afferent semicircular canal fibers are not modulated in the alert animal during OKN and OKAN (Keller, 1976; Büttner & Waespe, 1981). Instead, OKAN is probably lost as a result of abolition of tonic afferent input to the velocity storage mechanism after the receptors are destroyed. This is of considerable interest in that it indicates that the vestibular labyrinth plays an important role in determining how activity originating in the visual system is processed in the central vestibular system.

A subset of labyrinthectomy, much more difficult technically in the mammal, is to cut the nerves of the individual canals or otolith organs. Benjamins and Huizinga (1928) among others, utilized it elegantly to show that ocular counterrolling in the pigeon depends on the saccules. There has been little research on effects of individual canal nerve section in mammals. Suzuki and colleagues demonstrated that horizontal but not vertical OKAN is lost after the lateral canal nerves are cut (Cohen et al., 1983). This suggests that tonic activity arising in individual canals is important for maintaining velocity storage in the plane of that canal. The vertical canal nerves have not been separately sectioned, although the singular

nerve that innervates the posterior canal has been interrupted on one or both sides in humans for treatment of paroxysmal positional vertigo (Gacek, 1974). There appear to have been no studies of the VOR after such lesions. The effects of utricular nerve section on the velocity storage mechanism are not known. After lesions of the utricular nerve and saccular macula, horizontal OKN and OKAN were unaffected (Takahashi et al., 1977a). However, there was an effect of these lesions on the response to off axis rotation (Igarashi et al., 1980) and vertical OKN and OKAN (Igarashi et al., 1978b).

In contrast to labyrinthectomy or canal nerve section, Ewald (1892) devised an operation to interrupt the flow of endolymph within the membranous canals (Plombierungsmethode). Ewald's technique, as described in his classic monograph of 1892, entailed making a small hole in the wall of the bony canal after the adjacent sinus had been coagulated between two specially prepared ligatures. Only the perilymphatic space was entered, and the membranous canal remained intact. To plug the canal tiny bits of an amalgam of gold and quicksilver were stuffed into the hole until the bony canal was filled and the flow of perilymph was stopped. On the next day after the plug had set, a fine handsaw was used to cut through the plugged canal. Histological control showed that, in time, the plug became permanent with overgrowth of the cut ends of the bony canal and fusion of the ends of the membranous canal into blind sacs.

After unilateral canal plugging, pigeons had relatively little change in their normal behavior (in contrast to effects of unilateral labyrinthectomy). Ewald notes: "Immediately after the operation they fly back to their accustomed place on the roof of the institute. No trace of disease is to be observed in standing, walking or flying". There was a transient change in the response to rotation over the first week. Wing-beats were fewer during rotation when animals were rotated to the ipsi- than to the contralateral side. However, this difference rapidly disappeared.

The technique that is most commonly used to plug the semicircular canals in mammals at present is a modification of that used by Ewald in the pigeon; it was introduced by Money and Scott

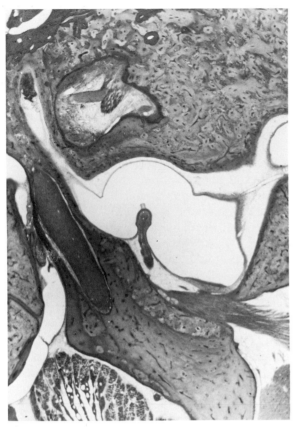

*Fig. 6.* Normal appearing ampulla of the horizontal semicircular canal of a squirrel monkey. The arm of this semicircular canal (upper left) has been plugged with bone dust (courtesy of Jerry Laufer and Ken Money).

(1962). The bony canal is interrupted by grinding across it and the membranous canal with a fine diamond burr. Bone bits fill the open ends of the canal and fuse to provide a solid barrier to perilymph and endolymph flow. The crista and the ampullae appear normal after such lesions (Fig. 6). The tonic discharge of the afferent fibers is maintained at the preoperative level, although there is no response to angular acceleration in the plane of the canals which have been plugged (Goldberg and Fernandez, 1975b). The maintenance of the tonic discharge implies that ionic differences in the endolymph and perilymph must also be maintained. More recently, canal plugging has been used to isolate the input to central vestibular neurons from a variety of peripheral receptors (Schor & Miller, 1982; Baker et al., 1982). The importance of canal plugging in the context of the present discussion is that OKAN, which represents

the state of the velocity storage integrator, is preserved after plugging (Fig. 8B) (Cohen et al., 1983). This allows one to study the response of the velocity storage integrator to activation of the otoliths in the absence of an input signal from the lateral canals.

A process comparable to canal plugging, which has been utilized for the otolith organs, is to destroy the otoconia, rendering the organ functionless. It has usually been accomplished by opening the labyrinth (Maxwell, 1923; Versteegh, 1927; Benjamins & Huizinga, 1928), but this may lead to infection and more widespread damage. An alternate procedure is to centrifuge animals until the otoconia are dislodged from the hair cells (Witmaack, 1909; Hasegawa, 1931; deKleyn and Versteegh, 1933; Parker et al, 1968). This technique is used infrequently, probably for several reasons: the high accelerations that are necessary to separate the otoconia may cause damage to other systems, and the dislodged otoconia cannot easily be removed from the labyrinth. It is also difficult to apply this technique to larger animals (Parker, 1968). Nevertheless, based on differences in the effects of canal plugging and canal nerve section, there should be a difference in the sequelae of otoconial removal and otolith organ nerve section.

In the sections that follow, several ocular compensatory responses will be described that are elicited by multidimensional vestibular stimuli. These are stimuli that simultaneously activate several parts of the labyrinth. Such stimuli include off-vertical axis rotation (OVAR) and pitch while rotating, which will be considered in detail. These stimuli are multidimensional in that the excitation is not limited to a single canal pair, or to the semicircular canals or otolith organs alone. In each case specific labyrinthine lesions have been important in determining which parts of the peripheral labyrinth are activated by these stimuli and in answering questions about how the peripheral labyrinth couples to the oculomotor system through the velocity storage mechanism.

## 4. Off-vertical axis rotation: physiology and effects of lesions

When subjects are rotated in darkness about a space-vertical axis, nystagmus is produced whose

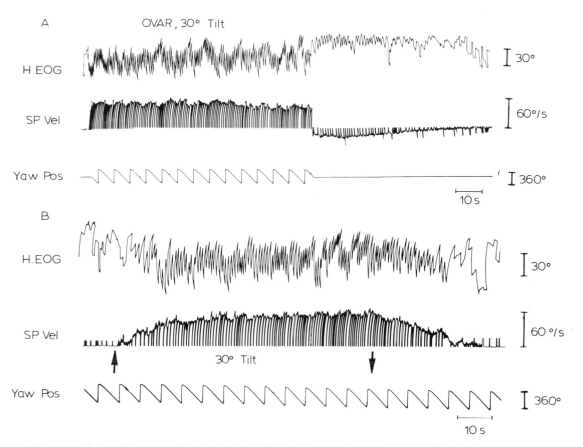

*Fig. 7.* A. Nystagmus induced by a step of head velocity of 60°/s in darkness about an axis tilted 30° from the vertical. The top trace is the horizontal EOG, the second trace is horizontal slow phase eye velocity and the third trace shows position about the monkey's yaw axis. The position trace reset after each 360° of rotation. B. Nystagmus induced by tilting the yaw axis 30° from the vertical during rotation in dark after the per-rotatory slow phase velocity had declined to zero. The moment of tilt is given by the upward arrow. After reaching a steady state eye velocity the axis of rotation was tilted back to the vertical at the downward arrow; eye velocity again declined to zero. The steady state eye velocities were comparable in A and B; OVAR, off vertical axis rotation (from Cohen et al., 1982).

slow phase velocity is initially close to the velocity of the stimulus (Fig. 1A). However, as rotation continues, slow phase velocity and the sensation of rotation both decline to zero over 30–60s (Mach, 1875) (Fig. 1A). The results are quite different if the subject is rotated about an axis tilted from the vertical (off-vertical axis rotation, OVAR). In humans, both nystagmus and the sensation of rotation persist for the duration of stimulation (Guedry, 1965; Benson & Bodin, 1966). In the monkey the initial ocular response to a step in velocity about a tilted axis is similar to that for rotation about a vertical axis (Raphan et al., 1981). However, slow phase velocity does not decline during OVAR, but is maintained at close to unity gain (eye velocity/stimulus velocity) for sti-

mulus velocities up to 50–60°/s for as long as the stimulus continues (Fig. 7A) (Young and Henn, 1975; Raphan et al., 1981). At the end of rotation post-rotatory nystagmus is either weak or absent. Thus, the addition of a rotating gravity vector with regard to the head has a striking effect on the oculomotor system in that it maintains compensatory eye movements against angular head rotation, an effect that is produced in darkness without involvement of the visual system.

There has been some controversy about the origin of the labyrinthine activity responsible for off-vertical axis nystagmus. Guedry (1965) originally postulated that such activity arose in the otolith organs, but Benson and Bodin (1966) thought that the response might originate as a result of a 'roller pump' action of gravity on the semicircular canals. Although theoretically possible (Steer, 1970), there are a number of objections to the roller pump hypothesis. First, inactivation of the semicircular canals by plugging or disease, while causing a loss of response to rotation about a vertical axis, does not abolish the continuous nystagmus during OVAR (Correia & Money, 1970; Graybiel et al., 1972). Second, activity of semicircular canal afferents is not related to changes in eye velocity during OVAR (Goldberg & Fernandez, 1981, 1982; Raphan et al., 1983b). Finally, if the utricular nerves are cut, they cause a loss of the response to OVAR (Janeke et al., 1970). From a study of the dynamics of the nystagmus induced by OVAR and of unit activity of otolith afferents during OVAR (Guedry, 1965; Goldberg & Fernandez, 1981, 1982; Raphan et al., 1981; Raphan et al., 1983b), it has been postulated that the central nervous system senses the sequential activation of otolith hair cells by the rotating gravity vector and creates a velocity signal that drives the oculomotor system.

The central processing for the nystagmus induced by off-vertical axis rotation is largely unknown. It is clear that activation of the semicircular canals is not necessary for the appearance of steady state nystagmus during OVAR. If animals are rotated in darkness until the nystagmus disappears and the axis of rotation is then tilted, nystagmus immediately reappears (Fig. 7B). It rises to a steady level that is held for as long as rotation continues. When the axis of rotation is brought back to the vertical, slow phase velocity declines over a time course similar to that of per- and post-rotatory nystagmus in darkness and OKAN (Figs. 1A, B, 7B).

The sustained slow phase velocity during OVAR suggests activation of the velocity storage integrator. This is also suggested by the slow rise and fall of slow phase velocity when the animals are tilted away from the vertical or back to the vertical while rotating. In accord with this, afternystagmus following rotation is much weaker when subjects are stopped in an off-axis position (Fig. 7A), than after rotation about a vertical axis in darkness (Benson & Bodin, 1966; Guedry, 1965; Igarashi et al., 1980; Raphan et al., 1981). Moreover, the maximum eye velocity of the post-

rotatory nystagmus after OVAR is reduced by the amount of eye velocity during the steady state nystagmus (Raphan et al., 1981). Thus, it seems likely that, in response to OVAR acting on the otolithic hair cells, a velocity signal is created which couples to the same velocity storage mechanism that is activated by lateral semicircular canals and the visual system to drive the eyes. This activity maintains the response during rotation and cancels or reduces the post-rotatory response coming from the semicircular canals at the end of rotation.

Lesion studies of the semicircular canals and semicircular canal nerves support this theoretical construct. After all six semicircular canals were plugged, nystagmus was no longer induced by steps of velocity about a vertical axis in darkness (Fig. 8A) (Cohen et al., 1983). However, OKN and OKAN were present (Fig. 8B). The charge and discharge of OKAN were normal, indicating that the velocity storage mechanism was functioning. During steps of velocity about off-vertical axes in darkness, the rapid rise in eye velocity at the onset of stimulation was lost (Fig. 8C, arrow) but, in agreement with Correia and Money (1970), continuous unidirectional compensatory horizontal nystagmus was induced as rotation continued. Superimposed on the steady state slow phase eye velocity were oscillations that were phase-locked to the animal's head position as in the normal animal (Fig. 7) (Guedry, 1965; Benson & Bodin, 1966; Young & Henn, 1975). The rise time of the buildup in slow phase velocity after canal plugging (Fig. 8C, D) was similar to that seen in a normal animal if the axis of rotation was tilted from the vertical after post-rotatory nystagmus had decayed to zero (Fig. 7B). Thus, inactivation of the semicircular canals by plugging abolished the high frequency components of the VOR response. However, low frequency components of the VOR that were elicited by OVAR, and which are presumably dependent on the otolith organs, were left intact, as was OKAN.

There were several differences in the response to OVAR before and after semicircular canal inactivation by plugging. Modulation in slow phase velocity, phase locked to head position, was more prominent after canal plugging (Fig. 8C, D) than in the normal animal (Fig. 7) and, as noted by

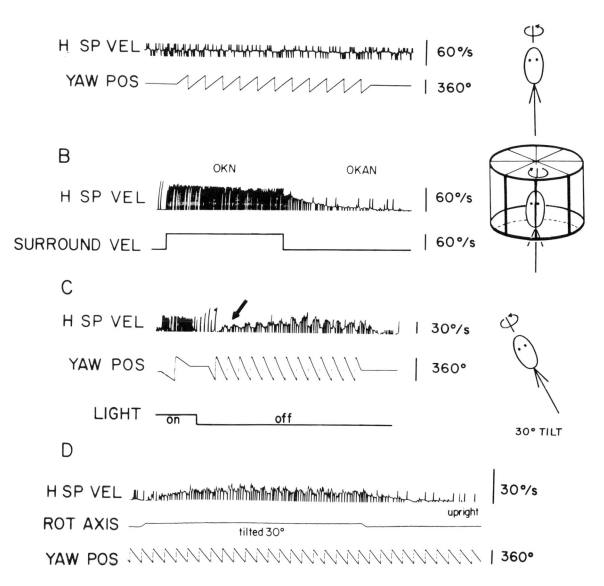

*Fig. 8.* Eye movements of a monkey with all six semicircular canals plugged. A. There was no response to rotation about a vertical axis in darkness. B. Both OKN and OKAN were induced by surround rotation at 60°/s. C. Response to steps of angular velocity about a yaw axis tilted 30° from the vertical at 30°/s in light (left), and at 90°/s in darkness (center). The response on the left is a calibration response combining OVAR and optokinetic stimulation. When the animal received the velocity step in darkness (center), there was no initial rapid rise in eye velocity (arrow). Instead the response built slowly to a peak velocity of about 30°/s. At the end of rotation it outlasted the stimulus by several seconds. D. Nystagmus induced by tilting the axis of rotation 30° while the animal was rotating in darkness. The rise time of the nystagmus induced by rotating the animal in the tilted position (C) was similar to the rise time of the response induced by tilting the axis during rotation (D). However, the decline in slow phase velocity when the animal was tilted back to the vertical (D) was longer than when the animal was stopped in the tilted position (C). The top trace in each panel shows differentiated horizontal slow phase velocity (H SP Vel). Velocities due to saccades have been rectified or manually reduced. The 2nd trace in A and C and the 3rd in D shows the monkey's yaw position. The traces reset after each 360° of rotation. The 2nd trace in B shows surround velocity, i.e., the speed of the optokinetic drum. In D the second trace shows the position of the axis of rotation with regard to the horizontal axis. The condition of the lights (on or off) is shown in C in the 3rd trace (from Cohen et al., 1983).

136

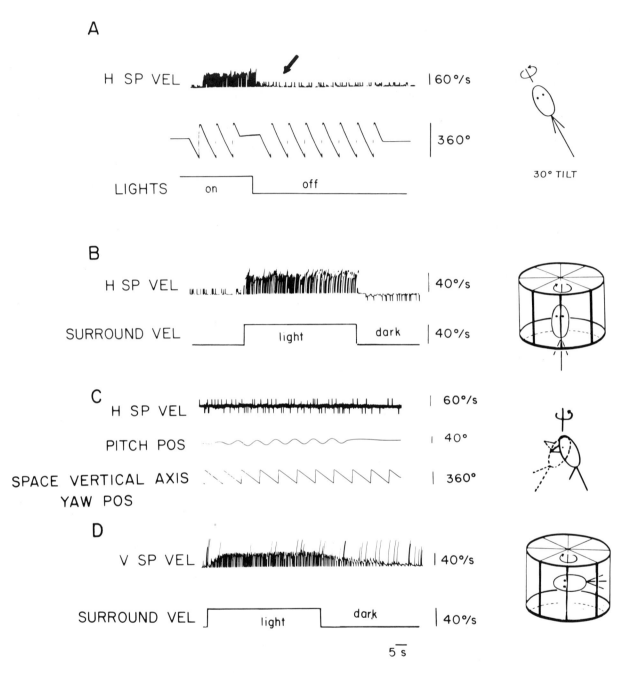

*Fig. 9.* A. Slow phase eye velocity of a monkey during rotation in light (left) and in darkness (center) at 60°/s about an axis of rotation tilted 30° from the vertical after the lateral canal nerves had been sectioned. The response in light was OKN. There was no sustained nystagmus induced by rotation in darkness (arrow). However, there were small changes in horizontal eye position dependent on head position with respect to gravity during OVAR. B. OKN induced after the lateral canal nerves were sectioned was characterized by a sudden rise in slow phase velocity to a peak level, and a sudden fall in eye velocity at the end of stimulation. There was no OKAN. C. There was no steady state nystagmus induced by pitch while rotating. D. Despite the loss of horizontal OKAN, downward OKN and OKAN induced with the animal in the 90° roll position (right side down) were normal (from Cohen et al. (1983) and Raphan et al. (1983a)).

Correia and Money (1970), the gain of the steady state response was reduced. Steady state eye velocity during OVAR did not exceed 30°/s, which was about half the value in the normal animal (Fig. 7) (Raphan et al., 1981). The cause for the drop in gain is not known. Despite these differences, characteristics of the nystagmus induced by OVAR before and after the canals were inactivated were similar. The post-rotatory nystagmus was shorter after stopping in tilted positions (Fig. 8C), than if it declined by bringing the animal to the upright position (Fig. 8D). This shortening of the post-rotatory nystagmus also occurs in the normal state (Guedry, 1965; Benson & Bodin, 1966), and there is a suggestion that it disappears after the utricles and saccules are destroyed (Igarashi et al., 1980).

In contrast to canal plugging which preserved OKAN, section of the lateral semicircular canal nerves abolished horizontal OKAN (Fig. 9B) (Cohen et al., 1983). This is similar to the effects of bilateral labyrinthectomy (Cohen et al., 1973; Uemura & Cohen, 1973). Horizontal OKN could still be induced by movement of the visual surround after bilateral lateral canal nerve section (Fig. 9B), but there was an immediate jump in eye velocity to the steady state value and no subsequent slow rise as in the normal animal (Fig. 1B). Steady state eye velocities were limited to about the contribution of the direct optokinetic pathways. Eye velocity fell promptly to zero at the end of stimulation when the animal was put into darkness, and there was no primary OKAN, i.e., OKAN in the same direction as the preceding OKN (Fig. 9B). Despite the loss of velocity storage for horizontal nystagmus, velocity storage for vertical nystagmus was maintained after lateral canal nerve section. The time course and gain of upward and downward OKN and OKAN were the same as in the normal animal (Fig. 9D) (Matsuo et al., 1979; Matsuo & Cohen, 1984). Vertical vestibular nystagmus induced by steps of velocity about a vertical axis with the animal in the 90° roll position on its side was also normal.

In association with the loss of velocity storage for horizontal nystagmus after lateral canal nerve section, sustained nystagmus could no longer be induced by rotating animals in darkness about axes tilted from the vertical (Fig. 9A, arrow).

During OVAR there were position-related oscillations in vertical and horizontal eye position, suggesting that the otolith organs were functioning. Histological examination was consistent with this. The otolith organs appeared normal, but the lateral canal ampullae had degenerated (Suzuki, unpublished observation). Despite the intact otolith organs, sustained eye velocities could not be evoked by OVAR, as in the normal animal (Fig. 7A) or after canal plugging (Fig. 8A). This supports the hypothesis that an intact velocity storage mechanism for horizontal nystagmus is critical for processing information for horizontal eye velocity during OVAR. These experiments provide additional evidence that the same velocity storage integrator that is activated during OKN, vestibular nystagmus and visual-vestibular interactions is the mechanism through which the otolith organs couple to the oculomotor system to produce compensatory nystagmus.

It was previously shown that labyrinthectomy abolishes OKAN for nystagmus in all directions (Cohen et al., 1973; Uemura & Cohen, 1973), but it was not clear where in the labyrinth the activity responsible for OKAN arose. The canal nerve section experiments identify the lateral semicircular canal nerves as the site of origin of activity that maintains velocity storage for horizontal nystagmus. In agreement with this, otolith ablation does not affect horizontal OKAN (Takahashi et al., 1977b). On the other hand, activity arising in the lateral canals does not appear to affect storage related to vertical nystagmus (Fig. 9). This suggests that velocity storage in the CNS is probably best represented by a multidimensional system with specific states of that system being maintained by activity arising in receptors and nerve fibers of specific semicircular canals.

## 5. Contribution of the vertical canals to horizontal nystagmus: nystagmus generated during pitch while rotating

Although the lateral canals are the primary effectors for generating horizontal nystagmus from the vestibular system, the vertical canals also receive a component of acceleration during normal lateral head rotation. Thus, they should also contribute to compensatory horizontal eye movements.

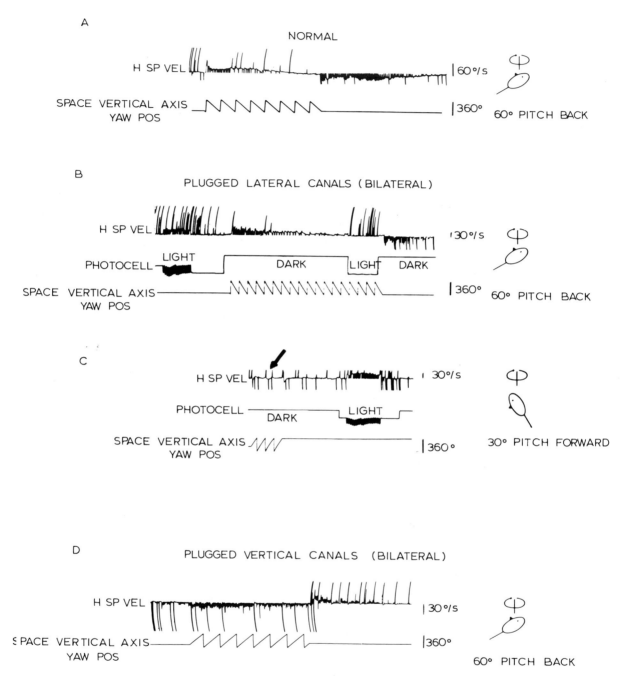

*Fig. 10.* A. Horizontal slow phase eye velocity (top trace) induced by rotation about a vertical axis with the monkey statically pitched 60° (feet up), so that the plane of the horizontal canals was approximately orthogonal to the plane of rotation. The bottom trace shows yaw position about a space-vertical axis. The position traces reset after each 360°. The inset shows a representation of the animal's head position and the axis of rotation. B, C. Lateral canal-plugged animals. In B a calibration response to rotation at 30°/s in light is shown on the left. On the right is the response to rotation in darkness. Despite the inactivation of the lateral canals a prominent horizontal component was elicited with the animal pitched 60° back. C. This component disappeared when the head was tilted forward so that rotation was given in the plane of the lateral canals (left arrow). A calibrating OKN response of 30°/s is shown on the right. D. After the anterior and posterior canals were inactivated by plugging, the horizontal component of motion could no longer be elicited with the animal in the 60° tilted back position (from Raphan et al, 1983).

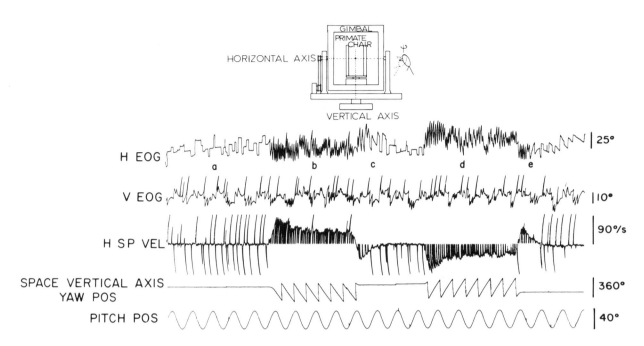

*Fig. 11.* Inset. Diagram of apparatus used for sinusoidal pitch while rotating. The gimbal rotates about a horizontal axis providing the pitch motion. Independently, the platform rotates about the vertical axis. The primate chair can be turned in its mount to provide pitch, roll or a combination of the two. To the right of the platform is a representation of a monkey sinusoidally pitching while rotating to the left. Eye movements induced by sinusoidal pitching alone (a), by sinusoidal pitching while rotating to the left (b) and to the right (d), and during post-rotatory nystagmus (c, e). The top trace is the horizontal EOG, the second trace is the vertical EOG, the third trace is horizontal slow phase velocity and the fourth trace is platform position (space vertical axis yaw position). The position trace resets after each 360° (from Raphan et al, 1983a). The fifth trace is pitch position.

This contribution can be demonstrated in the normal subject by rotating the head about a space-vertical axis with the head tilted 60° back, so that the lateral canals receive little or no acceleration. Under these circumstances a prominent horizontal component of eye movement is induced (Fig. 10A). That this component originates in the vertical canals is shown by its preservation after the lateral canals have been plugged (Fig 10B, center) (Kubo et al., 1981c; Baker et al., 1982; Boehmer & Henn, 1982). When the head is tilted forward after lateral canal plugging, so that the lateral canals are in the plane of rotation and the orthogonally placed vertical canals receive no acceleration, the horizontal component of nystagmus disappears (Fig. 10C, arrow). Moreover, when the vertical canals are inactivated by plugging but the horizontal canals are left intact, no compensatory horizontal nystagmus is induced when the subject is rotated after being pitched 60° back (Fig. 10D).

The vertical canals can also contribute to

steady state nystagmus when they are dynamically activated during rotation about a vertical axis. If an animal is sinusoidally pitched about a horizontal axis in darkness without rotating, vertical compensatory nystagmus is induced in the pitch plane, but no horizontal nystagmus is induced (Fig. 11a). However, if animals are rotated about a vertical axis as they pitch, horizontal nystagmus is induced that persists for the duration of stimulation (Raphan et al., 1981, 1983a). A diagram of the monkey receiving sinusoidal pitch while rotating is shown in the inset of Fig. 11, and the response to such stimulation in the traces below. At the onset of rotation (b, d) the horizontal component of eye velocity rises rapidly to the velocity of rotation. Rather than decaying to zero, as would occur in the absence of pitch, slow phase velocity is held at, or decays to, a steady state value that is maintained for as long as rotation continues. The direction of the horizontal component of the nystagmus is compensatory, so that rotation to the

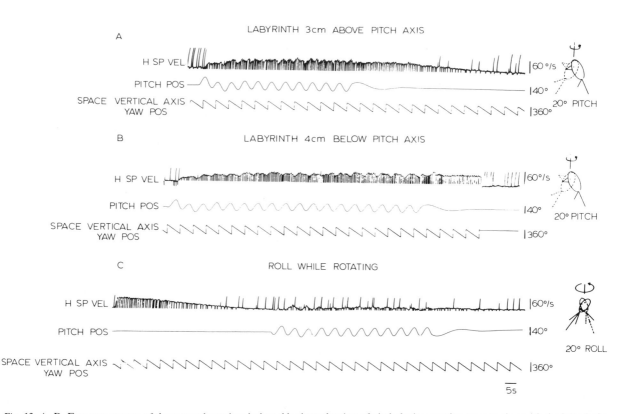

*Fig. 12.* A, B. Eye movements of the normal monkey induced by introduction of pitch during continuous rotation with the labyrinths 3 cm above the pitch axis (A) and 4 cm below it (B). Before recordings began in A and B, the monkey was rotated about a vertical axis in darkness until the horizontal nystagmus had disappeared. Then as rotation continued, pitch was introduced. This caused nystagmus to reappear with a compensatory horizontal component that rose slowly to a steady state value which varied according to pitch position. When pitch was discontinued, the nystagmus decayed to zero (A). If rotation was suddenly stopped during the decay after cessation of pitch, the stored velocity interacted with the post-rotatory nystagmus to reduce or cancel it (B). The characteristics of the steady state nystagmus were identical regardless of whether the labyrinths were above (A) or below (B) the pitch axis. C, left, step of velocity about a vertical axis in darkness, demonstrating time constant of per-rotatory nystagmus in the absence of pitch or roll. Right, sinusoidal roll while rotating about a horizontal axis caused only weak horizontal nystagmus. Compare the steady state horizontal nystagmus in C to that in A and B (from Raphan et al, 1983a).

left causes slow phase eye velocity to the right (Fig. 11b), and rotation to the right causes slow phases to the left (Fig. 11d).

The steady state velocity of the nystagmus induced by pitch while rotating is independent of the pitch period over a range of approximately 5 to 20 s. Instead it is proportional to rotational velocity for speeds up to about 50°/s, where eye velocity saturates. This is similar to the level of saturation of eye velocity observed during off-vertical axis rotation (Raphan et al., 1981).

At the end of rotation post-rotatory nystagmus is induced which decays to zero with a time constant of 3–5 s (Fig. 11c, e). This is considerably shorter than the 12–15 s time constant of per- or

post-rotatory nystagmus without pitching (Fig. 1A). As with nystagmus induced by off-vertical axis rotation, the peak velocity of the post-rotatory nystagmus (Fig. 11c, e) was considerably less than the initial velocity of the per-rotatory nystagmus (Fig. 11b, d). The change in velocity at the start of rotation was equal to the change in velocity when rotation was stopped. This indicates that activity related to horizontal slow phase eye velocity had been stored during pitching while rotating, and that the stored activity was used to diminish the post-rotatory nystagmus when the animal stopped rotating.

The charge and discharge characteristics of the stored velocity during pitch while rotating were studied by introducing, or stopping, pitching during rotation about a vertical axis in darkness after the horizontal nystagmus induced by the onset of the step had disappeared (Fig. 12). If pitching was introduced during rotation after eye velocity had decayed to zero, horizontal compensatory nystagmus immediately reappeared. Its slow phase velocity rose to a steady state level that was approximately equal to the velocity of rotation (Fig. 12A, B). Cessation of pitch during continued rotation (Fig. 12A) was followed by a slow decay of horizontal slow phase eye velocity to zero. If rotation was suddenly stopped, the horizontal post-rotatory nystagmus was cancelled (Fig. 12B). The rising and falling time constants of nystagmus induced by pitch while rotating (Fig. 12A, B) were similar to those of per- and post-rotatory nystagmus (Fig. 1A), OKAN (Fig. 1B) and OVAR (Fig 7B). All of these data suggest that the same storage integrator is charged by each of these various stimuli.

Each part of the labyrinth is activated by pitch while rotating. The lateral and vertical canals are excited by the rotation about a vertical axis and by their movement into and out of the plane of rotation. The otolith organs are excited by the changing attitude of the head with regard to gravity, and both the canals and the otoliths by the Coriolis force (Coriolis, 1844). The Coriolis force on the canals would be small in comparison to the force due to changes in angular acceleration as the canals move into and out of the plane of rotation. In addition, the Coriolis force would change sinusoidally without a DC component (Weaver, 1965; Valentinuzzi, 1967). Therefore, a Coriolis force acting on the semicircular canals probably does not contribute significantly to the continuous response. In support of this, if animals are rolled while rotating, the lateral canals move into and out of the plane of rotation in approximately the same way as during pitch while rotating. However, much less (Fig. 12C, right) or no steady state horizontal nystagmus was elicited during roll while rotating. This indicates that the lateral canals are not primarily responsible for generating the steady state nystagmus during pitch while rotating. It is more likely that most of the activity that produces this nystagmus arises either in the vertical canals or the otolith organs.

With regard to activation of the otolith organs, they are continually reoriented with regard to gravity during pitch. In addition, the macula is also moving in a rotating frame of reference. This would induce a Coriolis force on the macula which is perpendicular both to the direction of rotation and to the direction of movement of the macula according to a right-handed cross product (Coriolis, 1844). This could result in a force field rotating relative to the utricular macula, which in turn would induce a traveling wave in its cellular structure similar to that found during OVAR. However, the direction of the Coriolis force would vary depending on whether the otoliths were above or below the horizontal axis.

When the labyrinths were moved above and below the pitch axis, steady state eye velocity and the charge characteristics of the nystagmus were always compensatory and did not vary (Fig. 12A, B). Moreover, the steady state eye velocity was linked to speed of rotation, not to pitch frequency, over a range of approximately 0.05 to 0.2 Hz. Thus, variations in the Coriolis force acting on the otolith organs did not significantly affect the continuous nystagmus. This makes it unlikely that the interaction of the Coriolis force and gravity on the otoliths was the primary mechanism that produced the continous nystagmus during pitch while rotating. By exclusion, it suggests that activity originating in the vertical canals was an important factor in generating the response.

Canal plugging experiments provided decisive support for this idea. After the lateral canals were inactivated by plugging, sustained horizontal nystagmus was still induced if animals were pitched during rotation (Fig. 13A). The characteristics of this nystagmus were similar to those of nystagmus induced by pitch while rotating in the normal animal with several exceptions. The cycle-to-cycle modulation in slow phase eye velocity was deeper than in the intact animal (Compare Fig. 13A to Fig. 12A,B) and was similar to the deep modulation in slow phase velocity dependent on position during off-vertical axis rotation in canal plugged animals (Fig. 8C, D). As with OVAR the steady state velocity induced by pitch while rotating after canal plugging was approximately half of that induced in the normal animal. This strongly suggests that, *in contrast to OVAR which is primarily*

142

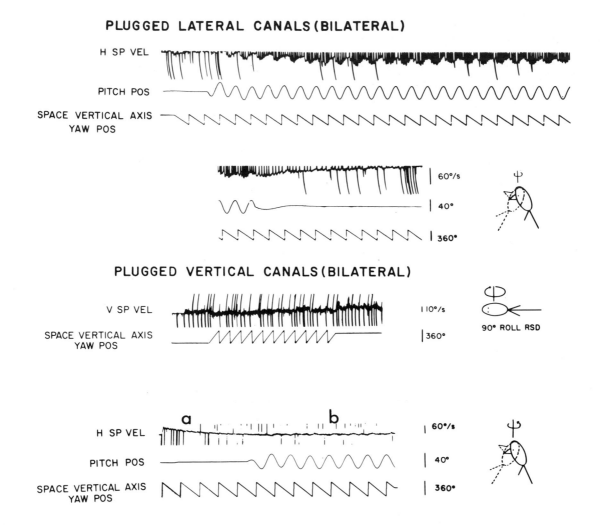

**Fig. 13.** A. Horizontal nystagmus elicited by pitch while rotating after the lateral canals were plugged. B, C. Anterior and posterior canals plugged animals. B. Rotation about a vertical axis with the animal in the 90° roll, right side down position elicited no nystagmus. C, left. Rotation about a vertical axis with the animal upright in darkness induced horizontal per-rotatory nystagmus with a normal time constant (a), but as shown on the right (b), there was no response to pitch while rotating (from Raphan et al, 1983a).

*due to activation of the otolith organs, pitch while rotating had activated the vertical canals to induce the steady state horizontal nystagmus.*

After the anterior and posterior canals were plugged on both sides, leaving the lateral canals intact, there was no response to rotation about a vertical axis with the animal rolled 90° right side down (RSD) (Fig. 13B). As the horizontal canals were intact, the step response to rotation about a vertical axis with the animal in the stereotaxic or 30° tilted-down position was normal (Fig. 13Ca).

However, during pitch while rotating there was no sustained unidirectional nystagmus (Fig. 13Cb), although there were cycle-to-cycle modulations in eye position related to pitch cycle.

As with nystagmus generated by OVAR, an intact velocity storage mechanism was critical for producing the response to pitch while rotating. After the horizontal canal nerves were sectioned and the velocity storage mechanism for horizontal nystagmus was inactivated, sustained horizontal nystagmus could not be elicited by pitch while rotating (Fig. 9C). This was in spite of the fact that both the vertical canals and velocity storage associated with vertical nystagmus were intact (Fig. 9D). Thus, an intact velocity storage mechanism for horizontal nystagmus is essential to produce the continuous nystagmus during pitch while rotating.

## 6. Comments

Experiments have been reviewed that show that the mechanism in the VOR, that stores activity related to slow phase eye velocity in the horizontal plane, integrates input from the visual system, each of the semicircular canals and otoliths to produce accurate compensatory eye movements to the level of saturation of the velocity storage mechanism. Although the evidence is not yet available, it is likely that second order Type I and Type II horizontal vestibular nuclei neurons, similar to the cell shown in Fig. 2, are excited during off-vertical axis rotation and pitch while rotating in the same way as during OKN. If correct, these neurons should have firing rates during these stimuli that are proportional to head velocity to the level of saturation of the velocity storage mechanism. In monkeys this is about 60–90°/s (Cohen et al., 1977; Waespe & Henn, 1977a,b; Raphan et al., 1979). In humans it is about 15°/s (Cohen et al., 1981; Koenig & Dichgans, 1981). Moreover, these neurons should carry the bulk of the activity that generates slow phase eye velocity during steady state nystagmus produced by these complex vestibular stimuli. This would necessitate powerful convergence from every part of the labyrinth onto horizontal Type I and Type II neurons. Such convergence has been demonstrated from both canals and otolith organs (Duensing & Schaefer, 1959; Curthoys & Markham, 1971; Schor, 1971, 1974; Baker et al., 1982; Schor & Miller, 1981, 1982). How a steady velocity signal is generated by sinusoidal activation of the otolith hair cells, what the neural basis for velocity storage might be, and exactly how these various inputs activate the storage mechanism are still unknown.

There are several conditions under which Type I and Type II neurons do not reflect steady state eye velocity during slow eye movements. These include OKN, ocular pursuit and conflict stimulation. In each, direct and indirect visual-oculomotor pathways contribute to the response. The direct visual oculomotor pathways and the pathways for ocular pursuit primarily engage circuitry through the flocculus, and they do not appear to have a strong effect on Type I and Type II vestibular nuclei neurons. After flocculectomy each of these types of slow eye movements is attenuated. It becomes difficult for the subject to pursue, to have a rapid rise in OKN, or to visually suppress the VOR. Then unit activity in the vestibular nuclei is approximately proportional to eye velocity under all circumstances.

The original function of storage as conceived by Ter Braak (1936) and Mowrer (1937) was to cancel post-rotatory nystagmus after prolonged periods of rotation in light. The experiments reported in this paper bear out this initial impression, but suggest that the velocity storage mechanism has a greater function: namely to serve as a focus for superposing a variety of sensory inputs that signal motion and provide the central nervous system with a coordinate basis for interpreting continuous movement of the head relative to the environment. During locomotion, frequencies of angular head movement do not ordinarily invoke velocity storage, although it could be pathologically excited in disease states. The global nature of the involvement of velocity storage in a wide variety of vestibulo-ocular reflexes indicates that it must play an important role in postural and ocular stabilization.

### Acknowledgements

This work was supported by NIH Research Grants EY 04148, NS 00294, Core Center Grant EY 01867, PSC-CUNY FRAP Award 6-63231 (T.R) and a grant from the Young Men's Philanthropic League (B.C.). We thank Mrs Inga Glasser for help in translation.

Adaptive mechanisms in gaze control
Facts and theories
Eds. Berthoz & Melvill Jones
© 1985 Elsevier Science Publishers BV (Biomedical Division)

# Chapter 9

# Plasticity in the vestibulo-ocular and optokinetic reflexes following modification of canal input

## G. D. Paige

*Department of Ophthalmology, U490, University of California, San Francisco, CA 94143, U.S.A.*

## 1. Introduction

The vestibulo-ocular reflex (VOR) maintains re-tinal image stability during head movements by generating conjugate eye movements that are equal and opposite to head rotations. The VOR behaves as a fast 'open loop' system and is there-fore without the resilient accuracy inherent in continuous feedback systems such as visual track-ing. How, then, is proper calibration of the VOR maintained throughout life despite potential changes in its neural and mechanical elements? A proposed solution is that a parametric feedback mechanism exists which utilizes visual error de-tection during head movements to induce sus-tained adaptations in VOR performance (Ito, 1975; Melvill Jones, 1977; Robinson, 1976). It is well known that prolonged optical modifications of vision (reversing prisms, magnifying lenses or mirrors), which generate retinal image instability during head movements, can induce long-term adaptive changes in the VOR (see Chapters 2 & 3). The question then arises: would the modification of vestibular input, as opposed to visual feedback, result in a comparable adaptation in the VOR?

The manipulation of vestibular input has been studied in the past. In one approach, the vestibu-lar endorgan or its peripheral nerve is destroyed on one side (labyrinthectomy or neurotomy). This alters the VOR in at least two important ways. First, the loss of normal peripheral afferent activity from one labyrinth produces a tonic vesti-bular imbalance with the head at rest. This tonic imbalance and its sequelae are progressively re-solved through an adaptive process known as ves-tibular compensation (Schaefer & Meyer, 1974). Unlike the optical paradigms referred to above, vestibular compensation entails lesion-induced plastic mechanisms following a destructive insult to the central nervous system (see Chapters 17 & 18). A second alteration in the VOR following labyrinthectomy is the loss of half the normal dynamic vestibular input during head move-ments. In contrast to the compensation of the tonic imbalance, correction of the dynamic deficit has never been clearly demonstrated. However, potential mechanisms which might modify dyna-mic VOR function may be altered or masked by the coexisting tonic effects.

An alternative and more appealing vestibular manipulation is provided by the canal plugging technique of Money and Scott (1962) (see Chap-ter 8). This method has the distinct advantage of mechanically inactivating a canal's response to angular acceleration without disturbing its neural innervation or tonic vestibular activity (Goldberg & Fernández, 1975b; Paige, 1983b). Thus, plug-ging the horizontal canal (HC) on one side would be expected to reduce the normal vestibular response to horizontal head rotation by half, while maintaining vestibular balance with the head at rest. An early investigation (Zuckerman,

1967) indeed demonstrated that unilateral HC plug reduced the horizontal VOR response to near 50% of normal without incurring the spontaneous vestibular nystagmus (VN) and postural abnormalities associated with labyrinthectomy. However, neither that nor several subsequent studies (Takahashi et al, 1977a; Baloh et al., 1977; Barmack & Pettorossi, 1981) showed evidence for adaptive recalibration of dynamic VOR responses. This seems curious in light of the clear enhancement of VOR responses described following adaptation to 2× magnifying lenses (Miles & Eighmy, 1980), which presumably provide the same visual-vestibular mismatch as a 50% reduction in vestibular input.

The apparent discrepancy led to a systematic reevaluation of potential VOR plasticity following unilateral HC inactivation in the squirrel monkey (Paige, 1983a,b). Included in these investigations was an assessment of the optokinetic reflex (OKR) and its interactions with the VOR. This is important because the VOR and OKR are known to share brain stem circuitry, including the vestibular nuclei (Waespe & Henn, 1977a). Modifications in the behavior of one reflex might therefore be expected to automatically entail alterations in the behavior of the other. In accord with this notion, adaptation to long-term optical manipulations are known to produce changes in both the VOR and OKR (Collewijn & Grootendorst, 1979; Lisberger et al., 1981). How such changes effect eye movement response characteristics when the VOR and OKR act together, i.e., during visual-vestibular interaction (VVI), is also of interest, since most natural head movements are made in the presence of a viewed surround or target.

## 2. Unilateral HC plug

The horizontal VOR, OKR, and their interactions were studied in eight squirrel monkeys before and after unilateral HC plug. Horizontal eye movements were recorded using the scleral search-coil technique (Robinson, 1963). A servo-controlled rate table was employed to rotate either the subject, a full field optokinetic drum, or both. This permitted an assessment of: (1) the VOR, by rotating the monkey in darkness; (2) the OKR, by rotating the lit drum around a stationary subject; (3) synergistic interaction of the VOR and OKR, by rotating the animal inside an illuminated stationary drum; and (4) antagonistic interaction of the VOR and OKR, by rotating the subject and the drum in tandem.

Sinusoidal stimuli were presented at nine frequencies in the range 0.01–4.0 Hz, at constant peak velocity of 40°/s (reduced to 20°/s at 4 Hz). At each frequency slow phase eye velocity (SPEV) was analyzed relative to head or drum velocity, yielding gain (peak SPEV/peak stimulus velocity) and phase (phase angle at peak SPEV relative to phase angle at peak stimulus velocity).

### 2.1. Vestibulo-ocular reflex

The gain of the normal squirrel monkey VOR is relatively constant over the entire frequency bandwidth tested and averages 0.86. Phase is near 0° from 4 to 0.1 Hz, but then rises with decreasing frequency below 0.1 Hz to reach an average of 40° at 0.01 Hz. Following HC plug, two modifications in VOR behavior occur — a generalized drop in gain which is capable of rapid recovery, and a deterioration in response characteristics at low frequencies which persists for weeks to months. For the VOR modeled as a first-order lead-lag system governed by the transfer function:

$$H(s) = G_v (sT_v)/(sT_v + 1) \qquad (1)$$

where $G_v$ is the VOR system gain, $T_v$ is the effective VOR time constant, and $s$ is the Laplace complex frequency; these modifications can be described as independent changes in $G_v$ and $T_v$, as presented below.

The VOR system gain ($G_v$) was estimated as the mean gain in a 'midband' region of the bandwidth (0.1–2.0 Hz) where phase was near zero and gain was nearly independent of frequency in all animals, both before (Paige, 1983a) and after (Paige, 1983b) HC plug. The $G_v$ obtained in this restricted region before HC plug averaged 0.85 ± 0.08 (mean ±SD). To illustrate changes in $G_v$ following HC plug, results are presented in normalized form. For each animal, gains at all frequencies were transformed into percentages of that subject's normal $G_v$. The mean in the midband region then served as an estimate of post-plug $G_v$ as a percentage of normal. A $G_v$ of 50%, for example, would then correspond to a VOR system gain of half normal.

Following HC plug, data were collected within 2 days, and after 1 week, 1 month, and 3 months. Since a concern in this study was to determine the potential role of VVI in the acquisition of VOR gain recalibration following HC plug, animals were treated differently with regard to VVI during the first post-plug week. This is depicted in Table 1, which summarizes VOR gain changes as a function of post-plug delay and according to whether normal VVI was permitted (+VVI) or prevented (−VVI) during the first week. The details are as follows.

*Table 1*

VOR midband gain ($G_v$) after unilateral HC plug

Normal VVI was either permitted (+VVI) or prevented (−VVI) during the first post-plug week

| | Acute | 1 Week | | 1 Month | 3 Months |
| | | −VVI | +VVI | | |
|---|---|---|---|---|---|
| $N$ | 6 | 4 | 4 | 7 | 4 |
| $G_v$ | 57±5% | 52±5% | 78±3% | 83±8% | 87±8% |

Immediately after HC plug, six subjects were placed in darkness with their heads fixed, thereby depriving them of normal VVI, while the remaining two animals were returned to their home cages where they could generate unrestricted head movements in a lit environment and therefore experience normal VVI. In the six VVI-deprived monkeys, $G_v$ averaged 57% of normal acutely (18−44 h) after HC plug (Table 1, Acute). Two of these monkeys were then returned to their home cages to allow normal VVI. By the end of the first week, $G_v$ climbed to 78%. The increase in VOR gain can occur rapidly, since in the two monkeys who were permitted normal VVI from the onset of HC plug, $G_v$ was the same after only 2 days as after 1 week, averaging 79%. Because this value was indistinguishable from that in the former two subjects, after one

week results from all four animals were pooled (Table 1; 1 week, +VVI). The remaining four subjects were denied normal VVI for the entire week after HC plug by either maintaining head fixation in light, darkness with the head free, or head fixation in darkness. $G_v$ in these monkeys remained persistently low, averaging 52% one week after HC plug (Table 1; 1 week, −VVI). This was true regardless of the method used to prevent normal VVI. When normal VVI was permitted over the next 3–4 weeks, $G_v$ in these previously deprived monkeys rose to match that of the other subjects who had experienced a full month of normal VVI. The pooled average $G_v$ one month after HC plug measured 83% (Table 1), obtained from all but one animal whose eye coil failed prematurely. In four monkeys studied 3 months after HC plug, $G_v$ increased to 87%.

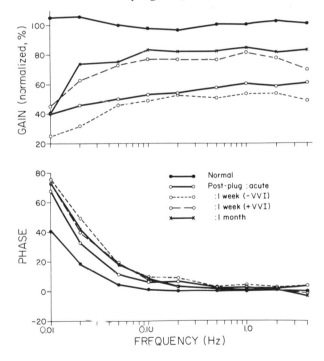

*Fig. 1.* Average VOR gains (normalized) and phases as a function of frequency at constant peak head velocity of 40°/s (20°/s at 4 Hz). The key codes experiments performed before (normal) and after (acute, one week, and one month) HC Plug. Visual-vestibular interaction (VVI) was either permitted (+VVI) or prevented (−VVI) during the first post-plug week. Data at 4 Hz from one unusual animal were eliminated due to a large change in gain and phase at this frequency relative to midband (0.1–2 Hz) values (from Paige, 1983b, with permission).

148

Thus, although most of the VOR gain recovery seen after HC plug takes place within days, some modest change continues for several months.

So far, only gains at midband frequencies have been considered in the interest of isolating changes in VOR system gain $(G_v)$. Attention now expands to a broader view of VOR response characteristics. Fig. 1 displays average gains and phases over the entire bandwidth from normal and post-plug experiments. Data were pooled as in Table 1. Note that for each experiment, gain and phase are nearly constant and independent of frequency above 0.1 Hz. This illustrates the point made above, that midband VOR response dynamics before and after HC plug are distinguished solely by differences in VOR gain. Below 0.1 Hz, a different phenomenon is observed. Following HC plug, phase lead rises more rapidly than normal with decreasing frequency (Fig. 1), accompanied by a decline in gain relative to that in the midband region. This deterioration in VOR responses at low frequencies occurred in all monkeys and was independent of VVI or changes in $G_v$; in Fig. 1, one week post-plug, note the similarity between the +VVI and −VVI phase curves in contrast to the obvious differences between their corresponding gain curves. The phenomenon can be described as a decrease in effective VOR time constant $(T_v)$. Values for $T_v$ were calculated according to the relation

$$T_v = \tan(90-\phi)/2\pi f,$$

where $\phi$ is phase lead at $f=0.01$ Hz (before HC plug) or 0.02 Hz (after HC plug). Average $T_v$ dropped from the normal 21 s to 13 s acutely after HC plug, and then to 9 s one week later. There was no significant recovery in $T_v$ after one month. However, in two of the four monkeys studied 3 months after HC plug, $T_v$ climbed to 14 s. Although this value is still less than normal, the potential for long-term recovery in $T_v$ is implied.

The linear dynamic range of the VOR was assessed before and after HC plug at a midband frequency (0.2 Hz), using five peak head velocities between 40 and 360°/s. Before HC plug, both gain and phase were nearly constant over the entire range of head velocities. Acutely after HC plug, gain and phase remained flat from 40 to

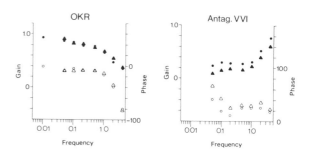

Fig. 2. Average gains and phases as a function of frequency for the OKR and antagonistic VVI before (circles) and one month after (triangles) HC plug. Solid circles and triangles correspond to gains; open circles and triangles, to phases. Responses were not routinely recorded at frequencies below 0.05 Hz. Normal OKR gain and phase at 0.01 Hz represent results from two monkeys. Other data represent six subjects in which a full complement of OKR and VVI responses were recorded before and after HC plug.

120°/s. However, VOR responses at 240 and 360°/s head velocity displayed a saturating nonlinearity which remained nearly unchanged after one month. Saturation appeared as a flattening of the peak SPEV response during half-cycles in which the remaining patent HC was maximally inhibited. The phenomenon may reflect a known saturating nonlinearity in peripheral canal afferent responses; namely, that given the average resting discharge rate of 90 spikes/s and average sensitivity of 0.5 (spikes/s)/(°/s) (Goldberg and Fernández, 1971), the average afferent fibre would be expected to cease firing during inhibitory head rotations exceeding 180°/s.

### 2.2 Optokinetic reflex

As mentioned in the Introduction, adaptive modifications in the VOR may be associated with related changes in the OKR, since the two reflexes are known to share common brain stem pathways. Therefore, the OKR was routinely tested before and after HC Plug, using both sinusoidal and constant velocity drum rotations.

OKR gains and phases from sinusoidal rotations are shown in Fig. 2 (OKR) as a function of frequency before (circles) and 1 month after (triangles) HC plug. Normal gain and phase at 0.01 Hz are near 1.0 and 0°, respectively. Gain declines with increasing frequency to reach 0.76 at 0.5 Hz, accompanied by a phase lag of under

10°. Gain falls while phase lag rises rapidly with increasing frequency above 0.5 Hz. One month after HC plug (Fig. 2, OKR, triangles) OKR responses were indistinguishable from normal in the frequency range 0.05–4.0 Hz. Additional rotations at 0.5 Hz and up to 80°/s head velocity also failed to reveal any post-plug changes in OKR responses.

That responses to sinusoidal rotations are the same after HC plug as before does not necessarily mean that the OKR is entirely unaltered by HC inactivation. The OKR is thought to represent the summed response of a slow and a fast process (Cohen et al, 1977; Lisberger et al., 1981). In the squirrel monkey, the OKR is consistent with the combination of a slow process effective from DC to around 0.03 Hz, and a fast process effective from DC to around 1 Hz (Paige, 1983a). Since the post-plug OKR was studied at frequencies greater than 0.03 Hz, the results predominantly reflect the behavior of the fast process. We can therefore only conclude that the fast OKR process is unaltered by HC plug. To determine if changes in the slow OKR process might occur after HC plug, constant velocity rotations were employed. Steady state DC responses to four drum velocities in the range 20–120°/s were recorded before and 1 month after HC plug. The higher velocities were needed to stress the limits of the OKR, since under more modest conditions, the OKR might effectively use visual feedback to mask the effects of even large alterations in its forward pathway (open-loop) gain. Fig. 3 displays DC gains (steady state SPEV/drum velocity) before and one month after HC plug. In both cases, DC gains are near unity at 20°/s and decline progressively with increasing drum velocity above 20°/s. However, DC gains are typically greater after HC plug than before (Fig. 3). Although the difference is small at lower drum velocities, it becomes steadily larger with increasing drum velocity. At 120°/s the difference averages 11% ($P<0.025$; two tailed $t$ test). Given that DC responses include both fast and slow OKR processes, and that the fast process is unaltered by HC plug, the data imply that the gain of the slow OKR process is enhanced following HC plug along with that of the VOR.

Another aspect of the OKR was addressed using constant velocity drum rotations. The VOR and OKR are thought to share a central velocity storage mechanism as part of their shared brain stem circuitry (Raphan et al., 1979; Chapter 8). This mechanism would account for the extended low frequency bandwidth of the VOR relative to its canal input (Skavenski and Robinson, 1973; Paige, 1983a) and for the phenomenon of optokinetic afternystagmus (OKAN) (Raphan et al., 1979). OKAN is a persistent response in darkness following prolonged optokinetic stimulation and is one manifestation of the slow OKR process. If the post-plug decrease in effective VOR time constant described above were the result of a deterioration in the velocity storage mechanism shared by the VOR and OKR, then one might expect a comparable drop in OKAN time constant. This was not generally the case.

OKAN was evaluated by extinguishing the light after 30 s of drum rotation at 40°/s. Initially, SPEV dropped slightly, and then decayed roughly exponentially to baseline. The time constant of decay, taken as the delay for SPEV to fall by 63%, averaged 19 s before HC plug. No significant change in OKAN time constant occurred acutely after HC plug, and in four subjects no change had developed after one month. This is in contrast to the universal decline seen in the effective VOR time constant. One possible explanation for the discrepancy is that the VOR and OKR do not share a common velocity storage mechanism, as concluded by others (Skavenski et al., 1981). Alternatively, the post-plug decline in

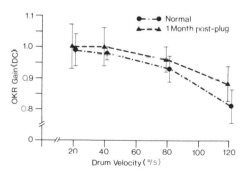

*Fig. 3.* Average OKR steady-state D.C. gains as a function of drum velocity during constant velocity rotation before (circles) and one month after (triangles) HC plug (*n*=6).

effective VOR time constant may be due to a modification in some VOR element distal to a shared velocity storage circuit. Since this circuit is thought to include the vestibular nuclei (Waespe & Henn, 1977a; Raphan et al., 1979), such a modification would presumably effect peripheral canal afferent dynamics, and may be mediated by the efferent vestibular system. Although adaptive gain changes are not manifested in peripheral afferent responses at midband frequencies (Miles & Braitman, 1980), potential changes in afferent low frequency response characteristics have not been studied. Of potential relevance is the observation in anesthetized squirrel monkeys that peripheral afferent responses to vestibular efferent stimulation contain slow and fast components, with the former having time constants of 5–20 s (Goldberg & Fernández, 1980).

## 2.3 Visual-vestibular interactions

Since modifications in both the VOR and OKR occur following HC plug, the question then arises: might these changes be accompanied by alterations in the mechanisms underlying their interactions? To answer this question, eye movement responses were recorded during sinusoidal rotations of the monkey within a stationary lit drum (synergistic VVI) and during combined synchronous rotation of the animal and drum (antagonistic VVI).

Prior to HC plug, responses during synergistic VVI dispayed nearly constant gain and phase, near unity and 0°, respectively, over the entire frequency bandwidth (0.01–4 Hz). Thus, eye movements compensate nearly perfectly for head rotations under conditions of synergistic VVI. This assures nearly perfect gaze (eye position in space) and retinal image stability during most natural head movements. One month after HC plug, this gaze stability is slightly poorer. Response gain in the region 0.01–1.0 Hz is flat but averages 6% lower than normal, while phase remains near zero. Gain declines while phase lag rises slightly with increasing frequency above 1 Hz (Paige, 1983b).

Response gain and phase during antagonistic VVI are illustrated in Fig. 2 as a function of frequency before (circles) and one month after

(triangles) HC plug. In both cases, gain at 4 Hz matches that of the VOR in darkness. This is to be expected, given the poor OKR response at this frequency (Fig. 2, OKR). As frequency decreases and the fast OKR process becomes more robust, better suppression of the VOR is apparent and gain declines rapidly to reach a relatively flat region between 0.5 and 0.1 Hz (Fig. 2, antag. VVI). Gain then declines with decreasing frequency below 0.1 Hz, which presumably reflects additional suppression as the slow OKR process comes into play. The phase curve shows a 20–40° lead between 4 and 0.5 Hz. Phase lead then dips to a minimum at 0.2 Hz before rising with decreasing frequency below 0.2 Hz. Results obtained one month after HC plug are qualitatively similar to normal but display smaller gains and greater phase leads at all frequencies (Fig. 2, antag. VVI).

Although the above findings seem to suggest that the response dynamics of synergistic and antagonistic VVI are altered after HC plug, they nevertheless behave as linear combinations of isolated VOR and OKR response characteristics (Paige, 1983b), as is the case in normal monkeys (Paige, 1983a). The quantitative changes described simply reflect known modifications arising in the VOR and OKR after HC plug.

## 3. Bilateral HC plug

To determine whether VOR recalibration following unilateral HC plug was due to the enhancement of input from the opposite patent HC or to changes involving other potential sources, such as vertical canals or somatic inputs, the second HC was plugged in four monkeys several months after the first. Subjects were tested in darkness at 0.2 Hz, 120°/s. Acutely after the second HC plug, a VOR-like response was consistently observed whose gain averaged 8% of normal. Rotations with the monkeys placed in a variety of pitch, roll and excentric off-axis positions failed to provide a clear canal or otolith end-organ etiology for this residual response. Whatever its cause, the 8% residual gain cannot account for the VOR recovery observed after unilateral HC plug, which climbed from 57 to 87%. That phenomenon must be due to the enhancement of horizontal rotatory information from the remaining patent HC, which probably occurs centrally (Paige, 1983b). However, the residual response after bilateral HC plug might explain why gain was 57% instead of 50% acutely after unilateral HC plug.

To determine whether 'VOR' gain following the second HC plug would be subject to adaptive modifications, monkeys were tested after 2–4 weeks in the presence of normal VVI. Response gain remained low, averaging 13%. Thus, in the absence of HC function, a large deficit remained in the animals' ability to maintain a stable retinal image during passive horizontal head movements. Adaptive mechanisms which might have improved compensatory eye movements, such as cross-axis effects from the vertical canals (Schultheis & Robinson, 1981) or somatic influences (Dichgans et al., 1973a), are apparently quite limited.

These limitations may not apply during active head movements. Following the second HC plug, a different kind of adaptive 'VOR' plasticity was observed — the development of post-saccadic return eye movements in the absence of head movements (Paige, 1980). These are smooth eye movements occurring immediately after saccades and in the opposite direction (Fig. 4B). They were not observed before or after unilateral HC plug (Fig. 4A). The return eye movements were small or absent acutely after the second HC plug but were prominent 2–4 weeks later (Fig. 4B). The phenomenon is not due to the animals' inability to maintain excentric fixation, since examples can be found in which saccades stop short of midline and the return eye movements then carry the eyes excentrically (Fig. 4B, arrows). Furthermore, the return eye movements are brief and typically leave the eyes at a stable excentric plateau. The most likely explanation for these unusual eye movements is that they represent a preprogrammed component of eye-head coordinated gaze shifts. Normally, a voluntary gaze shift includes a saccadic eye movement to a target followed by a head movement in the same direction. During the head movement, the VOR counter-rotates the eyes and thereby maintains gaze and image stability (Bizzi et al., 1972a,b). In the absence of VOR function, the head movement would be expected to

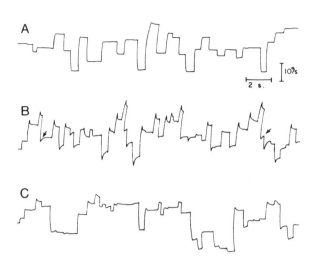

*Fig. 4.* Spontaneous shifts in gaze (eye position in space) one month after HC plug on one side (A), and 2 weeks after a second HC plug on the opposite side (B and C). In A and B the head was fixed, but in C the head was free. The arrows in B point to examples of smooth post-saccadic eye movements which are directed away from the midline position. See text for details.

drive the eyes away from the target, resulting in a gaze overshoot (Dichgans et al., 1973a). One adaptive strategy to prevent gaze overshoot is for the animal to preprogram a post-saccadic return eye movement to counter the head movement — to synthesize a replacement for the VOR during gaze shifts. In accord with this notion, when the head was freed 2–4 weeks after the second HC plug, gaze was reasonably stable between saccades, and no post-saccadic overshoots were seen (Fig. 4C). When head movements were prevented, but presumably still programmed by the animal, the isolated return eye movements were revealed (Fig. 4B). This phenomenon has been reported in rhesus monkeys following bilateral destruction of the labyrinth (Dichgans et al., 1973a). The current results show that the same phenomenon occurs following the loss that the same phenomenon occurs following the loss of canal function without the destructive anatomical insult incurred by labyrinthectomy. This point is discussed by Berthoz in Chapter 12.

## 4. Discussion

After unilateral HC plug, VOR gain drops to nearly half normal but recovers rapidly in the presence of normal VVI. If normal VVI is prevented following HC plug, by depriving the animal of either head movement or vision, VOR gain remains low. These findings demonstrate that adaptive VVI-dependent recalibration occurs in the VOR following direct modification of its canal input. Several features of this phenomenon warrant emphasis.

First, the acquisition of VOR recalibration requires some aspect of visual feedback during head movements. The effect is independent of laboratory manipulation or conditioning and follows from experiences generated by the animal.

Second, VOR gain recalibration is generalized over a broad spectrum of head velocities and frequencies, up to at least 360°/s and 4Hz, respectively. This is commensurate with head movements encountered during normal behaviour, which can exceed 500°/s and 5 Hz (Skavenski et al., 1979; Pulaski et al., 1981). The generalization of gain recalibration distinguishes the adaptive plasticity after HC plug from that seen after prolonged conditioning with reversing prisms. The latter effect is most robust at lower head velocities and frequencies and diminishes with increasing velocity or frequency (Melvill Jones & Davies, 1976; Miles & Eighmy, 1980) (see Chapter 2).

Third, post-plug VOR gain recalibration is accompanied by a parallel modification in the slow OKR process gain, while the fast OKR process gain remains unaltered. This is in accord with Lisberger et al. (1981), who demonstrated parallel modifications in the gain of the VOR and slow OKR process, but not the fast OKR process, in rhesus monkeys adapted to 2× or 0.5× lenses. The adaptive modifications induced by HC plug and 2× lenses are similar. Both phenomena are consistent with the notion that the plastic changes in the VOR and slow OKR process are produced by parametric modifications in a central element shared by the two systems (Paige, 1980; 1983b; Lisberger et al., 1981).

Why has VOR gain recalibration following unilateral HC plug or labyrinthectomy not been observed in the past? One reason is that many studies have allowed at least 10 days after surgery before assessing VOR function, and most of the recalibration would have already taken place by then. Another factor is that most studies have used limited low-frequency or acceleration-step rotations. Any gain recalibration which had occurred may have been missed because of the opposing effects that an increase in VOR system gain ($G_v$) and a decrease in VOR time constant ($T_v$) have on gain at low frequencies. For example, note in Fig. 1 the similarity between acute and one month post-plug gains at 0.01 Hz despite the clear difference seen in the midband region. These problems aside, there is no ready explanation for why VOR gain remained near half normal in studies employing broadband stimuli in rabbit (Baarsma & Collewijn, 1975; Barmack & Pettorossi, 1981) and cat (Zuckerman, 1967; Maioli et al., 1982). The possibility that species differences may play a role is unappealing since, at least in the cat, the potential for VOR gain to increase following adaptation to 2× lenses has been demonstrated (Demer, 1981).

Following unilateral HC plug, another alteration develops in the VOR independently of gain recalibration — the deterioration of response characteristics at low frequencies, which can be described as a decrease in effective VOR time constant ($T_v$). A possible etiology for the decline in $T_v$ might be that a subtle plug-induced injury to the HC had occurred, resulting in a slight vestibular imbalance between the two sides at rest. This would have simulated a rotatory stimulus which may have 'habituated' the VOR at low frequencies, just as happens after repeated long-duration accelerations (Paige, 1980; Jäger & Henn, 1981a). A behavioral correlate of vestibular imbalance is a spontaneous vestibular nystagmus (VN). A small VN was indeed observed acutely after HC plug, whose SPEV was directed toward the plugged side (Paige, 1983b). The VN disappeared over several days, given visual experience. A similar imbalance phenomenon on a grand scale follows unilateral labyrinthectomy (Schaefer & Meyer, 1974). Aside from the well-known postural abnormalities incurred, a marked VN with SPEV toward the injured side is present, along with a drop in effective VOR time constant (Baarsma & Collewijn, 1975; Wolfe & Kos, 1977; Maioli et al., 1982). The VN and postural effects decline over weeks to months in the presence of visual experience (Courjon et al., 1977; Putkonen et al., 1977), but the time constant remains unchanged for months to years (Wolfe & Kos, 1977; Olson et al., 1981; Maioli et al., 1982). This is not the case following HC plug, since considerable recovery of $T_v$ was observed in two of four monkeys studied after 3 months.

## 5. Summary

The vestibulo-ocular reflex (VOR), the optokinetic reflex (OKR), and their interactions were studied before and after unilateral horizontal canal (HC) plug. Two independent changes occur in the VOR following HC plug: (a) a drop in VOR gain which recovers rapidly, provided that monkeys are permitted normal visual-vestibular interaction (VVI); and (b) a deterioration in response characteristics at low frequencies, consistent with a decrease in effective VOR time constant. The latter occurs regardless of VVI and VOR gain recovery and progresses over several days. The time constant may recover, but only after several months. OKR responses are in keeping with the notion that they represent a combination of fast and slow processes. Results after HC plug suggest that the gain of the slow OKR process rises along with that of the VOR. Response characteristics of synergistic and antagonistic VVI behave as linear combinations of VOR and OKR response characteristics both before and after HC plug. Changes in VVI arising after HC plug simply reflect modifications in VOR and OKR response characteristics.

## Acknowledgements

I thank Drs. J.M. Goldberg and C. Fernández for the use of their laboratory and for their support. This research was supported by National Institutes of Health Grant NSO1330 and National Aeronautics and Space Administration Grant NGR–14–001–225. The author was supported by National Institutes of Health Grant T32–GM07281; Medical Scientist Training Program.

Adaptive mechanisms in gaze control
Facts and theories
Eds. Berthoz & Melvill Jones
©1985 Elsevier Science Publishers BV (Biomedical Division)

# Chapter 10

# Adaptation to modified otolith input

## L.R. Young

*Man-vehicle Laboratory, Department of Aeronautics and Astronautics, M.I.T., Cambridge, MA 02139, U.S.A.*

## 1. Introduction

The otolith organs in the human non-auditory labyrinth detect the orientation of the head with respect to the vertical and initiate postural reactions of the trunk, head and eyes. They are intimately involved in perception of spatial orientation. Although they also respond to angular acceleration (Benson & Barnes, 1978), their primary functional role is as linear accelerometers (Young, 1984). Since no instruments are able to distinguish between the inertial reaction forces associated with linear acceleration and those due to gravity, the otolith organs are capable only of signalling head orientation with respect to the net specific force vector (gravity minus acceleration) which, in a given steady state always points in the direction adopted by a damped pendulum. Any ambiguity between head tilt with respect to the vertical, and rotation of the specific force vector associated with acceleration, must be resolved through previous knowledge of the situation or complementary information received from other sensory systems. Although the utricular and saccular otolith organs respond to high frequency (above 1 Hz), as well as low frequency, stimuli (Fernandez & Goldberg, 1976a,b), it is the low frequency or quasi-static portion of their response which is primarily used for orientation. A review concerning linear motion perception has been presented by Berthoz and Droulez (1982).

The otolith organs are certainly not the only sources of information concerning the direction of the vertical. Vision often provides this information, as does proprioception, and especially local tactile pressure sources. To a great extent, these sources of redundant information can substitute for missing or altered otolith cues. Even labyrinthine-defective patients with relatively little residual otolith function can operate normally under most conditions. For example, Graybiel et al. (1967) showed that when labyrinthine-defective subjects were required to set a line to the perceived horizontal as they were tilted at various angles from the upright, they were able to do so, with considerable underestimation, but with some consistency. However, when these same subjects were asked to repeat the test in an underwater situation, in which local tactile cues concerning the vertical were removed, their ability to judge the horizontal disappeared almost entirely. For normal subjects, there was only a slight decrement in their performance underwater.

The influence of otolith stimulation upon eye movements has been recognized for many years, although studied much less intensively than the semicircular canal generated vestibulo-ocular reflex. The principal eye movements associated with otolith stimulation are: static eye deviation (including doll's eye movements); linear acceleration-induced vertical or horizontal nystagmus (L-nystagmus); and torsional eye movements. The linear acceleration-induced nystagmus is independent of any rotation of the gravitoinertial vector.

It consists of smooth (compensatory) eye movements opposite to the acceleration, interrupted periodically by fast beats in the direction of the acceleration. Although it could conceivably result from the linear acceleration sensitivity of the semicircular canals, this possibility has been largely eliminated by the canal plugging experiments of Correia and Money (1970). The typical L-nystagmus sensitivity in man is of the order of 10°/s/g, increasing with the frequency of the linear acceleration oscillation. It is quite labile, often difficult to detect, and frequently absent for vertical oscillations (Correia et al., 1965). Furthermore, the development of compensatory eye movements and L-nystagmus in response to linear acceleration depends upon the axis of the head being stimulated, as well as on the orientation of this axis with respect to the vertical. Vidic et al. (1976) demonstrated that normal subjects can maintain reasonably effective fixation at a nearby imagined stationary point during horizontal motion with the head erect in the dark, but that compensation is successively less effective during vertical motion along the lateral axis, during horizontal motion along the longitudinal axis, and finally during vertical motion with the head erect. In this latter case, it is primarily the saccular rather than the utricular otolith system which is stimulated. Furthermore, the influence of mental set and the distance away from the subject of an imagined fixation point is crucial, even more so than for the vestibulo-ocular reflex to rotation. When the imagined fixation point is brought closer to the subject, the gain of the compensatory eye movement increases. Influence of otolith stimulation on OKN slow phase velocity (Buizza et al., 1980) and on tracking of acoustic targets (Buizza et al., 1979) indicate that otolith influence on eye movements is processed through indirect pathways concerned with multimodal interaction.

Ocular counterrolling represents a direct reflex response to otolith stimulation. Torsion of the eye around the line of sight may be produced by optokinetic, semicircular canal or otolith stimulation. Only the latter is properly referred to as ocular counterrolling, as it produces a movement of the eye compensatory to 'roll motions' of the head to the side in the frontal plane. For static displacements these movements are generally small in humans, and typically compensate for only approximately 10% of the head movement (Kompanajetz, 1928; Miller, 1962; Woellner & Graybiel, 1959; Cohen et al., 1970; and others). The frequency response of ocular counterrolling to sinusoidally varying linear accelerations was investigated by Hannen et al. (1966), by Diamond et al. (1979) using constant velocity roll about a horizontal axis, and by Lichtenberg et al. (1982) using horizontal linear acceleration. The sensitivity of ocular counterrolling decreases markedly at frequencies above approximately 0.3 Hz and the phase lag between the stimulus and the ocular torsion increases with increasing frequency. The reduced static counterrolling observed in subjects with documented otolith system abnormalities, as well as direct experimental evidence (Smiles et al., 1975) supports the link between otolith function and ocular counterrolling. In the case of a normal head tilt to the shoulder, the optokinetic drive from the rotating visual field and the torsional vestibulo-ocular reflex from the vertical semicircular canal add to the transient ocular torsion, but the static effect is predominantly attributable to otolith stimulation.

## 2. Adaptation to the absence of normally functioning otolith organs

In an attempt to determine the relationship between the degree of otolith function as measured by ocular counterrolling and a functionally important parameter, we explored the capability of labyrinthine defective (LD) subjects to identify the onset and direction of horizontal linear accelerations (Young & Graybiel, 1985). Those LDs who had vestibular loss consequent to streptomycin treatment were identified separately. The subjects were placed in a linear motion cart seated in a webbed-back chair with head supported on a cushioned headrest and strapped firmly to the chair with a shoulder harness (Young & Meiry, 1968). The simulator was hooded to prevent visual cues concerning motion in a precursor of the 'space sled' experiments carried out in conjunction with the Space Shuttle flights of the 1980s. The cart was accelerated at constant acceleration starting from rest, with the

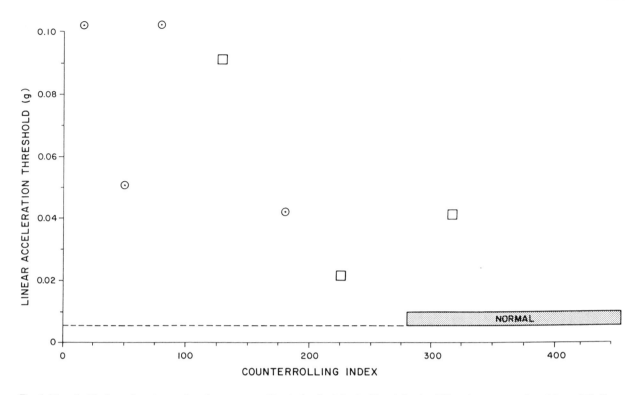

*Fig. 1.* Threshold of acceleration and ocular counterrolling index for labyrinthine defective (⊙) and streptomycin subjects (□) (from Young and Graybiel, 1985).

direction and magnitude of the acceleration radomized. The general pattern was, as for normals, that the time to detect accelerations varied according to the formula

$$a(t_{\mathrm{d}} - t_{\mathrm{o}}) = \text{constant},$$

where $a$ is the acceleration magnitude, $t_{\mathrm{d}}$ is the time to detect, and $t_{\mathrm{o}}$ is the minimum reaction time (Melvill Jones & Young, 1978). Surprisingly, the LDs were frequently capable of detecting quite low levels of accelerations but with a high likelihood of indicating the wrong direction. This is reminiscent of findings on normal subjects for accelerations longitudinally in the vertical axis, then attributable primarily to stimulation of the saccular rather than the utricular otolith organs (Malcolm & Melvill Jones, 1970; Melvill Jones & Young, 1978). When the response of the LD's was measured in terms of a quantitative assessment of threshold (the acceleration level required to achieve 75% correct detection of direction), a clear correlation was found. As shown in Fig. 1,

those subjects who had a very low ocular counterrolling index also showed a higher threshold of acceleration for correct detection of motion direction (ocular counterrolling index is defined as the average counterrolling, in minutes of arc, for a tilt of 50° left and right, and has a mean of 344 arc minutes in normal subjects (Graybiel, 1974). Thus, even though these LD's were eventually able to substitute visual and tactile cues for normal postural regulation and locomotion, the tactile/proprioceptive cues were not capable of filling in for the missing otolith cues in detecting low levels of linear acceleration.

## 3. Otolith organ response during brief weightlessness

Weightlessness is the term commonly employed, somewhat imprecisely, to the condition of free-fall in the absence of any retarding forces. The linear acceleration of a body is then equal to the gravitational acceleration. Under these conditions, the specific force is zero and any linear accelerometer, including the otolith organs, produces a null reading or, even worse, a meaningless indication of direction of acceleration. We all commonly experience weightlessness, for fractions of a second, each time we run or jump, and for several seconds at a time on trampoline or during a dive. Gravity sensitive information from the otolith organs is useless during these periods, just as it is of no help to the cat in righting itself once it has been dropped. Fortunately, for these brief durations of weightlessness, the semicircular canals normally provide sufficient angular position information to permit adequate regulation of gaze, head and body posture. During extended free fall, such as occurs in space flight or during parabolic aircraft maneuvres, however, the period of inadequate otolith information far exceeds the dominant long time constant of the semicicular canal (10–12 s), and a reinterpretation of vestibular signals concerning posture, gaze and spatial orientation is required.

Consider, for simplicity, the simple act of tilting one's head to the right shoulder on the surface of the earth and in weightlessness. When performed in the laboratory, all sensory and motor signals agree. The otolith organs signal both a transient linear acceleration to the right and a tonic minimally adapting signal that the direction of the vertical is shifted toward the right ear, in head coordinates. The vertical semicircular canals confirm a transient clockwise head rotation, and both signals lead to a compensatory counterclockwise ocular torsion (as seen from behind the subject). Because the static ocular torsion amounts to only about 10% of the head movement, the entire visual image on the retina rotates, also confirming the head tilt. Because the head tilt normally shifts the center of mass, it will result in an increase in pressure on the right foot and initiate postural reactions to prevent falling. Finally, all of the sensory signals are consistent with any postulated corollary discharge information associated with the initiation of a voluntary head movement. Now consider the same head movement in weightlessness. All of the signals are as on the earth with the exception of the otolith organs and the changed tactile pressure. The otolith organs will still signal

the transient linear acceleration and deceleration, but will give no indication of static orientation of the head before or following the head movement. Tactile cues will either be absent or indicate only transient responses. The nervous system must now deal with the novel situation in which the otolith organs continue to function normally but, because of a vastly altered environment, the interpretation of the signals they generate must be changed from that of 'gravity receptor' to that of an indicator of transient movements. This novel situation of conflict between semicircular canals and vision-versus-otolith signals is the basis of the 'conflict theory of space motion sickness' described below. Evidence of adaptation to the altered environment is primarily indirect at this time and relates to the alleviation of space motion sickness after several days in weightlessness, and the retention of certain maladaptive postural patterns indicating altered usage of otolith signals for a short while after return from space to earth. Although some preliminary indication of changes in the peripheral end-organs during spaceflight have been recorded (Bracchi et al., 1975), there is currently insufficient evidence to even speculate on the site or extent of otolith system adaptation to extended weightlessness.

## 4. Ocular torsion under varying *G* levels

The magnitude of compensatory ocular counterrolling normally increases with the angle of head tilt up to a maximum of about 60° of roll (Miller, 1962; Diamond et al., 1979). The magnitude of the peak ocular counterrolling depends both on the angle of head tilt and the magnitude of the lateral gravitoinertial force. Thus, a head tilt with respect to the specific force vector in a centrifuge would produce a higher level of counterrolling than in one *g*. Similarly, head tilt in a reduced gravity environment, such as those achieved during aircraft flight, produce reduced ocular counterrolling (Miller & Graybiel, 1965). Even for the LDs, ocular torsion depends upon the angle of head tilt and total *g* level, indicating either residual otolith function or an increasing use of nonotolith information for driving ocular torsion.

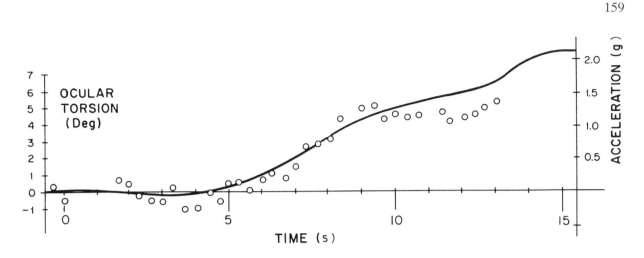

*Fig. 2.* An example of ocular torsion induced by the gradual onset of lateral gravitoinertial force following a period of approximately 25 s of free fall in the KC-135 aircraft. Subjects were positioned such that the force was exerted in the lateral direction (y-axis). Solid line indicates acceleration of aircraft. Solid circles indicate angle of torsion measured in each frame of photographic data (from Arrott, 1982).

## 5. Ocular counterrolling during weightlessness

Ample evidence has been accumulated to show that ocular counterrolling depends on an intact otolith system, and that it is stimulated by components of linear acceleration or gravity acting laterally on the head. Lichtenberg et al. (1982) demonstrated, using sinusoidal lateral horizontal accelerations, that the frequency response of the acceleration ocular counterrolling system achieved by pure sinusoidal variation of the lateral component was essentially the same as that obtained by slow, constant velocity roll about a horizontal axis. Arrott (1982) further demonstrated that, over the range of peak accelerations from 0.1 to 0.8 $g$, this system is reasonably linear. One important question had remained unanswered — whether or not the ocular torsion was in response to rotation of the net gravitoinertial vector with respect to the head, or simply to the variability of the lateral component of this vector. Benson and Barnes (1978), among others, had demonstrated that the compressive as well as lateral components of specific force influenced ocular counterrolling.

To determine the answer to this question, a series of experiments were performed in NASA's KC–135 airplane, which flew in parabolic flights to yield transitions from 2 $g$ through 1 $g$ to 0 $g$ and

back to 2 $g$. By positioning a subject lying on his side on the floor of the aircraft, facing the front, the transition from the 25 s of weightlessness into the 2 $g$ pullout provided the required linear acceleration pattern to answer this question (Young et al., 1981). The net gravitoinertial force changed from zero to the appearance of an increasingly long vector directed laterally during the transition from 0 $g$ to 2 $g$. At no point did this vector rotate. If ocular torsion were to be dependent upon compensation for rotation of this vector, it should not appear, whereas if it were dependent primarily on just the lateral component of specific force, it should take place. The results of the experiments clearly indicated that ocular torsion develops even without any rotation of the specific force vector and that its magnitude is roughly proportional to the magnitude of the applied $g$ force up through 2 $g$.

The total sensitivity of ocular counterrolling, calculated by the ratio of ocular torsion at any instant to the $g$ force present at that moment, and neglecting dynamic responses was slightly less than 4°/$g$, which is only about two-thirds of that which is observed during ocular counterrolling in a 1$g$ field. It is conceivable that the lack of a compressive component, which further deflects the otolithic membrane once it has been moved in response to the lateral specific force, accounts for

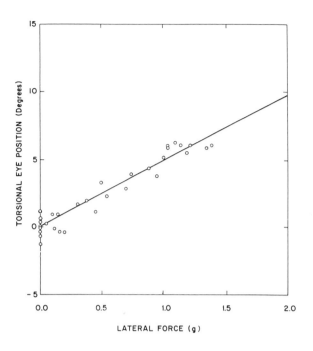

*Fig. 3.* An example of ocular torsion plotted versus lateral acceleration for the onset of force from zero *g* in parabolic flight. This regression line has a sensitivity of 4.85°/*g*, and *r* = 0.96 (from Arrott, 1982).

this difference. A typical case showing the time course of lateral acceleration on ocular counter-rolling, measured three times per second, and lateral *g*, beginning at the end of a parabola, is shown in Fig. 2. The approximate linearity of the individual response is shown in Fig. 3 (Arrott, 1982). The typical correlation coefficient is about 0.9 and the OCR sensitivity among the 29 trials on eight subjects ranged from 2.4°/*g* up to 7.4°/*g*. The average across all subjects was 3.4°/*g*.

## 6. Substitution of tactile cues for otolith cues

It has been mentioned that LDs show a remarkable degree of return of spatial perception ability and postural control following rehabilitation. Increased utilization of non-otolith graviceptive information, including important tactile cues, appeared to account for this recovery. Tests carried out in the parabolic flight program dealt with the influence of tactile cues upon perception of self-motion and ocular torsion. Tactile cues were produced by increased pressure on the soles of the feet, either by pressing down against a foot restraint, or by the use of stretched elastic cords which pulled from a harness about the subject's upper torso to fixed points on the floor. Pressure under the feet was created to approximately equal that associated with standing erect in a 1 *g* field. The influence of tactile cues in the absence of otolith graviceptive information was clear for the case of the psychophysical measurements of visually induced sensation of self-rotation in the roll plane (vection) while watching a rotating dome. Tactile cues did, to a large extent, fill in for the missing otolith cues, with significant increase of vection latency and decrease of its magnitude. Thus, the pressure served as a useful reminder that the feet define a direction which tends to be associated with 'down' (Young et al., 1981; Young, 1982; Dichgans et al., 1972). On the other hand, no clear influence of tactile cues upon ocular torsion was noted. Ocular torsion in this case was developed by optokinetic stimulation from the rotating dome. It is possibly of significance that the nervous system is capable of utilizing tactile cues during the short-term absence of otolith graviceptor information for the purpose of judgements of spatial orientation, but that it does not take advantage of these cues for the lower (brain stem) level regulation of ocular torsion.

## 7. Space motion sickness

Space motion sickness forms part of the general pattern of the space adaptation syndrome. This latter term includes the panoply of physiological reactions to extended weightlessness, including complex renal, cardiovascular and hematological changes which occur during adaptation to weightlessness (Johnston & Dietlein, 1977). Space motion sickness has occurred in nearly half of all astronauts and cosmonauts in recent spacecraft. The onset of symptoms typically occurs during the first hours on orbit, although it may be delayed until the second day, and normally does not last more than about 3 or 4 days. Space sickness symptoms appear to be brought on by active head movements, and may be triggered by disorienting visual scenes, such as appearance of a new portion of the spacecraft or observation of an 'inverted earth'. Symptoms include drowsiness, nausea, salivation, pallor, changes in skin temperature, and vomiting (Oman, 1982b).

There have been some attempts to explain the symptoms of space motion sickness on the basis of fluid shifts toward the head and pressure redistribution in weightlessness. The most popular theory, as yet unproven, is the 'sensory motor conflict' theory. According to this, the occurrence of any kind of motion sickness depends upon the production of conflicting cues, either a conflict between sensory systems or between one sensory system and the expected response based upon an internal model reacting to the commanded voluntary head movement (Benson, 1977; Oman, 1982a; Reason & Brand, 1975). According to the conflict theory, each time that a pitch or roll head movement is made in weightlessness, a conflict is created between (a) the corollary discharge and the semicircular canals and visual system, which react normally, and (b) the responses of the otolith system, which does not confirm a change in static head position. The course of adapting to weightlessness, and thereby overcoming the symptoms of space motion sickness, presumably involves a reorganization of spatial orientation. In particular, otolith cues must be either reinterpreted or inhibited. An appropriate reinterpretation would be to restrict otolith signal use to the high frequency range, which still correctly transduces rapid head movements, and substitute visual and tactile cues for quasi-static low frequency otolith cues concerning steady state spatial orientation.

The exploration of this hypothesis and the search for evidence of otolith system adaptation at various levels of gaze and postural stabilization form a basis for many of the space flight vestibular adaptation experiments scheduled for the 1980s. Among these, a series of interrelated experiments were performed on the four science crewmembers of the Spacelab-1 mission. This 10 day spaceflight, carried out in December of 1983, encompassed extensive pre- and post-flight evaluations of otolith function and postural stability, as well as inflight measurements of adaptation to weightlessness.* These experiments emphasized otolith system adaptation in terms of visual-vestibular interactions and otolith-spinal reflexes. Reactions of the postural system were measured by electromyographic recordings, which will be analyzed to determine any changes with respect to preflight ground measures. The visual vestibular interaction tests were carried out in the 'rotating dome' apparatus. Crewmembers viewed a patterned dome, fully filling their visual field, which rotated at speeds from 30 to 60°/s, inducing sensations of self-motion and ocular torsion. The visual effects, in terms of the psychophysical measure of perception of self rotation, were considerably stronger on orbit than on the ground. Furthermore, substitution of tactile cues on the feet for the missing otolith cues, which had some effect on the inhibition of visually induced motion early in the flight, appeared to be inadequate and greatly subservient to visual cues later on in the mission. Immediate post-flight postural reactions showed severe disturbances which lasted for several days. These appeared both as difficulty in standing on rails and in reacting to sudden postural disturbances.

## 8. Conclusions concerning human adaptation to prolonged weightlessness

Several facts are clearly established concerning human spatial adaptation to weightlessness, but they do not yet provide sufficient background to develop a solid theory. It is clear that normal otolith function is disrupted, and illusions of inversion take place during the early days of spaceflight for most subjects (Matsnev et al., 1983). It is equally true that for some and possibly most space travelers, the disorientation and symptoms of space motion sickness that occur early in the flight are related to head movements, and possibly to the generation of unusual otolith signals. It is also clear that after a number of days in weightlessness, the symptoms and illusions disappear and the crewmembers become extremely versatile

---

*These MIT-Canadian experiments were conducted by Drs. K.E. Money, C.M. Oman, D.G.D. Watt and L.R. Young, as well as Dr. B. K. Lichtenberg serving as a Payload Specialist.

and agile in their body movements. Even a casual observation of the facility with which first-time space travelers move provides evidence of a remarkable degree of sensory motor readaptation. It is tempting to relegate all of this improvement in motor control to sensory adaptation or to substitution of visual and tactile cues for the quasi-static otolith cues. However, it is certainly possible that the adaptation is one of motor learning, and that, even in the presence of reduced sensory feedback, the motor system is operating efficiently by the use of an ensemble of newly developed 'motor programs' for the purpose of locomotion in weightlessness. Finally, it is apparent that a certain degree of post-flight maladaptive behavior is present, resulting both in postural instabilities and vertigo. This observation indicates the likelihood of an internal sensory motor rearrangement based upon an altered central nervous system utilization of otolith cues during weightlessness.

# Section IC

## Multimodal nature of the adaptive responses

Adaptive mechanisms in gaze control
Facts and theories
*Eds. Berthoz & Melvill Jones*

# Chapter 11

# Studies of adaptation in human oculomotor disorders

## D. S. Zee[a] & L. M. Optican[b]

*[a]Departments of Neurology, Ophthalmology and Neuroscience, John Hopkins Hospital, Baltimore, MD 21205 and Clinical Branch, National Eye Institute, Bethesda, MD 20205, and [b]Laboratory of Sensorimotor Research, National Eye Institute, National Institutes of Health, Bethesda, MD 20205, U.S.A.*

## 1. Introduction

In the past decade, a major focus of basic ocular motor research has been upon the adaptive processes by which the brain maintains optimal motor performance. Both during normal development and aging as well as in the face of disease and trauma, mechanisms operate to detect inappropriate motor responses (dysmetria) and to recalibrate sensory input-motor output relationships accordingly. Two important clinical implications derive from such an adaptive capability.

First a lesion within a subsystem directly controlling eye movements will manifest itself as such only immediately after the neurological insult. Subsequent adaptive compensation for the resulting dysmetria will progressively tend to mask the lesion's specific effects.

Secondly, the adaptive repair process itself may be disrupted by a neurological lesion in any of its component parts, for example, the 'error' inputs that signal a need for 'repair', the central networks that calculate the necessary readjustments, and the outputs that carry corrective commands to the subsystem that ultimately drives the ocular motor neurons. It follows that lesions within the adaptive networks can, in themselves, create oculomotor abnormalities. Moreover, in some cases, pathological inactivation of the adaptive mechanism might produce clinical abnormalities by causing reversion to a prior state of clinical 'disrepair' which had previously been rehabilitated by a (then) functionally active adaptive mechanism. Indeed such unmasking might even reveal disabilities that are not the outcome of a previous lesion, but represent inherent idiosyncratic inadequacies of a given individual.

In this chapter, we review recent clinical studies aimed at identifying and elucidating adaptive effects in human neuro-ophthalmological disorders. As an outcome it will be seen that clinical disorders provide a fruitful source of material and ideas for further understanding of both the behavioral significance and neurophysiological mechanisms of the normal adaptive process. From a clinical standpoint a knowledge of adaptive processes and the effects of their participation in, or inactivation by, pathological disorders is becoming essential for proper understanding and diagnosis of many neurological conditions.

## 2. Vestibulo-ocular reflex dysmetria

The vestibulo-ocular reflex (VOR) has served as a model for studying the adaptive capacities of the ocular motor system (see Chapters 2 & 3). Experimentally, the VOR can be made to seem inappropriate using optical devices such as reversing prisms (which cause the seen world to appear to move in the same direction as the head), or magnifying (or minifying) spectacles, or by coupling image motion in one plane to head rotation in another. In response to such optically imposed retinal image motion, the amplitude (or gain), direction and phase of the VOR can be readjusted so that slow phase eye movements compensate for any type of image motion that occurs during movement of the head.

In clinical situations, too, such adaptive mechanisms are called upon to ensure optimal VOR performance. For example, the patient who receives a new eye glass prescription must recalibrate the VOR gain to compensate for the minifying or magnifying effects of the new spectacles. Likewise, adaptation is critical for patients with peripheral vestibular lesions since afferent signals no longer reliably reflect the actual position or motion of the head in space.

On the other hand, more central lesions of the adaptive mechanisms themselves may interfere with proper maintenance of VOR parameters. In some instances, such lesions may lead to *mal-adaptive* repair which actually creates an ocular motor disorder. The following section examines a number of situations where an appreciation of adaptive capabilities is essential for understanding a particular clinical disorder.

### 2.1. Abnormal vestibulo-ocular reflex gain

#### 2.1.1. Adaptation to altered visual input

The need for adaptive modification of the gain of the VOR is illustrated by the patient who undergoes a cataract extraction and then must wear an aphakic spectacle correction. The new magnification factor of the corrective lens necessitates an increase in the gain of the VOR. The visual discomfort that such patients experience during the first few days of wearing their new spectacles reflects, in part, the time it takes to readjust their VOR gain. The distortion caused by the prismatic effects of such high magnification spectacles may also contribute to the patient's symptoms (Fonda, 1981) (see also Section 5.1). While the VOR gain has never been measured in patients after cataract extraction, Hale and Strachan (1981) reported that aphakic patients who had unusual difficulty 'adapting' to their new glasses also showed poor smooth pursuit and im-

paired VOR suppression. These latter findings suggest cerebellar and especially floccular dysfunction (Zee, 1982), although they also appear in old age. Since the flocculus is also involved in adaptive control of the gain of the VOR, Hale and Strachan inferred that such patients had lost the ability to adaptively increase their VOR gain. It would be useful to actually measure the VOR gain (and pursuit capacity) in patients before and after cataract extraction and to compare the results in those patients who wear contact or intraocular lenses with those patients who wear spectacles. Only the latter would need to change the gain of their VOR since their corrective lenses move with the head not with the globe.

#### 2.1.2 Abnormal VOR gain with cerebellar lesions

Disturbed VOR gain control is often a feature of cerebellar lesions. Patients with, for example, the Arnold-Chiari malformation — a congenital hindbrain abnormality involving the vestibulocerebellum — often have persistent oscillopsia (illusory movements of the environment) during head movements because of an inappropriate gain of the VOR. The values are variable and may even be greater than 1.0 (Zee et al., 1974). The VOR gain may vary from patient to patient because different individuals may have different 'innate' values of VOR gain. The cerebellar lesions, then, by removing the adaptive control mechanism, would uncover a different 'default' value in each individual. Experimental work in animals, including the monkey (Optican et al., 1980) has shown that the flocculus and paraflocculus are necessary for normal adaptive control of the gain of the VOR (see also Chapter 14). Not unexpectedly, the flocculus and paraflocculus are typically involved in the Arnold-Chiari malformation. Other patients, with chronic unexplained imbalance and vertigo associated with persistent caloric testing abnormalities, have also been found to have associated cerebellar lesions (Rudge & Chambers, 1982). Presumably these patients have lost their ability to adapt to a peripheral vestibular lesion because of cerebellar deficits.

Yagi et al. (1981) compared the capacity of normal versus cerebellar-lesioned patients to adjust the gain of their VOR. These investigators measured the VOR gain, in darkness, before and after their subjects had worn left-right reversing prisms for one hour. The patients with cerebellar lesions had a smaller decrease in VOR gain than normal subjects. This study illustrates the clinical potential of testing a patient's capacity for adaptive modulation of the gain of their VOR. Such a test might be diagnostically useful in patients who have unexplained vestibular symptoms. Furthermore, by studying adaptive VOR gain control in patients with various neurological lesions, more might be learned about the anatomical and physiological substrate of VOR adaptation in normal human beings.

## 2.2. Unilateral loss of labyrinthine function

When faced with the destruction of one labyrinth, the central nervous system must do more than simply readjust the gain of the VOR so that it is appropriate during head rotation in either direction. It must also correct for the bias created by the imbalance between the spontaneous discharge rates of the left and right vestibular nuclei (see Chapters 9, 17 and 22). This vestibular imbalance causes spontaneous nystagmus, even when the head is still and may lead to a 'directional preponderance' (the gain being higher in one direction than in the other) when the head is rotating. Directional preponderance, however, also reflects the loss of the contribution (either an increase or decrease in discharge) of the defective labyrinth to the 'push-pull' mechanism by which differences between the activity of the left and right vestibular nuclei drive the eyes in a compensatory slow phase. To nullify the spontaneous nystagmus, the resting discharge rates of the vestibular nuclei must be equalized. To eliminate the directional preponderance during head rotation the spontaneous nystagmus must be removed and the relative sensitivity of the vestibular nuclei to head rotation in opposite directions must be readjusted. Rebalancing of the spontaneous rate of discharge of the vestibular nuclei is usually prompt and relatively complete, although a small amount of spontaneous nystagmus in darkness may persist for years after a unilateral loss of labyrinthine function (Fisch, 1973). On the other

hand, repair of asymmetry during head rotation appears to be a slower process and significant directional preponderance in the VOR (as measured in darkness) often persists (Barnes, 1979b). The directional preponderance appears to be more prominent at low frequencies of rotation.

Two additional types of vestibular nystagmus, *Bechterew nystagmus* and *recovery nystagmus*, are clinically important and must be properly interpreted so as not to lead to misdiagnosis. They each reflect the action of the mechanisms that adapt for unilateral labyrinthine dysfunction (see Chapters 2, 18, and 22). *Bechterew nystagmus* occurs after successive destruction of both labyrinths but with an intervening interval during which compensation for the first lesion takes place. The second lesion produces unidirectional nystagmus even though there is now no input from either labyrinth. Bechterew nystagmus has recently been reported in a human patient (Zee et al., 1982a).

*Recovery nystagmus* occurs when, after an initial insult to one labyrinth, recovery takes place and some peripheral labyrinthine function is restored. Due to the rebalancing between the vestibular nuclei in response to the initial insult, subsequent recovery in the periphery leads to a new central imbalance and consequent nystagmus with the slow phase directed away from the affected labyrinth (McClure et al., 1981).

## 2.3. Bilateral loss of labyrinthine function

An even more challenging problem for the central nervous system is to compensate for a complete bilateral loss of labyrinthine function. Here, no vestibulo-ocular reflex exists to modulate and alternative strategies to compensate for head movements must be invoked. Dichgans et al. (1973a) recorded eye-head coordination in monkeys before and after bilateral labyrinthectomy. They identified three major adaptive strategies used to help improve gaze accuracy during head movements: (1) potentiation of the cervico-ocular reflex; (2) preprogramming of compensatory slow phases in anticipation of intended head motion; and (3) decrease in the saccadic amplitude-retinal error relation selectively during combined eye-head movements to prevent gaze overshoot.

These same adaptive mechanisms have been identified in human beings after bilateral loss of labyrinthine function (Gresty et al., 1977; Kasai & Zee, 1978) but in association with several additional adaptive strategies. They include: (1) substitution of small saccades and quick phases in the direction opposite to head rotation in order to augment inadequate compensatory slow phases; (2) extension of the range of frequencies over which the visual following reflexes can function (but within the limits of pursuit system stability see Section 4); (3) use of the effort of spatial localization, as judged by imagining targets in total darkness, to increase the gain of compensatory slow phases; and (4) use of predictive strategies to improve gaze stability during tracking of targets jumping periodically or during self-generated tracking between two stationary targets. Where in the nervous system each of these adaptive strategies is elaborated is unknown (see also Chapter 12).

## 2.4 Disorders of vestibulo-ocular adaptive mechanisms

*Periodic alternating nystagmus* is a horizontal nystagmus that alternates direction every few minutes. It probably is an example of a vestibular disorder that reflects the combined action of several different adaptive mechanisms which, in pathological situations, become 'maladaptive' and produce an inappropriate spontaneous nystagmus (Leigh et al., 1981). Periodic alternating nystagmus is especially common with acquired neurological lesions in the region of the caudal cerebellum and dorsal medulla. It has also been reported in blind patients with no other evidence of neurological disease and as a toxic side effect of certain medications.

Periodic alternating nystagmus has been attributed to exaggeration of a normal vestibular response — the reversal phase of post-rotatory nystagmus — shown by intact individuals. The normal response in darkness to a sustained rotational stimulus (velocity step) is a primary vestibular nystagmus that slowly dies away with a time constant of about 15 s. A weaker, secondary response then follows with slow phases in the opposite direction. This reversal phase has been attributed to a vestibular adaptive repair process that would, in a pathological situation, such as acute destruction of one labyrinth, act to nullify persistent, unidirectional nystagmus (Malcolm & Melvill Jones, 1970).

Kornhuber (1959) speculated that the reversals of periodic alternating nystagmus were an exaggerated form of the normal reversal phase of post-rotatory nystagmus. Using this idea, Leigh et al. (1981) postulated that periodic alternating nystagmus arises because of three factors. First, there is an instability in the brain stem neural networks that generate the slow phases of vestibular and optokinetic nystagmus. This instability is due to an inappropriately high gain within a postulated positive feedback loop in the vestibulo-optokinetic system (Robinson, 1977). (The function of this feedback loop is both to increase the vestibulo-ocular reflex time constant and to produce optokinetic afternystagmus. These responses lead to better image stabilization both during and after sustained head movements, see Chapter 8.) The reason for the increase in gain in the positive feedback loop is not clear. It may relate to lesions in the vestibulocerebellum or the region of the vestibular commissure; both structures are usually involved in patients with periodic alternating nystagmus. Secondly, the development of periodic alternating nystagmus depends upon the action of the adaptive network that normally acts to nullify prolonged, unidirectional nystagmus, i.e., the mechanism that produces the reversal phase of post-rotatory nystagmus. Thirdly, periodic alternating nystagmus persists because of an inability to use visual information (retinal image slip) for long-term adaptive adjustments of the gain within the brain stem vestibular-optokinetic pathways. This latter abnormality may be due to lesions within the vestibulocerebellum. Thus, one can analyze and interpret periodic alternating nystagmus in the context of the variety of adaptive control mechanisms used to modulate the gain and phase of the VOR, and to maintain the equilibrium between the spontaneous activity of the right and left vestibular nuclei.

One might ask why some blind patients, without other evidence of neurological disease, also show periodic alternating nystagmus. Such patients may have an inherently high gain within their vestibular-optokinetic positive feedback loop. Normally, the gain would be adjusted downward by the cerebellum. When visual feedback is lost, however, the cerebellum receives no error signal to activate its adaptive mechanisms. Thus, a patient's performance may revert back to a 'default' value that, in particular individuals, might be too high and consequently lead to periodic alternating nystagmus. In one patient who developed periodic alternating nystagmus after becoming blind, subsequent restoration of vision led to relief of periodic alternating nystagmus (Cross et al., 1982). A similar line of reasoning may apply to the periodic alternating nystagmus that appears in patients who are overmedicated with, for example, phenytoin, an anticonvulsant. The drug, which is known to disturb cerebellar functions, may create periodic alternating nystagmus because of a depressant effect on the vestibulo-cerebellum. Blind patients typically show other ocular motor abnormalities that resemble those due to acquired cerebellar lesions (Leigh & Zee, 1980). Again the cerebellum is deprived of error signals that may lead to inappropriate or ineffective adaptive modulation of ocular motor performance.

Another result of disturbed vestibulo-ocular adaptive control may be so called 'perverted nystagmus' (Toupet & Pialoux, 1981). This abnormality refers to the finding of vertical, torsional or obliquely directed nystagmus, rather than a primarily horizontal response, during caloric testing. (It is not known if inappropriately directed slow phases also occur during rotational testing in such patients. They probably do.) Perverted nystagmus may reflect a disorder of the adaptive mechanism that ensures that the VOR appropriately combines information from the horizontal and vertical semicircular canals to produce a compensatory eye rotation in a plane parallel to that of the head rotation (see Chapters 20 & 21).

Finally, another form of nystagmus – rebound nystagmus – has been linked to adaptive mechanisms mediated by the vestibular nuclei (Hood, 1981). This nystagmus appears when the eyes are returned to the primary position after a prolonged period of attempting to hold eccentric gaze. Slow phases are directed in the direction of prior eccentric gaze and the nystagmus dies out in 5–15 s. Rebound nystagmus is most prominent in patients with cerebellar lesions but also occurs, to a lesser degree, in normal individuals after prolonged eccentric gaze if the lights are turned off (eliminating smooth pursuit and other fixation mechanisms) when the eyes are returned to the primary position.

It has been suggested that rebound nystagmus is the result of a bias developed in the attempt to hold an eccentric position of gaze (Yamazaki & Zee, 1979). The bias in effect resets the 'primary position' of gaze toward the position where the eyes are being held most of the time. The time course of decay of the bias is reflected in the disappearance of rebound nystagmus. Hood (1981) suggested that the vestibular nuclei are the source of this bias.

## 3. Saccadic dysmetria

### 3.1. Ocular muscle weakness

Kommerell and colleagues (1976) first demonstrated that the saccadic system of human beings can adapt to ocular muscle weakness. Eye movements were recorded in patients with partial, unilateral abducens nerve palsies who, for reasons of slightly better visual acuity, habitually viewed with their paretic eye. With the paretic eye viewing, saccades made by the paretic eye were accurate, even those directed toward the side of the muscle weakness. Saccades made by the covered, nonparetic eye were much larger and were followed by post-saccadic drift. When the subject was forced to view the target with the strong eye, by transiently covering the paretic eye, the saccades made by the strong eye were dysmetric. Saccades directed toward the side of the lesion overshot the target (implying an increase in the size of the saccadic pulse of innervation) and saccades made in either horizontal direction were followed by post-saccadic drift directed away from the side of the paralysis (implying a mismatch between the saccadic pulse and step of innervation). (See Chapter 4 for a discussion of the neural control signals underlying saccadic eye movements.) The results of Kommerell et al. (1976) suggested that saccadic innervation had been readjusted, to both eyes because of Her-

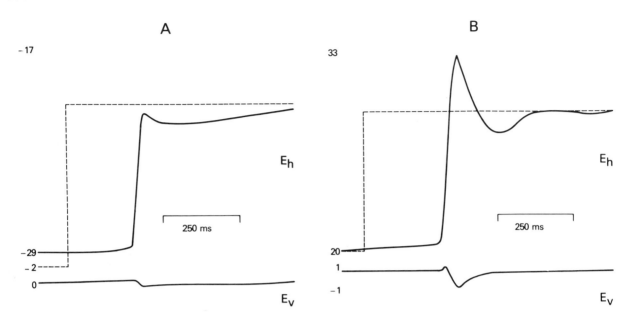

*Fig. 1* Orbital position dependence of adaptation to saccadic dysmetria. Eye movements were recorded by the magnetic field search coil technique in a patient with a complete *right* lateral rectus palsy who had been habitually viewing out of his *right* eye for 9 days (left eye patched). Shown here are the movements of the left eye (right eye covered) as it viewed the target. The position of the eye (solid lines) and target (dashed lines) are shown. For each record, the scale in degrees is shown on the ordinate with the top two numbers indicating horizontal position and the bottom two numbers vertical eye position. Positive numbers are for upward and rightward positions. Eh = horizontal eye position, Ev = vertical eye position. In A a saccade made in a left orbital position is shown, and it appears relatively normal. In B a saccade made in a rightward orbital position is shown, and it is hypermetric with post-saccadic drift. This 'dysmetria' reflects the adaptive changes in saccadic neural drive used to overcome the weakness in the left eye.

ring's Law of equal innervation, in an attempt to improve the performance of the habitually fixating but paretic eye.

Next, by long-term patching of their paretic eye, these patients were forced to habitually view with their non-paretic eye. After 3 days, saccades made by the nonparetic eye had become accurate without post-saccadic drift. To test the accuracy of saccades made by the paretic eye, the patch was transiently switched and its saccades were now found to be hypometric — they undershot the target. These findings confirmed the idea that the central nervous system can change the saccadic neural drive in order to best meet the visual needs of the habitually viewing eye.

Abel and co-workers (1978) performed a similar experiment in a patient with a third nerve palsy to learn how saccadic amplitude is increased. They showed that the duration of the saccade was increased but that the peak velocity-amplitude relationship for saccades made by the normal eye

was unchanged. They surmised that the duration but not the height of the saccadic pulse had increased. If the latter had taken place, which would have meant an increase in the frequency of discharge during the saccadic pulse, there would have been a change in the saccade velocity-amplitude relationship. This was not observed. Thus, the adaptive adjustment of saccadic amplitude appears to depend on changing saccade duration not saccade velocity.

We recently examined a patient with a unilateral abducens nerve palsy and studied the relationship of saccadic adaptation to orbital position and direction of eye movements (Optican et al., 1982). Fig. 1 illustrates the results in a patient with a complete right lateral rectus palsy. The left eye had been patched for 9 days forcing the patient to habitually view with his paretic, right eye. To assess adaptive innervational changes the patch was temporarily switched to cover the right eye and the movements of the left eye were re-

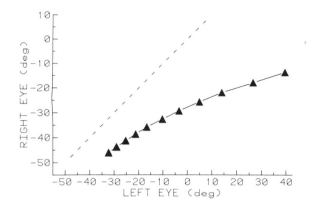

Fig. 2. Static eye-position curve in a patient with a right lateral rectus palsy. Eye position was determined using the Lancaster red-green test. The subject wore red-green goggles and used a red light (seen by the right eye only) to match the position of a green light (seen by the left eye only) moved by the examiner. The positions of the two lights were measured and plotted on a graph. To control the state of accommodation, the subject was instructed to focus on a red grid which could only be seen (as black) by the eye viewing with the green filter. The dashed line represents perfect ocular alignment. When there is no difference between the strength of the two eyes, the slope of the static eye position is 1.0. Note that the slope of the curve is close to 1.0 for leftward orbital positions but decreases as the eyes are moved toward rightward orbital positions.

corded as it viewed the target. We could then infer innervational changes from the movements of the normal left eye. For rightward saccades made in the left part of the orbit, the amplitude of the saccade was nearly normal and there was only a small amount of post-saccadic drift (Fig. 1A). For rightward saccades made in the right part of the orbit, the amplitude of the saccade was too large and there was a large amount of post saccadic drift (Fig. 1B). Thus, the adaptive changes in saccadic innervation were orbital position dependent.

We could also correlate changes in saccadic innervation directly to abnormal lateral rectus forces. The latter could be inferred by plotting a static eye position curve (right eye versus left eye) using data from the Lancaster red-green test. This curve (Fig. 2) reflects the relationship between the degree of ocular misalignment and the position of the eyes in the orbit. Note that in far left

gaze, where the effect of the right lateral rectus palsy is least, the curve has a slope close to 1.0 indicating nearly equal strength in the two eyes. Little adaptation would be needed for saccades made in left orbital positions (compare Fig. 1A). In right gaze, though, the slope of the curve is much less than 1.0 indicating a significant difference in strength between the two eyes. Hence larger adaptive changes are necessary for saccades made in right orbital positions (compare Fig. 1B).

### 3.2. Myasthenia gravis

The adaptive cababilities of the saccadic system are also exemplified by patients with myasthenia gravis, a disorder of neuromuscular transmission that does not affect the central nervous system. If a myasthenic patient with a severe degree of ophthalmoparesis is given an anticholinesterase inhibitor, such as edrophonium, to relieve the neuromuscular blockade, his saccades may suddenly become much larger. When the patient is then required to fixate a target, the eyes may oscillate about the position of the target because the patient cannot make a saccade small enough to acquire it (Zee & Robinson, 1979; Schmidt et al., 1980). The reason is, of course, that the anticholinesterase inhibitor, by relieving the eye muscle weakness, unmasks the increased saccadic neural signal that had been programmed by the central nervous system to overcome the peripheral muscle weakness. Now, for a given retinal error (the distance between the peripheral retinal location of the image of a target and the fovea), the saccadic neural signal is too large. This increase in the gain of the saccadic system creates saccadic hypermetria (overshoot) and, when the gain is 2.0 or greater, sustained macro-saccadic oscillations occur. This latter term refers to sequences of hypermetric saccades, separated by an intersaccadic interval of several hundred ms, that cause the eyes to oscillate about the position of the target. The introduction of saccadic hypermetria with edrophonium is a sensitive bedside test for myasthenia gravis and is easy to detect clinically because of the subsequent oppositely-directed corrective saccade.

172

### 3.3. Internuclear ophthalmoplegia

Saccadic adaptation has also been implicated in the recovery of patients with internuclear ophthalmoplegia (INO). This syndrome is due to a lesion of the medial longitudinal fasciculus (MLF). Patients with INO show a weakness of adduction on the side of the lesion during versional (but not vergence) eye movements. There is often an accompanying nystagmus in the contralateral eye when gaze is directed away from the side of the lesioned MLF. Feldon and co-workers (1980) recorded eye movements in patients with INO and found that the duration of the saccadic pulse of innervation was increased for saccades directed away from the side of the lesioned MLF. They attributed this change to an adaptive strategy for improving saccadic accuracy. The hypometria created by the inability to adequately innervate the medial rectus could be corrected by increasing the duration of the saccadic pulse. Baloh et al. (1978) suggested that the abducting nystagmus in the contralateral eye reflects the same adaptive process. Doslak and colleagues (1980), on the other hand, suggested that recovery of adduction in INO is consequent to return of function of MLF axons rather than to any adaptive changes. Unfortunately, in none of these studies of patients with INO were the habitual viewing conditions controlled by patching first one and then the other eye. Only in this way can one be sure that an ocular motor response reflects adaptation to the visual disturbance created by the ocular motor dysmetria.

### 3.4. Disorders of adaptive mechanisms

Just as disorders of VOR adaptive mechanisms lead to inappropriate VOR responses, disorders of saccadic adaptation mechanisms lead to abnormal saccades. For both systems, the cerebellum plays an important role in maintaining orthometria (see also Chapter 4). An enduring saccadic dysmetria is a classical neuro-ophthalmologic sign of cerebellar dysfunction, though specific patterns of dysmetria are idiosyncratic from patient to patient (Zee, 1982). The latter finding, like the variable changes in VOR gain in patients with cere-

bellar lesions, perhaps reflects the idea that cerebellar lesions lead to a default to an inherent state of ocular motor dysmetria that is peculiar to each patient. Unlike the VOR, however, different structures within the cerebellum mediate the control of the pulse and step components of the saccadic neural command (see Chapter 4). Thus, lesions within the dorsal vermis and underlying deep nuclei lead to disorders of control of the saccadic pulse; lesions within the flocculus lead to disorders of control of the saccadic step and hence the pulse-step match. Saccadic pulse dysmetria and post-saccadic drift, respectively, are the ocular motor signs consequent to lesions in these regions.

Extreme saccadic pulse hypermetria creates macro-saccadic oscillations (see Section 3.2) which can occur in patients with cerebellar lesions, especially the dorsal vermis and underlying fastigial nuclei (Selhorst et al., 1976). Macro-saccadic oscillations reflect both an increase in, and inability to adaptively modulate, the saccadic system gain.

### 4. Pursuit dysmetria

Unlike vestibulo-ocular and saccadic dysmetria, there have been virtually no studies of the mechanisms by which the central nervous system adapts for pursuit dysmetria. We have recently studied this problem in a patient with a chronic, unilateral right *abducens nerve palsy*. We recorded the effects of habitual viewing with the paretic eye on smooth pursuit responses (Optican et al., 1982). By recording the movements of the normal left eye, before and after prolonged patching of the normal eye, we could assess adaptive pursuit capabilities. We found that the initiation of pursuit in the 'open loop' period (the first 130 ms of eye movement before visual feedback has time to influence the motor response) showed an adaptive increase in innervation that was orbital position dependent. This is illustrated in Fig. 3 which shows the tracking responses of the good left eye attempting to smoothly follow the target. Pursuit tracking to the right beginning in left orbital positions was relatively normal (Fig. 3A). For tracking in right orbital positions, the gain of the pursuit system was increased causing the left

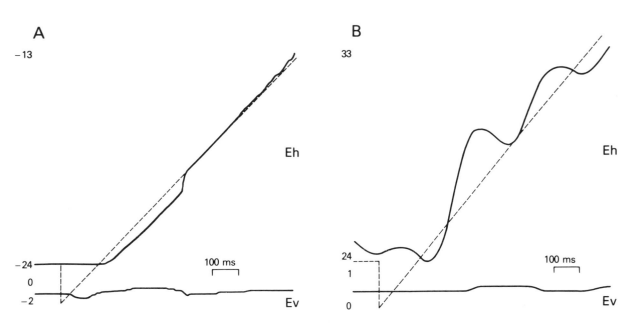

*Fig. 3.* Orbital position dependence of adaptation to pursuit dysmetria. Identical experimental conditions to those described in Fig. 1, except the target (dashed line) here moves in a step-ramp pattern. In A, rightward pursuit beginning from a leftward orbital position is seen to be normal. In B, rightward pursuit beginning from a rightward orbital position is shown. There is pursuit overshoot and an approximately 3 Hz oscillation. The eye is oscillating slightly even during the fixation period before the target begins to move.

eye to overshoot the target (Fig. 3B). These position specific changes in pursuit neural drives could be related to the muscle forces reflected in the static eye position curve (Fig. 2). In rightward orbital positions, pursuit system gain increased so much that when the patient was forced to track using the good eye smooth pendular oscillations at a frequency of about 3 Hz appeared (see Fig. 3B). This finding suggests that some types of pathological pendular oscillations might arise from an inappropriately increased pursuit system gain.

## 5. Ocular misalignment

### 5.1. Phoria adaptation (see also Chapter 5)

The term 'phoria' refers to the relative position of the visual axes of the eyes when only one eye is viewing the target. In this condition, disparity-induced (fusional) vergence is in abeyance and accommodative-induced vergence alone influences ocular alignment. The term orthophoria indicates that the visual axes of both eyes are aligned on the target even though only one eye is viewing the target. When viewing a distant target, orthophoria indicates that the visual axes are parallel. Eso- and exphoria refer to convergence and divergence of the visual axes, respectively. The phoria is usually measured clinically with the alternate cover test. The patient is instructed to fixate a target and then the cover is alternately switched from one eye to the other. Any corrective refixational movements, which reveal the presence of eso- or exophoria, are noted. Prisms of increasing power are then introduced in front of one eye until the eyes do not move when the cover is switched. The strength of the prism then indicates the amplitude of the phoria.

If a normal subject, viewing binocularly, wears a prism in front of one eye for more than 10 or 15 s the amplitude and sense of his phoria begins to change depending on the prism's characteristics. The change is such that if the phoria were measured with the prism on, it would revert back to its original value. For example, take a subject who normally has a 2° esophoria when viewing a distance target. If a 2° base out prism is placed in front of one eye and then his phoria is measured, its value will be zero. After a period of binocular viewing, with the prism on, however, his phoria, measured with the prism on, will again become a 2° esophoria. If the prism is then removed and the phoria measured immediately, its value will be about 4° of esophoria. If the subject then views binocularly, without any prism, the esophoria will revert to its original value of 2°. This change in ocular alignment is termed phoria (or prism) adaptation and represents a realignment of the visual axes of the eyes when measured in the absence of fusional drives.*

Phoria adaptation is not simply a mechanism to maintain orthophoria since when normal subjects wear a prism the eyes are realigned toward any inherent deviation (eso- or exophoria) the subject may have (Schor, 1983; Henson & Dharamshi, 1982). The subject's deviation may even pass through orthophoria on the way back to the initial alignment. The function of phoria adaptation is not exactly clear, although in most cases it does act to relieve the stress upon fusional convergence mechanisms that would otherwise lead to increasing fixation disparity.** Phoria adaptation is probably stimulated by a sustained, disparity-induced, fusional vergence response; it does not occur in response to monocular accommodative vergence drives. Schor (1979b) has presented a model to explain the interaction between disparity-induced fusional vergence and the phoria adaptation mechanism.

Henson and Dharamshi (1982) showed that phoria adaptation was orbital position dependent. They had subjects wear a prism in front of one eye and then the subjects, while viewing binocularly, maintained one position of gaze. Phoria adaptation was found to be greatest when the eyes were tested in that particular position of gaze. There were progressively decreasing amounts of adaptation as the eyes were tested away from the adapting position. (Compare this position specific phoria adaptation with frequency specific VOR adaptation (see Chapter 21).) In a related experiment, Henson and Dharamshi (1982) used a combination of contact lenses and spectacles to cause the prism strength to vary as a function of eye position. They found that phoria adaptation also varied with eye position provided the ratio of the change in prism strength to the change in eye position was small. No adaptation occurred when the ratio was as high as 0.24. Both these experiments illustrate that the ocular motor system can adapt to small amounts of ocular misalignment even when the deviation is nonconcomitant, i.e., varies with orbital position.

The effects of a phoria adaptation mechanism can also be revealed by prolonged monocular viewing in normal subjects (Marlow, 1921). Both concomitant (the ocular deviation is independent of orbital position) and nonconcomitant deviations may emerge when normal subjects patch one eye continuously for a period of time. An illustration of this phenomenon is shown in Fig. 4.

Thus, phoria adaptation is a mechanism that, within limits, helps to ensure that ocular alignment is maintained in the face of changes in orbital mechanics caused by normal development, aging and disease. This may be one way that Herring's Law of equal innervation is maintained through a wide range of orbital positions (see also Westheimer, 1982). Phoria adaptation also ensures compensation for the prismatic effects of spectacles used to correct patients with anisometropia. So called 'spread of comitance', in which the ocular deviation caused by an ocular muscle paresis changes from nonconcomitant to concomitant may be, in part, a manifestation of this same adaptive mechanism.

## 5.2. Clinical studies

Phoria adaptation can be counterproductive in a patient with strabismus who is fitted with prisms

---

*Note the similarity between phoria adaptation and the mechanism creating rebound nystagmus (see Section 2.4.). The former reflects a disconjugate bias that resets ocular alignment. The latter reflects a conjugate bias that resets the 'primary position' of gaze.

**Fixation disparity refers to small errors of fusional vergence that do not cause diplopia since they do not exceed Panum's fusional limits. Increasing disparity is associated with increasing fusional effort.

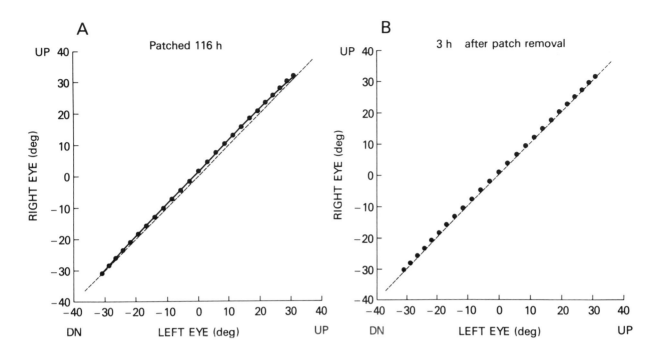

*Fig. 4.* The effect of prolonged monocular occlusion upon vertical ocular alignment in a normal subject. Eye position was determined using the Lancaster red-green test. (See legend of Fig. 2 for details.) For this graph, five measurements were taken at each position and the average standard error of the mean was only 0.1°. (The radius of the circle depicting data points is 0.75°.) After 116 h of monocular viewing (right eye patched) there was a small right hyperphoria (and tropia — the subject experienced vertical diplopia). The deviation was nonconcomitant, being greater on upgaze with a maximum value of 1.5° (A). After 50 min of binocular viewing the vertical diplopia disappeared. A repeat Lancaster red-green test then showed a smaller (about 0.6°) essentially concomitant, right hyperphoria (B).

to relieve diplopia. Phoria adaptation may overcome the effect of the prismatic correction and cause diplopia to reemerge. In clinical jargon, this is called 'eating up a prism'. On the other hand, patients with asthenopia (visual fatigue, blurred or double vision) who have poor phoria adaptation may be relieved of their symptoms with prisms.

North and Henson (1981) used a test of phoria adaptation to evaluate a group of patients with asthenopia. Most symptomatic subjects had abnormal horizontal phoria adaptation, at least in one direction, with the abnormality being greatest when viewing at the distance where the symptoms were most severe. Vertical phoria adaptation was usually intact. There was a poor correlation, however, between adaptive capability, the direction and amplitude of the phoria, vergence amplitudes and the presence of fixation disparity. Schor

(1979a) also found abnormal phoria adaptation to base out (but not base in) prisms in three patients with intermittent esotropia. It would be interesting to extend these types of studies to patients with acquired neurological disorders of binocularity, e.g., divergence paralysis, skew deviations. Are they also disorders of phoria adaptation? Similarly, do adults who suddenly become symptomatic from a pre-existing but previously well compensated stabismus do so because of a breakdown in their phoria adaptation mechanism?

What is the neuroanatomical substrate for phoria adaptation? Milder and Reinecke (1983) studied a group of patients with cerebellar disease and found decreased phoria adaptation. This raises the question: which specific part of the cerebellum might mediate phoria adaptation? We only know that the flocculus is probably not involved. Experimentally, in two monkeys, with bilateral floccular ablations, phoria adaptation was found to be within the normal range (Judge, Miles & Zee, unpublished observations).

## 6. Conclusions

This review has emphasized the importance of considering adaptive mechanisms in the evaluation of patients with ocular motor disorders. Clinicians now realize they must understand how normal adaptive control mechanisms work in order to distinguish between the primary effects of a lesion and the secondary effects due to adaptive control. Lesions of the adaptive control mechanisms themselves may lead to ocular motor syndromes mimicking those of lesions elsewhere in the central nervous system. Furthermore, specific testing of ocular motor adaptive capabilities may become a potent clinical tool in the evaluation of patients with persistent unexplained visual and vestibular symptomatology. For the basic scientist, too, the results of clinical studies of adaptive control are important. Much can be inferred about the normal function of adaptive mechanisms when patients with brain lesions are carefully studied and the results cautiously interpreted.

## Acknowledgements

We acknowledge the support of NIH Grants EY01849 and EY00158. Vendetta Matthews prepared the manuscript.

Adaptive mechanisms in gaze control
Facts and theories
*Eds. Berthoz & Melvill Jones*
© 1985 Elsevier Science Publishers BV (Biomedical Division)

**Chapter 12**

# Adaptive mechanisms in eye-head coordination

## A. Berthoz

*Laboratoire de Physiologie Neurosensorielle du CNRS, 15, rue de l'École de Médecine, 75270 Paris, Cedex 06, France*

## 1. Introduction

The main purpose of eye-head coordination is the control of gaze. Gaze can be defined as the direction of the optical axis with respect to space. However, gaze control does not require the same type of eye-head coordination in every species because the anatomy of the eye and head, the relation between head, body and limbs, as well as the properties of the visual systems, vary from one species to another. The development of a head seems to have been one of the main changes which occurred when the vertebrates appeared. Gans and Northcutt (1983) propose that the head of vertebrates is an addition to the existing body of the protochordates. According to these authors it allowed a basic change in feeding behaviour from filter feeding to prey catching. It accompanied the expansion of the neural tube and the development of paired and external special sense organs. If one follows this theory, the development of a head was very early related to the need to orient to a prey, although predator fishes may orient the body to catch a prey and many species 'orient' not to become a prey!

The evolution of the eyes and their relation to the vestibular system are described by Simpson and Graf in Chapter 1. The main anatomical changes which have occurred in the eye-head systems are the following.

(a) Migration of the eyes in the head from a lateral to a frontal position.

(b) A modification of the geometrical relationship between biomechanical properties of the eye, the head and the body, which has, for example, led to an increasing alignment of the neck vertebral axis with gravity, probably due to two requirements operating at the same time: on one hand the necessity to maintain the plane of the so-called 'horizontal' canals in a plane perpendicular to gravity, and on the other hand the development of bipedal locomotion and upright stance in humans.

The study of the repercussion of phylogenetic constraints on eye-head coordination remains an open field but would represent a fascinating area. It is most probable that throughout phylogeny, central modifications of neural control for eye-head coordination has occurred in relation with the evolution of the geometry and biomechanics of the neck. However, even in humans, only few studies have been devoted to biomechanical studies of the head-neck system (see Viviani & Berthoz, 1975; Reber & Goldsmith, 1979; Zangemeister et al., 1981a,b).

The physiological mechanisms underlying eye-head coordination have probably also been adapted to the behaviour (prey-catching, locomotion, flying, swimming, etc.) of each species. The study of adaptive processes in this case will therefore be much more complex than it is for the vestibulo-ocular reflex (VOR). In fact, remarkably few studies have been devoted to these processes in spite of a large body of clinical knowledge on head-eye coordination deficit (see the recent reviews by Zee, 1977; Gresty & Halmagyi, 1979). Whenever they are available, experimental results have revealed, as will be evident in the present review, a great complexity of mechanisms ranging from 'simple' parametric gain adjustments to rather ill-defined 'motor programs' or novel 'strategies' which can be observed during the basic stabilizing reflexes (VOR, VCR, etc.) during orienting behaviour, or after lesions (see recent review by Bizzi, 1981; and symposium books containing relevant material: Fuchs & Becker, 1981; Lennerstrand et al. 1982; Roucoux & Crommelinck, 1982).

In the following sections several topics will be reviewed. First, we shall follow the main stages of phylogenetic development of eye-head coordination. Our purpose will not be to make an extensive comparative study of the subject but rather to take some specific examples in order to develop a thematic argument along the following lines.

As a starting point it seems reasonable to assume that eye-head coordination is generally subserved by *identifiable neural subsystems* (e.g., compensatory or stabilizing reflexes such as VCR, CCR, VOR, OKR or subsystems responsible for orienting behaviour such as the saccadic system and pursuit). Presumably these have appeared in an ordered phylogenetic succession, probably beginning with the VCR and culminating with pursuit, best represented in the primates. In addition, at any given stage of evolution, needs for physiological adaptation have been imposed when animals were faced with one or several of the following situations: (a) the normal moment-to-moment demand for changes in subsystem behaviour during the course of everyday activity; (b) peripheral or central lesions; and (c) abnormal demands resulting from novel environmental pressures. In the latter case one may guess that an individual would first try to use a *combination of existing subsystems already represented in the normal motor 'repertoire'* of the species. If this should succeed and if the need for change were maintained over a prolonged period of time, the continued redeployment of these subsystems would then lead to *plastic* changes whose goal would be to stabilize a new set of controlling parameters in the subsystems and their interactions. If this were not enough, further changes would be developed creating new *cooperative functions* in available neuronal networks which

*may* or *may not* lead to plastic changes.

To understand this complexity we need to identify the participating subsystems: hence our primary concern with comparative aspects of eye-head coordination, in spite of its apparently rather academic implications. This review will therefore attempt to give some examples of the basic organization of eye-head coordination in normal conditions for some terrestrial animals (frog, rabbit, cat, monkey), although it should be noted that birds also offer fascinating aspects which will not be dealt with here. From time to time we shall turn to adaptive consequences of pathological interference when this introduces some evidence concerning specific mechanisms. We shall also summarize some recent findings concerning adaptation to environmental factors and present some of our own results obtained mainly in collaboration with G. Melvill Jones and D. Guitton.

## 2. Eye-head coordination in some terrestrial animals

### 2.1. Preponderance of head movements in the frog

Like all species, the frog shows *stabilizing* or *orienting* patterns of behaviour. When posture is perturbed by movement of the animal's base, compensatory (stabilizing) reflexes of vestibular or optic origin are set into action (see Chapters 17 & 18). When the animal wants to orient to a target it also makes coordinated eye and head movements. Both types of movements will now briefly be described because the frog is a good example of an animal with a restricted repertoire of subsystems.

### 2.1.1. Stabilizing reflexes

The frog can stabilize its head or eye in space by vestibulo-ocular (VOR) or vestibulo-collicular (VCR) reflexes and can stabilize a moving image on the retina by the optokinetic reflex (OKR). The eye and the head of the frog can both be driven by monocular optokinetic stimulation without body rotation (Birukow, 1937; Dieringer & Precht, 1982a) as in most species with an unspecialized fovea (Tauber & Atkin, 1968).

However, fast phases of vestibular or optokinetic nystagmus are, as in the fish, asymmetric (Dieringer et al., 1982).

Compensatory eye and head movements can be induced in the frog by passive rotation of the body of the animal around any head axis. Recent measurements made by Dieringer and Precht (1982a) on *Rana temporaria* show that during sinusoidal earth vertical axis body rotation in the plane of the horizontal canals, the stabilization of gaze is mainly accomplished by *head* turning rather than eye rotation with gains between 0.8 and 0.9 (ratio of head velocity to body velocity) in the frequency range 0.025 to 0.5 Hz. These gains have been obtained when the rotation was made in the light and therefore visual (optokinetic) and vestibular signals combined to produce the compensatory head movement. The optokinetic component is dominant at low frequencies and the vestibular component at high frequencies.

### 2.1.2. Orienting behaviour

In general it seems that the frog makes, at rest, virtually no spontaneous eye movements (Autrum, 1959). Saccades have a very small amplitude (less than 2°). Frogs rely obviously more on the head than the eye to orient to a target (Comer & Grobstein, 1981) as they do to stabilize their gaze as we have seen above. Their eye saccades have, for a given amplitude of eye displacement, the longest duration (about five times) and lowest velocities of all vertebrates studied so far (Dieringer et al., 1982). An extensive description of the frog's head and eye fast movements has been given by Dieringer et al. (1982) (Ch. 17).

### 2.1.3. Compensation of vestibular lesions

Trabal et al. (1980) and Dieringer and Precht (1981) have described the compensation of bilateral labyrinthine lesions in the frog. Compensation takes 2 or 3 months. There is an interesting dissociation between optokinetically driven head movements which are impaired and do not recover and the vestibulo-collicular reflex which does not recover because absence of labyrinth but is replaced gradually, probably by a proprioceptive input from neck or body. However, the authors have not studied the possible contribution of central 'programs' suggested by similar experiments on primates and man (see sections below).

### 2.2. Eye-head coordination in the rabbit

### 2.2.1. Stabilizing reflexes

During passive rotation in darkness the vestibulo-collicular reflex allows the rabbit to produce compensatory head movements which, combined with the vestibulo-ocular reflex, allow stabilization of gaze. In addition, a cervico-ocular reflex (COR) can be demonstrated by trunk rotation. Although some debate has arisen on this reflex (Gresty, 1976), it seems that it is anti-compensatory i.e., it deviates the eye in the direction of head motion when the head is turning with respect to the trunk). Although one may have believed that during active motion of the trunk with respect to the head, it may have been useful to recalibrate the VCR and VOR, the COR has a very small gain in the normal animal (0.03–0.067 between 0.1 and 0.2 Hz according to Fuller, 1980a). No data is available concerning the role of this low gain system for recovery of vestibular lesion in the rabbit. (It may in fact belong to orienting reflexes). In addition to VOR and VCR the rabbit has also a powerful optokinetic system which has been extensively studied (see Chapter 3).

### 2.2.2. Orienting behaviour

The coordination between eye and head movements in the rabbit has been thoroughly described by Collewijn (1977a). The animal with a freely moving head makes spontaneous saccades as well as synchronous eye-head movements whose characteristics resemble those of the primate. When the head is fixed, however, rabbits rarely make saccades, and all eye movements, such as fast phases of nystagmus, are accompanied by a head torque induced on the holding device (Fuller, (1980b). This suggests a high degree of coupling between eye and head neuronal mechanisms and a rather poor or absent mechanism for uncoupling.

The fact that the rabbit has a visual streak rather than a fovea probably accounts for the absence of any micro-saccades and corrective saccades and probably explains the absence of pursuit mechanism in this animal which follows

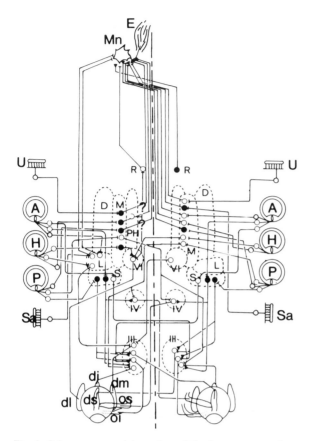

**Fig. 1.** Schema summarizing a few of the known connections between the vestibular receptors, the extraocular muscles and the neck muscles. It appears that the disynaptic vestibular projection to the neck motoneurons is as specific as it is for the extraocular muscles (note that the drawing of connectivity for the vestibulo-ocular pathways is extremely simplified compared to what is now known of the real collateral distribution of second order neurons). The reticulo-spinal system projecting to the neck, which is complex, has been reduced to only one pair of neurons (R) supposed to belong to the medial reticulo-spinal pool because they are the most probable candidates to mediate the 'oculo-collicular coupling' recently described by Roucoux et al. (1982b), Berthoz et al. (1982) and Vidal et al. (1982, 1983a). Note that it is hypothesized in this diagram that the common source for the eye position (or gaze) signal to both the abducens nucleus and the reticulo-spinal neurons is the prepositus nucleus although this is only speculative. R neurons have been located caudal to the vestibular nucleus only for the sake of graphical clarity. White unfilled neurons are excitatory. Black filled neurons are inhibitory. (By courtesy of P. Denise). P, H, A, posterior, horizontal, anterior semicircular canals; U, utriculus; Sa, sacculus; S, M, L, D, superior, medial, lateral, descending vestibular nuclei; III, IV, VI, oculomotor, trochlear, abducens nuclei; dm, ds, dl, medial, superior, lateral recti; oi, os, inferior, superieur obliques; Ph, prepositus hypoglosi nucleus; R, reticulo spinal neurons; Mn, motoneurons; E, extensor neck muscle.

'interesting' things only with a succession of saccades. Otherwise the amplitude-velocity and duration-duration characteristic of rabbit's saccades were found by Collewijn (1977a) to be very similar to those of the primate. There is not study available on eye-head coordination during adaptive processes in the rabbit although this animal has been extensively used for the study of VOR plasticity.

## 2.3. Eye-head coordination in the cat

The cat's eyes are placed in the head in a near to frontal position. Although mainly a nocturnal animal with no fovea but an "area centralis", the cat has a visual system which shares many features with the primate visual system. Head-eye coordination is very elaborate in this animal which uses a combination of stabilizing reflexes (VOR, VCR, COR, CCR) (see review in Peterson and Goldberg, 1982) (Chapter 3) and orienting movements (Blakemore and Donaghy, 1980; Guitton & Douglas, 1981; Roucoux et al., 1981; Harris, 1980; Fuller et al., 1983; Guitton et al, 1984). It is out of the scope of the present paper to review the detailed properties of these subsystems. However, it is relevant to our theme to summarize some recent findings which illustrate the existence of several possibilities for adaptive mechanisms to be brought into action.

### 2.3.1. Stabilizing reflexes

*Vestibulo-ocular reflex (VOR).* The VOR in the cat has been extensively studied (review in Wilson & Melvill Jones, 1979) (Chapters 2 & 3). The purpose of the VOR is to stabilize a visual image on the retina and in the cat (as in man) VOR gain is coupled with the vergence system (Blakemore & Donaghy, 1980). A recent suggestion has bearings on both the understanding of the basic organization of the horizontal VOR and the question of eye-head coordination. The suggestion is that type I, 'horizontal' second order neurons projecting from the medial vestibular nucleus to the contralateral abducens nucleus (i.e., excitatory vestibular neurons which constitutes the second neuron of the disynaptic vestibulo-ocular reflex arc) also project down to the spinal cord as well as to several other brainstem nuclei (McCrea et al.,

1980; Berthoz et al., 1981b; Isu et al., 1984). The exact projection sites are not known. This suggests on one hand a tight coupling between eye and head and also provides a potential alternate route for the VCR pathway in addition to specific vestibulo-spinal neurons. A few of the neurons involved in both VOR and vestibulo-spinal relations are shown in Fig. 1.

*Vestibulo-collicular reflex (VCR)*. In the decerebrate cat the VCR has been quantified by many authors following the first attempts to apply dynamic analysis to these reflexes (Berthoz & Anderson, 1971a,b; Billoto et al., 1982; Ezure & Sasaki, 1978; Schor & Miller, 1981). Recent results indicate that in the alert cat this reflex is itself under modulatory control of an ipsiversive oculo-collicular coupling mechanism (Vidal et al., 1982, 1983a; Berthoz et al., 1982; Roucoux et al;. 1982b) which will be discussed in the next section.

*Cervico-ocular reflex (COR)*. The cervico-ocular reflex in the cat seems to have a low or negligible gain (0.15 at 0.08 Hz and 0.2 at 0.6 Hz trunk rotation in the alert cat according to Fuller, 1980a). It is thought not to play a decisive role (see also Peterson and Goldberg, 1982) except, maybe, for very slow rotations for which the VOR has a varying gain. This does not, however, preclude a basic role of neck proprioception in the central control of gaze in adaptation (see below the evidence obtained in the monkey).

Image stabilization on the retina is also achieved by the optokinetic reflex described in other chapters in this volume. (Chapters 3 & 7).

## 2.3.2. Orienting behaviour

Orienting behaviour of eye and head in the cat is determined both by acoustic and visual targets. The cat is able to make both head and eye movements at velocities as high as 500–600°/s. (Guitton et al., 1984). Saccades are, for a given amplitude, slower than in the monkey but paradoxically their amplitude is greater when the head is moving than when it is fixed (Haddad & Robinson, 1977; Blakemore & Donaghy, 1980; Guitton et al. 1984). Guitton et al. (1980) and Roucoux et al. (1980) have recently proposed a model which describes the basic mechanisms underlying the fixation reflex in the cat and focuses on the role of the superior colliculus. The interesting aspect of this model, for our purpose, is that it suggests the existence of different 'modes' or 'strategies' of eye-head coordination depending upon the eccentricity of the target in space with respect to the head. Three main subcircuits are considered, which correspond to three different 'modes' of eye-head coordination.

*2.3.2.1. Mode 1 or 'coordination by addition of saccade and VOR'* (Fig. 3). This mode would occur in the cat for gaze shifts smaller than 25°. Foveation can be achieved by an eye saccade without head movement, but in practice cats with a freely moving head nearly always make a head movement with the saccade. This is similar to what was described by Bizzi et al. (1971) (see below) in the monkey. The VOR is operating at a gain close to one before, during and after the saccade. It must be said that this suggestion is in contradiction with the observation made by McCrea et al. (1980) and Berthoz et al. (1981b), which indicates that activity of type I second order neurons subtending the VOR, and potentially the VCR, is strongly decreased during saccades. Type I vestibular second order neurons terminating in the Abducens nucleus also probably project to the spinal cord. This makes it likely that the VOR is at least partially suppressed during the saccade even in this mode unless the suppression occurs at spinal cord level and the VCR simply looses access to neck motoneurons by some as yet undefined mechanism. (The VCR *has* to be suppressed during an active head rotation.) However this point is still open and no definitive statement should be made at this stage. The results of Whittington et al. (1984) in the monkey and of Guitton et al. (1984) in the cat suggest that VOR is not suppressed during the saccade.

It is interesting to note that, in their model, Roucoux et al. (1980) predicted that an eye position signal had to be inserted in the head control loop for this mode I which requires a transformation of retinotopic to craniotopic coordinates downstream from the superior colliculus. Vidal et al. (1982) have in fact confirmed this prediction by discovering that the activity of the dorsal neck muscles in the alert cat whose head is fixed is closely correlated with the ipsilateral horizontal

182

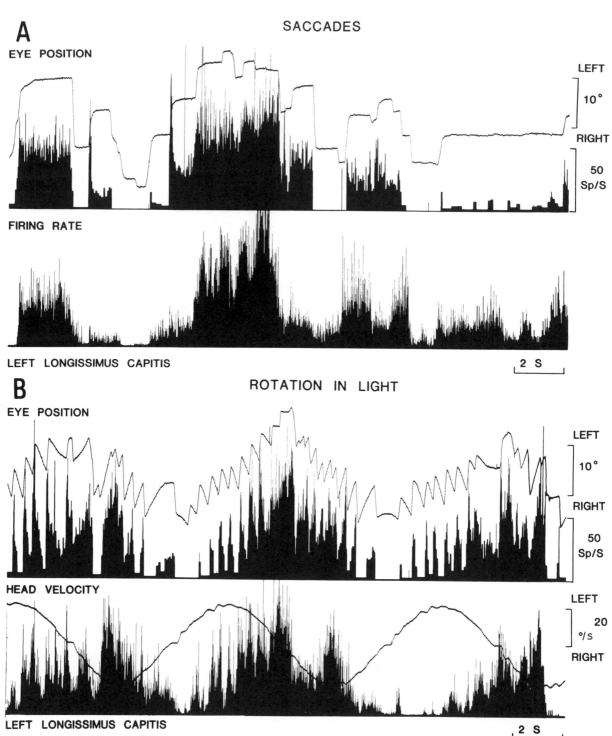

*Fig. 2.* Instantaneous firing rate of a 'burst-tonic' reticular neuron recorded in periabducens area in the alert, head fixed cat. A. Firing pattern during spontaneous fixations. From top to bottom, horizontal component of eye position, firing of the neuron, rectified integrated EMG activity of the left longissimus capitis muscle. B. Firing pattern during sinusoidal head rotation in the light. From top to bottom, horizontal component of eye position firing rate of the neuron, head velocity trace partially overlapping the integrated rectified EMG activity of the left longissimus capitis muscle (from Vidal et al., 1983a).

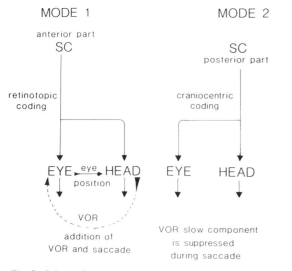

MODE 1                    MODE 2

anterior part
SC                        SC
                          posterior part

retinotopic               craniocentric
coding                    coding

EYE ►eye► HEAD     EYE        HEAD
      position

VOR

addition of               VOR slow component
VOR and saccade           is suppressed
                          during saccade

*Fig. 3.* Schematic representation of the main signal processing properties of the two modes of eye-head configuration in the cat as hypothesized by Roucoux and Crommelinck. (By courtesy of these authors.)

component of eye position. Crommelinck et al. (1982) have also shown that the horizontal eye position signal is present in head free conditions. These findings suggest the existence of a *tonic ipsiversive system* linking the abducens nucleus to the motoneurons of the neck. Berthoz et al. (1982) and Vidal et al. (1983a) have suggested that a reticulo-spinal system would mediate this influence and we suggest that it could be called 'oculo-collicular coupling or synergy'. (Figs. 1 and 2). In the cat this coupling exists for all types of eye movements (fixations, vestibular and opto-kinetic nystagmus). Berthoz and Grantyn (1985) have suggested that reticulospinal neurons subserving that coupling also project to the facial nucleus and probably control an eye-ear-head synergy for orienting. It was confirmed by Wilson et al. (1983) that all compartments of the Splenius muscle show the same behaviour. This coupling is also present in the monkey (Lestienne et al.,) (1984), and Bennett and Savill (1889) had predicted it for humans. Darlot et al. (1985) have shown that this horizontal eye movement signal in neck muscles is blended with the VCR in the frontal plane with a quasi-linear algebraic summation of the two signals (VCR and ipsilateral eye position) during passive head rotations.

This mode would be controlled, according to the model of Roucoux et al. (1980), by the anteri-

or part of the superior colliculus. The output of the colliculus would provide a target position.

*2.3.2.2. Mode 2 or 'coordination by suppression of VOR'.* According to Roucoux et al. (1980) when the target lies outside the 25° range, the signal indicating target eccentricity which is coded in the retinotopic coordinate is transformed at collicular level into craniocentric (in head coordinates) coordinates by adding an efferent copy signal of actual eye position (Fig. 3). The VOR should be suppressed during the saccade but is turned on at the end of the saccade with a gain of one. This suggestion is consistent with the results of McCrea et al. (1980) and Berthoz et al. (1981b). The intermediate zone of superior colliculus would mediate these movements.

This clear distinction between two modes has recently been challenged by Guitton et al. (1985) who have suggested an alternative model of eye-head coordination, in which visually triggered saccades are combined with vestibular quick phases in the context of an extended version of Robinson's local feedback model. Fuller et al. (1983) have even suggested that the amplitude of gaze beyond which summation exists seems to be stochastic.

The most interesting point for the general hypothesis that we have proposed at the onset of this chapter, and for the following considerations concerning humans, is the conclusion of Fuller et al. (1983) that "whatever the origin of alternating eye movements during single step gaze shifts, at the end of the shift the gaze landed accurately on its goal. This accurate landing sometimes occurred in complete darkness... Therefore it seems that the brain can estimate the actual position of gaze with respect to its intended position. The vestibular input may contribute in two ways: not only by driving compensatory eye movement (VOR) but also by providing an internal signal used to compute actual gaze positions... VOR became operative once the intended shift of gaze was complete" (p.249).

This lengthy quotation is fundamental for our perspective because the vestibular input is then not only the origin of a reflex (as hypothesized by Bernstein, 1967, who spoke of the 'two functions' of sensory receptors), but is also essential for the

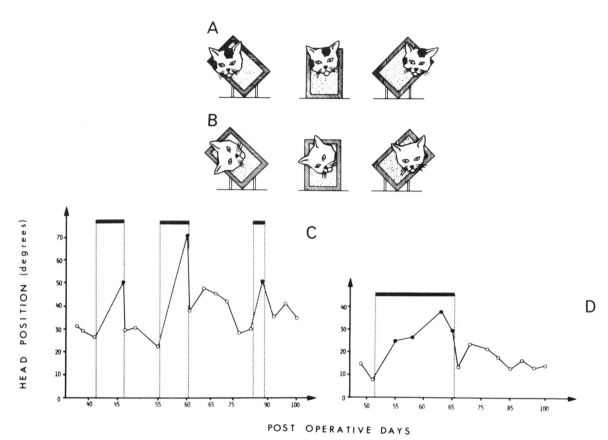

*Fig. 4.* Sensory substitution for head posture control by vision after hemilabyrinthectomy in the cat. A,B. Experiment set-up used to test postural symmetry in the cat (redrawn from original photographs). A. Normal cat. Note incomplete righting of the head when the body is tilted (to the right, $+45°$; or to the left, $-45°$). B. Right hemilabyrinthectomized cat 2 days after operation. Each photograph was analyzed by tracing the inter-ocular axis on the cat's face, and by measuring its angulation with respect to the physical horizontal. Values obtained for a given position (e.g., horizontal, $0°$) were averaged for each session. C,D. Decompensation of head tilt in the dark in two partially compensated cats. In this diagram the values (a) of head-tilt obtained in the three body positions ($+45°$, $0°$, $-45°$) have been averaged.

Open symbols, data taken in the light; dark symbols, in the dark. Areas limited by dotted lines indicate the duration and the position in postoperative time of dark periods. Animal illustrated in C was put in the dark during two periods of 5 days ($42^{nd}$–$47^{th}$, and $55^{th}$–$60^{th}$ postoperative days) and one period of 2 days ($87^{th}$–$89^{th}$ days). Photographs were taken only at the end of the episode, i.e., a few minutes before turning the lights on. Animal illustrated in D was put in the dark for a 14 day period ($51^{st}$–$65^{th}$ postoperative days). Photographs were taken throughout the period (from Putkonen et al., 1977).

central computation of an 'intended' and an 'actual' gaze direction (this idea was also proposed by Chun & Robinson (1978); Lestienne et al. (1981); Mays & Sparks (1980); Roucoux et al. (1980). The mechanisms of adaptation will therefore, in the cat, be themselves dependent upon much more complex processes than a single synaptic rearrangement in a disynaptic reflex pathway.

*2.3.2.3. Mode 3: Body turning.* Lastly, the model supposes that, when a visual target cannot be foveated by an eye and head movement because it is too eccentric, the body is turned. This body turning could be mediated through the most posterior part of the superior colliculus. However, the question of when body turning is used is also a complex problem because involvement of body turning may be imposed by other factors than mechanical limits.

In conclusion, it is interesting to note that this model explicitly suggests that the three modes of orienting possibly subserved by the three parts of the colliculus (anterior, intermediate and posterior), represent the successive steps of eye-head coordination development. The posterior colliculus would be the remainder of the archaic, and phylogenetically oldest, direct control of body movements during orientation in fish, reptiles and lower amphibians (Ewert, 1967). The anterior colliculus would correspond to a more recently developed structure for the execution of saccades, dissociated from head movements, which is particularly developed in primates and humans.

The cat has therefore a repertoire of several mechanisms with which it can modify the gain of compensatory reflexes, switch them off temporarily, or change the modes of head eye coordination. At the present time it is convenient (although probably not exhaustive) to summarize by saying that the cat has two extreme possible strategies.

(a) A 'compensatory' one in which the animal stabilizes gaze in space. In this highly automatized mode the various compensatory reflexes are at play. They can, however, be modulated or even suppressed depending upon where the cat is directing its gaze with respect to its body. (This modulation or suppression can be performed by a signal of eye position sent to the vestibular nuclei, for example, or to the neck.) The eye or gaze signal present in all the stations of the reflex neuronal network allows an automatic correction of reflex gain depending on the intended and actual gaze.

(b) An 'orienting' strategy in which synergistic activation of eye and head is made with both phasic and tonic activities. Phasic activity of the neck is probably mediated by the tecto-bulbo-oculomotor and tecto-bulbo-spinal system (Grantyn and Berthoz, 1983; Grantyn & Berthoz, 1985).

It seems that when an adaptive change is required, the first response of the animal could be to *compose* a combination of the available very rich repertoire of these modes and capabilities without first using any plastic change; unless, as stated in the introduction, required to *stabilize*

and retain the constructed combination, or to create a durable new set of modes.

### 2.3.3. Adaptive processes

*2.3.3.1. Recovery from vestibular lesions.* The recovery after peripheral block was studied by Baker et al. (1982). After canal plugging in the cat the cervico-ocular gains did not increase very much (0.06–0.08 at 0.5–2 Hz horizontal rotation in dark). However, this modest contribution of the COR to recovery may be dependent upon the experimental situation. Two weeks after plugging, some signs of a build up of compensatory eye movements by preprogramming were observed (Fig. 1D of their paper).

In fact remarkably little work has been done on adaptive processes in eye-head coordination in the cat. Putkonen et al. (1977) have studied the compensation of head posture following hemi-labyrinthectomy (see Fig. 4) and have described the important role of vision in the recovery of normal head posture, but have not related this process to eye movements. However, in the light of recent findings of Vidal et al. (1982, 1983a,b) and Berthoz et al. (1982) it is possible that part of the role attributed to 'vision' is in fact dependent upon the tonic oculo-collicular coupling system discovered by these authors.

An hypothesis could be that, after hemilabyrinthectomy, in darkness head posture asymmetry is due to two combined factors: (a) an unbalanced vestibulo-spinal influence, and (b) an asymmetry of eye position which induces an additional unbalance through the reticulo-spinal pathways mediating the tonic oculo-collicular coupling (Berthoz et al. 1982; Vidal et al. 1983). When the animal is in the light, visual cues help the animal to recenter the eye in the orbit decreasing the effect of the oculo-collicular coupling.

### 2.4. Eye-head coordination in the monkey

The monkey is a foveated animal in which all the compensatory reflexes described in the cat are operating (VOR, VCR, COR, OKR). The subsystems involved in oculomotor control for this species are described in Chapters 3, 8 & 16, they will therefore not be reviewed here.

### 2.4.1. Orienting behaviour

#### 2.4.1.1. Cooperation of saccades and vestibulo-ocular reflex.
Eye-head coordination in the monkey has been extensively studied by Bizzi and his colleagues (Bizzi et al., 1971, 1972a,b; Morasso et al., 1973) and reviewed by Bizzi (1981). An essential result is that, in the simplest case, called the 'triggered mode' (when a target is flashed at the periphery of the visual field and the monkey is trained to make a combined eye and head movement to orient gaze in the direction of the target), a stereotyped sequence of events occurs. First the brain computes target eccentricity in craniotopic coordinates and gives a phasic motor order to *both* the head and eye motor systems to execute the appropriate saccade; the eye starts first due to its small inertia and high dynamic muscle properties, the head follows. When the head starts to rotate the eye saccade is still developing and the VOR reduces its peak amplitude and recenters the eye in the orbit with a gain of approximately one.

Often a monkey will orient in anticipation of a stimulus. In this case, called by Bizzi the 'predictive mode', the relation between head and eye is complex, and the head often starts to move before the eye.

In addition to these two phasic modes of orienting, Lestienne et al. (1984) have shown recently that, during spontaneous gaze changes with head fixed, the tonic horizontal eye position signal which had been found in the cat (Vidal et al., 1982, 1983a) is present. This tonic synergy of eye and head is clearly shown by the parallel course of head torque in the horizontal plane and horizontal eye position, and it indicates that the coupling mechanism which links eye position to ispilateral neck muscles in the rabbit and cat is probably also present in the monkey. Kubo et al. (1981a,b) have also shown that, during OKN or vestibular stimulation, there is a synergy between horizontal eye position and head torque (or EMG). However, by contrast with lower species, the monkey can obviously decouple this linkage and, during a saccade both the 'vestibulo-collicular' and the 'oculo-collicular' reflexes can be suppressed.

#### 2.4.1.2. 'Central programming'.
A major finding which is essential to understand adaptive mechanisms in gaze control is the fact that the final head and eye positions have been shown by Bizzi et al. (1976) to be dependent upon a so-called 'central program' which is set in advance in the case of visually triggered movements, and which does not depend upon neck proprioceptive signals during the movement. Central programming and storage of pursuit has also been demonstrated by Lanman et al. (1978) who in an elegant experiment, showed that if a monkey pursues a visual target with the head, and if the head rotation is suddenly braked by a motor, the eye immediately starts to pursue the target with a latency (15 ms) too short to involve any visual feedback (minimum 50–60 ms). The authors concluded that a central process called 'calculation of perceived target velocity' was generating and controlling the smooth pursuit. Eckmiller and Mackeben (1978) also showed that when the light is turned off during the pursuit of a sinusoidally moving target in the monkey, abducens motoneurons continued to be modulated for a few seconds at a rate which is adequate to pursue the now absent target with the 'adequate' velocity. This finding would point to a pursuit velocity storage mechanism which may keep stored centrally the dynamics of target velocity in the *absence of any physical stimulus*, and utilise this memory for preprogramming of gaze shifts. (see Chapters 3 & 13).

We shall now see how this repertoire of capabilities is used by the monkey to respond to adaptive challenge due to lesions of the peripheral vestibular nerve.

### 2.4.2 Recovery from vestibular peripheral lesions

#### 2.4.2.1. Sensory substitution and adaptive strategies.
The accomplishment of a precise orientation of gaze to a target is heavily dependent, in the monkey, upon the vestibular system which allows an automatic regulation of eye position depending on head movement. However, if this clever way of preventing the brain from having to worry about what the head is doing is impaired by labyrinthectomy, the CNS has to find a substitute process. Dichgans et al. (1973a) showed that, following bilateral vestibulectomy in *Macaca mulata* monkeys, the compensatory eye move-

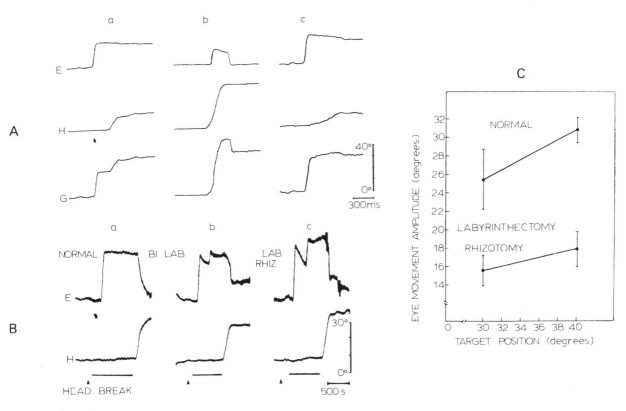

Fig. 5. A. Strategies of eye-head coordination in the first days following labyrinthectomy. Eye movements (E). Head movements (H). Gaze movements (G) represent the sum of E plus H. (a) Delayed initiation of head movement; (b) coordination achieved almost exclusively with the head; (c) reduction in head velocity. B. Evidence of centrally programmed compensatory eye movements. Eye movements (E); head movements (H); arrow indicates target light; lower line indicates unexpected stopping of head movements. (a) Intact normal monkey. Note lack of compensatory eye movement. (b) Bilateral labyrinthectomized monkey. Note centrally programmed compensatory eye movement. (c) Labyrinthectomized animal subjected to C1–C6 dorsal rhizotomy. Note increase in compensatory eye movement. The eye movement after release of the head break only in A fully matches the head movement, whereas in B and C a saccade is triggered. Vertical scale indicates eye calibration. C. Comparison of saccade amplitude during head movement in the intact monkey (upper line) and in a labyrinthectomized and rhizotomized monkey (lower line). Note that saccades made during head movement also in the intact monkey are shorter than inter-target intervals (for further explanation see Morasso et al., 1973) (N = 25 for each data point) (from Dichgans et al., 1973).

ments disappeared immediately and then recovered, reaching, within 7 weeks, 90% of the control value. Three mechanisms seem to underly this recovery (a summary of their results is shown in Fig. 5).

(a) Firstly, an increase in the gain of the cervico-ocular reflex. This reflex has normally a very small contribution to the compensatory eye movements. Dichgans et al. (1973) have calculated a gain of about 0.02–0.03 for *Macacca mulata*, and Fuller, (1980a), on another primate (the bush baby), a gain of 0.015–0.024 between 0.08 and 0.6 Hz. However this reflex allowed of compensation of head movements with a gain of 0.3,

55 days after the lesions (see Fig. 6 of their paper which illustrates this remarkable time course of potentiation of the neck-ocular loop following passive head rotation).

(b) Secondly, in the first post-operative days, a variety of combinations of eye and head movements which were obviously 'tried' by the monkey (they are illustrated in Fig. 5A).

(c) Thirdly, preprogrammed compensatory eye movements. These preprogrammed movements appeared within the first day after lesion (Fig. 4B), their amplitude was 1–12° (for a 30–40° gaze change) and their duration 200–400 ms. They were further enhanced when labyrinthec-

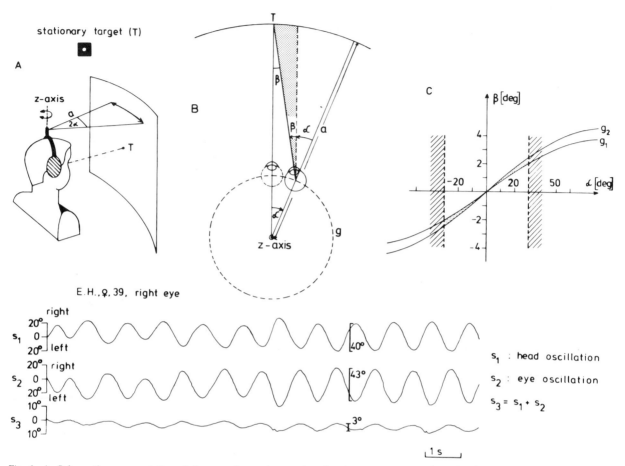

Fig. 6. A. Schematic representation of the experimental procedure for the measurement of eye-head coordination and retinal slip during oscillatory head movements about the vertical, z-axis with fixation of a stationary target. B. Geometrical representation of the different angles of head and eye rotation required in order to maintain fixation on the target during head oscillation. For an accurate determination of eye-head coordination, it is necessary to calculate the required additional rotation of the eye ($\beta$) which results from the different axis of rotation of eye and head. C. $\beta$ as a function of angular head displacement for a distance of 1.2 m between z-axis and fixaton target. $\alpha$ = Angle of head rotation; $\alpha + \beta$ = angle of eye rotation; $\beta$ = additional angle of eye rotation; g = head circumference ($g_1$ = 0.51 m, $g_2$ = 0.61 m); $a$ = target-z-axis distance ($a$ = 1.2 m). D. Records of head ($S_1$) and eye ($S_2$) oscillations at 1 Hz. The algebric sum $S_1 + S_2 = S_3$ gives retinal slip which in this particular case was 3° (from Wist et al., 1983).

tomy was combined with rhizotomy (cervical deafferentations including suppression of the cervico-ocular reflex). However their amplitude had no clear relation with amplitude of head movement. In addition, the monkey clearly was using 'adaptive strategies' such as the reduction of saccadic amplitude for a given gaze change (see Fig. 5C) (this prevented the gaze overshoot and there-

fore compensated for the absence of VOR saccade interaction).

Kubo et al. (1981a) have studied the effect of lateral semi-circular canal plugging on eye-head coordination in squirrel monkeys. They analyzed horizontal eye and head nystagmus during optokinetic stimulation. They showed that the slow phase of head nystagmus during OKN decreases after canal plugging and suggest that repeated measurements of head and eye velocity may provide a useful tool of functional compensation after vestibular lesion. Igarashi et al. (1983) also investigated a rather forgotten area of the cerebellum which may have important functions in eye-head coordination: the uvula and modulus. After uvulonodular lesion they found marked alterations in several aspects of eye-head coordination.

*2.4.2.2. Role of early post-lesion activity.* The above observation of the various active attempts made by a monkey on the first post-operative days are important because they demonstrate the *choice* of solutions that the animal is making, but also they suggest an important role for *post-lesional activity*. Although they were not dealing with eye-head coordination specifically, Igarashi et al. (1975, 1979) have drawn attention to the very fundamental role of *early post-lesion activity* for the completion of compensation as tested by eye movements or equilibrium tests. Similar emphasis has been put forward by Xerri and Lacour (1980) and Lacour et al. (1976), who showed that activity after labyrinthectomy considerably increases the speed of recovery of vestibulo-spinal mechanisms. It could be hypothesized, following the line of thoughts proposed in the introduction of this chapter, that activity allows a more complete and efficient organization and tuning of the adequate combination of subsystems. By exploring combinations of *available subsystems*, activity allows also the identification of appropriate *plastic* changes to be made. It is also most probable that central rewiring, when necessary, is facilitated by activity, a fact known to be true for the development of direction specificity in the visual system.

## 3. Eye-head coordination in humans: reflex plasticity and/or orchestration of available repertoire of subsystems?

### 3.1. Normal properties of eye-head coordination in humans

Eye-head coordination in humans has been stu-

died in a great variety of conditions in which either the goal of the gaze shift or the type of stimulus was different. We shall distinguish several conditions. Some of them have already been defined for the monkey, others are specific to experimental situations used by investigators in human studies (although they could of course have been used in the monkey). It is of great importance to distinguish clearly these different situations because different combinations of adaptive mechanisms may be specific for each of them. We shall not review here the basic properties of the oculomotor subsystem in the human. They are discussed extensively in Chapters 2, 3 & 11.

Most of the available results on eye-head coordination concern eye and head rotation in the *horizontal* plane during *active* or *passive* movements either in *light* or in *darkness*, in adults (Melvill Jones, 1964, 1966; Gresty, 1974; Gresty & Ell, 1982; Barnes & Somerville, 1978; Barnes, 1979a; Tomlinson et al., 1980; Uemura et al., 1980; Zangemeister & Stark, 1981, 1982; Zangemeister et al., 1981,a,b, 1982) or in children (Funk & Anderson, 1977; Roucoux et al., 1982a). We shall summarize the findings obtained in two main situations.

(a) Compensatory eye-head movements which are necessary if a subject maintains gaze on an earth fixed target. The geometrical aspects of this situation are shown in Fig. 6. Collewijn et al. (1982) have also described these characteristics.

(b) The orienting eye-head movements accomplished when the subject shifts his gaze from one target to another.

### 3.1.1. Passive or active head rotation with maintenance of gaze to an earth fixed target (compensatory or stabilizing mode)

If a subject maintains his gaze fixed to an earth stationary visual target and turns his head in the horizontal plane, the eye rotates in the head with a compensatory movement of exactly opposite direction and velocity to that of the head (Figs. 6 & 8). This *compensatory* movement can be produced by the VOR, the pursuit system or by the cervico-ocular reflex. The role of these compensatory mechanisms has been studied in two conditions: oscillatory or single head movement.

*3.1.1.1. Oscillatory head movements.* When a

subject moves his head in the horizontal plane a perception of visual world motion called 'oscillopsia' (see review in Bender, 1965; Atkin and Bender, 1968; Wist et al., 1983) is produced when retinal slip becomes too great or when central disorders prevent perceptual stabilization. Normally, however, stabilization in the light is excellent for rather rapid head oscillations. Recently, it has been shown that in *darkness*, during active head shaking in the horizontal plane, and imagining an earth fixed target, the gain of the VOR is 0.9–1.1 according to Tomlinson et al. (1980) and 0.92 according to Jell et al. (1982) up to frequencies of 4 or 5 Hz (see also Collewijn et al., 1983). This compensation by the VOR is not as good during *passive* whole body rotation (Benson 1970). The increase of VOR efficiency during *active* head movement could be due to the cervico-ocular reflex, but Meiry (1971) and Barnes and Forbat (1979) have shown that the gain of this reflex is very small (0.05 during passive body rotation between 0.2 and 1.3 Hz with head fixed as reported by the latter authors). VOR gain is also dependent upon target distance (Biguer & Prablanc, 1981). In addition, even with retinal slip of up to 20′ of arc for Skavenski et al. (1979) and 4°/s for Steinman and Collewijn (1980), perceived stability was not impaired. Development of gaze fixation and pursuit during eye-head coordination have recently been studied by Roucoux et al. (1982a; 1983). They have shown that, although in young infants (5 weeks) fixation is accompanied by several small hypometric saccades, after a few weeks eye-head coordination seems basically the same as in the adult. It also seems that after a few weeks of age the eye-head coordination pattern during pursuit does not change with age.

*3.1.1.2. Single head movements.* One can therefore expect that, during a single head movement in darkness or in light, the VOR gain will be about one, and that even for rather high velocities the stabilization of gaze will be efficient. This particular pattern will be discussed in the next section.

*3.1.2. Passive or active head rotation to a new direction of gaze (orienting behaviour)*
*3.1.2.1. Rotation in darkness.* If instead of being instructed to keep 'looking' at an initial target the subject is told to shift his gaze to a new target in the direction of head movement, an orienting pattern of eye-head coordination is observed, both in the passive or active head movement. (*Passive* head movement can be induced by body rotation or by head rotation on the trunk. In humans, given the low contribution of the cervico-ocular reflex, the two situations yield similar general patterns.) When the head starts moving, passively or actively, and the subject is instructed to orient his gaze to an earth fixed eccentric *imagined* target, a compensatory eye movement is first produced by the VOR with a gain of about one in most subjects (Fig. 9A). After a latency which depends upon the experimental conditions, a single or several saccades (or quick phases) are initiated in the anticompensatory (same direction as head movement) direction. This saccade, which is also present in the cat, has been described by Melvill Jones (1964) and Henriksson et al. (1974) following sudden onset or arrest of passive body rotation in dark. Barnes (1979a) has calculated the latencies of onset of the first saccade (see Table 1) in different conditions. Uemura et al. (1980) have obtained numbers which are in the same range for closed loop conditions.

*Table 1*

Mean time lag between eye and head movements for head rotation in the horizontal plane and for the following conditions: (1) passive head rotation in darkness; (2) active head rotation in darkness; (3) active head rotation to a visual eccentric target flashed before start of head movement (open loop condition); (4) active head rotation to a visual eccentric target continuously present (closed loop condition). Positive numbers indicate that eye saccade starts after onset of head movement (from Barnes, 1979a).

|  | Latency (ms) | S.D. (ms) |
|---|---|---|
| 1. Passive head rotation in darkness | 140 | 85 |
| 2. Active head rotation in darkness | 78 | 78 |
| 3. Target flashed condition (open loop) | 30 | 57 |
| 4. Continuous target presentation in the light (closed loop) | − 1 | 58 |

The saccade rarely precedes active head movement in darkness (Melvill Jones and Berthoz, unpublished observation) and never precedes passive head movement. Sometimes it can start simultaneously with the head movement in darkness. Barnes (1979a) has suggested that during voluntary movement in darkness the saccade may be initiated by a central command, an hypothesis which is identical to the one proposed by Bizzi for the monkey. The hypothesis was therefore made by Barnes (1979a) that "in the absence of adequate retinal information the vestibulo-ocular reflex could provide an estimate for future head position". Other parameters of the eye-head sequence have been analyzed. Most authors agree that total head displacement at the end of the first saccade is proportional to gaze displacement in all conditions (slope 1°/s; intercept 1°). Bard et al (1982) have found a great variability and suggested a classification in 'head movers' and 'non head movers'. This linkage between saccade and head movement does not seem to be present in newborns during passive head movements (who show the doll's eye phenomenon) and is reduced in blind persons (Henriksson et al., 1974). It is present, however, in newborns during active head movements (Roucoux et al., 1983).

*3.1.2.2. Rotation in the light.* When the subject is asked to orient suddenly to a visual target, the basic pattern of eye-head coordination in humans is essentially the same as in monkeys, (Fig. 10A). The latency of the 'leading' saccade is given in Table 1 for the open (with visual feedback) and closed loop conditions. Head velocity is proportional to gaze displacement (Slope 1.2°/s per degree; intercept 12.6°). There is no significant difference between the two visual conditions (open and closed loop) for the head-gaze displacement relationship, but a greater difference in timing of head movement and eye saccades for continuously present and flashed targets: when the target is continuously present, the latency between target onset and eye saccades ranges from 243–383 ms for gaze angles of 15 and 75°, whereas the range is 317–396 ms when the target is flashed (open loop) (Barnes, 1979a).

Zangemeister and Stark (1982) have recently described, for fast voluntary closed loop orienting eye movements, the main characteristics of eye-head motion patterns in the case of predictable visual target jumps. They propose to present the data in the form of a *gaze latency* diagram which is a plot of eye movement onset latency (with respect to target onset) versus head movement onset latency. They found that, following the trigger signal, eye movement and head movement onsets were co-varying but were dependent upon a number of factors, such as predictability, fatigue, frequency of target jumps, etc. Latencies found by these authors are similar to latencies measured by Barnes (1979a) also in a closed loop condition. The variability of these latencies was also described by Funk and Anderson (1977) in children. All authors take this variability as a sign of a high capability of humans to dissociate eye and head movements.

*3.1.3. Eye-head coordination during pursuit*

Very little is known about pursuit of moving targets by eye and head in man, although it is a very common motor behaviour. Collewijn et al. (1982a,b) have recently studied this problem following the earlier studies of Fleming et al. (1969), Shirachi et al. (1978) and Gresty and Leech (1977). In the horizontal direction with the target moving in an unpredictable way, they show that the quality of pursuit is equally good (about 1.5° error) when the subject uses mainly his eyes or his head, except that pursuit with the eyes becomes poor when target excursion is greater than 30–40°. VOR suppression is often incomplete, as was also noticed by Gresty and Leech (1977) and is frequency dependent (Barnes and Sommerville, 1978) (see also Bard et al., 1982).

*3.2. Compensation of vestibular deficits*

Among all pathological deficits which have been shown to impair eye-head coordination (see reviews in Zee, 1977, Gresty & Halmagyi, 1979, Cohen, 1981, Gresty, 1982, Lennerstrand et al., 1982, Roucoux & Crommelinck, 1982, Pfaltz, 1983, Wist et al. 1983) peripheral vestibular deficit is a particularly interesting case because it suppresses, as we have seen previously, the main automatic mechanism for recentering the eye during head movement.

192

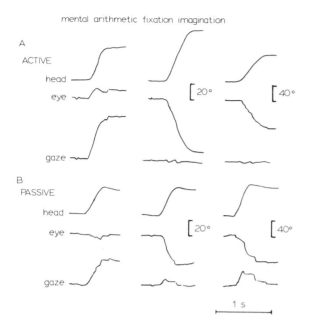

mental arithmetic   fixation   imagination

A
ACTIVE
head
eye
                                           [20°          [40°

gaze

B
PASSIVE
head
eye
                                           [20°          [40°

gaze

1 s

*Fig. 7.* Compensation of the vestibulo-oscular reflex in labyrinthectomised patients. Horizontal eye and head movements in a patient during active or passive head rotation under three conditions: (a) mental arithmetic (M.A.), subject performs mental arithmetic; (b) fixation, subject attempts to keep gaze on a stationary visible target; (c) imagination, in total darkness subject attempts to maintain gaze on the imagined location of the fixation target. A. Active head rotation made on command. In the mental arithmetic paradigm a saccade is usually made synchronously with the head movement and gaze is inadequately stabilized. With fixation of the visual target and, remarkably, using imagination in total darkness stability is nearly perfect. B. Passive, non-predictable head rotations. Long latency and low gain of the passively induced cervico-ocular reflex are noted in the M.A. paradigm. With imagination in darkness, the cervico-ocular reflex is potentiated with the velocity of compensatory slow phases near the velocity of the head. Saccades are also used to correct position errors, even in total darkness (from Kasai & Zee, 1978; redrawn from original publication). Notice saccades on eye records.

Although it is known that peripheral vestibular lesion induces strong deficits in the tonic posture of the head in humans and animals (see Chapter 17), and it has been suggested that vision in the cat plays a role in the recovery of normal head position (Putkonen et al., 1977), only recently has there been systematic quantified studies of the influence of vestibular deficits on eye-head coordination. Zee (1977) in his review concerning patients with cerebellar disorders, congenital motor apraxia and labyrinthine defective patients, gives,

a particular emphasis to a group of three subjects with complete loss of vestibular function due to childhood meningitis. In these patients, compensation from vestibular lesions was adequate but not always as complete as the one reported by Dichgans et al. (1973) for the monkey. More recently Takahashi et al. (1981) found that compensatory eye movements in patients with bilateral labyrinthectomy amount to 38–40% of compensatory movements found in normal subjects performing mental arithmetic. For instance, during active head shaking in darkness, the compensatory eye-head gain ranged from 0.2 to 0.58 at 0.67 Hz. Kasai and Zee (1978) reported, for similar conditions, 0.5–0.96 at 0.5 Hz for 40–50° of head oscillation amplitude. For patients with unilateral lesions, compensatory gain for movements towards the intact side was similar to the normal, and for movements to the lesioned side it was similar to the bilateral labyrinthectomized patients.

Such compensatory gain has to be due to nonvestibular mechanisms. The *cervico-ocular reflex* is a possible candidate (Botros, 1979) if one recalls the result of Dichgans et al. (1973) in the monkey. However, it seems that in man this reflex makes a modest contribution to the recovery. Zee (1977) reports a gain of 0.27 and 0.5 at 0.5 Hz during body rotation for two patients without labyrinth, head fixed in darkness, while doing mental arithmetic. These numbers should be compared with remarkably high gains of 0.88 and 0.97, respectively, measured in the same patients during active head movement with imagined targets in darkness at the same frequency. A similar result was reported by Barnes (1979b) in labyrinthine defective patients.

All authors agree on the fact that patients use various strategies to compensate for the absence of labyrinth: corrective saccades, in particular, seem to be often used during head shaking or orienting movements, together with quick phases which are in the opposite direction to the head movement, and therefore are also opposite in direction to the head movement and the 'leading' saccade or quick phase described by Melvill Jones (1964). The question is, therefore, to know if the saccade normally triggered during active or passive head movement in darkness is reversed by labyrinthine defective patients to substitute for an absent VOR, or if a novel 'saccade-like' or 'pursuit-like' eye movement is produced by another mechanism. That the latter is true is indicated by several other results (see Section below).

Modifications of the saccadic system also involve a clear recalibration of saccade amplitude and of target location during active head turning (a result similar to the one of Dichgans et al. (1973) in the monkey). Such a use of the saccadic system to substitute for the pathological loss of pursuit has been found in amblyopic patients by Ciuffreda et al. (1979) and in hemianopic patients by Meienberg et al. (1981) and Zangemeister et al. (1982). The latter authors noted that, during orienting movements to the blind hemifield, patients with homonymous hemianopia made 'synkinetic' head and eye staircase movements or immobilized the head. It is interesting to recall that this strategy (using the saccadic system) was associated with a differential change of VOR gain, i.e., an increase during gaze shifts towards the blind hemifield, and a decrease in the other direction. This complex strategy involves probably central processing at a higher level than the brain stem mechanisms. An indication that complex central processing is taking place is given by increased latency for head movements in these patients (see Fig. 7).

An elegant way to demonstrate central 'programming' is to brake the head in the course of its movements. Morasso et al. (1973) and Kasai and Zee (1978) have used this technique and demonstrated, in labyrinthine defective patients, that the compensatory eye movement continued to develop in the absence of any visual or vestibular drive after head blockage. This finding is similar to the observations made by Melvill Jones et al. (1983) after wearing reversing prisms (see below).

Finally, adaptive processes occurring after lesions, can be evidenced by the variations of the amount of perceived image motion (oscillopsia). These problems have been discussed extensively by Wist et al. (1983) and will therefore not be reviewed here.

## 3.3. Adaptation to environmental changes

When visual world motion is modified by optical means, it is necessary to reorganize the pattern of eye-head coordination for either stabilization of gaze or orienting. Two main experimental devices have been used with which eye-head coordination was studied: magnifying lenses and reversing prisms. Lenses produce change in apparent visual motion velocity in all directions without any change in perceived direction; dove prisms produce a reversal of apparent visual motion in the horizontal and frontal (torsional) plane with no change in the vertical sagittal plane.

### 3.3.1. Change induced by magnifying lenses

Gauthier and Robinson (1975) have explored in humans the changes in active VOR induced by wearing 2.1x magnifying lenses for 5 days. This work is reviewed in Chapter 2. More recently Collewijn et al. (1983) studied the effects of relatively small changes in the visual magnification factor introduced by ordinary spectacles. They measured the time course and completeness of VOR adaptation, differences between active and passive rotation in the light and the dark, and differences between the two eyes. Subjects made head oscillations in the frequency range between 0.33 and 1.33 Hz. The subjects wore magnifying or reducing spectacles of low optical power for periods of 40 min to 24 h. They observed a very rapid adaptation (within 30 min). Differential adaptation to unequal demands for the two eyes proved to be very hard or impossible. They concluded that retinal slip, although it is the initial driving force, may not be the prime adaptive factor, and agree with the hypothesis of Miles and Lisberger (1981) who proposed that a substitute would be the pursuit system.

"The burden of compensation is transferred in this time (during adaptation course) to the VOR, possibly to relieve the pursuit system from a routine stabilization task which would require constant effort and keep it free to pursue targets moving independently of the head" (Collewijn et al., 1983, p. 284).

### 3.3.2. Short and long term adaptation in eye-head coordination during prism reversal adaptation

When a subject wears reversing prisms the VOR operates in the wrong direction and image stabilization on the retina in the horizontal plane

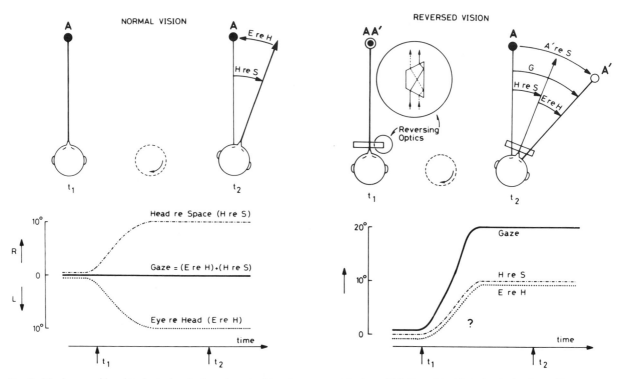

*Fig. 8.* Ideal eye and head trajectories during a transient head movement during which the subject is instructed to keep his gaze on a stationary target. A. Normal case. Head and eye trajectories are of opposite direction and amplitude. This corresponds to a VOR gain of one. B. During prism wearing. Due to reversed vision, eye movement has to be of the same direction and amplitude as head motion. Target moves at twice head velocity (from Melvill Jones & Berthoz (unpublished)).

requires dramatic rearrangements whose features and implications are reviewed in Chapter 2. During active head movements the various eye-head coordination patterns which have been described above also have to be modified (see Fig. 8). The corresponding adaptive processes have been studied behaviourally on human subjects in several experiments which will now be reviewed. Emphasis will be put in this section on the remarkable ability of the central nervous system to generate adequate adaptive behaviour using parametric changes of reflex activity plus a combination, or orchestration, of available oculomotor or oculo-cephalo-motor subsystems to achieve the adaptive goal.

### 3.3.2.1. *Is the optokinetic system or pursuit contributing to rapid movements?* A good example is given by Melvill Jones and Gonshor (1982) who studied thoroughly the modification of active ocu-

lomotor behaviour in three subjects who wore dove prisms for 17, 29 and 49 days, respectively. The main conclusions of this study (see also Chapter 2) were that:

(a) the dynamics of pursuit, by head fixed subjects, of a visual target oscillating horizontally at frequencies up to 4 Hz was unchanged (typically the gain decreased from one to about 0.8 between 0.3 and 1 Hz, and dropped quickly to 0.1 at 4 Hz exactly as in control tests performed on the same subject);

(b) saccadic amplitude-duration characteristics were unchanged;

(c) when the adapted subjects were instructed to shake their head sinusoidally while stabilizing gaze in space (head oscillating at 1.75 and 3 Hz while fixating an earth fixed target) a substantial VOR gain decrease was observed. It was associated with perceptual blurring. However, VOR gain was found to be frequency dependent.

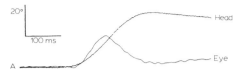

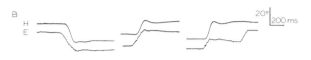

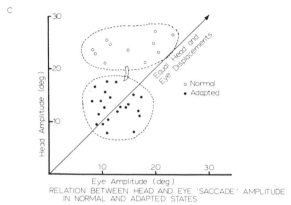

*Fig. 9.* Eye and head movements in the horizontal plane in a subject who wore reversing prisms for 19 days. A. Normal eye-head coordination during active head rotation in the dark. The typical sequence of movement is composed of an initial VOR (which is here very short) followed by a saccade in the same direction as the head motion. The VOR has in this case a gain of nearly one as judged by the clearly opposite trajectories of head and eye. B. Adapted response after 7 days of reversing prism wearing (Active rotation in the dark). Note the fact that although the subject does not see the reversed target image motion the VOR gain is practically zero. C Relation between head and eye saccade amplitudes in normal and adapted states. The eye saccade which has an amplitude smaller than head movement in the normal case tends to have an amplitude similar to head movement in the adapted state (from Melvill Jones & Berthoz, 1981, unpublished).

The nature of the processes underlying adaptation was studied by temporarily removing the prisms and testing eye movements during head shaking in the adapted subjects. At a head shaking frequency of 0.5 Hz, in spite of a *normal* visual motion because prisms were removed, the eye movements remained *reversed* relative to the normal VOR. This result was most surprising because at this frequency pursuit should have been able to achieve fixation. At 3 Hz, in the same conditions, the response was attenuated but not reversed, although 'pursuit' could not (according to classical results on normal subjects as well as control tests on the same subject) be efficient at this frequency. When prisms were put on and head shaken at 3 Hz, a drastic change in phase occurred. Change in phase of the ocular response occurred. This implies, that, at a frequency too high for effective visual tracking, vision played a critical role in changing the eye movement. An analogous effect is the visual restoration of VOR gain, from 1.3 in darkness to 1 in light, when a monkey is oscillated at 4 Hz (Kelly, 1978).

This finding may seem to contradict the usual conception that visual motion direction is a 'slow' system (acting on perception or postural control only below approx. 1 Hz). It is, however, compatible with observations made on rapid effects of vision on postural reaction shown by Nashner and Berthoz (1978), reviewed in Berthoz et al. (1979); and also with recent observations by Kawano and Miles (1983) on the contribution of vision to the pursuit of a rapidly shifting visual scene.

Melvill Jones and Gonshor (1982), after 'dissecting' the adaptive response into two putative components (a simple gain change and a 'complex' frequency dependent change), suggest that a "novel kind of adaptive effect" could thus be at play, manifest as an adaptively enhanced access of vision to control of the VOR, a suggestion recently substantiated by Ferran et al. (1984).

*3.3.2.2. Adaptive modification of the vestibulo-ocular reflex during transient head rotation, or the power of strategies.* An interesting question is whether long term vision reversal produces adaptive reversal of the VOR during rapid stepwise rotation of the head. We have investigated (Berthoz et al., 1981a,c; Melvill Jones & Berthoz, 1981; Berthoz & Melvill Jones, 1981) long term adaptive modifications in a human subject who wore horizontally reversing dove prisms continuously for 19 days. Eye-head coordination was tested by passive and active transient head movements in the horizontal plane either in darkness or in the light.

During *active head movements in darkness* we observed, after 19 days of prism wearing, a novel

196

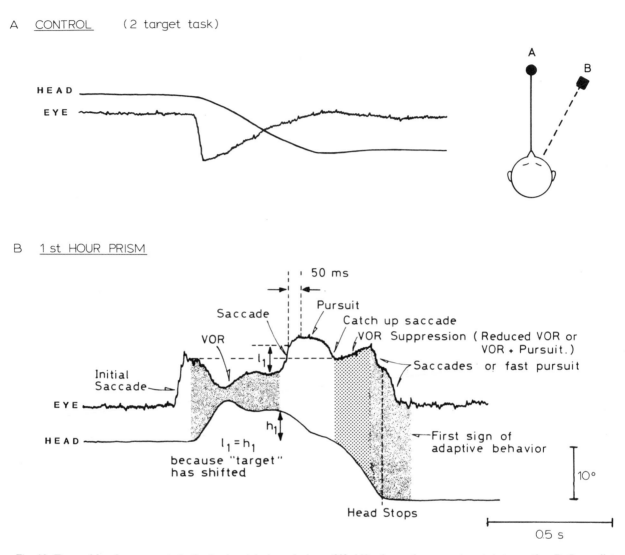

A   CONTROL   (2 target task)

B   1st HOUR PRISM

50 ms

Saccade
Pursuit
Catch up saccade
VOR Suppression (Reduced VOR or
VOR + Pursuit.)

VOR

Saccades or fast pursuit

Initial
Saccade

EYE

$l_1$

$h_1$

HEAD

First sign of
adaptive behavior

$l_1 = h_1$
because "target"
has shifted

10°

Head Stops

0.5 s

*Fig. 10.* Eye and head movements in the horizontal plane during a 20° shift of gaze from one target A to another B. Immediate adaptation to prism wearing. A. Typical sequence of normal eye and head movements. Note that the subject makes a 20° saccade towards the target B followed by a head movement. The VOR slows the saccade and induces a compensatory eye movement. B. Sequence of eye and head movements during one of the first attempts of the same subject wearing reversing prisms. Note that the initial saccade is to the direction of the reversed image, and that after trying a few of the combinations belonging to his oculomotor repertoire the subject succeeds in performing a head and eye movement in the same direction by a succession of rapid eye movements with an apparent suppression of VOR. This constitutes the first sign of adaptive behavior after only a few minutes of prism wearing. (From Melvill Jones et al., 1983, unpublished).

form of rapid eye movement whose amplitude, direction and velocity in the orbit closely paralleled the amplitude and velocity of the head movement relative to space (Fig. 9B). As such, it would be suitable for following the reversed moving image on the retina if the movement were made in the light and if the subject was instructed to keep gaze fixed on the visual target viewed

through the prisms, i.e., it looked like a reversed VOR. However, this movement had a variable, often negative latency, and VOR did occur infrequently with a reduced gain but normal direction. The fact that VOR was reduced in gain but not reversed was demonstrated by *passive head rotation in darkness* during which VOR gain (eye velocity versus head velocity) ranged from 0.27 to

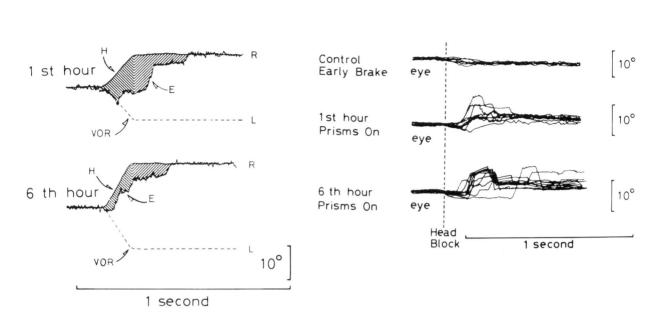

*Fig. 11.* Typical eye and head movements of a subject wearing reversing prisms for 6 h. A. Short term adaptation of the eye movements in this subject during a stabilizing combined eye and head (E, H) horizontal movements keeping gaze on a stationary target (case B of Fig.     ). The dashed line indicates the control VOR before prism wearing. Note that there is an initial small VOR. The gain of this initial segment for this subject was 0.97 (range, 0.94–1.05) for control values, 0.87 (range 0.1–0.91) after one hour, and 0.17 (range 0–0.56) after 6 hr of prism wearing. The initial VOR is followed by a sequence of saccades and smooth eye movements in the same direction as head movement (adapted response). R, rightward; L, leftward. B. 'Program' revealed by breaking the head (head block) movement immediately before the head starts. A sound signal indicates to the subject that he has to make a head movement. The same sound signal triggers a mechanical break which stops the head from moving. In spite of the absence of head motion, and therefore of retinal slip of target image, the adapted subjects makes an eye movement (central progam?) similar to the one shown in A (from Melvill Jones et al., 1983, unpublished).

0.48 as compared to normal values which range from 0.75 (S.E. 0.03, n = 20) to 1.01 (S.E. 0.03, n = 18) according to Barnes (1979a).

Development of this compensatory rapid eye movement in a direction opposite to the normal VOR during the initial 10 days of vision reversal suggests that it might represent an adaptively modified 'saccade' preprogrammed to coincide with the head movement. This point will be discussed in more detail below.

During *active head movements in the light* the subject was asked to shift her gaze from the mid-position to one of the targets located 10° on each side of the sagittal plane while wearing the prisms: the right of the subject is seen through the prisms on the left, it moves to the right when the subject moves the head to the right to visually catch the target. The VOR is, therefore, non-

functional and the subject has to develop an adapted motor coordination. A variety of motor patterns were observed in this case. Three of them were frequent: (a) suppression of VOR and blockage of eye position in the orbit; (b) a saccade to catch the target before the head movement followed by a rapid 'saccade-like' movement of the type described above, which allowed the eye to follow the acquired target; (c) an attenuated VOR which brought the eye towards the moving target and was followed by a rapid visual pursuit of the target.

These results demonstrate that eye-head coordination adaptation to prism reversal is not accomplished by a plastic reversal of VOR but by the addition of a partial or complete reversible suppression of the *VOR which is itself replaced by an adequate combination and sequencing of ex-*

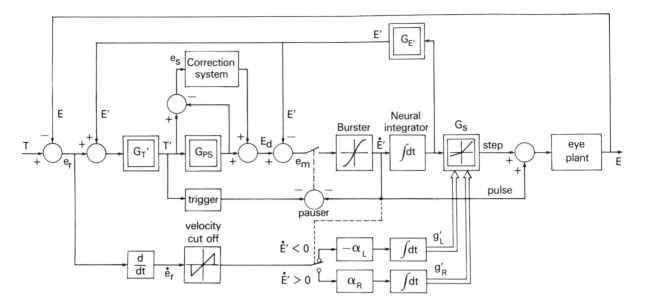

*Fig. 12.* Schematic diagrams of an adaptive control system that adjusts both pulse and step gains (based on Optican, this volume, and Optican, 1982). Signal pathways are shown as single solid lines. Switch controls are shown as dashed lines. Variable gain elements are shown as double boxes. Double line pathways adjust variable gain elements (see text) (by courtesy of L. Optican).

*isting types of movements available from the normal oculomotor subsystem repertoire of the subject.*

That this is the case is also suggested by the results of another study (Melvill Jones et al., 1983) which concerned the development of this adaptation during the first 6 h of reversed vision in two subjects. Horizontal eye-head coordination was tested by active head movements either in the light or in darkness. The task was to maintain fixation on the reversed (moving) image of a single earth fixed target during a voluntary change of head position. Fig. 10B gives a remarkable example of a record taken within the first few moments of prism wearing, it shows that the subject used, a succession of oculomotor subsystems to accomplish the visual stabilization task. Records taken within the first 6 h proved the adaptive process to be merely a refinement of this immediate strategy (Fig. 11).

Typically, during the first hour of reversed vision, the induced eye movements were composed of three phases (Fig. 11A): (a) a short period of VOR where gain was markedly reduced within the first few trials; (b) a 'catch up' saccade in the direction of the reversed image movement (i.e., same direction as that of the head) whose latency was compatible with visual triggering; (c) a smooth rapid eye movement which could either resemble a further reduced 'VOR' or occur in the reversed direction, sometimes reaching velocities similar to that of the head and resembling the 'saccade-like' movement of the previous long term subject (Fig. 9B). In general, within 6 h many of the effects seen after 19 days were present although eye and head velocity were not as smoothly parallel.

Some elements in the adaptive strategy described above are therefore designed within the first moments of adaptation. The most important finding is that this process, when operative, seems to be a centrally constructed scheme independent of sensory reafference (not an on-line servo process). This was evidenced by braking the head movement in the middle of the intended trajectory (Fig. 11B). Prevention of intended head movement was followed in both 1st and 6th hour test by a smooth rapid eye movement in the appropriate direction, being synchronous with the intended prolongation of head movement. This suggests a newly established central motor 'program or scheme'. As for the reduction of VOR it could easily be produced by a simple change in mental set known to allow reduction of VOR from 0.9 to 0.2 by simply imagining a head fixed target (Barr et al., 1976; Melvill Jones et al., 1983).

These findings in humans are strikingly similar to those made by Dichgans et al. (1973) in the monkey, who observed such strategies on the first day after labyrinthectomy; and those of Kasai and Zee (1978) in labyrinthine defective subjects. We think however that the term 'program' is probably not really adequate to specify the exact nature of the processes underlying these strategies.

### 3.4. Adaptive role of the saccadic system, a factor involved in adaptation or vestibular compensation for eye-head coordination

A very striking observation made both in lesioned monkeys and human patients, or after prism wearing, which has repeatedly been referred in this review is the use *of saccades as substitute of the slow phase of the VOR* by humans or primates whenever it is absent or needs to be reversed.

As described in Chapter 4, the saccadic system can produce adapted saccades probably by modulating either the pulse or the step of the saccade generating neuronal network. A schematic diagram of an adaptive control system that adjusts pulse and step gains is shown in Fig. 12. The following description is from Optican (personal communication); it is placed here to support the hypothesis of the use of the saccadic system as a substitute for the VOR.

$T$ is the position of the target, and $E$ is the position of the eye, in spatial coordinates. Their difference is the position error in retinal coordinates ($e_r$). A considerable amount of signal processing is needed to generate a saccade. First, the brain's best estimate of current eye position, ($E'$) is added to the retinal error, to convert from retinal to spatial coordinates. This value is scaled by the variable gain element ($G_{T'}$) to obtain $T'$, the brain's estimate of where the target is in space. To make a saccade the continuous controller in the brain stem (made up of the burst, pause and integrator cells) must be given a desired eye position ($E_d$) and a starting trigger. $E_d$ is obtained by multiplying $T'$ by $G_{ps'}$, the gain of the primary

saccade. When $E'$ is subtracted from this signal an estimate of the motor error ($e_m$) is obtained. When the trigger inhibits the pause cells, the burst cells are disinhibited and begin generating the pulse of innervation needed to drive the eyes against the viscous drag of the orbital tissues. This burst ($\dot{E}'$) is the neural correlate of eye velocity. When it is integrated and scaled by the variable gain element ($G_{E'}$) it gives rise to a neural correlate of eye position ($E'$) based on an efference copy of the saccadic innervation. Because $E'$ is in the feedback loop around the burst cells, as the burst is generated the motor error signal ($e_m$) is continuously reduced, and the burst automatically cuts off when the eye is on target. The output of the neural integrator is weighted by another variable gain element ($G_s$) to obtain the step of innervation needed to hold the eye still against the elastic restoring forces of the orbit. The sum of the pulse and step of innervation is fed to the extraocular muscles and, when filtered through the dynamics of the ocular motor plant, determines the eye position ($E$).

If the pulse and step of innervation are not exactly matched to the dynamics of the ocular motor plant, the eye will drift exponentially after a saccade. To compensate for this the brain must be able to adjust the gain element ($G_s$). Since all parts of the image on the retina will have the same slip after the saccade, it is sufficient to look at the retinal slip following each saccade. Since the direction of the change in the step gain depends on both the direction of the slip and the direction of the antecedent saccade, two gains must be controlled, one for leftward ($g'_L$) and one for rightward ($g'_R$) saccades. This is done by differentiating the retinal error signal to obtain retinal slip ($\dot{e}_r$). After clipping out the very high slip velocities due to the saccade itself, the retinal slip is integrated in one of two integrators, depending on the direction of the antecedent saccade. The factors $\alpha_L$ and $\alpha_R$ determine the rate at which the step gains ($g'_L$ and $g'_R$) can be adjusted.

If the pulse of innervation is not correct, the eye movements will be dysmetric. Adjusting the size of the pulse is much more complicated than controlling the step gain, because after the saccade there is no simple error signal. In this model a position error signal is obtained from a correction system. The correction system's ultimate goal is to adjust $G_{T'}$, the gain of the target position estimate. This will then cause the brain stem generator to automatically make saccades of the correct size. If the nervous system is performing saccadic signal processing in spatial coordinates, however, adjusting $G_{T'}$ is not easy. From the point of view of the brain, the saccadic system is actually operating in an open loop fashion, since the internal feedback of efference copy ($E'$) effectively cancels the physical feedback of eye position ($E$). Hence it is unable to detect any absolute position errors. To get around this problem, the correction system introduces a perturbation of known size into the desired eye position signal. The size of this perturbation is determined by $G_{ps}$, which is less than one. The difference between this scaled signal and $T'$ is then the size of the expected retinal error immediately after the saccade ($e_s$). After the comparison between the actual retinal error ($e_r$) and the expected error the correction system updates the desired eye position signal ($E_d$), causing a corrective saccade to be generated. The difference between $e_r$ and $e_s$ can be used to adjust the gain of the target position in space ($G_{T'}$).

Two other variable gain elements are needed to keep the saccadic system operating correctly. The gain of the primary saccade appears to be stringently regulated, and hence is represented by a double box. The reason for keeping $G_{ps}$ less than one may be to force the post-saccadic retinal error into the same hemisphere of the brain that determined the target before the saccade. This would reduce the time it takes for the correction system to determine the post-saccadic error, and would thus reduce the probability that an error was due to motion of the target. Finally, the gain element ($G_E$) is needed so that the efference copy ($E'$) accurately represents eye position. For example, if disease processes lower the gain of the extraocular muscles to one half, then the gain of the target estimate ($G_{T'}$) would be raised to two. This causes the eye to move the correct amount reducing retinal error to zero. However, if the efference copy signal were not also scaled, E' would reflect the doubled gain of the target estimate, making it appear as if the target had moved. Hence the brain must be capable of reg-

ulating $G_{E'}$, whose desired value is always equal to the gain of the ocular motor plant, and is thus the reciprocal of $G_{T'}$ (end of Optican's comments).

It could therefore be speculated that the rapid smooth 'saccade-like' eye movement seen in subjects after prism wearing is merely a particular saccade obtained by modification of the step gain inducing an exponential post-saccadic ocular drift, or a slowed down pulse-driven saccade as compensatory movement. In addition the records of Kasai and Zee in Fig. 7. (imagination) could be explained by a sequencing of saccades. This would require that, somewhere in the network, information concerning head velocity is fed in order to adequately tune the step gain to produce a saccade whose velocity would be equal to that of the head. It could also be that both eye and head are driven by an internal signal of intended head or eye position, as supposed by Bizzi (see previous section), and evidenced by Fuller et al. (1983), in the monkey, the cat, or suggested by various evidence in man (see Chapter 13). It is probable that this constructed eye movement requires some long term training.

Whatever the precise mechanisms, adaptation in this case would therefore require two simultaneous processes: one leading to the use of a modified saccade, the other modifying the head velocity itself in order to give this parameter a value compatible with the adaptive capabilities of the saccadic system.

Suggestions along this line have been made previously by Kommerell et al. (1976) for patients with abducens palsy, and Meienberg et al. (1981) for patients with homonymous hemianopia. Theoretical speculations which suggest the detailed operation of this adaptive mechanism are described not only by Optican (Chapter 4) but also be Bahill et al. (1975 a,b, 1978). The ability of the brain to produce an internally generated smooth rapid eye movement to substitute for an inadequate VOR is therefore remarkable. That this is akin to a 'program' is shown by the invariance of this pattern in head braking experiments (Melvill Jones et al., 1983)

The following chapter (Melvill Jones & Berthoz) will provide an illustration of the internal nature of these adaptive modifications by demonstrating that VOR gain changes can be induced by mental training.

### 3.5 Adaptation of eye-head coordination to microgravity

All of the previous results have concerned eye-head movements in the horizontal plane. In this plane the VOR depends mainly upon the semicircular canals to measure head angular rotation. In the vertical planes the otoliths, which sense not only linear acceleration but also the components of gravity in the plane of the maculae, contribute significantly to the VOR (see Chapters 2 & 10). In conditions of microgravity such as *spaceflight* this contribution is reduced and a serious decrement of VOR gain can be expected (see also Chapter 2, Fig. 8). This is probably an important cause of *space-sickness*. To investigate the adaptation of the vertical VOR in microgravity we performed, for the first time, an experiment during the flight of Spacelab I (von Baumgarten et al., 1984) in which we measured head and eye movements during head pitch. The results suggest that the VOR gain during pitch head movements returns to a normal gain after a few days of flight (possibly even much earlier). The first day after flight another quick readaptation occurs. These measures have been very preliminary and the tests will be repeated in subsequent flights in 1985. According to the hypothesis developed in this chapter we can expect substitutions of other reflexes such as the cervico-ocular reflex but also a potential contribution of the saccadic system and even, as will be described in the next chapter (Chapter 13), complex rearrangements which will have to be analyzed.

### 4. Conclusions

The hypothesis proposed in the introduction is verified by reviewing the available evidence, i.e., adaptive mechanisms in eye-head coordination in the case of *environmental* or *peripheral modifica-tion* consist of (a) combination of oculomotor or cephalomotor subsystems which are available in each species, and (b) *stabilization* of adequate *strategies* by mechanisms which are not known to us yet.

When a sensory cue is deficient, another cue from another sensory modality providing adequate information can be substituted. But *substitution* is not in any way the only solution. Very often there will be a central construction of an *intended motion signal* which may provide a *non-sensory* central cue. This signal itself will be the result of some kind of 'program' or, as proposed by Droulez et al. (1984), topological representation, which will specify which sensory cue has to be used and organize the sequencing of subsystems contributions. This reorganization of systems is probably partly responsible for the 'distributed' aspect of activity after vestibular compensation in the cat (Llinás & Walton, 1979b). It also suggests that higher processes involving the cerebral cortex are at play as recently shown by Sasaki and Gember (1982) in the prefrontal cortex (see also Chapter 15, p. 230), and by Van der Steen et al. (1984) who studied recovery of eye head coordination after lesion of the frontal eye fields in the monkey. One role of the cerebellum in this view could be "to provide co-operation between the synergisms and adapt them to the environment" as suggested recently by Arshavsky et al. (1983).

In other words, before looking for modifiable synapses in the brain or making models of variable gain elements, it seems necessary to identify firstly which, in the repertoire of subsystems, have been selected as adequate, and how they are used in time and space. Subsequently one can search for the modified elements required if these combined subsystems (saccadic, pursuit, OKN, VOR, etc.) are used with parametric adjustments within the usual range of physiological values. Only if it is not the case should some structural changes be suspected, or if some *permanence* has to be maintained.

Adaptive mechanisms in gaze control
Facts and theories
*Eds. Berthoz & Melvill Jones*
© 1985 Elsevier Science Publishers BV (Biomedical Division)

# Chapter 13

# Mental control of the adaptive process

G. Melvill Jones[a] & A. Berthoz[b]

[a]*Aerospace Medical Research Unit, Department of Physiology, McGill University, Montréal, Québec, Canada H3G 1Y6, and*
[b]*Laboratoire de Physiologie Neurosensorielle du C.N.R.S., Paris, France*

## 1. Introduction

At first sight it would seem almost self-evident that vision should play an essential role in the adaptive rearrangement of gaze control. Indeed the preceding chapters have described a variety of such rearrangements induced by altering specifically the visual component of integrated multipathway systems. We have seen that magnifying and diminishing lenses combined with head movement to produce, respectively, augmentation or reduction of the dark-tested VOR; that vision reversal produces alterations specific to the planes of optical inversion; that orthogonal cross-coupling of visual and vestibular stimuli changes the vector of VOR responses; that new strategies of head-eye coordination emerge when altered vision modifies their normal interaction; that the accommodation-vergence system adapts to visual rearrangement between these two separately innervated mechanisms; that vision is necessary for activation of the adaption which occurs after unilateral canal plugging. Even emergence of the adaptive mechanism itself requires exposure to real visual experience during early development.

Nevertheless, it has been known for many years that the input-output characteristics of the VOR are subject to major moment-to-moment fluctuations depending on non-visual factors, such as state of 'arousal' (e.g., Melvill Jones & Sugie, 1972) and mental set (e.g., Collins, 1962). More recently, it has been found that the influ-

ence of 'mental set' depends explicitly upon the subject's conscious choice of intended visual goal (Barr et al., 1976; Sharpe et al., 1981; Baloh et al., 1984). The dramatic effect of changing goals is illustrated in Fig. 1 (reproduced from Barr et al., 1976). It shows the distribution of ocular gain (eye velocity/head velocity) as a function of frequency for five different conditions, two in the light and three in the dark. Note particularly the wide separation of filled squares and filled circles, which represent the *dark*-tested VOR gains of a subject trying to 'look', respectively, at *earth*-fixed and *head*-fixed targets during head rotation. Evidently, given a constant vestibular input, we can substantially modulate our oculomotor output according to our conscious assessment of the prevailing functional need, even without the aid of visual feedback. This raises the interesting question of whether consistent alteration of the mentally chosen goal could alone produce adaptive alteration of internal parameters controlling VOR gain, bearing in mind that with the aid of vision this certainly can be done.

This question incidentally bears on the currently controversial issue of whether retinal afferent signals derived from a slipping retinal image are necessary for activation of the adaptive process. One hypothesis (Ito, 1972, 1982a; see also Chapter 14) calls for afferent responses from retinal image slip detectors to be compared with concurrent vestibular afferents for the activation of adaptive changes suitable for effective reduction of the im-

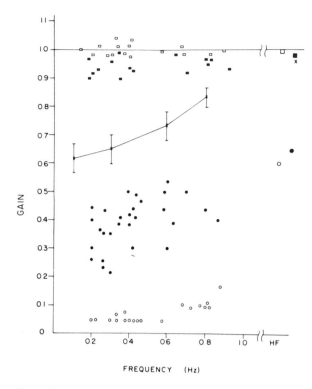

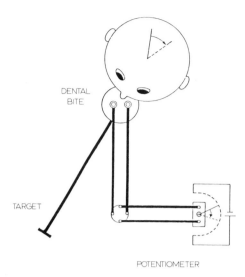

Fig. 1. Dependence of ocular gain (eye vel./head vel.) upon intended goal. Filled points obtained during rotation in the dark (VOR) when trying to 'look' at an earth fixed (squares) or head fixed (circles) target. Corresponding open points obtained with real visual targets. The drawn curve shows the intermediate effect of mental arithmetic, which has no goal-directed relevance for the oculomotor system (reproduced from Fig. 3 of Barr et al., 1976).

Fig. 2. Recording system for measurement of active rotational head movement during mental fixation on a head fixed target. Note that the parallel arm device (a miniature drawing board arm) ensures selective exclusion of translational movement so that only the angular component of head movement is recorded, yet the system is not constrained to a fixed axis of rotation in space (reproduced from Fig. 1A of Melvill Jones et al., 1984).

& Precht, 1981; Miles & Eighmy, 1980), would non-visual suppression produce by mental effort alone bring about a similar adaptive effect?

## 2. Experimental approach

Human subjects were seated on a conventional servo-controlled rotating chair, surrounded by an earth-fixed cyclindrical drum covered inside with a colourful scene of New York city at dusk. The head could either be fixed to a dental bite attached to the turntable (for passive stimuli) or to a bite attached to an angular head movement recorder and a light weight head-fixed target (for active head rotation relative to the stationary body), as in Fig. 2. Before beginning an experiment the subject, with head still, was familiarized with this head fixed target in the light. Then, with the turntable stationary, an attempt was made to continue looking at the target during a total of 3 h of self-paced and *actively* generated head oscillations conducted in complete darkness. When working hard at the

age slip. On the other hand Miles and Lisberger (1981b), basing their arguments on observations of Miles et al. (1980a,b; see also Chapter 3) concluded that, at least in the primate, the 'working' comparison is made between the vestibular input and an efferent feedback copy of the concurrent oculomotor output, rather than the visual consequence of that output.

The present chapter reviews a recent experimental study which addressed these questions by using the ability of mental VOR suppression (filled circles of Fig. 1) to produce prolonged alteration of sensory-motor relations in the reflex without the aid of vision (Melvill Jones et al., 1984). Specifically, since prolonged *visual* suppression of reflex output adaptively attenuates the inherent VOR gain (Ito et al., 1974a,b; Keller task this is a tiring procedure, and intermittent rest periods were allowed, during which the subject could relax and incidentally refresh the visual memory of the real target assembly. Of course during rest periods in the light the head was not allowed to move. Although the frequency and amplitude of active head rotation was not controlled, subjects usually chose comfortable periodic movement between about 1.0–0.2 Hz and over an amplitude range of about 5–60°.

VOR gain was measured before and after the 3 h period of its non-visual suppression, using a test regime similar to that of Gauthier and Robinson (1975), in order to evoke realistic goal-directed conditions for these primary tests. The method is illustrated in the results of Fig. 3. First, the stationary subject fixated a stationary foveal target on the stationary drum. Then, whilst still trying to 'look' at the target, the lights were extinguished (shaded area) and the head rotated rapidly through 20–40° about a vertical axis. Immediately after cessation of movement the lights were switched on again and the subject refixated the now visible target. Thus, the eye movement in darkness represents the VOR obtained during a mental set calling for its operation at unity gain (filled square at top and right-hand side of Fig. 1). When present, the refixation saccade (S in Fig. 3) represents the degree of failure to achieve this goal. Bearing in mind the active nature of the forced suppression, these tests were performed with both passive (chair rotation) and active head movements, to discriminate between adaptive changes in VOR per se (passive tests) and the introduction of programmed and/or neck dependent influences (active tests).

In view of the perceptual correlates of VOR changes induced by altered visual stimuli, (Gauthier & Robinson, 1975; Gonshor & Melvill Jones, 1980; Oman et al., 1980) it seemed important to attempt measurement of this correlate also. For this, the single visual target was lapped on either side by a circumferential scale marked in degrees and the subject asked to estimate from this both the direction and magnitude of apparent movement of the drum after switching on the light. Normally, after VOR alteration there are striking illusions of world movement associated with head rotation.

## 3. Alteration of VOR gain

The degree of adaptive change produced in VOR gain is illustrated in Fig. 3, which compares ocular responses to passive step changes of head position before (control) and after (adapted) the 3 h period of mental suppression. In section A we see the reflex compensatory eye rotations produced by three successive passive head rotations in the dark. In control conditions the eyes were usually close to being on target when the lights went on, although there was a normal (see Fig. 3B) tendency for intermittent small undershoots to be followed by small corrective saccades. In marked contrast, the adapted state, seen on the right-hand side, produced consistently large undershoots, followed by correspondingly large saccadic corrections of gaze back onto target. Fig. 3B shows superimposed and time expanded traces of head and eye movement which demonstrate the same adaptive phenomenon more clearly.

*Table 1*

Mean adaptive effects of 3 h mental VOR suppression, tested under passive and active conditions of head rotation (see Fig. 3) obtained from the same three subjects in each condition (data from Melvill Jones et al., 1984)

| Test condition | VOR gain = $(T-S)/T$ | | | | % gain attenuation | $P$ |
| | Control | (n) | Adapted | (n) | | |
|---|---|---|---|---|---|---|
| Passive | 0.92 | 52 | 0.82 | 63 | 10.9 | ≪ 0.001 |
| Active | 0.96 | 50 | 0.85 | 59 | 11.4 | ≪ 0.001 |

The cumulative results in Table 1, calculated as in the legend of Fig. 3, show that a highly significant reduction of gain occurred as a result of the non-visual mental suppression exercise, as tested with both passive and active head movements. The conclusion was equally valid for individual as well as for cumulative mean values. Also noteworthy is the fact that there was no significant difference ($P > 0.1$) between passive and active attenuations, indicating that the primary adaptive alteration was restricted to the dark-tested VOR, rather than the introduction of programmed suppression or some form of adaptively activated cervico-ocular influence.

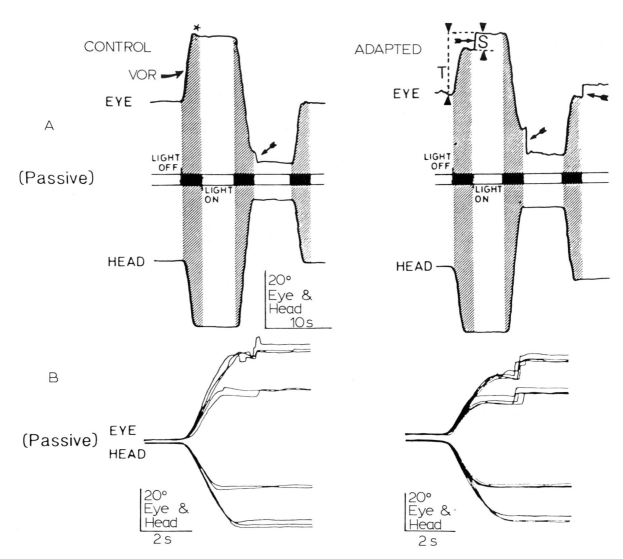

*Fig. 3.* Eye and head movements recorded during the standard test regime, obtained before (control) and after (adapted) 3 h of mental VOR suppression in the dark. A. Samples of ocular response to three successive passive step changes of head angle, each conducted in darkness (shaded bands), with the subject trying to maintain ocular fixation on the earth fixed target. Inadequacy of VOR leads to a corrective saccade (S) shortly after switching on the lights. Since, after refixation, the total eye excursion (T) is equated to total head excursion, VOR gain = (T–S)/T and the estimate is self calibrated. Note the greatly enlarged corrective saccades in the 'adapted' state, reflecting the systematic adaptive reduction of VOR gain, even though the subject's conscious goal is to achieve unit gain throughout these tests. B. Superimposed traces for 20° and 40° (passive) head movements obtained in control and adapted conditions. Note the normal tendency for some slight degree of undershooting in control conditions (compare the normal tendency for saccadic undershooting noted and discussed in Chapter 4), and the consistently reduced VOR compensation leading to enlarged corrective saccades in the adapted state (selected data from Fig. 2 of Melvill Jones et al., 1984).

These findings clearly show that external visual stimulation of the retina is not a necessary condition for the production of a modified reflex. It is of course important to note that the results do not exclude the efficacy of real visual stimuli. Indeed, the 10% reduction of gain produced in these experiments is relatively small compared to the 25–30% change to be expected during 3 h of vision through reversing dove prisms (Melvill Jones & Mandl, 1979); or indeed compared to the very

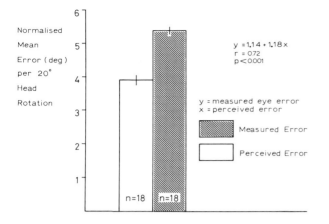

*Fig. 4.* Correlation of adaptively induced perceptual and oculomotor errors. Bars give standard error of mean. Note that the mean perceptual error tended to be less than the oculomotor error, possibly reflecting the fact that some undershooting (see Fig. 3) occurs in normal control subjects, who do not perceive world movement when turning the head. The linear regression equation demonstrates a highly significant correlation between trial by trial estimates of perceptual and motor errors.

rapid changes induced by vision through prescription spectacle lenses, recently reported by Collewijn et al. (1983) (see also Chapter 3). Furthermore, it is quite possible that 'spontaneous' mosaics of light-dark patterns, 'seen' in the dark, could have contributed in some way; although the failure of after images to enhance mental VOR control noted by Barr et al. (1976) does not encourage this view. Rather, the findings would seem to support the hypothesis proposed by Miles and Lisberger (1981), whereby comparison of the vestibular afferent response with internal recurrent feedback of oculomotor performance activates the adaptive mechanism. Very recently, Lisberger et al. (1984) have adduced further evidence in support of this hypothesis by demonstrating substantial adaptive change in monkeys who successfully suppressed (or augmented) their VOR by tracking a small foveal target in the absence of optokinetic stimulation.

Perhaps in reality multiple processes are at play, as would be suggested by the admittedly simplistic model proposed by Barr et al. (1976, their Fig. 6). This model invokes the concept of a

central 'spatial localization calculator' (SL) receiving inputs from (i) retinal error detectors, (ii) a motor efferent feedback signal, and (iii) the vestibular afferent input. The output of the calculator is then used to inject a corrective command into the oculomotor system. Given this arrangement, then it might be the corrective command signal which ultimately 'teaches' the adaptive mechanism to produce changes of internal neural parameters controlling gain. Barr et al. (1976) proposed that, in the absence of vision, it is the vestibular pathway through SL which "appears to be modulated non-visually by the subjects' efforts to stabilize their eyes in a fixed or moving frame of reference".

## 4. Perceptual correlates

An interesting possibility suggested by Barr et al. (1976) is that one recreates, in SL, a neural signal which represents the *percept* of target position relative to the head. In this case we should expect to find perceptual correlates of the modified motor response, as was reported by Gauthier and Robinson (1975) when they adaptively enhanced VOR by means of vision through magnifying spectacles.

It is, therefore, particularly intriguing to enquire whether the adaptive gain reduction produced by mental effort alone was associated with correlated alteration of perceived self motion. Fig. 4 shows how, in one subject tested as described above, a clear relationship emerged between adaptively induced perceptual and oculomotor 'errors'. The figure compares the two kinds of (normalized) error as they emerged from a single series of 18 trials, conducted after the 3 h period of mental VOR suppression. The linear regression equation inset in the figure reveals a tight ($P < 0.001$) correlation of the two variables, with a slope of 1.18, indicating that the motor error tended to be greater than the perceptual one, as seen in the figure. Perhaps this difference between mean perceptual and motor errors might be accounted for by the fact already pointed out (and seen in Fig. 3B), that normal subjects tend to undershoot their visual target, and yet perceive a stationary world when moving the head.

## 5. Concluding remarks

The above findings make it clear that activation of an adaptive response is not restricted to error activated feedback control of central parameters referenced to the real physical world of the external environment. Apparently internal neurally coded reference signals can also serve an effective role. Additional insight produced by the present result focuses on the teasing fact that it seems possible to change those internal reference signals by application of mental effort alone. And furthermore, the induced change carries with it a correlated perceptual change: which in turn argues for recalibration of conscious perception through conscious mental effort. Evidently, on the one hand we need real physical contact with the external world to restrain our internal system from adversely modifying itself. On the other hand one may guess that it is only by this means (i.e., adaptive homeostasis through sensory-motor contact with the physical world) that it is possible to retain an adequate level of perceptual veracity; which smacks of the 'positivist' views of earlier natural philosophers (e.g., Mach, 1886; English translation, 1959). Perhaps the well known adverse perceptual effects of prolonged sensory deprivation in humans (e.g., Bexton et al., 1954) could be accounted for along these lines? Speculating more wildly, perhaps some forms of psychiatric disorders of perception might prove to be accountable in terms of disordered adaptive mechanisms, which thereby fail to maintain an adequate level of perceptual veracity with respect to the physical world.

# Part II

## Internal Processes Underlying Adaptation

# Section IIA

## Neuronal mechanisms

Adaptive mechanisms in gaze control
Facts and theories
Eds. Berthoz & Melvill Jones
© 1985 Elsevier Science Publishers BV (Biomedical Division)

# Chapter 14

# Synaptic plasticity in the cerebellar cortex that may underlie the vestibulo-ocular adaptation

## M. Ito

*Department of Physiology, Faculty of Medicine, University of Tokyo, Bunkyo-ku, Tokyo, Japan 113*

## 1. Introduction

Since its demonstration in human subjects (Gonshor & Melvill Jones, 1971, 1976a,b), adaptiveness of the vestibulo-ocular reflex (VOR) has attracted attention as a model of neural plasticity. The hypothesis that the cerebellar flocculus is the site of adaptiveness of the VOR has been put forward independently on the ground of intimate neuronal connections between the flocculus and the VOR arc (Ito, 1970, 1972, 1974). This "flocculus hypothesis of the VOR control" views the flocculus as a modifiable sidepath element attached to the VOR arc for the purpose of adaptive adjustment of the overall dynamic characteristics of the VOR under altered visual-vestibular environments (Fig. 1). The hypothesis matches the modifiable neuronal network model of the cerebellum (Marr, 1969; Albus, 1971), and is in accordance with the experimental demonstration that flocculectomy removes the adaptiveness of the VOR in rabbits (Ito et al., 1974b, 1982a; Nakao, 1983) and cats (Robinson, 1976).

Since these earlier findings, several lines of supportive evidence for the flocculus hypothesis of the VOR control have been accumulated through dissection of neuronal connections, analysis of neuronal activity and measurements of dynamic characteristics of eye movement. I recently reviewed these lines of evidence (Ito, 1982a), but more evidence has now become available. Direct evidence for the postulated synaptic

plasticity in the cerebellar cortex, which has been lacking for a decade, was eventually provided (Ito et al., 1982a; Ito & Kano, 1982; Ekerot & Kano, 1984). Neuronal activity in the flocculus correlated with adaptive changes of the VOR was confirmed not only in rabbits (Dufossé et al., 1978a) but also in monkeys (Watanabe, 1984). Theoretical approach along the line of the Marr-Albus model yielded Fujita's (1982a) adaptive filter model of the cerebellum which, when incorporated into a model of the oculomotor system, successfully reproduced the adaptive behavior of the VOR (Fujita, 1982b). This article introduces these recent developments.

## 2. Synaptic plasticity in the cerebellar cortex

In conceiving a modifiable neuronal network model of the cerebellar cortex, Marr (1969) assumed that the synaptic connection from parallel fibers (axons of granule cells) to Purkinje cells is modifiable in transmission efficacy, and that this modification is effected by conjunctive activation of a parallel fiber and a climbing fiber converging onto the same Purkinje cell dendrite (Fig. 2). Marr (1969) originally suggested an enhancement of the synaptic efficacy, but Albus (1971) later preferred the idea of a depression when formulating a similar model. The following several series of experiments on the cerebellar cortex of decerebrate rabbits demonstrated a prominent long-term depression to occur in parallel fiber-

214

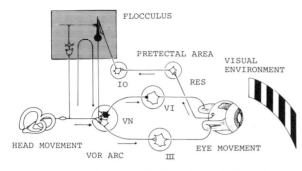

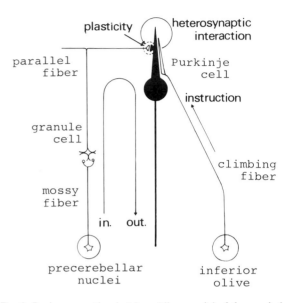

*Fig. 1.* Neuronal diagram of the flocculo-vestibulo-ocular system in the rabbit. III and VI, oculomotor and a abducens nuclei. It illustrates the possible mechanism of the vestibulo-ocular adaptation; the vestibular mossy fiber–granule cell–Purkinje cell pathway through the flocculus acts as a modifiable sidepath to the VOR arc, and the modification of the sidepath is effected by retinal error signals conveyed through the pretectal area (inferior olive, IO) climbing fiber pathway. The retinal error signals (RES) monitor mismatching of the VOR to the visual environment.

*Fig. 2.* Basic assumption in Marr-Albus model of the cerebellum. Note that the neuronal connections in Fig. 2 apply to the floccular part of Fig. 1.

Purkinje cell synapses when activated in conjunction with climbing fibers.

Throughout these experiments, Purkinje cells were identified by initiation of two distinctive types of spikes, *complex* and *simple*. Complex spikes represent activation of Purkinje cells directly by climbing fiber signals, whereas simple spikes reflect activation by mossy fiber signals indirectly mediated via granule cells and other cortical neurons (Eccles et al., 1966; Thach, 1968). Simple spikes discharge at a relatively high rate (around 50 Hz) and serve as the major output signals of Purkinje cells. Complex spikes, by contrast, discharge at a low (around 1 Hz) irregular rate and make only a subsidiary contribution to Purkinje cell output. The distinctively different behavior of the two types of spikes are in accordance with the view that mossy fibers provide the major input signals to be converted in the cerebellar cortex to Purkinje cell output, whereas climbing fibers provide instruction signals for reorganization of the mossy fiber input–Purkinje cell output relationship.

### 2.1. Conjunctive stimulation of mossy fibers and climbing fibers

In the first series of experiments (Ito et al., 1982c), responsiveness of floccular Purkinje cells was tested by applying single pulse stimuli to a vestibular nerve which projects to the flocculus as mossy fiber afferents. These stimuli excited Purkinje cells with a latency of 3–6 ms via granule cells and parallel fibers. Similar excitation was seen commonly also among putative basket cells. Firing index for these excitations was calculated from the number of spikes initiated, above the spontaneous firing level, during 100 sweeps repeated at the rate of 2 Hz. Conjunctive stimulation of climbing fibers and mossy fibers was performed by applying a 4 Hz stimulus to the inferior olive (site of origin of climbing fibers) and a 20 Hz stimulus to a vestibular nerve, simultaneously, for a period of 25 s, thus delivering 100 climbing fiber impulses and 500 vestibular mossy fiber impulses to the flocculus. As 4 Hz was the maximum discharge frequency in floccular climbing fibers under natural stimulus conditions of alert rabbits this was chosen (Ghelarducci et al., 1975). 20 Hz is a moderate discharge frequency for a vestibular nerve during head rotation.

It was thus demonstrated that a conjunctive stimulation effectively depresses the vestibular mossy fiber responsiveness of flocculus Purkinje cells (Fig. 3). While the depression diminishes in about 10 min, there is usually a slow phase of

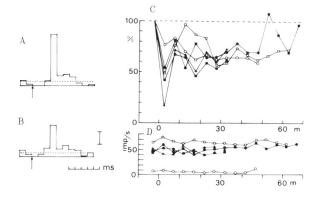

*Fig. 3.* Effects of conjunctive vestibular-olivary stimulation on vestibular mossy fiber reponsiveness of flocculus Purkinje cells. A and B, peristimulus histograms for *simple* spike discharge of a Purkinje cell. Arrows mark the moment of stimulation of a vestibular nerve. A, before and B, after a conjunctive stimulation. C, ordinate, firing index of Purkinje cells in stimulation of a vestibular nerve. Abscissa, time after conjunctive stimulation. Note that results from five Purkinje cells are plotted with different symbols. D, spontaneous firing rates measured simultaneously with C. Note that spontaneous firing rates are not affected significantly by conjunctive stimulation (Ito et al., 1982c).

weak depression which lasts for more than one hour. This effect was obtained specifically in response to stimulation of the vestibular nerve which was involved in the conjunctive stimulation. No such depression occurred in response to the other vestibular nerve. These observations clearly indicate that the effect of a conjunctive stimulation is not due to general depression in Purkinje cells; it is specific to a site or sites in the mossy fiber–granule cell–Purkinje cell pathway involved in the conjunctive stimulation.

Conjunctive stimulation of climbing fibers and mossy fibers did not affect the responsiveness of putative basket cells to mossy fiber inputs. Inhibition or rebound facilitation elicited in Purkinje cells by vestibular mossy fiber signals was not affected at all by the conjunctive stimulation. Field potentials recorded in the granular layers and white matter of the flocculus were not affected either. These responses represent impulse transmission in the mossy fibers and cortical network, with the exception of the parallel fiber-Purkinje cell synapses. Therefore, it was concluded that the signal transmission at a parallel

fiber-Purkinje cell synapse undergoes a long term depression after conjunctive activation with the climbing fiber impinging on the same Purkinje cell.

Repetitive stimulation of a vestibular nerve at a rate of 20 Hz may mimic naturally occurring vestibular nerve inputs during angular head acceleration. When the number of impulses, evoked during 20 Hz stimulation for 2.5 s above the spontaneous firing level, was measured as an index of the responsiveness of the Purkinje cell to vestibular mossy fiber inputs, a similar long term depression could also be demonstrated after conjunctive stimulation of the vestibular nerve and the inferior olive (Ito, 1982c).

## 2.2. Conjunctive stimulation of parallel fibers and climbing fibers

In the second series of experiments (Ito & Kano, 1982), parallel fibers were stimulated directly through a glass microelectrode placed in the molecular layer. Application of brief pulses (0.2 ms duration) of 20–60 μA excites a narrow beam of parallel fibers along which double-peaked negative field potentials are recorded with another microelectrode. The first peak represents volleys conducting along parallel fibers and the second peak the postsynaptic excitation thereby evoked in dendrites of Purkinje and other cells of the cerebellar cortex. When the parallel fiber stimuli were paired with stimuli to the inferior olive with a time delay of 6–12 ms and repeated at a rate of 4 Hz for one or 2 min, the second peak often exhibited a relatively small but significant depression which lasted for more than one hour.

When the recording microelectrode was placed in the Purkinje cell layer, activation of single Purkinje cells by parallel fiber volleys could be observed (Ekerot et al., 1983; Ekerot & Kano, 1984). Conjunctive stimulation of a parallel fiber beam and the inferior olive regularly produced a prominent depression of the responsiveness of Purkinje cells to the parallel fiber stimulation (Fig. 4). The depression usually developed in two steps, with an early phase lasting for about 10 min and a late phase for the succeeding period of more than an hour. Some Purkinje cells could be excited through two separate parallel fiber

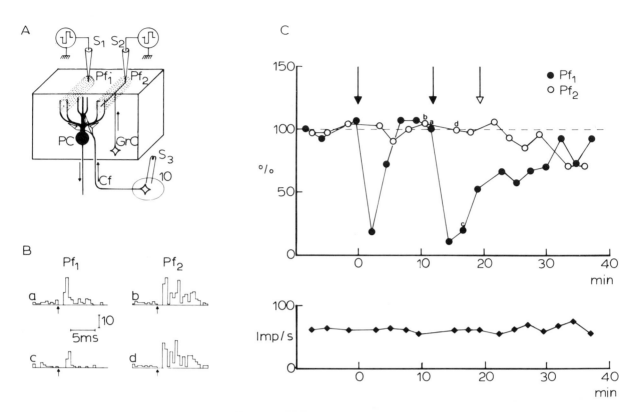

*Fig. 4.* Effects of conjunctive parallel fiber–climbing fiber stimulation on postsynaptic action of parallel fibers. A shows experimental arrangements for stimulating two fascicles of parallel fibers ($Pf_1$, $Pf_2$) and climbing fibers while recording from a Purkinje cell. B, peristimulus histograms similar to Fig. 3A,B, but with parallel fiber fascicles stimulated at the moments indicated by arrows. Upper, before and lower, after conjunctive stimulation of $Pf_1$ and climbing fibers. C plots firing index for stimulation of $Pf_1$ and $Pf_2$. Lower diagram shows spontaneous firing rate of the tested Purkinje cell (by courtesy of Drs. Ekerot and Kano).

beams. When one of the two beams was stimulated in conjunction with the inferior olive stimulation, responsiveness of the Purkinje cell to that parallel fiber beam was specifically depressed, while the responsiveness to the other beam remained unchanged. This is in agreement with the observation made by stimulating two vestibular nerves (see above).

The depression detected in the molecular layer field potential in the molecular layer is usually small (10–20%) and often difficult to detect, in contrast to the regular occurrence of a prominent depression in unit spike responses of Purkinje cells. This discrepancy may be explained by the heterogenous origin of the molecular layer field potentials in not only Purkinje cells but also basket, stellate and Golgi cells. It may also be due to

a non-linear relationship between the excitatory synaptic currents and, thereby, induced membrane excitation. Another possibility to be entertained is that the conjunctive activation of parallel fibers and climbing fibers depresses not only the synaptic chemical transmission mechanisms, as demonstrated below, but also excitability in the local postsynaptic membrane.

## 2.3. Mechanism of long term depression

In the third series of experiments (Ito et al., 1982c), parallel fiber stimulation was replaced by iontophoretic application of glutamate which is a putative neurotransmitter of parallel fibers (Hacket et al., 1979; Sandoval & Cotman, 1978). Application of glutamate and aspartate normally

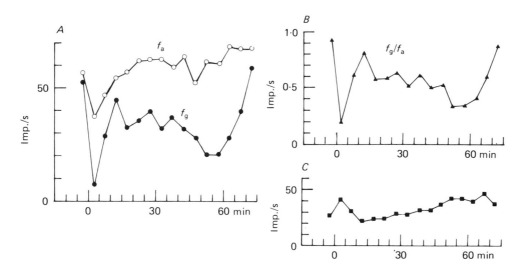

*Fig. 5.* Effects of conjunctive application of L-glutamate with climbing fiber impulses. A, discharges evoked in a Purkinje cell by iontophoresis of L-glutamate ($f_g$, 2.9nA) and L-aspartate ($f_a$, 99nA). B plots the time course of changes in the ratio of $f_g/f_a$. spontaneous firing rates. At the zero time, glutamate was applied with 2.9nA for 25 s, together with 4 Hz climbing fiber stimulation, (Ito et al., 1982c).

excites Purkinje cells. Application of glutamate in conjunction with 4 Hz stimulation of climbing fibers was found to depress very effectively the glutamate sensitivity of Purkinje cells; aspartate sensitivity, tested as control, was depressed to a much lesser degree. The depression diminished in about 10 min, but this recovery was followed by a slow depression lasting for an hour (Fig. 5). Close similarlity in time course of this slow depression of glutamate-responsiveness to the long term depression of parallel fiber–Purkinje cell transmission suggests that the site of the long term depression is postsynaptic, rather than presynaptic, and probably involves glutamate receptor mechanisms in Purkinje cell dendritic membrane.

Hebb (1949) assumed that coincidence of presynaptic and postsynaptic impulses plays a key role in producing a plastic change of synaptic efficacy. However, this seems not to be the case, because (1) parallel fiber volleys which excite Purkinje cells do not produce by themselves any sign of plastic change in parallel fiber-Purkinje cell synapses, (2) iontophoretic application of glutamate which by itself excites Purkinje cells does not modify glutamate sensitivity of Purkinje cells, and (3) climbing fiber impulses are effective at the low rate of 4 Hz, implying that postsynaptic im-

pulses evoked by climbing fiber activation do not play a major role in producing the long lasting depression. The above third argument does not exclude the possibility that a very long lasting plateau potential produced in Purkinje cell dendrites by climbing fiber activation (Ekerot & Oscarsson, 1981) plays a role in producing the depression.

Mechanisms of the long term depression in parallel fiber–Purkinje cell synapses have yet to be investigated, but several possibilities may be raised. First, since climbing fiber activation of Purkinje cells appear to involve a voltage dependent increase of calcium permeability of the dendritic membrane (Llinás & Sugimori, 1980), it is probable that intradendritic calcium of Purkinje cells increases significantly following climbing fiber impulses. This could in turn facilitate the desensitization, i.e., the process which renders postsynaptic receptor molecules insensitive to neurotransmitter molecules, just as has been suggested to occur in neuromuscular junctions (Miledi, 1980; Ekerot & Oscarsson, 1981). Second, one may imagine that the increased intracellular calcium acting from inside, and the parallel fiber transmitter molecules acting from outside, conjointly cause in some way a change in the shape of the dendritic spines on which parallel fibers make synaptic contact. On theoretical grounds (Rall, 1974; Koch & Poggio, 1983), one may speculate that constriction at the neck of the spines may account for the decreased synaptic efficacy during the long term depression. A third possibilitiy is that climbing fibers liberate a chemical substance which reacts with both subsynaptic receptor molecules and parallel fiber neurotransmitter, thereby rendering the receptors insensitive to the parallel fiber neurotransmitter (Ito et al., 1982c), just as thyrotropin-releasing hormone (TRH) reduces glutamate sensitivity of cerebral cortical neurons without affecting aspartate sensitivity (Renaud et al., 1979).

It is an important future task to find which of these possibilities is the case. In view of the recent data by Ekerot and Kano (1984), the last possibility for a chemical climbing fiber substance seems unlikely, because abolition of the climbing fiber-evoked plateau potentials in Purkinje cell dendrites by cortical inhibition results in diminution of the long term potentiation. This observation implies that the plateau potential representing calcium entry plays an essential role in effecting the long term potentiation, thus favoring the above first and second possibilities.

## 3. Response modification in floccular Purkinje cells underlying VOR adaptation

An essential concept of the 'flocculus hypothesis of the VOR control' is that the vestibular mossy fiber responsiveness of floccular Purkinje cells is modified by reference to retinal error signals conveyed by the visual climbing fiber pathway (Fig. 1). This proposition was supported by the observation in rabbit flocculus that *simple* spike responsiveness of floccular Purkinje cells was altered in the directions consistent with predictions from the 'flocculus hypothesis' (Dufossé et al., 1977). However, investigation in monkey flocculus failed to detect such a neuronal correlate to the VOR adaptation (Miles et al., 1980a,b), and consequently a model of the VOR system was proposed with a modifiable element placed not in the flocculus but in an unspecified region of the brain stem (Miles & Lisberger, 1981b).

The conflict between rabbit and monkey data,

though, apparently is due to a different manner of sampling floccular Purkinje cells adopted for yielding them. Crucial from this respect is the fine structural and functional parcellation that exists within the flocculus. In rabbits, at least five zones have been specified to have different efferent connections to vestibular and cerebellar nuclei and, accordingly, to have different functional involvement (Yamamoto, 1978; Ito et al., 1982b). Similar zonal structures of the flocculus have been recognized also in cats (Voogd & Bigaré, 1980; Sato et al., 1982a,b) and monkeys (Balaban et al., 1981; Watanabe & Balaban, 1983). Only one of these zones is related to the horizontal VOR through its connections to relay cells for this reflex in the vestibular nuclei (Ito et al., 1977). This particular zone, conveniently called the H-zone, can be identified by local electrical stimulation which causes horizontal abduction of the ipsilateral eye (Dufossé et al., 1977). It is obvious that, for the purpose of finding neuronal correlates with adaptation of the horizontal VOR, H-zone Purkinje cells should selectively be investigated. This is particularly so because Purkinje cells in other zones are also responsive to vestibular stimuli. If Purkinje cells are sampled from various zones in mixture, any change specific to the H-zone Purkinje cells would be obscured by behavior of other types of Purkinje cells which is often opposite to that of H-zone Purkinje cells (Dufossé et al., 1978). Taking this warning into consideration, Watanabe (1984) reinvestigated monkey's flocculus and uncovered a remarkable modification of *simple* spike vestibular responsiveness of H-zone Purkinje cells during the VOR adaptation.

As shown in Fig. 6, *simple* spike discharge of H-zone Purkinje cells is modulated sinusoidally during sinusoidal head rotation on the horizontal plane. The modulation may be in phase, or 180° out of phase, with the head velocity (B and C). When a monkey was subjected to continuous rotation for one hour with the surrounding screen moving either out of phase or in phase with the turntable, the VOR gain was increased or decreased adaptively. Correspondingly, the response patterns of H-zone Purkinje cells were modified: from in phase to out of phase (B) in parallel with an increase of the VOR gain, and from out of phase to in phase (C) in parallel with

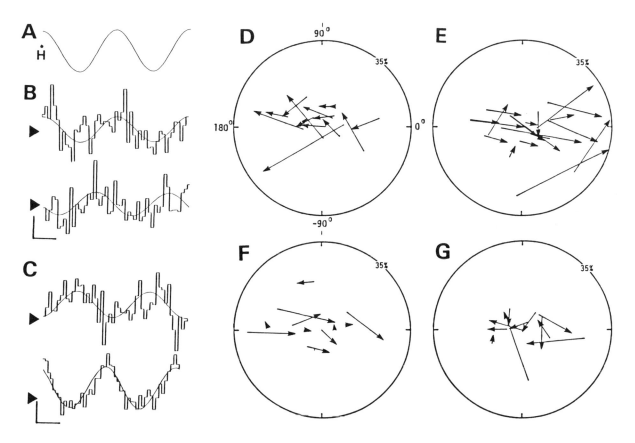

*Fig. 6.* Modulation of *simple* spike discharge of Purkinje cells of monkey's flocculus induced by horizontal head rotation in darkness. A shows the time course of head velocity ($\dot{H}$) change (0.3 Hz by 50°/s peak-to-peak). B shows *simple* spike density histograms taken from one and the same Purkinje cell in response to head rotation in darkness. Upper trace, before, and lower trace, after horizontal VOR gain decreased adaptively. C shows similar data for another Purkinje cell, before and after adaptive increase of horizontal VOR gain. Calibration, 1 s (horizontal) and 10 pulses/s (vertical). Filled triangles mark spike frequency of 60 pulses/s. In D–G, arrows represent changes in modulation pattern of each Purkinje cell before and after horizontal VOR adaptation on polar diagrams. D and E show the changes induced in Purkinje cells of the H-zone, and F and G in those of other zones: D and F, under stimulating conditions for VOR gain increase; E and G, for VOR gain decrease (Watanabe, 1984).

a VOR gain decrease. In the polar diagram of Fig. 6D,E, points plotted in the quadrant for ±45° represent modulation of in phase type, while those in the quadrant for −180°±45° imply modulation of out of phase type. Those in other quadrants are of intermediate types. Fig. 6D,E thus demonstrates that an adaptive increase of the VOR gain is accompanied by shift of the points in the in phase to out of phase direction, while an adaptive decrease of the VOR gain is associated with shift of the points in the out of phase to in phase direction.

As discussed earlier (Lisberger & Fuchs, 1974;

Ito, 1975), the in phase-modulating signals of inhibitory Purkinje cells cancel the excitatory action of vestibular afferent signals onto relay cells of the VOR, as the latter is also modulated in phase with head velocity. By contrast, out of phase-modulating signals of inhibitory Purkinje cells would cooperate with the in phase modulating excitatory vestibular signals on VOR relay cells. Consequently, the in phase type of Purkinje cell responses would have an action of depressing, and the out of phase type an action of facilitating, the VOR. Thus, the changes in Purkinje cell responses illustrated in Fig. 6A–E are consistent with the view that changes in the vestibular responsiveness of H-zone Purkinje cells are causal to the VOR gain changes.

Since, however, floccular Purkinje cells receive eye velocity signals via mossy fiber afferents (Lisberger & Fuchs, 1978a,b), a possibility remains that the observed changes in Purkinje cell reponses are merely an effect secondary to changes in eye velocity due to adaptive VOR gain changes. This possibility has been examined and *excluded* by evaluating that the actual eye velocity inputs to rabbit flocculus are minor relative to vestibular inputs (Miyashita, 1984), and also by demonstrating that adaptive changes in monkey flocculus still occurred even after elimination of eye velocity signals by lesions of vestibular nuclei (Watanabe, 1984).

## 4. Adaptive filter model of the cerebellum

The Marr-Albus model of the cerebellum is essentially a pattern-recognizer; it does not give a sufficient account for processing of temporal patterns of time-analog signals which frequency-modulated nerve impulses convey in the nervous system. Fujita (1982a) recently combined the Marr-Albus type of learning principle with the adaptive filter theory and formulated a new model which is capable of setting its input–output relationships for temporally coded mossy fiber signals by learning. In Fujita's model (Fig. 7A), the mossy fiber-granule cell-Golgi cell network converts an input signal to a subset of varied phase lag versions. This phase-converter action is based mainly on a leaky integrator property of the Golgi cell circuitry. These output signals of parallel fibers are gathered together through adjustable synaptic weights to form a final output signal of a Purkinje cell. The synaptic weights are assumed to alter by coincidence of signals of a climbing fiber and a parallel fiber. It has thus been shown mathematically that outputs of a Purkinje cell ($y(t)$ in Fig. 7A) converge to the desired responses ($c(t)$), as the climbing fiber for this Purkinje cell keeps signaling the deviation of the actual Purkinje cell outputs from the desired ones.

Fujita (1982b) incorporated the adaptive filter

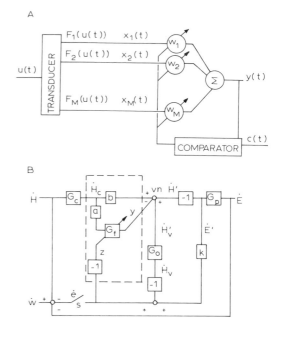

*Fig. 7.* Adaptive filter model of the cerebellum. A, structure of the model; $u(t)$, input signal; $x_j$ ($j=1,2.\ldots.M$), intermediate signals of parallel fibers at time $t.X_j(t)=F_j(u(t))$. $F_j$ denotes the function of a transducer to the $j$-th output signal. The output $y(t)$ is determined by the sum of $w_jx_j(t)$. $c(t)$, given desired signal (Fujita, 1982a). B, a linear interaction model of the VOR and the optokinetic eye movement. The area enclosed by a broken line denotes an incorporated model of the cerebellum and the related pathways. $G_f$, flocculus; $y$, floccular output; $z$, visual climbing fiber input; $vn$, vestibular nuclear relay; $\dot{H}$ head velocity; $\dot{W}$, velocity of visual field movement; $\dot{e}$, retinal error signal; $s$, switch simulating the visual pathway which is to be opened in darkness; $\dot{E}$, eye velocity; $\dot{E}'$, internal feedback signal for eye velocity. $\dot{H}_v$, the visual system's estimate of head velocity in space (Fujita, 1982b).

model of the cerebellum into a linear control model of the oculomotor system, just as the flocculus in the VOR arc, as shown in Fig. 7B. This flocculus model receives horizontal canal signals through the vestibular mossy fiber afferents, and retinal slip signals through the visual climbing fiber afferents, and it alters its signal transfer characteristics for the vestibular mossy fiber inputs in the direction to minimize retinal slip signals during the VOR. The model of Fig. 7B reproduced faithfully adaptive modification of the VOR in both gain and phase, as shown in Fig. 8 in comparison with the data of Gonshor and Melvill

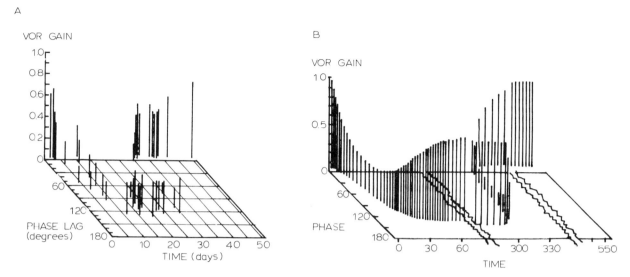

*Fig. 8.* Simulation of the VOR adaptation with Fujita's model. A, experimental data by Gonshor and Melvill Jones (1976b). Three-dimensional display of the VOR gain and phase changes as functions of time. B, simulation results illustrated similarly to A (Fujita, 1982b) (see also Chapter 2).

Jones (1976b). This simulation study is justified by the recent experimental evidence for the learning principle of Marr-Albus model as introduced above, and provides an excellent theoretical support for the 'flocculus hypothesis of the VOR control'.

## 5. Comments

There now seems to be enough reason to believe that the flocculus hypothesis of the VOR has a general applicability. This situation encourages further investigations toward complete understanding of the roles and mechanisms of the cerebellum in adaptation and learning in general. It is important to study in more detail properties of the long term potentiation at parallel fiber–Pur-

kinje cell synapses. The entire time course of this depression has yet to follow, and its possible relationship to permanent memory should be clarified. The idea that the H-zone of the flocculus acts as a modifiable sideparth to the horizontal VOR arc may be expanded to a general principle that each small area of the cerebellum acts as a modifiable sidepath for various reflex arcs and central control systems. The postulated action of the flocculus to calibrate the VOR with reference to retinal error signal may be generalized such that each modifiable sidepath of the cerebellum acts to calibrate reflex actions and central controls with reference to control error signals. Such calibrator action may secure the preciseness and smoothness of controls for which the cerebellum has been assumed to play the key role.

**Adaptive mechanisms in gaze control**
Facts and theories
*Eds. Berthoz & Melvill Jones*
© Elsevier Science Publishers BV (Biomedical Division)

# Chapter 15

# Cerebellar function and the adaptive feature of the central nervous system

## R. Llinás & A. Pellionisz

*Department of Physiology and Biophysics, New York University Medical Center, New York, USA*

## 1. Introduction

The cerebellum has been known for more than 100 years as the organ for motor coordination (Flourens, 1842; Holmes, 1939). This remarkably uniform structure is composed of two main regions, the cerebellar cortex and the cerebellar nuclei which together constitute a functional unit, the 'cerebellar system'. The inputs to this system are of two distinct morphological classes, the mossy and climbing fibers which enter via the cerebellar peduncles, project towards the cerebellar cortex and, on their way, give collaterals to the cerebellar nuclei. The axons of these latter nuclei represent the main output of this system back to the CNS (Ramón y Cajal, 1911) while the intracerebellar corticonuclear projection is represented by the axons of the Purkinje cells. The cerebellum has been quite successfully studied with all the armaments available in neuroscience and, thus, may be considered the region of the CNS most completely investigated and described, both by experimentalists and theorists (cf. Llinás & Simpson, 1981). The basic question remains, however, as to the manner in which present knowledge relating to this cerebellar system is to be transformed into an understanding of motor coordination. Accordingly, in this brief essay we wish to assess the degree of recent advancement towards such an understanding. Some comments will also address the issue of its alleged role in 'motor learning'.

## 2. Cerebellar modelling and theory

The goal of theoretical brain research is not the modeling of any specific part of the CNS per se but rather the development of general theories of brain function that may serve as heuristic tools for the synthesis of at least some of the available analytical data. The choice of the cerebellum as an initial paradigm was clearly related to its striking morphological simplicity, which permitted the construction of quantitative models. Added to this advantage was the considerable knowledge available relating to the electrophysiology of single elements, and that concerning the properties of the cerebellar circuits which they form (Eccles et al., 1967; Llinás, 1969; Palay & Chan-Palay, 1982). Thus, models of cerebellar function, while aiming at resolving particular issues relating to 'motor coordination', also provided a possibility of expanding them into a theory of general brain function. Indeed, in our own case, such modeling (Pellionisz et al., 1977) furnished the impetus for the development of a formal brain theory (Pellionisz & Llinás, 1979b; 1980, 1982a). The cerebellum had the further advantage of providing an excellent model for addressing several basic questions relating to the parallel nature of CNS organization and to the adaptive features of the CNS in general. While such functional principles had also been recognized in connection with the visual system (Lashley, 1942), motor coordination provided a clear and physically accessible example of the collective cooperative character of CNS function (Llinás 1974).

## 3. From analytical details to global function

At a descriptive level, it has long been evident that cerebellar ablation leads to a dysmetric decomposition of movements both in space and in time, in addition to an abnormal level of muscle tone (Holmes, 1939). However, until rather recently insufficient data and lack of formal analysis made impossible the forging of such knowledge into a general conception of the manner in which the cerebellum, as a neuronal system, coordinates movements. Being a motor coordinator with little to do with 'higher brain functions', the cerebellum has always been a lackluster target for the philosophers of mind. And yet, from a general point of view, the lack of a clear understanding of how such a limited brain function as motor coordination emerges from the CNS serves as a reminder of the conceptual backwardness of neuroscience.

## 4. The present challenge

Reviewing the many opinions and partial hypotheses presently available concerning cerebellar function (cf., Llinás & Simpson, 1981; Pellionisz, 1984b), it would be difficult to assert that no general synthesis theories for such cerebellar function have been proposed. Indeed, a problem may be that there are *too many* views, compelling scientists either to make a difficult choice in favoring one, or to learn to navigate with a non-cohesive 'set of maps'. For example, while some of the available representations leave the time dimension out (Marr, 1969), others feature only this aspect (Braitenberg & Onesto, 1961). Still others yield hardware-implementable schemes (Albus, 1971) based on a theory which, however, "did not..tell one how to go about programming a mechanical arm" (Marr, 1982), and featuring *learning*, rather than coordination, as the main cerebellar function.

It appears desirable, therefore, to search for unifying representations, rather than for fragmented sets of partial explanations. Indeed, modeling of cerebellar function must be primarily con-

cerned with motor coordination and an essential first step in such development may be to deal with such coordination by means of vectorial coordinates. Vectorial representations within the brain, however, must be expressed in the CNS' own reference frames, intrinsic to the body, rather than in the conventional extrinsic Cartesian frames. This, in turn, necessitates a sufficiently general formalism to handle non-orthogonal coordinates and, in addition, to define the reference-frame invariant properties of vectorial transformations of general coordinates.

The above line of argument led to the tensor network theory of the CNS, and to its application to cerebellar modeling (Pellionisz & Llinás, 1979b, 1980, 1982a). The key concepts involved in featuring the cerebellum as a tensorial coordination-device are summarized in Fig. 1. The scheme presents the cerebellum in the context of the vestibulo-collicular sensorimotor system, suggesting how vestibular sensory signals are transformed into neck-muscle motor signals. Such a system may serve to compensate, for instance, for a passive turn of the head, produced by a tilt of the body. The compensation would be implemented by an active head rotation using the neck musculature. For a successful compensation, the turn of the head must be expressed by a set of sensory input signals and the implementation will in turn utilize a set of motor output signals. The multivariable vectorial sensory and motor expressions are both assigned to the same 'physical object', to be defined here as the initial deviation of the head and the successive compensatory movement back to the initial head position, with only a sign difference between the passive turn and its active compensation.

Mathematically speaking, a 'physical object' such as a head turn can be vectorially expressed in any frame of reference, whereby the relation amongst different vectorial expressions is tensorial — nevertheless, the question of how the CNS achieves a transformation of a vectorial expression from a sensory to motor frame is not trivial. The core of the problem is that the frames of reference, intrinsic to the body, are different from one another, and are not limited to the three-dimensional orthogonal Cartesian systems. For instance, in Fig. 1A the contractions of the alpha, beta and gamma neck muscles generate a head-turn around axes which clearly constitute a non-orthogonal system. Some other frames intrinsic to CNS function, while not visible, have also been found to be non-orthogonal (Simpson et al., 1981a) (see also Chapter 1).

The general question of how the CNS transforms a vectorial expression of an external physical invariant from one frame to another is complicated by the fact that many motor systems may be of higher dimensionality than the sensory input. This increase in dimensionality is symbolically depicted in Fig. 1. in the simplest possible form as a *two*-dimensional sensory and a *three*-dimensional motor system. This simplification was made here in order to illustrate the transformations by two-dimensional pictograms, and yet maintain the overcomplete character of the multivariable motor system compared to the sensory apparatus. While the vestibulo-collicular system is of considerably higher dimensionality (from six sensors to dozens of motor effectors, even if only gross functional units are counted — and obviously of much higher dimensionality in the CNS' intrinsic *neuronal* terms), the abstract problem of coordination is evident even in the simplified symbolic scheme. Although the expression of an invariant that is given by a lower dimensional vector is mathematically also possible in a higher dimensional space, the problem is that such an overcomplete expression is not unique.

The central problem of coordination is: "based on what paradigm does the CNS arrive at a single executed vectorial expression from an infinite number of possibilitites?" This general problem is rarely considered since CNS systems are most often reduced to single variable control-loops (e.g., horizontal canal to horizontal extraocular muscle system; Robinson, 1968). Lately, with the barrier of single dimensionality broken, the former multivariable approaches (e.g., Krewson, 1950) are thriving again (see in this volume). However, when the multidimensional approach is restricted to three-dimensions throughout the system, then there is no coordination required for implementing such a non-overcomplete transformation. In addition, such dimensional reduction requires an arbitrary 'pairing' of the six extraocular muscles in order to confine the system into a

three-dimensional motor scheme (Robinson, 1982) (Chapter 20). A solution to the problem of overcompleteness is nevertheless possible by means of the generalized inverse of the covariant metric tensor serving as a contravariant metric (Pellionisz, 1983a,b). Quantitative examples for the generalized inverse paradigm were given both for an abstract sensorimotor system (Pellionisz, 1984a) and for the VOR (Chapter 19).

A second problem is raised by the fact that the CNS may use non-orthogonal frames of reference. In such systems there are two kinds of vectorial expressions assigned to a single physical invariant. Sensory information is interpreted as the covariant and motor execution as the contravariant vectorial representation of the same physical invariant (cf., Pellionisz & Llinás, 1980). Therefore, a second question arises: "how can the CNS transform covariants into contravariant vectors?"

And a third, and most general question: "how does the CNS transform vectorial representations from one frame of reference, e.g., sensory, to another, e.g., motor?"

All these questions are addressed by the scheme in Fig. 1. That these functions might not be executed in one step has been discussed in detail (Pellionisz & Llinás, 1980, 1982a). For example, while a sensory to motor transformation is an unavoidable fact, a covariant embedding of the sensory input will yield, of necessity, the *covariant* vectorial version of such input which we denote an intention. Such covariant embedding does allow the transformation of a sensory vector even into an overcomplete motor frame of reference, but such transformation generates a vectorial form which is inappropriate for correct motor implementation. Thus, step I (Fig. 1B) serves the function of coordinate-system transformation, while step II (Fig. 1C) is a metric-type cerebellar transformation that converts the covariant motor intention vector into the physically implementable contravariant form.

As a first step, a two-dimensional vectorial sensory expression of a rotation (such as shown by solid triangles) will be transformed via the $c_{jk}$ transformation matrix into a three-component motor vector expression. A physical summation of the components of this covariant intention vector would, however, be of the wrong amplitude

# COORDINATION via the Cerebellum Acting as a Metric Tensor of the Motor Geometry

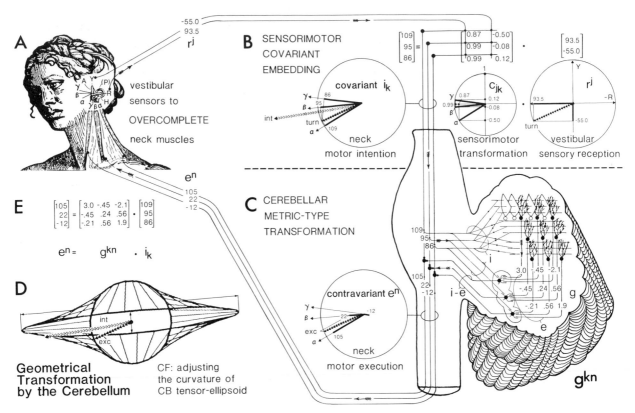

*Fig. 1.* Representation of the geometrical concept and formalism of tensor analysis in its application to cerebellar coordination in a simplified head turn sensorimotor scheme. A: Sensorimotor system of head stabilization. Initial head position is momentarily disturbed by a head turn produced by passive tilt of the body. Anterior (A) and horizontal (H) vestibular canals decompose such head turn, around an axis in the plane of the paper, into roll (R) and yaw (Y) vectorial components of the $r^j$ reception vector. Posterior canal (P) is rendered inactive in the situation depicted. The alpha, beta, gamma neck-muscles, activated by the three-component execution-vector $e^n$, turn the head around respective axes (all lying in the plane of the paper) and re-establish head position. Numerical expressions in the figure are in arbitrary units (shown rounded), negative representing a lowering of the spontaneous firing frequency. Note that the YR sensory- and the alpha, beta, gamma motor-frames are different the latter being higher dimensional (overcomplete). B. Transformation from two-dimensional sensory vector into three-dimensional motor frame of reference. The vestibular $r^j$ is transformed to neck motor intention vector $i_k$, via the sensorimotor transformation matrix $c_{jk}$. Note that such embedding, while it can be executed from lower to higher dimensional spaces, yields covariant vectorial expression. Its components would not physically add to yield the required turn, but would yield dysmetric performance with wrong amplitude and direction (labelled *int*). C. Cerebellar transformation of covariant intention ($i$) to contravariant execution ($e$) via the neuronal network acting as the metric tensor of the motor space ($g^{kn}$). With cerebellar ablation the motor intention ($i$) would be directly executed into an ataxic performance. The mossy fiber-granule cell-Purkinje cell corticonuclear network, comprised as matrix $g$, acts as the space-time metric tensor of the motor space. Stacks of Purkinje cells, marked with open and full circles, represent 'temporal lookahead modules'. The execution vector $e$ projects, via inhibitory Purkinje cells, to cerebellar nuclear cells. Together with excitatory mossy fiber collaterals, the vector leaving the cerebellar nuclei is $i$-$e$ and, in the brain stem nuclei, becomes $i$-$(i$-$e)$=$e$, execution vector. This motor execution vector (exc) will turn the head with the appropriate magnitude and direction. D. The distortion of intention vectors (compared to the required execution) necessitates the cerebellar geometrical transformation. Not only is there an amplitude difference between intention and execution, but such 'gain' is directionally different: about 2 along the bigger axis of tensor ellipsoid, while about 0.2 along the shorter axis. In addition, there is a direction-deviation between intention and execution, except along the axes of tensor ellipsoid. Such distortion of head-turn vectors along a circle into an ellipsoid of intent is geometrically compensated by the cerebellar transformation. E. Reference frame independent tensorial expression, and particular vector-matrix representations of cerebellar transformations, to complete the 2D pictograms, the network-implementation and the verbal description. The abstract notation defines the function of cerebellum as a covariant to contravariant transformation

and direction (see in Fig. 1 *int* differing from *turn*).

We would like to emphasize that for representational convenience the complexity of Fig. 1. has been reduced to the minimum. Indeed, in addition to the reduction of the dimensionality of an overcomplete multidimensional system (two to three), the vestibular frame is depicted as being orthogonal; thus the $r^j$ sensory vector here is both covariant and contravariant. As shown earlier (Pellionisz & Llinás, 1982a) (see also Chapter 19), the covariant embedding procedure is fully valid in general (non-orthogonal) frames as well. However, in the latter case, if the sensory reference frame is oblique, an additional *sensory metric transformation* would also be required since the covariant embedding procedure requires a contravariant sensory vector to be transformed into a covariant motor intention. Since the step of sensory metric transformations is elaborated elsewhere (Pellionisz & Llinás, 1982a) (Chapter 19), it is omitted here.

In the second step (Fig 1D), the general conceptual interpretation of cerebellar function is, then, a geometrical transformation not unlike the 'mirror analogy' (Llinás, 1974). The circle of possible rotations, distorted into a tensor ellipsoid of corresponding intentions, is shaped by the cerebellum into the original circle of executions. From this conceptual point of view, the generation and modification of cerebellar network function would be aimed at adjusting the curvature of the cerebellar tensor ellipsoid via the climbing fiber system (cf., Pellionisz & Llinás, 1982a).

## 5. Assessment of status quo

In comparing the various attempts at a synthesis of cerebellar function, it is clear that the tensor approach is compatible with an array of former hypotheses, although some of their basic assumptions have had to be considerably reinterpreted.

For instance, the modifiable character of CNS function is a prominent target of various conceptual interpretations. While Ito (1982b) stresses learning as an important cerebellar function, he appears to agree that the primary and secondary roles of the cerebellum are motor coordination and timing. As is emphasized in this Chapter, plasticity must be a property of all subsystems of the CNS, especially during development. This is particularly clear when coping with circumstances such as the increase in body size during growth. It may be an error, however, to mistake the development of a function for the function itself. For example, if the cerebellar function is a geometrical transformation of covariants into contravariant activity vectors (determining a relation between a circle and a tensor ellipsoid), the dynamic adjustment of the curvature of this ellipsoid may be a role that the climbing fiber system plays in coordination. This is, however, quite a different notion than the assumption that the role of the cerebellum is motor learning and that such learning is due to the heterosynaptic depression of parallel fiber activity by climbing fiber activation.

The need for an integrative view of the function of CNS subsystems is another central issue. Integrative cerebellar theories cannot exclude any prominent aspect of the total coordination function. A theory that is restricted to only one or two aspects of coordination, brilliant as it may be (e.g., the 'timing' notion of Braitenberg & Onesto, 1961), serves only as a transient, sharply focused, flash on a detail. Overly narrow representations usually have to be considerably reinterpreted if they are eventually to be fitted into a model with enough power to illuminate a much broader perspective.

A special example of this is the above mentioned notion of timing. Originally, the cerebellum was suggested to perform a clock function (Braitenberg & Onesto, 1961). This view assumed that the CNS uses reference frames with separable space and time, as in classical mechanics. By pointing out that such separation in the CNS is impossible, spatial and temporal coordination was explained as a metric function in a unified space-time frame (Pellionisz & Llinás, 1982a).

Other attempts at space-time integration have also been made, for instance, by supplementing

---

(raising the lower covariant index into an upper contravariant one), no matter what particular motor frame is used. The numerical representation, different for each given frame, yields a particular quantitative description of the general function (modified from Pellionisz, 1984b).

the 'learning device' paradigm with the time dimension. Attributing the temporal properties of cerebellar function to the Golgi cell-interneuron system (Fujita, 1982a), however, raises the problem that some cerebella (e.g., in amphibia) exhibit marked temporal dynamism (Freeman, 1969; Llinás et al 1971), even though the Golgi cell-interneuronal system is hardly found in these species (Hillman, 1969).

A trend towards unification, starting with the integrating of different aspects of the function of the cerebellum into a coherent model, cannot stop at the boundaries of this subsystem. Indeed, an old question stares us in the face: "can we make a real systems approach to cerebellar function without modeling the whole motor system?" (Eccles et al., 1967). A particularly serious challenge to brain theorists and modelists is, therefore, to integrate separate models of different subsystems of the CNS; for instance, to merge models relating to motor coordination (cerebellum) with those relating to sensory centers (tectum) in order to generate a unified view of how sensory input is transformed into the motor execution. Tensor network theory of the CNS integrates cerebellar theory into a multisensory-multimotor system by considering the function of the superior colliculus in relation to the cerebellum (Pellionisz, 1983a).

Specifically, the major aspects of compatibility of tensor theory of cerebellar coordination with former notions are as follows.

*(a) Morphological and physiological features.* Nontrivial properties of cerebellar neurons and neuronal networks are meaningfully incorporated into a coherent conceptual scheme. For instance, the observation that stacks of Purkinje cells exhibit different derivative-type dynamic features (Llinás et al., 1971) led to the concept of 'temporal lookahead-modules' (Pellionisz et al., 1977; Pellionisz & Llinás, 1979b).

*(b) Lateral inhibition scheme.* Szentágothai's (1963) concept, the surrounding of these modules with basket cell inhibition, is reinterpreted as the lateral inhibition serving to protect and enhance the 'lookahead-modules' (Pellionisz & Llinás, 1979b).

*(c) Timing properties of the cerebellum.* The pioneering notion of timing (Braitenberg & Onesto, 1961) is unified into a spacetime representa-

tion via the predictive space–time metric tensor (Pellionisz & Llinás, 1982a).

*(d) Synergy-control.* The classical notion by Bernstein (1947) is formally developed into describing co-activated groups of muscles as commanded by motor vectors, expressed in oblique reference frames intrinsic to the muscles, skeletal system and CNS (Pellionisz & Llinás, 1980).

*(e) Coordination.* The fundamental clinical observation (Holmes, 1939) that cerebellar ablation leads to motor dysmetria is conceptually and formally elaborated into the interpretation of cerebellar function as the metric-type transformation of covariant intention into contravariant execution (Pellionisz & Llinás, 1980, 1982a).

*(f) Adaptive gain control and plasticity.* Adaptability is seen not as the function itself, but as a feature of the evolvement of the function, which is motor coordination. While the cerebellum has been assumed to yield a scalar variable gain (Ito, 1970; Robinson, 1975a), the cerebellar tensor ellipsoid indicates that there is an infinite number of such 'gains' (if one insists on this misuse of the term 'gain'). Moreover, each such 'gain' represents a multidimensional distortion of both *amplitude* and *direction*; the distortion is direction-dependent both in its scalar magnification factor and its hitherto overlooked refraction angle, resembling 'phase'. Instead of studying the alteration of a single scalar 'gain', both theoretical analyses and experimental studies of the adjustments in the metric type function are now possible.

## 6. Role of cerebellum in motor adaptation

Finally, some points must be made relating to the interpretation of the cerebellum as a 'learning machine'. Over the last 20 years, since the initial formulation of Brindley (1964) and Grossberg (1964), elaborated by Marr (1969) and Albus (1971), that the cerebellar cortex functions as the site for motor memory, much effort has been dedicated to this hypothetical function of the cerebellum (cf., Ito, 1980). The main motive for identifying cerebellar function with motor learning has been a peculiarity in the synaptic organization of the cerebellar cortex. It concerns the rather specialized nature of the two afferents to the Purkinje cell, the central neuron in this cortex. Indeed, because the climbing fiber system and the mossy fiber-granule cell system form extremely different morphological arrangements on the dendrites of this neuron, it has been assumed that these two types of contact embody two quite distinct operational characteristics. Accordingly, the above authors postulated that the climbing fiber with its widespread coverage of the dendritic tree has the unique function of modification, by heterosynaptic action, of the synaptic efficacy of parallel fiber input activated within a certain time window. This modification is assumed to last over a protracted time, providing a mechanism for the acquisition of motor skill. The central experimental basis in support of this assertion, made most recently by Ito et al. (1982c), has been that activation of climbing fiber and parallel fiber inputs to a particular Purkinje cell, within a particular time interval, causes a marked and sustained decrease of the parallel fiber excitation onto that particular neuron. This heterosynaptic depression of the parallel fiber Purkinje cell synapse was then interpreted as the mechanism by which the cerebellar cortex is modified by experience in order for the animal to acquire motor skills. On the other hand, attempts to reproduce the same effects by the more sensitive intracellular methods have failed to indicate any such change (Llinás et al., 1981). However, this experimental discrepancy, which will be ultimately resolved with better recording techniques, is really not the central issue. Rather, two fundamental questions must be raised with respect to this specific learning hypothesis.

(1) does the climbing fiber system play a more profound role than heterosynaptic modulation?

(2) does heterosynaptic depression fit into an interpretation of cerebellar function as (a) a motor coordinator or (b) a pattern recognition device?

As for the first point, several lines of experimental evidence have suggested that the climbing fiber system arises as an afferent pathway in its own right. Thus, recent results suggest that the inferior olive (IO) is organized in such a way that clusters of neurons tend to fire in a close to synchronous manner (Bower and Llinás, 1982, 1983) and that such firing is produced by the elec-

troresponsive properties of the IO neurons in conjunction with their electrotonic interactions (Llinás & Yarom, 1981a,b). Furthermore, the inferior olivary system has been shown to be activated by sensory stimuli such as retinal slip (Simpson, 1979), motion of limb joints (Rubia & Kolb, 1978), vestibular stimulation (Ferin et al., 1971;), and neck afferent activation (Berthoz & Llinás, 1974). In addition, when the IO is activated electrically (Boylls, 1978; Barmack, 1979) or with drugs such as harmaline (de Montigny & Lamarre, 1973; Llinás & Volkind, 1973), particular stereotypic movements occur (cf., Llinás & Simpson, 1981). It must also be remembered that the climbing fiber system sends collaterals to the cerebellar nuclei indicating a clear throughput via the cerebellar nuclear efferents. It can be argued, therefore, that any hypothesis relating to the function of cerebellum which negates the functional role of an afferent system as salient as the olivocerebellar input in the continuous process of motor coordination is, of necessity, at least incomplete if not downright inadequate.

The second question posed above raises a significant criticism of the 'learning hypothesis' relating to the manner in which the assumed modification of the parallel fiber system by the climbing fiber afferents may serve as information storage. Indeed, before considerable effort is invested into finding experimental validation for particular assumptions to support the cerebellar learning hypothesis, such a conjecture should be put into proper perspective with regard to motor coordination. Such a general perspective of the learning paradigm has not been produced so far.

## 7. Role of the cerebellum in the acquisition of motor learning in intact animals

The question of the role of the cerebellar cortex in motor learning has been considered experimentally at other than cellular levels. The question focused clearly once the cerebellum became, at least in theory, the 'center' for the acquisition of new motor patterns. This assumption reached such impetus that a paper on "the cerebellum as a motor repair shop" was published by Robinson (1975c), which suggested that motor compensation following peripheral or central nervous system damage was implemented by altered cerebellar function. Research in our laboratory on this matter had related to the role of the cerebellum in vestibular compensation following unilateral vestibular lesion in the rat (Llinás et al., 1975). The results following surgical or X-ray lesions of the cortex, or following lesion of the climbing fiber system (either complete or partial), all indicated that acquisition of vestibular compensation in the rat requires the presence of an intact inferior olive and of cerebellar nuclei, but does not require the cerebellar cortex. Furthermore, when only the climbing fiber system in this structure was lesioned, animals showed an inability to compensate. This could be viewed as the climbing fiber system being required for acquisition of such compensation. However, following the acquisition of compensation, damage of the inferior olive produced an immediate disappearance of the compensated state. This indicated, then, that the presence of the inferior olive was required for the *acquisition* and the *maintenance* of this motor adaptation. Evidently, motor adaptation requires the olivocerebellar system probably as *part* of the pathway which produces the compensation. Furthermore, in rats with partial IO lesions, the climbing fiber system could support vestibular compensation. However, harmaline which affected the remaining portion of the olive produced disappearance of the compensation, which returned after the effect of the drug had worn off, indicating that compensation required a continued prevalence of the appropriate action of the olivary neurons. These results do indicate that the olivocerebellar system is clearly essential in the acquisition of motor compensation, but do not demonstrate, on their own, that such motor learning takes place at the level of the inferior olive. Similar conclusions drawn from the same experimental paradigm were recently reported concerning adaptation of the VOR following momentary disconnection of the inferior olive by tetrodotoxin. The results were striking enough to generate disenchantment with the hypothesis of cerebellar learning (Demer & Robinson, 1982).

A different set of studies, putting the cerebellum in the context of the motor system at large, concerned the development of movement in monkeys (Sasaki & Gemba, 1982). Results indicated that acquisition of motor commands probably takes place in the prefrontal cortex and that the cerebellum is of importance mainly as a throughput for the acquisition of motor response in the time range of 510 ms. In agreement with our previous studies, such research indicates that the acquisition of a motor task, while damaged by cerebellar ablation, is less impaired if only the cerebellar cortex is damaged, underlining again the central importance of the cerebellar nuclei in the overall function.

Finally, in an elegant set of experiments by Lincoln et al. (1982) and McCormick et al. (1982), it has been demonstrated that the classical conditioned eyelid/nictitating membrane response may be specifically blocked by cerebellar nuclear damage. These conditioned responses are obliterated when the dendate and interpositus cerebellar nuclei are destroyed, but are only partly modified, following exclusive cerebellar cortex damage. All of the above data strongly indicate that the cerebellar system probably functions as an important throughput via the inputs and outputs of the cerebellar nuclei. The cerebellar cortex, on the other hand, seems to modulate this particular nuclear throughput on the basis of information coming through the cortex as the movement takes place. This view is in accordance with the idea that cortical function sets motor intentions in the context of the position and functional state of the motor system.

In our view, any motor 'learning' first relates to the adjustment of intended movements, probably arising from the prefrontal cortex (see Sasaki & Gemba, 1982) which are then refined by a trial and error process. Such intended movements, as covariant versions of the final movement, would be relayed to the cerebellum to be translated into executable (i.e., contravariant) motor coordinates. To be capable of properly implementing such transformation, all parts of the cerebellar system, and in particular the cerebellar nuclei, apparently play an important role in the organization of movement. It follows, therefore, that damage to the cerebellar nuclei has a devastating effect, both in the process of motor acquisition and in motor coordination. Nevertheless, this does not mean that learning actually occurs at the cerebellar nuclear level.

## 8. Is the cerebellum capable of any form of plasticity?

When considering the role of the cerebellum, the authors (together and in separate publications) have emphasized the issue of motor coordination. Tensor network theory suggests that the cerebellum serves as a covariant to contravariant metric tensor, i.e., that an internal functional geometry of the motor hyperspace is embodied in the cerebellar circuitry. However, in order to develop and perfect such transformations, the cerebellum as a system must be capable of plasticity, just as the rest of the CNS. Indeed, as a living organism changes its dimensions (e.g., body size) during development, the internal metric of the system must change with them in order to maintain or improve a coordinated functional state. This is particularly clear during embryonic development, when the intrinsic coordinate systems are developed at the same time as the emergence of their internal CNS representation embodied in the simultaneously developing neuronal networks. In fact, the role of tremor during development has been suggested as a biological basis for establishing the internal reference frames that allow sensory-motor transformations (Llinás, 1984).

Plasticity may then be related to the function of both mossy and climbing fiber inputs and may be a distributed function relating to a very subtle set of changes involving a very large number of neurons during development. This would undoubtedly involve the cerebellar system if one assumes that the cerebellum is the place where the covariant-contravariant transformations subserving the conversion of motor intention into proper motor execution take place.

Our views on cerebellar plasticity relate then to that degree of subtle change required for developing and perfecting a metric tensor that embodies the internal functional geometry and not as a depository of specific patterns of activity required for the learning of a particular motor sequence. A system must have sufficient plasticity to be able to modify its functional geometry such that the coordination of *all* possible movements is perfected. According to our view, plasticity in the cerebellum exists to allow the *development of coordination*, but not the learning of particular movements.

### Acknowledgements

Research was supported by United States Public Health Service grant NS13742 from the National Institute of Neurological and Communicative Disorders and Stroke.

Adaptive mechanisms in gaze control
Facts and theories
*Eds. Berthoz & Melvill Jones*
©1985 Elsevier Science Publishers BV (Biomedical Division)

# Chapter 16

# Cooperative functions of vestibular nuclei neurons and floccular Purkinje cells in the control of nystagmus slow phase velocity: single cell recordings and lesion studies in the monkey

W. Waespe & V.Henn

*Department of Neurology, University Hospital, 8091 Zürich, Switzerland*

## 1. Introduction

Ever since scientists have recognized that head movements induce eye movements, speculations about mechanisms have been put forward. Purkinje (1820) assumed movement of the brain and fluid shifts to be responsible. The anatomical structures involved were unknown until the semicircular canals of the labyrinth were recognized as special sense organs to detect angular head accelerations (Goltz, 1870; Breuer, 1874; Crum Brown, 1874; Mach, 1875). The decisive next step was the description of the three neuron reflex arc — the vestibulo-ocular reflex (VOR) (Lorente de Nó, 1933). Head rotation induces a signal in the primary vestibular neurons of the eighth nerve, and secondary neurons in the vestibular nuclei transmit this signal directly to motoneurons in the oculomotor nuclei (Fig. 1A). However, already Lorente de Nó (1933) recognized the functional importance of other, polysynaptic pathways via the cerebellum and reticular formation: "That the vestibular impulses really have at their disposal different anatomic paths is demonstrated by the fact that no labyrinthine excitation necessarily sets up a determinant reaction." In a similar way Mowrer (1935, 1937) speculated about the role of the vestibular nuclei during visual-vestibular interaction.

In the following decades clinical and experimental evidence accumulated showing that both the vestibular nuclei and the flocculus of the vestibulo-cerebellum have important functions in the generation and suppression of nystagmus during visual-vestibular interactions. In recent years analysis of nystagmus slow phase velocity, and recordings of single cell activity in the alert animal, have yielded a wealth of quantitative data. Based on these data, models have been built and experimental results simulated on the computer (Robinson, 1977a,b; Raphan & Cohen, 1981; Buizza & Schmid, 1982; for review see Henn et al., 1980) (see also Chs. 8, 19, 20, 21 & 22). It became clear that nystagmus generation cannot be reduced to activity in the basic three neuron reflex arc only. Activity in this reflex has probably only explanatory value in the anesthetized animal or comatose patient if the head is passively rotated and tonic eye deviations are seen. In all other situations, when nystagmus is present, many more neuron populations in the brain stem and cerebellum are involved. The analytical problem emerges to determine causal relationships between different neuron populations. Logical analysis and computer simulation showed that input-output relations (head acceleration vs. eye position) cannot be described by one single operator. Rather different integrators, switches, sum-

234

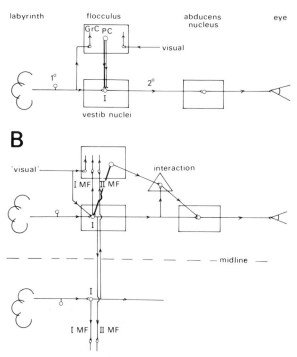

**A**

labyrinth      flocculus      abducens      eye
nucleus

GrC PC

visual

1°      2°

I

vestib nuclei

**B**

'visual'      interaction

I MF   II MF

I

—— midline ——

I

I MF | II MF

*Fig. 1.* Scheme of pathways important in visual-vestibular interaction. A, Ito's hypothesis (1976, 1982a); B, hypothesis based on results in the monkey. In A the primary vestibular fibers from the labyrinth (1°) project to secondary type I vestibular neurons (2°) which project directly to neurons of the abducens nucleus. Primary vestibular fibers project also to the flocculus, and their signal reaches the Purkinje cell (PC) via Granule cells (GrC). The visual system projects to the flocculus either via mossy fibers (MFs) or directly on P-cells via climbing fibers (not shown). In B the three neuron reflex arc is unchanged. The main projection from the vestibular system to the flocculus originates from type I central vestibular neurons from the vestibular nuclei of both sides. There is a separate 'visual' input to the flocculus and to the vestibular nuclei. This input denotes an input carrying an image slip velocity signal and/or a signal derived from it. Floccular P-cells project directly on secondary vestibular neurons (heavy line) as in A, and also to target cells of unknown localization where their signals interact with signals from central vestibular neurons (denoted as 'interaction'). The heavy projection is thought to be important for long term, and the thin projection for immediate, adjustments of the VOR and OKN. The velocity-to-position integrator is omitted (Skavenski & Robinson, 1973). Compare with Figs. 1 & 2 of Ch. 14.

ming points, etc., are required to build a minimal network capable to perform the necessary signal transformations. Activity changes in many of

these internal elements cannot be directly correlated to input or output parameters such as head acceleration or eye velocity, as they represent the state of internal operators. Computer simulation helped to formulate the logical problem and to identify logical gaps. However, it is still necessary anatomically and physiologically to determine how a certain operation is implemented on a neuronal basis. The following review will summarize the analyses of eye movement recordings and of single cell activity in the vestibular nerve, vestibular nuclei and the flocculus in monkeys during visual-vestibular interactions. One important restriction is that all measurements refer to the horizontal plane only. The coding of direction other than horizontal has only recently been addressed (Robinson, 1982; Goldberg & Fernandez, 1981; Henn et al., 1983) (Chapters 2 & 20).

The activity changes of single neurons will be examined in relation to the stimulus parameters and to slow phase eye velocity (Fig. 3). Such an approach relies on quantitative analyses of single unit recordings in trying to establish logical links of input-output relations. In order to obtain evidence of a causal relationship between events in different neuron populations and eye velocity, focal lesions were applied to selectively block elements in this network. With this approach we hope to be able to separate the contributions of different cell populations in the generation or suppression of nystagmus. We will show how activity of single cells in the vestibular nuclei and the flocculus can behave very differently in response to the same head acceleration depending on whether and what visual stimulus is present, whether the animal will have nystagmus or suppresses it, and on the individual history of an animal which can change vestibular time constants over wide ranges. This will lay the groundwork for some speculation about the mechanism of adaptation.

## 2. Various types of nystagmus and combined visual-vestibular stimulation

### 2.1 Vestibular nystagmus (VN)

VN in the horizontal plane is induced by rotation

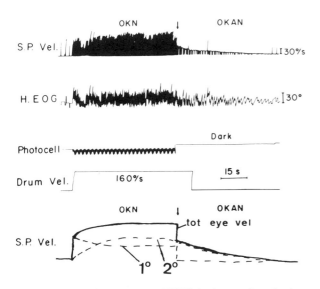

*Fig. 2.* Optokinetic nystagmus (OKN) in the monkey. In descending order from top: velocity of horizontal eye movements (SP Vel), downward arrow marks the time when the lights are turned off and OKN continues as optokinetic afternystagmus (OKAN) in darkness; horizontal eye position (H.EOG); photocell signal marking the period of optokinetic stimulation; velocity profile of the optokinetic drum (acceleration 2600°/s², constant velocity 160°/s); Lower, scheme to explain how the 'direct' (1°), and the 'indirect' (2°) pathways contribute to nystagmus velocity (tot eye vel).

of the monkey with its head fixed about a vertical axis in darkness. After an acceleration impulse, nystagmus slow phase velocity declines progressively. The time course of this declining response is roughly exponential and is characterized by a dominant time constant ($T_c$). After one time constant the eye velocity had declined to 37% of its initial value. $T_c$ ranges between 10 and 40+ s (Raphan et al., 1979; Buettner et al., 1978; Waespe & Henn, 1979b; Waespe et al., 1980). The time constant of VN slow phase velocity is thus longer than that of the cupula which is 5-6 sec in the monkey (Goldberg & Fernandez, 1971; Büttner & Waespe 1981). The variation in the time constant is largely due to different states of habituation and can decrease with repetitive vestibular stimulation (Jaeger & Henn, 1981a; Raphan et al., 1979).

## 2.2. Optokinetic nystagmus (OKN)

OKN is induced by rotation of a patterned wholefield visual surround around the stationary monkey. Its direction is usually defined by the direction of its fast phases. It is composed of two processes: a rapid initial change in slow phase eye velocity followed by a slower rise to a steady state level (Cohen et al., 1977) (Fig. 2). The initial fast rise reaches 40–80% of the steady state velocity. Pathways responsible for the fast rise are referred to as 'direct' visual-oculomotor pathways (Cohen et al., 1977) or as the smooth pursuit system (Robinson, 1981b). Pathways responsible for the slower changes in eye velocity during OKN and for the occurrence of optokinetic after-nystagmus are referred to as 'indirect' visual-oculomotor pathways (Cohen et al, 1977; Raphan et al, 1979; Waespe et al, 1983) or as the optokinetic-system (Robinson, 1981b). A key element in the 'indirect' pathways is a velocity storage mechanism shared with the vestibular system.

## 2.3. Smooth pursuit eye movements

These are defined as slow movements in foveated animals generated by a single target object moving in front of the animal. Peak velocities exceed 100°/s in the monkey (Lisberger & Fuchs, 1978a). Determining factors are the velocity and eccentricity of the target object relative to the fovea. Smooth pursuit eye movements show no substantial after-effects.

## 2.4. Optokinetic afternystagmus (OKAN)

OKAN is the continuing nystagmus in darkness after optokinetic stimulation. Eye velocity decreases sharply in the first second after lights off to a velocity from which it declines slower over a much longer time course (Fig. 2). The amount of the initial fast decay in eye velocity is dependent on the preceding stimulus velocity, and increases with higher stimulus and OKN velocities (Cohen et al., 1977). Up to a velocity of 60°/s it is very small. The maximal value to which the eye velocity decays in the first second after lights off is called the saturation velocity of the OKAN (Cohen et al., 1977). In our monkeys it ranged between 50 and 80°/s (see also Lisberger et al., 1981), but values up to 120°/s have been reported (Cohen et al., 1977). Primary OKAN beats into the same direction as the preceding OKN. Its slow phase velocity declines with a similar time course as VN and $T_c$ ranges between 10 and 40 s. Primary OKAN may be followed by secondary OKAN which beats into the opposite direction. With increasing duration of stimulation and with repetitive optokinetic stimulation the duration of primary OKAN becomes shorter and the strength and duration of secondary OKAN increases (Brandt et al., 1974; Büttner et al., 1976; Waespe & Henn, 1978b; Cohen et al., 1977; Koenig and Dichgans, 1981).

## 2.5. Combined nystagmus

This is induced by rotation of the monkey within the space-stationary visual surround. Within limits its slow phase velocity is nearly compensatory and reflects stimulus velocity at each instance of stimulation (Waespe et al., 1980). The vestibular contribution to nystagmus is responsible for an adequate phasic response during high accelerations while the optokinetic system contributes to the sustained nystagmus response during periods of constant velocity rotation.

## 2.6. Conflict stimulation

This refers to yet another mode of visual-vestibular interaction. In this mode the whole-field visual surround is mechanically coupled to the turntable and both are rotated into the same direction. The conflict is that the labyrinths detect a motion into one direction which is not supported by information from the visual system as no visual displacement takes place. The vestibular nystagmus is either completely suppressed or attenuated and its time constant is shortened to between 2 and 6 s. When nystagmus cannot be completely suppressed at high stimulus accelerations image slip into the same direction as actual motion is present. This is opposite to the image slip direction during acceleration into the same direction inside a stationary surround (combined nystagmus).

## 2.7. VOR suppression

This refers to the situation whereby an animal attempts to fixate a small light spot maintained in the center of its visual field, while both animal and light spot are rotated in otherwise complete darkness.

## 3. Neuronal activity in the vestibular nerve

Primary vestibular neurons connect the semicircular canals with secondary neurons in the vestibular nuclei. Horizontal canal neurons have a high resting discharge of almost 100 imp/s on average (Goldberg & Fernandez, 1971; Keller, 1976; Büttner & Waespe, 1981). These neurons are modulated in a bidirectional manner with activation during acceleration towards the ipsilateral and inhibition during acceleration towards the contralateral side. This behavior had been defined as a type I response by Duensing and Schaefer (1958). After a pulse of acceleration activity returns to the resting discharge level with a time constant of 5.7 s in the anesthetized squirrel monkey (Goldberg & Fernandez, 1971) and 5.9 s (range 3–7 s) in the alert Rhesus monkey (Büttner & Waespe, 1981). The neurons are not modulated during optokinetic stimulation (Keller, 1976; Büttner & Waespe, 1981). As a consequence the modulation of primary vestibular neurons is not influenced during angular rotation by concomitant visual stimuli. These neurons are also not modulated with fast eye movements (Keller, 1976; Büttner & Waespe, 1981). The response of primary neurons to the above described different stimuli is schematically drawn in Fig. 3. The signal is carried to central vestibular neurons (Fig. 1). Whether it also reaches the flocculus is still controversial (Korte & Mugnaini, 1979).

## 3.1. Effects of vestibular nerve lesion

Different techniques with similar results have been used to interrupt the information transmission in the vestibular nerve: labyrinthectomy (mechanical destruction of the labyrinth), or neurectomy (surgical cutting of one or all branches of the nerves from the labyrinth). Beyond the lack of a vestibular response in such animals there is one important modification of visually in-

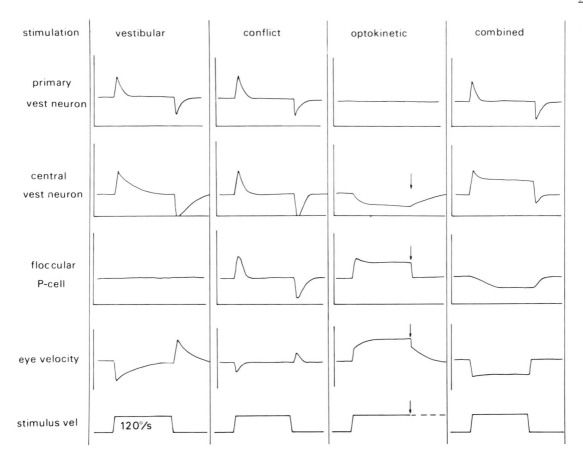

*Fig. 3.* Scheme of the activity in primary and central type I vestibular neurons, floccular P-cells and nystagmus slow phase velocity during different modes of stimulation (velocity steps of 120°/s to the ipsilateral side). Downward arrows indicate the time when lights are turned off and nystagmus continues as OKAN.

duced eye movements: OKN is slowed down and less regular, and primary OKAN is abolished (Cohen et al., 1973). As primary vestibular neurons do not code visual information about motion, the effect of labyrinthectomy on OKN and OKAN must be an indirect one. One possibility is that secondary vestibular neurons degenerate together with the primary neurons. A more likely possibility is that secondary neurons need the continuous high frequency input in order to function normally and to maintain their own resting discharge which is almost 50 imp/s on average. This interpretation is supported by the results of canal plugging which does not lead to such changes of OKN or OKAN (Cohen et al., 1982) (see also Ch 9). With this technique the canals are

surgically plugged so that during acceleration no pressure gradient can build up (Ewald, 1982; Money & Scott, 1962). Primary fibers then continue to display their high continuous resting discharge but without modulation during vestibular stimulation.

## 4. Neuronal activity in the vestibular nuclei

Neurons responding to angular acceleration in the horizontal plane are commonly classified as type I and type II neurons (Duensing & Schaefer, 1958). Neurons with a threshold to angular acceleration below $5°/s^2$ were investigated and will be referred to as central vestibular neurons (Fig. 4). They are also modulated during horizontal optokinetic sti-

238

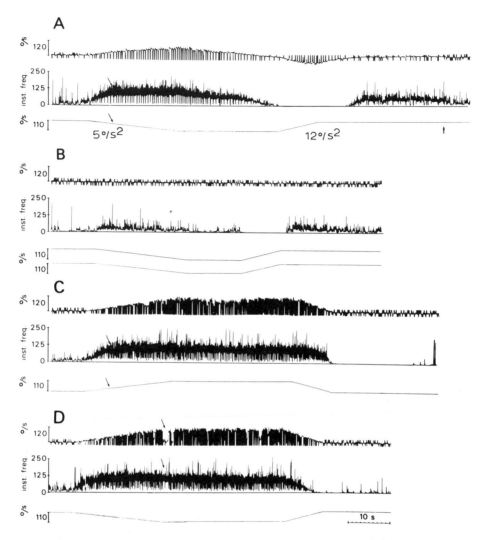

*Fig. 4.* Instantaneous activity of a type I neuron in the vestibular nuclei during vestibular (A), conflict (B), optokinetic (C), and combined (D) stimulation. Upper part of each subfigure: eye velocity (fast phases are clipped at an arbitrary level); instantaneous activity (imp/s); stimulus velocity (acceleration 5°/s²; constant velocity 110°/s), A–D respectively. The neuron is inhibited with saccades to the ipsilateral side and shows a weak burst with movements to the contralateral side. There is also a weak eye position signal. Neuronal frequency increases during vestibular stimulation to the ipsilateral (A) and during optokinetic stimulation to the opposite side (C). Note that during the acceleration the frequency reaches a steady state level already at a velocity of about 30–40°/s (arrow in A and C). During deceleration in C the frequency starts to decay sharply at a velocity of about 30°/s. During conflict stimulation (B) neuronal modulation is strongly reduced and there is no nystagmus. Note in D that activity is maintained although nystagmus temporarily decreases over several seconds due to a momentary drop in alertness (arrow). In this and subsequent figures unit activity is shown unfiltered as instantaneous frequency. The compressed time scale variability seems to be high which is mostly due to short-lasting changes of activity during rapid eye movements. In this example the neuron pauses with rapid nystagmus phases to the ipsilateral side, most clearly seen in A where activity is interrupted with each nystagmus beat.

mulation in a direction specific way (Waespe & Henn, 1977a;b). Type I neurons increase their frequency during vestibular stimulation to the recording side, and during optokinetic stimulation to the contralateral side (Fig. 4A,C). In both situations nystagmus to the recording side is elicited. During stimulation into opposite directions type I neurons are inhibited. Type II neurons show a mirrorlike behavior. Qualitatively all central vestibular neurons give the same responses, quantitatively they differ in their dynamics (Waespe & Henn, 1979a,b). The response after vestibular acceleration during rotation at constant velocity is characterized by a dominant decaying time constant ($T_c$) which is similar to that of vestibular nystagmus (VN) and in the range between 10 and 40+ s (Fig. 4A). It is always longer than that found for neurons in the vestibular nerve (around 6 s). However, if the monkeys are anesthetized, the neuronal time constant shortens to values found for the primary vestibular neurons (Buettner et al., 1978).

Constant velocity optokinetic stimulation leads to maintained frequency changes which can be related to stimulus velocities up to 60°/s on average. At higher stimulus velocities frequency does not further change in contrast to slow phase velocity of OKN (Fig. 9A). During acceleration of the optokinetic stimulus, frequency changes follow instantaneous velocity of the visual surround up to acceleration values of 5–10°/s² on average. If lights are turned out during optokinetic stimulation, nystagmus continues as optokinetic after-nystagmus (OKAN). The slow change in eye velocity during OKAN is faithfully reflected in a similar slow frequency change of central vestibular neurons, but the initial fast drop is not (Waespe & Henn, 1977b).

In monkeys which have been trained to suppress OKN by fixating a single light point in front of them (stimulus velocity then is equal to image slip velocity), neuronal activity changes are less, about 60% of the response during OKN (Buettner & Büttner, 1979). The above shown modulation of neuronal activity during OKAN suggests that it can be related to eye velocity, but during other conditions, such as suppression of OKN, it can be related to the velocity of image slip.

Combined visual-vestibular stimulation leads to firing rates during acceleration which can be related to the instantaneous velocity over a larger range than with the visual or vestibular stimulus alone. Within a certain velocity range frequency changes are independent of the acceleration values (tested for values between 1.25 and 10°/s²). However, neurons show also saturation phenomena (Waespe & Henn, 1979b). Above a certain velocity, the change in frequency is minimal or neurons reach a constant firing level which is maintained during the remaining period of acceleration (Fig. 4D). During constant velocity stimulation the frequency is maintained at the same level as during optokinetic stimulation alone.

Conflict stimulation leads to peak frequency changes which are smaller as compared to vestibular stimulation alone. The effect is strongest at low accelerations (Fig. 4B) and minimal at accelerations above 20°/s² when nystagmus is still attenuated by more than 50%. For all accelerations, however, the dominant time constant of neuronal activity after an acceleration pulse is less than 8 s (Waespe & Henn, 1978a) which is close to the range of the time constant of primary vestibular neurons. During suppression of vestibular nystagmus by fixating a single light point (VOR suppression) peak modulation is not attenuated, even at low accelerations (Buettner & Büttner, 1979).

### 4.1 Fast eye movements

40–50% of the neurons show some modulation during fast eye movements, and about 20% in addition, some modulation with eye position (Fuchs & Kimm, 1975; Waespe et al., 1977). Most often neurons are inhibited with saccades in one or in all directions, and frequency increases with eye positions opposite to the on-direction of vestibular stimulation. Activity in neurons discussed here was always dominated by the vestibular or optokinetic response and in comparison the eye position modulation was negligible. There are other neurons with a modulation during fast eye movements and different eye positions, similar to neurons in the paramedial pontine reticular formation (PPRF) and the perihypoglossal region (Keller & Kamath, 1975). After PPRF lesions which lead to an abolishment of all rapid eye movements towards the ipsilateral side, fast eye movement modulation in this particular direction also disappears in the central vestibular neurons, thus identifying the PPRF as its source (Jäger et al., 1981). The quantitative distribution of the different types of cells in the vestibular nuclei cannot be determined from extracellular recordings in alert monkeys. Probably a high percentage of them project to oculomotor areas including the cerebellum, while neurons projecting to the thalamus are not modulated in such a way (Büttner & Henn, 1976).

## 4.2. Modelling

The frequency changes of central vestibular neurons during slow phase optokinetic nystagmus, the saturation at a stimulus velocity of 60°/s, and the modulation of these neurons during OKAN led to the hypothesis that activity of central vestibular neurons reflects the state of the 'velocity storage' mechanism. The Raphan and Cohen model (1981) (Chapter 8) simulates neuronal activity under all above described stimulus conditions.

The responses of central vestibular neurons to the different stimulus situations are drawn schematically in Fig. 3. The signals are carried monosynaptically to the abducens nucleus, to the flocculus (see below), and over polysynaptic brain stem pathways to other structures (Fig. 1B). At present it is unclear over which pathways the visual information reaches the central vestibular neurons in the monkey, and whether the signal within these pathways codes only image slip velocity.

In conclusion, the activity of central vestibular neurons changes monotonically in relation to nytagmus slow phase velocity during optokinetic stimulation as long as certain values of velocity and acceleration are not exceeded for the visual stimulus. Frequency changes of central vestibular neurons also accurately reflect OKAN velocities. However, neuronal activity changes can always be dissociated from the velocity of the eyes or the stimulus during combined, conflict and some modes of optokinetic stimulations. Consequently additional neuronal populations must contribute the generation or suppression of slow eye movements during these stimulus conditions.

## 5. Neuronal activity in the flocculus

### 5.1. Mossy fiber activity

Mossy fiber (MF) activity has been recorded from fibers, granule cells (Waespe et al., 1981; Miles et al., 1980a,b), or probably from MF terminals (Llinás, personal communication). Many MFs show a modulation similar to that of central vestibular neurons during all stimulation conditions (Waespe et al, 1981) (Fig. 5). Type I and II MFs are equally distributed. During vestibular stimulation the decaying time constant is as long as that of vestibular nystagmus, in the range of 10–40 s (Fig. 5A). During conflict stimulation peak modulation is strongly attenuated only at low (below 10°/s$^2$) but not at higher accelerations (40°/s$^2$), and $T_c$ is always short, lss than 8 s (Fig. 5B). During constant velocity optokinetic stimulation, frequency changes are maintained and neuronal modulation saturates at a velocity of 60°/s on average (Fig. 5C). During rapid velocity changes of the visual stimulus, neuronal frequency changes are slow, although eye velocity adjusts faster. During OKAN, frequency returns to resting discharge levels with a similar time course as eye velocity. The initial rapid drop in eye velocity at the transition from OKN to OKAN is not reflected in a similar rapid change in neuronal activity (Waespe et al, 1981). About 90% of the neurons are also modulated during fast eye movements and with different eye positions.

Since many of these features are found in type I eye movement-related central vestibular neurons, we postulate that type I and type II mossy fibers originate from type I eye movement-related neurons in the ipsilateral and contralateral vestibular nuclei, respectively. Both neuron populations have been shown to exhibit the same high sensitivity to vestibular and optokinetic stimulation. Based on physiological characteristics, such as time constants and lack of modulation during optokinetic stimulation, MFs originating from primary vestibular neurons have not been found in the flocculus (Lisberger & Fuchs, 1978a,b; Waespe et al., 1981). In addition there are other MF inputs modulated by visual signals (Noda, 1981; Waespe et al., 1981), or by parameters of fast eye movements and eye position. In these neurons the eye position signal dominates over a weak eye velocity signal during pursuit movements (Noda & Suzuki, 1978; Lisberger & Fuchs, 1978a,b; Miles et al, 1980a,b).

### 5.2. Purkinje cell activity

Purkinje cells (P-cells) described in this context were selected according to the modulation of their simple spike (SS) activity during optokinetic or during conflict stimulation. This amounts to

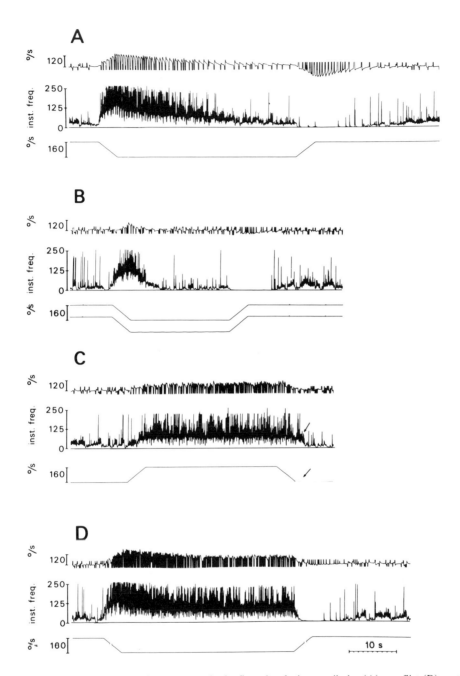

*Fig. 5.* Instantaneous activity of a type II MF input neuron in the flocculus during vestibular (A), conflict (B), optokinetic (C), and combined (D) stimulation. As in Fig. 4 this neuron is also modulated during saccades and weakly during different horizontal eye positions. Same format as in Fig. 4. Acceleration and deceleration 40°/s², constant velocity 160°/s. Neuronal activity increases during vestibular stimulation to the contralateral side (A) and during optokinetic stimulation to the ipsilateral side (C). Initially, at the beginning of optokinetic stimulation there is a delay of about 2 s until frequency starts to increase. During deceleration, resting discharge level is reached only 2–3 s after the end of deceleration (arrow), indicating storage. During conflict stimulation (B), neuronal activation is nearly as strong as during vestibular stimulation but the time constant ($T_c$) is short and nystagmus velocity is strongly reduced. In D, during combined stimulation, neuronal modulation during the acceleration is similar to that in darkness; during rotation at a constant velocity it is similar to that during optokinetic stimulation alone.

242

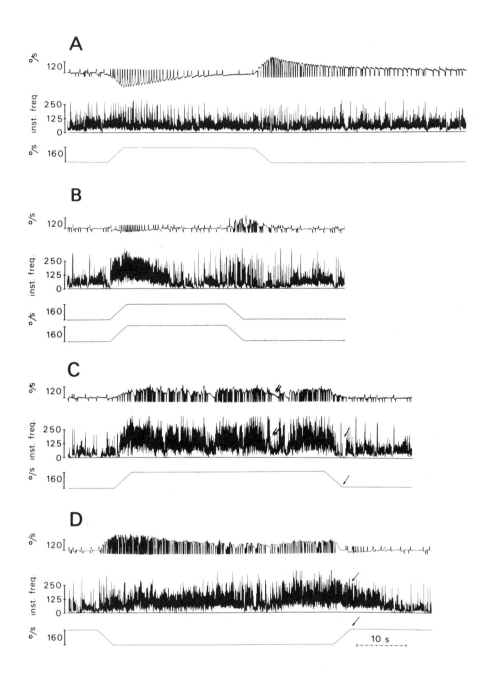

*Fig. 6.* Instantaneous simple spike (SS) activity of a floccular Purkinje cell (P-cell) during vestibular (A), conflict (B), optokinetic (C) and combined (D) stimulation. Same format and stimulation parameters as in Fig. 5. With saccades to the ipsilateral side there is an irregular burst activity, and with saccades to the opposite side frequency is reduced. During vestibular stimulation (A) there is no clear modulation in P-cell activity but there is a strong increase during conflict (B) and optokinetic stimulation (C) to the ipsilateral side. Note that in C peak frequency change is reached with the end of acceleration, and that resting discharge is reached before the end of deceleration (arrow). Whenever slow phase eye velocity decreases during constant velocity optokinetic stimulation, SS activity decreases also (double arrow in C). During optokinetic stimulation to the opposite side SS activity decreased (not shown).

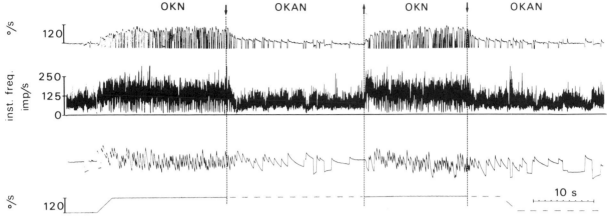

*Fig. 7.* Instantaneous simple spike activity of a P-cell during optokinetic stimulation to the ipsilateral side. In descending order from top: velocity of horizontal eye movements; SS activity (imp/s); horizontal eye position; and stimulus velocity (acceleration $40°/s^2$, constant velocity $120°/s$, downward arrow lights off, upward arrow lights on). Note the rapid frequency increase after lights on and decrease after lights off.

10–20% of the P-cells found in the flocculus. Other P-cells were not found to be modulated during this or other modes of visual or vestibular stimulation. In the responsive group, 40% of the P-cells are not modulated during vestibular stimulation in darkness (modulation less than $±10\%$ of the resting discharge, Fig. 6A); 60% show some modulation which is always less than during conflict stimulation (Fig. 6B). During conflict stimulation they are strongly modulated at an acceleration of $40°/s^2$ but are little, or not, modulated at 5 or $10°/s^2$ except for the most sensitive P-cells. SS activity is modulated during high constant velocity optokinetic nystagmus (above $30–60°/s$; Figs. 6C, 8, 9B, 10) or during a rapid change in optokinetic nystagmus velocity (above $5–10°/s^2$) (Figs. 6C, 7) (Waespe & Henn, 1981). During a transient reduction of eye velocity at stimulus velocities of 120 or $160°/s$ SS modulation also decreases (Fig. 6C). With lights off during OKN, SS activity returns within one second to the resting discharge level and is not further modulated during OKAN (Fig. 7). About 90% of these P-cells increase SS activity during both conflict and optokinetic stimulation to the same, i.e., the recording side. However, whereas optokinetic nystagmus beats with the fast phase to the contralateral side, during conflict stimulation nystagmus beats to the ipsilateral side. This demonstrates a clear dissociation between nystagmus direction and SS activity. In contrast, type I central vestibular neurons are activated during nystagmus which always beats to the ipsilateral side independently of whether activation is due to optokinetic, vestibular or conflict stimulation. Other paradigms also showed a dissociation between P-cell activity and nystagmus velocity, such as during OKN or OKAN. Therefore P-cells cannot code gaze velocity exclusively. The modulation of SS activity of flocculus P-cells during the different forms of stimulation is drawn schematically in Fig. 3.

### 5.3. Functional conclusions

Our hypothesis is that floccular P-cells are a link in the 'direct', and that the central vestibular neurons are a link in the 'indirect', visual-oculomotor pathways. This would explain why neurons in the vestibular nuclei and floccular P-cells are modulated in a complementary way during visual-vestibular stimulation, each neuron population having its own working range for optimal modulation. This hypothesis can be tested by placing a lesion in one structure and by observing the effects on nystagmus and on single cell activity in the other structure.

244

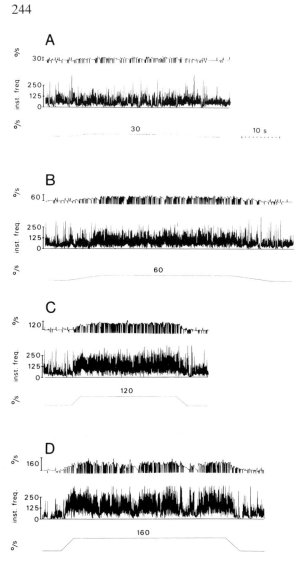

Fig. 8. Instantaneous simple spike activity of a floccular P-cell (same neuron and format as in Fig. 6) during optokinetic stimulation and OKN at velocities between 30 and 160°/s. SS activity is only modulated at stimulus velocities above 30°/s.

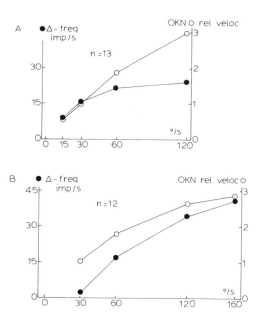

Fig. 9. Change in neuronal activity (left ordinate) of central vestibular neurons (A) and of P-cells (SS activity) in the flocculus (B) in relation to slow phase velocity of OKN (right ordinate) at different constant velocities of optokinetic stimulation (abscissa). Averaged values: 13 neurons in A, 12 neurons in B. OKN is normalized. Nystagmus velocity and unit activity dissociates for vestibular cells at high velocities, and for P-cells at low velocities.

Other hypotheses were derived from specialized experiments. Lisberger and Fuchs (1978b) and Miles et al. (1980a,b) postulate two necessary inputs to the flocculus, one originating in the labyrinths carrying a head velocity signal, and another one from the brain stem carrying an eye velocity signal. Their experiment was to test P-cells during pursuit eye movement and during VOR-suppression (monkeys fixated on a small light). P-cells exhibit a consistent modulation during

both conditions and they concluded that P-cells code gaze velocity (head minus eye velocity). More extended experiments in our laboratory show that these P-cells are also modulated during conflict stimulation (instead of a small fixation light the whole surround is illuminated) and high velocity optokinetic nystagmus (Fig. 10) (Büttner & Waespe, 1984). Although the P-cells are strongly modulated during sinusoidal smooth pursuit movements with peak velocities of 40°/s or less, not one was modulated during constant velocity OKN of the same velocity (Fig. 10). The same P-cells started to be modulated during OKN if its slow phase velocity was above 40–60°/s. We postulate that the drive for the constant slow phase velocity of optokinetic nystagmus consists of two parts. The signal for the velocity range from zero up to approximately 60°/s is contributed by central vestibular neurons, and that for velocities greater than 60°/s by the floccular P-cells. During a 40°/s constant velocity optokinetic stimulation, P-cells are not modulated, as the

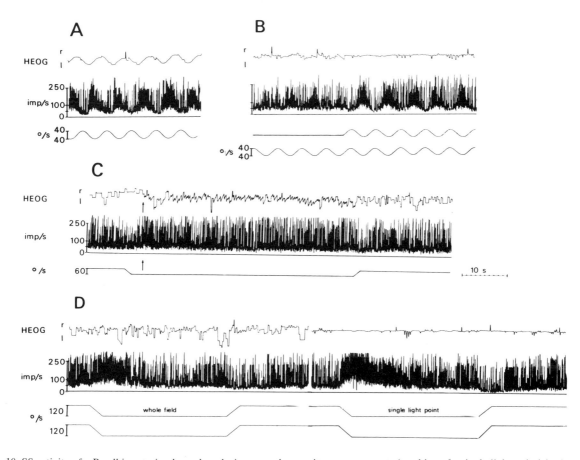

*Fig. 10.* SS activity of a P-cell in a trained monkey during smooth pursuit eye movements (tracking of a single light point) in A, and during vestibular stimulation and visual suppression of the vestibular nystagmus by fixating a single light point (VOR suppression) in B. In C the same P-cell during OKN at a stimulus velocity of 60°/s. In D on the left side conflict stimulation with the whole visual field rotating with the monkey; on the right VOR-suppression (acceleration 40°/s², end velocity 120°/s). Upper part of each subfigure: horizontal eye position; instantaneous SS activity; velocity of the visual stimulus; chair velocity, A–D, respectively. Upward arrow lights on. Note that the P-cell is only slightly modulated during vestibular stimulation (left part of B). Modulation is deeper during conflict stimulation (vestibular nystagmus not completely suppressed) and even more pronounced during VOR suppression (vestibular nystagmus is completely suppressed). The P-cell is not modulated during constant velocity OKN at 60°/s, but transiently at the beginning and end of stimulation. During all stimulus conditions, SS activity increases with stimulation to the ipsilateral side.

appropriate signal for nystagmus is mediated by central vestibular neurons. For the same eye velocity during pursuit movement, the signal is provided by the floccular P-cells. Such a signal has not been found in central vestibular neurons (Keller & Kamath, 1975).

Ito (1972, 1976, 1982a) (see Ch. 14) postulates one input to the rabbit's flocculus from the labyrinth and another one from the accessory visual system carrying a visual signal (Fig. 1A). P-cell output is thought to exert its influence mainly on secondary vestibular cells modulating the VOR. These experiments refer to the rabbit and have been performed to study short and long term adaptation. The results are not directly comparable to the above described results in the monkeys, as quantitative investigations of vestibular nuclei activity are still lacking in the rabbit (for further discussion see Waespe and Henn, 1985).

A decisive problem for any interpretation is

the lack of complete anatomical data in the monkey. A peripheral vestibular input to the flocculus had not been identified by physiological means. Theories which are based on a powerful peripheral vestibular input to the flocculus meet the obstacle that as yet all physiologically identified vestibular input seems to originate in the vestibular nuclei )Lisberger & Fuchs, 1978a,b; Waespe et al., 1981) (Fig. 1B), although a projection of the vestibular nerve to the flocculus is generally assumed to exist (monkey: Carpenter et al., 1972; cat: Brodal & Høivik, 1964). Recently Korte and Mugnaini (1979) have shown, in the cat, that probably only few primary fibers project to the flocculus. Another concept states that P-cells project to the vestibular nuclei to inhibit secondary neurons which in turn project to the oculomotor nuclei (Fig. 1A). However, activity changes of floccular P-cells during OKN, conflict stimulation, and smooth pursuit are not reflected by corresponding frequency changes in central vestibular neurons. Floccular P-cells for instance are able to change their SS activity to optokinetic stimulation more rapidly than central vestibular neurons. Especially, the firing pattern during conflict stimulation and OKN can only be interpreted if one assumes complementary rather than serial processing of information in floccular P-cells and central vestibular neurons. Our findings suggest a summing point of the outputs from central vestibular neurons and P-cells on separate target cells which have yet to be localized (Fig. 1B). Besides the projection to the lateral cerebellar nuclei and the γ-group, there is no evidence for other projections than to the vestibular nuclei in the monkey (Haines, 1977). In the cat a pathway to the nucleus prepositus hypoglossi seems to exist (Yingcharoen & Rinvik, 1983). Classical anatomical and electrophysiological work stresses monosynaptic connections and cannot estimate the functional importance of other polysynaptic pathways.

One faces the problem that recordings of single unit activity provide material for statistical correlations, but cannot decide about causal relations. Lesion experiments are notoriously difficult to interpret. Together with single unit studies, however, we think sufficient conclusions can be drawn to test predictions from different theories.

## 6. Bilateral flocculectomy and its effects on visual-vestibular interaction

The aforementioned activity of P-cells in the flocculus suggests that their modulation may be responsible for generating (a) high velocity OKN, i.e., above the OKAN saturation velocity of about 60°/s, (b) fast changes of OKN velocity, i.e., those exceeding 5–10°/s², and (c) suppression of VN during high acceleration conflict stimulation. These are the functions which are attributed, in the Raphan-Cohen model (1981), to the 'direct' visual-oculomotor pathways and in the Robinson model (1981b) to the 'smooth pursuit' pathways. Robinson's model predicts two further modes of action: (d) the generation of smooth pursuit eye movements; and (e) the suppression or cancellation of the VOR while animals foveate a single fixation light (VOR-suppression).

Attenuation of these specific functions in lesion experiments supports the hypothesis that the flocculus plays an essential role (Takemori & Cohen, 1974; Zee et al., 1981; Waespe et al., 1983). Lesions have been made surgically and have been fully described (Waespe et al, 1983). After bilateral flocculectomy the initial rapid increase in OKN velocity at the onset of stimulation is reduced by 60–90% and the slow increase in OKN velocity has a longer time course than normal (Fig. 11). This prolongation can be accounted for by the increased initial retinal slip velocity due to the reduced initial eye velocity. If adjusted for slip velocity the slow increase in OKN is similar before and after flocculectomy. OKN steady state velocities increase approximately up to the preoperative OKAN saturation velocities of 50–70°/s, but cannot reach higher values (Takemori & Cohen, 1974; Waespe et al., 1983). Monkeys are unable to follow adequately an acceleration of the visual surround of 5°/s² or more. Eye velocity, however, can be decelerated faster than accelerated, which points to an additional extra-floccular suppressing mechanism (Waespe et al., 1983). The transition of OKN to OKAN is smooth after flocculectomy at all stimulus velocities without, or with only a small, initial velocity drop (Fig. 11B,D). OKAN velocities and durations are essentially unchanged (Fig. 11). Flocculectomy has also little effect on gain and duration of the

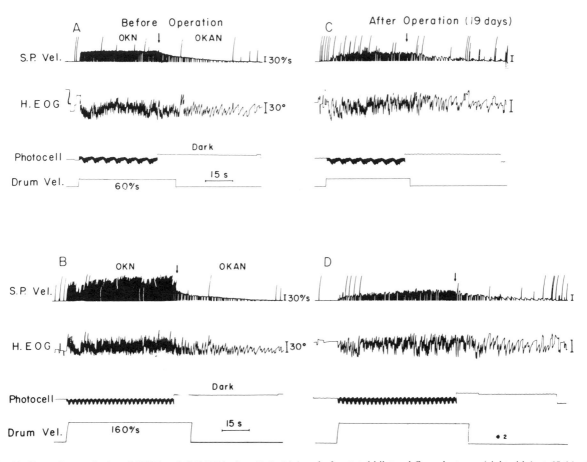

Fig. 11. Slow phase velocity of OKN and OKAN before (left side) and after total bilateral flocculectomy (right side) at 60 (A, C) and 160°/s (B, D) stimulus velocity. Upper part of each subfigure: nystagmus velocity; horizontal eye position; photocell signal indicating period of stimulation; velocity profile of the optokinetic stimulus, A–D, respectively. Downward arrows mark the time at which lights were turned off and nystagmus continues as OKAN. Note that after flocculectomy all rapid changes of nystagmus velocity are lost or severely reduced.

vestibular nystagmus (Zee et al., 1981). During conflict stimulation, time constants are still below 6–8 s but peak velocities cannot be attenuated during short pulses of high accelerations. On the other hand, at accelerations below $10°/s^2$ nystagmus is almost completely suppressed as in the normal animal. Unilateral flocculectomy has similar, but asymmetrical effects. OKN with slow phases to the operated side is more affected as is nystagmus during conflict stimulation with slow phases to the non-operated side.

Zee et al. (1981) specifically investigated pursuit eye movements and cancellation of the VOR by foveating a fixation light. Their monkeys, after bilateral flocculectomy, showed deficits in these tasks. Bilateral flocculectomy does not abolish all activity within the 'direct' visual-oculomotor pathways and one has to postulate that other brain stem or cerebellar structures contribute to these tasks.

## 6.1. Effects on the activity of central vestibular neurons

The activity of central vestibular neurons is qualitatively unchanged during vestibular, conflict and optokinetic stimulation after flocculectomy (Waespe & Cohen, 1983). During vestibular stimulation the decay time constant ($T_c$) is unchanged, during optokinetic stimulation neuronal activity increases up to a velocity of approximate-

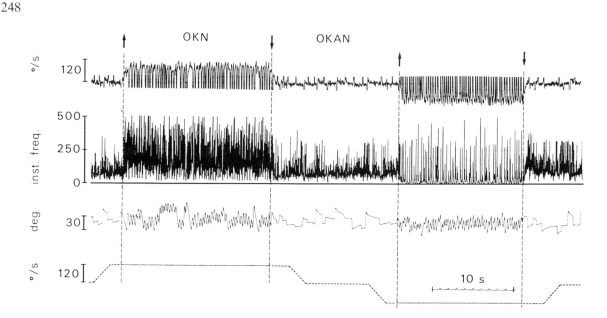

*Fig. 12.* Instantaneous SS activity of a floccular P-cell during optokinetic stimulation after bilateral vestibular neurectomy. In descending order from top: eye velocity; SS activity (imp/s); horizontal eye position; and optokinetic stimulus velocity, (upward arrow lights on; downward arrow lights off). Saccadic modulation of SS activity can be seen as pauses with right and bursts with left rapid nystagmus phases. SS activity increases during optokinetic nystagmus with slow phases to the ipsilateral side and decreases during nystagmus with slow phases to the contralateral side. Note that there is no OKAN.

ly 60°/s at which it saturates. During OKAN, neuronal activity accurately reflects the time course of nystagmus slow phase velocity. During conflict stimulation the time constant ($T_c$) is short. In summary, the effects of flocculectomy on nystagmus and single cell activity in the vestibular nuclei can be interpreted by assuming that the 'direct' but not the 'indirect' visual-oculomotor pathways are severely disrupted.

## 7. Effects of bilateral vestibular neurectomy on floccular P-cell activity

After bilateral labyrinthectomy or neurectomy maximal OKN velocities are reduced, OKAN is abolished and eye velocity no longer increases slowly after the initial fast rise during OKN (Cohen et al., 1982) (Fig. 12). But even after neurectomy monkeys can produce OKN with velocities up to 80–120°/s (Waespe, unpublished). These deficits can be attributed to a lack of activity within the 'indirect' visual-oculomotor pathways or the optokinetic system. The normally present high resting discharge of about 100 imp/s in the vestibular nerve is lacking, which is thought

to severely disrupt activity of central vestibular neurons which are then unable to transmit an eye velocity signal during OKN. Therefore, activity to generate nystagmus must mainly be mediated by the flocculus. SS modulation of P-cells in the flocculus during OKN is qualitatively unchanged after bilateral neurectomy (Fig. 12). Quantitatively however, P-cells are already modulated at low OKN velocities of 15 or 30°/s which is different from the normal monkey. The same P-cells are also modulated during smooth pursuit eye movements quantitatively in the same way as in the normal monkey. Modulation increases monotonically together with increasing OKN and smooth pursuit eye velocities. SS activity is not modulated by image slip velocity. A greater percentage of P-cells is modulated during OKN as compared to the normal monkey. The stronger modulation of P-cells during OKN after neurectomy is most likely the result of the inactivation of the MF input from central vestibular neurons. As OKN slow phases reach velocities as high as in the normal monkey, but with no contribution from the velocity storage, monkeys can use only the 'direct' visual-oculomotor pathways to produce

OKN after neurectomy: compared to the normal monkey one would predict a stronger modulation of P-cells during OKN, but the same modulation during smooth pursuit after neurectomy. This was actually found.

Thus, after neurectomy, which sets the OKAN saturation velocity to zero, floccular P-cells are modulated over the whole range of OKN velocities. Under these special circumstances, P-cell activity can be related to eye velocity under all stimulus conditions tested in our paradigms (Waespe et al., in preparation).

In conclusion, these results of single cell recordings before and after selective lesions support the hypothesis that floccular P-cells and central vestibular neurons process vestibular and optokinetic information in a complementary way. This further implies that floccular P-cells must have a projection to the oculomotor system by-passing central vestibular neurons (Fig. 1B). This complicates Ito's hypothesis as depicted in Fig. 1A. Resting discharge of central vestibular neurons is probably severely disrupted after neurectomy as indicated by the loss of OKAN. Floccular output mediating OKN and smooth pursuit, however, still reaches the oculomotor system which makes it unlikely that it is transmitted via central vestibular neurons.

The hypothesis of the existence of two dynamically different mechanisms in the generation of OKN and in the visual suppression of vestibular nystagmus has proven to be useful in the analysis of eye movements (cf., Chapter 8) and of the activity of different cell populations. Central vestibular neurons are mainly involved in the 'indirect', and floccular P-cells in the 'direct', visual-oculomotor pathways. In the analysis of the activity of single cells one has, however, not to adhere too strictly to this separation. There are central vestibular neurons which saturate at OKN velocities below or above the OKAN saturation velocity, and there are floccular P-cells which are modulated during OKN velocities below the OKAN saturation velocity. The lesion studies, however, favor the interpretation that floccular P-cells mainly contribute during OKN at velocities above the OKAN saturation velocity and during smooth pursuit at any velocity, but not during OKAN and the VOR in darkness. Central vestibular neurons

mainly contribute during OKN at velocities below the OKAN saturation velocity and during the VOR but not during smooth pursuit eye movements. So far we have no hypothesis about synaptic mechanisms of how signals are processed within these different pathways, and about the neuronal substrate for the 'velocity storage' mechanism. Furthermore, the target cells on which both pathways converge have not been localized.

## 8. Implications for adaptation studies

The flocculus constitutes a crucial link in inducing plastic changes of the VOR by altered visual input (Ito, 1972) (Chapters 2 & 14). There is no agreement yet concerning the possible mechanism for this phenomenon. Are the plastic modifiable elements localized within the flocculus itself (review: Ito, 1982a) or do floccular P-cells only carry an 'error signal' necessary for the induction of the adaptation process which takes place somewhere else (Miles & Lisberger, 1981b)? Ito's hypothesis is that the plastic changes take place in the floccular cortex through the activity of climbing fibers which modify the strengths of parallel fiber synapses on P-cell dendrites. According to Miles and co-workers the flocculus has an inductive role by providing visually derived signals indicating the existence and magnitude of errors in the VOR. Unclear are the pathways which transmit the 'error signal', and what the functional role of the direct connection of floccular P-cells to central vestibular neurons is. There seems to be no functional role for this direct connection in the immediate adjustment of the VOR by visual signals and in transmitting the signals for specific parameters of rapid changes or high velocity OKN as discussed in this review. The floccular projection to central vestibular neurons however, could be crucial during long term adjustments of the VOR. Signals of the same P-cells which are modulated during OKN, smooth pursuit and suppression of the VOR may at the same time constitute 'error signals' which are effective only when occurring either repetitively or continuously over long periods. Central vestibular neurons receiving such an 'error signal' may project back to the flocculus and may reduce this signal via a feedback loop. Lisberger and co-workers (1981) showed that, in the monkey, VOR gain adaptation is reflected by gain changes in the 'indirect' pathways only, supporting this hypothesis. With a VOR gain of 1.6 the OKAN saturation velocity is enhanced to 90°/s and for a VOR gain of 0.3 it is reduced to 30°/s. Lisberger and Miles (1980) specifically point out that they did not see changes in the 'direct' visual-oculomotor pathways. Our results suggest that adaptation of the OKAN should be reflected in the behavior of central vestibular neurons and P-cells. An increase in the saturation velocity of OKAN to 90°/s, for instance, should also increase the saturation velocity of central vestibular neurons during OKN, and the threshold for OKN modulation should be raised for floccular P-cells by the same amount. This reasoning further supports the general outline of our scheme in Fig. 1B. Lisberger and Miles (1980) found no significant differences in the sensitivity of type I central vestibular neurons in the MVn to vestibular stimulation in monkeys in which the VOR gain varied up to 4–5 times. The activity changes during OKAN were not tested. Keller and Precht (1979a) on the other hand found in the cat clear changes in the vestibular sensitivity of high gain type I and type II central neurons. These findings would support the hypothesis that the modifiable gain element is introduced before or at the level of the origin of the MF input which carries the vestibular signal to the flocculus (see Fig. 5 in Miles & Lisberger, 1981b).

Another experimental paradigm refers to balance control (Robinson, 1981b). Spontaneous nystagmus occurring after labyrinthine or eighth nerve lesions is compensated in normal cats, as well as in animals after removal of the vestibulo-cerebellum (Haddad et al., 1977). This recovery takes place even in the dark, but with a longer time course if the vestibulo-cerebellum had been removed. In the cat, during the first 90 min after eighth nerve lesions, otherwise normal animals reduce their spontaneous nystagmus by 50% in the dark, whereas animals with a previously removed vestibulo-cerebellum can do so only by 10% (Haddad et al., 1977). This also suggests a role in balance control for the vestibulo-cerebellum (Courjon et al., 1982; Jeannerod et al., 1981). After unilateral labyrinthectomy the flocculus ipsilateral to the lesion would receive only a type II MF input originating from contralateral type I and ipsilateral type II neurons in the vestibular nuclei. The flocculus contralateral to the lesion would receive only a type I MF input from corresponding neurons of both vestibular nuclei (according to the simplified scheme in Fig. 1B). The Type I and II MF input from the vestibular nuclei is changed after labyrinthectomy and this might be a basis for the balance control. Courjon et al. (1982) specifically investigated the dynamics of the recovery process in the VOR in the cat. If an animal had recovered from a labyrinthectomy, a flocculectomy introduced a transient spontaneous nystagmus and a transient asymmetry in the VOR gain. If the procedure was reversed, recovery from labyrinthectomy was severely delayed. Any such dynamic processes had not been investigated on a single unit level, therefore its mechanisms remains speculative.

Finally, the question of the localization of the modifiable element might be an elusive one. Llinás and Walton (1979b) (see also Ch. 15) pointed out how widespread alterations of glucose metabolism occur after labyrinthectomy. Lesion studies alone cannot answer the problem. Although the possibility to induce plastic changes in the VOR is lost after flocculectomy, this does not necessarily or exclusively place the modifiable element into the flocculus. In monkeys there may be a cell loss or inactivation of neurons within the vestibular nuclei after surgical flocculectomy (Waespe & Cohen, 1983). A similar cell loss has been documented for the inferior olive (Barmack & Simpson, 1980; Ito et al., 1980). Thus, localized surgical lesions can induce changes in remote parts of the brain. Pathophysiological mechanisms of the loss of adaptation after flocculectomy could include lack of P-cell output and retrograde degeneration of cells projecting as MFs or CFs to the flocculus. In spite of these difficulties in the interpretation of the results, the exploration of visual-vestibular interactions with a combined approach of lesion and single unit studies, seems for us a promising way to finally understand normal function.

Adaptive mechanisms in gaze control
Facts and theories
*Eds. Berthoz & Melvill Jones*
© 1985 Elsevier Science Publishers BV (Biomedical Division)

Chapter 17

# Neuronal events paralleling functional recovery (compensation) following peripheral vestibular lesions

W. Precht & N. Dieringer

*Brain Research Institute, University of Zürich, August-Forelstr. 1, 8029 Zürich, Switzerland*

## 1. Introduction

Ever since the pioneering work of Bechterew (1883) the functional recovery that follows peripheral vestibular lesions has attracted the interest of many neuroscientists. This intense interest over the past 100 years made the vestibular lesion model probably the best studied recovery model. Undoubtedly, the maintained interest in this model depends upon the fact that the spectacular symptoms which occur immediately after section of one vestibular nerve abate rather quickly, so that after recovery a naive observer often cannot tell a damaged from an intact animal, both at rest as well as during locomotion. Since the vestibular nerve and the hair cell receptor cells do not regenerate after lesions, all the compensatory processes leading to recovery of function must be generated by the central nervous system. The vestibular lesion paradigm, therefore, allows us to study the plastic as well as adaptive capacities of the nervous system in response to a well defined peripheral input. Further advantages of the vestibular lesion model are the following: (1) the extent of the lesion of the labyrinth or vestibular nerve can be precisely controlled and reproductible lesions can easily be made; (2) the normal function of the vestibular system and its interaction with other systems is easily studied both at behavioral and single unit levels; (3) the functional deficits and their recovery, e.g.,

postural asymmetries, vestibulospinal and vestibulo-ocular reflex behavior, are precisely measurable and quantifiable; and (4) the lesion-evoked symptoms are very similar in a large variety of species, offering the possibility to study similarities as well as differences in strategies of recovery.

Following unilateral vestibular neurotomy the central nervous system has to handle two distinct, although not completely independent, groups of functional deficits. Firstly, the symmetrical tonic influence exerted by the vestibular receptors and afferents on posture of head, body and eyes at rest is altered by the unilateral withdrawal of the resting activity of vestibular nerve fibers. Depending on the species studied, mean resting rates vary from 5 to 90 impulses/s (Precht, 1978). Sudden unilateral removal of resting activity results in an imbalance of the output of the vestibular nuclei to the oculomotor and spinal motor systems, causing a 'vestibular lesion syndrome'. It consists of severe postural asymmetries of head and body and strong eye and head nystagmus (for Refs. see Schaefer & Meyer, 1974). The nervous system, therefore, is forced to establish a new balance in the innervation of motor systems.

Secondly, as we shall see, vestibular unilateral neurotomy abolishes the interaction between the two labyrinths in dynamic reflex performance, and the resulting changes in reflex gains and symmetries call for adjustment.

In the following, the major recent advances in the field of recovery of function after unilateral vestibular lesion will be described and emphasis will be on neuronal correlates of recovery. Behavioral data will only be discussed in detail if they are of relevance for available single unit data. The chapter first deals with studies performed in mammals, mainly cat, rat and guinea pig, and then describes the findings obtained in submammalian vertebrates, mainly the frog. As will be seen, differences in the normal organization of vestibular and optokinetic circuitry between higher and lower vertebrates will require different strategies at the neuronal level to obtain the same goal, i.e., recovery of overall vestibular functions.

## 2. Studies performed in mammals

To date, the most thoroughly studied species is undoubtedly the cat in which recovery of both canal and otolith reflex systems have been studied, both behaviorally and at the single unit level. In addition, some combined data are available from studies in rat and guinea pigs particularly as far as recovery of balance and otolith functions are concerned.

Almost without exception, single unit work so far is restricted to the description of central vestibular nuclear neuron activity following complete unilateral vestibular lesions. Although this initial choice of the recording site is conceptually reasonable, given both the integrative and relay nature of the vestibular nuclei (VN) and their importance for muscular tone, it is by no means the only structure that should be studied in conjunction with compensation.

### 2.1. Semicircular canal system after lesion

All studies dealing with the recovery of balance and gain in the canal system have been restricted to measurements of the performance of the horizontal canal system following unilateral lesions of all afferents. Furthermore, it is only the horizontal canal system of the *cat* that has been studied both behaviorally and at the single unit level; therefore, in the following, the emphasis will be on the results obtained in this species.

### 2.1.1. Recovery of canal balance; behavioural studies

As in most other species, section of the whole vestibular nerve or removal of all vestibular end organs leads acutely to a strong, primarily horizontal, ocular nystagmus beating with its quick phase to the intact side, and a head nystagmus may initially accompany eye nystagmus (Kreidl 1906; Camis, 1912, 1930; Magnus, 1924; Spiegel & Demetriades, 1925; Money & Scott, 1962; Precht et al., 1966; Moran, 1974; Haddad et al., 1977; Courjon et al., 1977; Robles & Anderson, 1978; Precht et al., 1981; Maioli et al., 1983). In addition, tonic vertical and torsional changes in eye and head position have been observed in various species (cf., Schaefer & Meyer, 1974) although such changes have not been explicitly stated or studied in the cat.

Since in all the above studies the whole vestibular nerve and/or labyrinth has been damaged one wonders which of the symptoms can be ascribed to removal of the canals. In the cat only one study has attempted to section selectively the horizontal canal nerve (Mair & Fernandez, 1966). These authors report that the lesion-evoked symptoms were very similar to those obtained after whole nerve section. They presented careful histological controls showing that no other receptor organs but the horizontal crista were affected by the lesion. Of course, it is possible that the surgical intervention with the horizontal canal nerve caused some transient functional damage of nearby utricular fibers so that the symptomatology initially observed would resemble that of a complete lesion of the nerve. Since no selective utricular nerve lesions have been performed in the cat we can not separate the above lesion symptoms into those caused by canal or macular deafferentation. As for the ocular imbalance it may, however, be assumed that nystagmus is primarily caused by lesion of the canals, whereas the small changes in static eye position may be ascribed to macular deafferentation.

In the cat as well as in other species (rat: Llinás & Walton, 1979b; guinea pig: Jensen, 1979a) including man (Fisch, 1973) ocular nystagmus abates rather quickly and with similar time courses after the lesion, i.e., even when measured in the dark, there is only a slight nystagmus (ca.

5°/s slow phase velocity as compared to some 40°/s initially) present after the first p.o. week (Precht et al., 1966; Haddad et al., 1977; Courjon et al., 1977; Maioli et al., 1983). The recovery of ocular balance in the cat apparently requires the presence of structured visual surround; if animals are kept in dark after the lesion nystagmus does not seem to disappear as readily (Berthoz et al., 1975a; Courjon et al., 1977).

Head tilt likewise greatly recovers over a period of ca. 7–10 days when recovery takes place in light (Putkonen et al., 1977).

In summary, in the cat lesion-evoked symptoms of ocular and postural imbalance recover almost to control values within the first postoperative week. Essentially similar results were obtained with other species although the time courses of recovery vary considerably from extremely short periods, e.g., hours for compensation of head tilt in the rat (Llinás and Walton 1979) to several weeks in the frog (see Section 3). Ocular balance however, is established with similar time courses in rat (Llinás and Walton 1979), guinea pigs (Jenson 1979a) and cats.

### 2.1.2. Resting activity of vestibular nuclear neurons after lesion

Given the relatively high resting rate of primary canal afferents in the cat (Blanks & Precht, 1978) *acute* removal of one labyrinth would be expected to reduce or abolish the resting activity of target neurons on the *deafferented* side, including those areas of the vestibular nuclei receiving horizontal canal afferents, i.e., the MVN and SVN (medial and superior VN, respectively). That this is, indeed, the case has been demonstrated in the cat by several authors (Gernandt & Thulin, 1952; Shimazu & Precht, 1966; McCabe et al., 1972). The probability of picking up resting discharges was much less on the destroyed than on the intact side. Many of the silent units, however, can still be driven by electrical stimulation of the transsected nerve (Shimazu & Precht, 1966).

On the *intact* side, resting activity of central horizontal canal neurons increases ca. two-fold (from a mean of 19–45 spikes/s) in awake $C_1$-transsected cats *immediately* after the lesion (Markham et al., 1977; Shimazu & Precht, 1966).

Since removal of the midline cerebellum (vermis and fastigial nuclei) did not significantly alter the above results, the observed increase in firing may be ascribed to disinhibition of vestibular neurons due to removal of commissural vestibular influences (Shimazu & Precht, 1966).

It may be concluded that the strong asymmetry in resting activity between deafferented and intact vestibular nuclei is caused by unilateral removal of background input normally arriving via the vestibular nerve and is further enhanced by the additional inhibitory or disinhibitory effects mediated via the vestibular and cerebellar commissure on neurons located in the deafferented or intact nuclei, respectively. This asymmetry in vestibular activity can explain the above described strong ocular and postural imbalance occurring acutely after the lesion. Since a similar ocular nystagmus and neuronal asymmetry may be obtained by transiently silencing the input from one horizontal canal by caloric or galvanic stimulations (Ried et al., 1984) the nystagmus observed after lesion may be primarily caused by removal of the canal input.

Studies dealing with the time course of resting activity during early stages of recovery from the lesion are scarce. McCabe et al., (1972) report electrical silence in both intact and deafferented sides (MVN) 1–2 days p.o. These data certainly do not agree with behavioral work which still reveals large asymmetries in ocular balance and, therefore, requires confirmation. The authors also claim that cerebellar removal in this early stage causes the resting activity on the intact side to return whereas activity remains low on the deafferented side. After one week, cats with intact cerebella are reported to show moderate resting activity on the intact, and no activity on the deafferented, side (McCabe et al., 1972). Again, these data are not in agreement with behavioral data showing almost complete recovery of balance.

By one month after the lesion results are clearer and supported by several studies (Precht et al., 1966; McCabe et al., 1972; Ried et al., 1984). In the most recent study (Ried et al., 1984), resting activity of horizontal canal neurons were recorded systematically on both intact and deafferented sides one month, or later, after unilateral lesion of the ganglion Scarpae as compared to labyrinth-intact cats studied in the same experimental conditions (light Ketamine anaesthesia, midline cerebellum removed).

In *control* animals the mean discharge rate of type I and type II vestibular neurons measures $22.4 \pm 14$ ($n=122$) and $27.5 \pm 14.6$ spikes/s ($n=34$), respectively. Most units were recorded in the rostral MVN.

In chronically *deafferented* cats the mean resting rate of type I units — the main output neurons — on the intact and deafferented sides were $17.4 \pm 13$ spikes/s ($n=48$) and $13.2 \pm 10.4$ spikes/s ($n=45$), respectively. There is no statistically significant difference between the two populations, but a significant difference exists between these values and those obtained in controls. Previously, a similar conclusion was reached for the deafferented side (Precht et al., 1966).

The above results require an important further specification. In comparing intact and deafferented sides systematically in each animal it was found that very few type I units were detected on the deafferented compared to the intact side (see Section 2.1.4), so that the overall populations of type I neurons on the two sides are highly asymmetrical. It is, of course, possible that many of the units showing resting activity but no response to rotation are, in fact, former type I units contributing to balance but no longer to response dynamics. If, however, many former type I neurons became silent in chronic animals, a strong imbalance in the bilateral vestibular nuclear output would exist, and the ocular balance observed in this stage must be brought about by structures other than the vestibular nuclei. That other brain regions are involved in balance control has long been known, and recently been suggested in the rat based on lesion and [14]C-labelled 2-deoxy-D-glucose studies (Llinás & Walton, 1979b).

In spite of these complications it still remains to be explained how some vestibular canal neurons regain a new resting rate during the recovery period. In peripherally damaged animals, in which only the receptors are removed and the ganglion Scarpae is left intact, one may assume that ganglion cells develop spontaneous activity. We have recently shown in the rat that this is not the case, even though ganglion cells survive the

lesion for long periods of time and transmit electrically evoked impulses to vestibular nuclear neurons (Sirkin & Precht, 1984). McCabe et al., (1972) performed various lesion experiments in chronically hemilabyrinthectomized animals and found no major changes in resting rates of MVN units following cerebellar and cerebral (decerebration) ablations, midline transsections of the brainstem, spinal lesions as well as SVN and LVN (lateral VN) lesions. However, such lesion experiments are difficult to reconcile with other findings (see Section 2.2). At present, the possibility that partially deafferented neurons are initially driven by the joint action of many of the remaining inputs is very likely, although the contribution of some gradual buildup of intrinsic activity cannot be excluded. Since balance does not return or is significantly retarded when animals are kept in dark after the lesion, the importance of visual, in addition to proprioceptive, input drives for the acquisition of balance and resting rate is indicated. Presence of vision could, however, simply act by enhancing locomotor activity of the compensating animal, thereby forcing the animals to use compensatory reflexes.

In the cat (Spiegel & Demetriades, 1925; Robles & Anderson, 1978) — unlike the rat (Llinás & Walton, 1979b) — a cerebellectomy performed in animals that had already compensated for unilateral vestibular lesions does not *decompensate* ocular balance. Decompensation is likewise not obtained by decerebration (Spiegel & Demetriades, 1925) indicating that visual and other descending input are not necessary for maintenance of balance. The only procedure consistently leading to a decompensation of balance consists in removing, in compensated animals, the remaining labyrinth. This so-called Bechterew phenomenon is the mirror image of the first lesion. Its occurrence also proves that the intact labyrinth cannot be the only source for resting activity on the deafferented side after the first lesion.

### 2.1.3. Recovery of canalicular reflexes: behavioural studies

To date, most of the quantitative work related to dynamic reflex recovery after unilateral vestibular neurotomy relates to the horizontal vestibulo-ocular reflex (VOR) behavior. Since the cat is

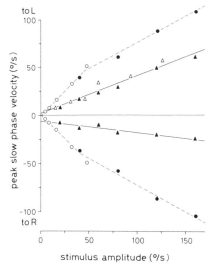

Fig. 1. Horizontal VOR measured in the dark in control and hemilabyrinthectomized cats. Note, in control animals, the occurrence of partial response saturation at about 50°/s stimulus velocity. A gain drop for responses in either direction and a marked asymmetry are the most prominent effects noted 3 days after unilateral deafferentation. ●, control steps; ○, control sines; ▲, 3 days postoperative steps; △ 3 days postoperative sines (from Maioli et al., 1983).

the only mammal in which both behavioral and single unit data have been obtained we shall restrict the discussion of VOR behavior to this species.

The VOR in the cat is a linear system within a certain range (Carpenter, 1972; Landers & Taylor, 1975; Robinson, 1976; Donaghy, 1980; Maioli et al., 1983). It is also well-known that the canal system works in a push-pull fashion, i.e., the VOR generated by head displacements depends on the reciprocal interaction of the two labyrinths. Whenever one canal is excited, the coplanar partner is disfacilitated. Since the magnitude of disfacilitation depends on the level of resting rate in vestibular neurons, we expect that, by increasing the stimulus, saturation will occur. The saturation will also depend on the velocity at which maximal recruitment of vestibular neurons is reached (Maioli et al., 1983). As shown in Fig. 1, eye velocity can match stimulus velocity with a gain close to unity up to ca. 50°/s. Further increase in stimulus magnitude still elicits linearly related responses, but with a much lower slope. Fig. 1 also shows that the responses are nicely symmetrical. The partial saturation point varies

among animals between 15 and 80°/s. From these findings it is clear that stimuli of small amplitude (below the saturation point) have to be used to study the effects of removal of one canal, because it is only at these amplitudes that the two canals maximally interact, and therefore, the largest changes may be expected.

*Acutely* following the lesion, VOR responses are superimposed on ocular nystagmus. Since the central resting activity on the deafferented side at this stage is close to zero, rotatory stimuli simply modulate, approximately symmetrically, the velocity of the spontaneous nystagmus, i.e., the nystagmus is not reversed. Already, 1–2 days p.o., a reversal of nystagmus is noted when stimuli are strong enough but the gain of the reversed response is lower (note change in velocity after reversal in Fig. 2, presumably because the contribution of the deafferented nucleus is still small and the disinhibitory efficacy of the intact nucleus is apparently not sufficient).

To quantify the VOR during rotation to the deafferented side, the gain (incremental gain) of VOR responses to stimuli strong enough to move the eyes opposite to that of the spontaneous nystagmus must be considered. In this case we, in fact, measure the capacity of the undamaged labyrinth to drive the eyes to the ipsilateral side through a decrease of its resting discharge. Fig. 1 gives a representative sample of the VOR responses measured before and 3 days p.o. In brief the following effects were noted: (1) a drop of VOR gain to stimuli to both directions is present, but the decrease is larger for stimuli to the deafferented side; (2) the decrease of the gain following rotation to the intact side is 50% or less compared to the gain of the non saturating responses in the controls; (3) no partial saturation is noted; and (4) a complete saturation of responses occurs on strong stimulations towards the deafferented side. In these cases the eye velocity is never higher than 50–60°/s, presumably because vestibular neuron activity on the deafferented side is saturated.

The time course of adaptive changes of VOR gain may be divided in three periods. In the first 4–5 days p.o. no clear improvement of either gain or symmetry of VOR was observed. The incremental gain following rotation to the *intact*

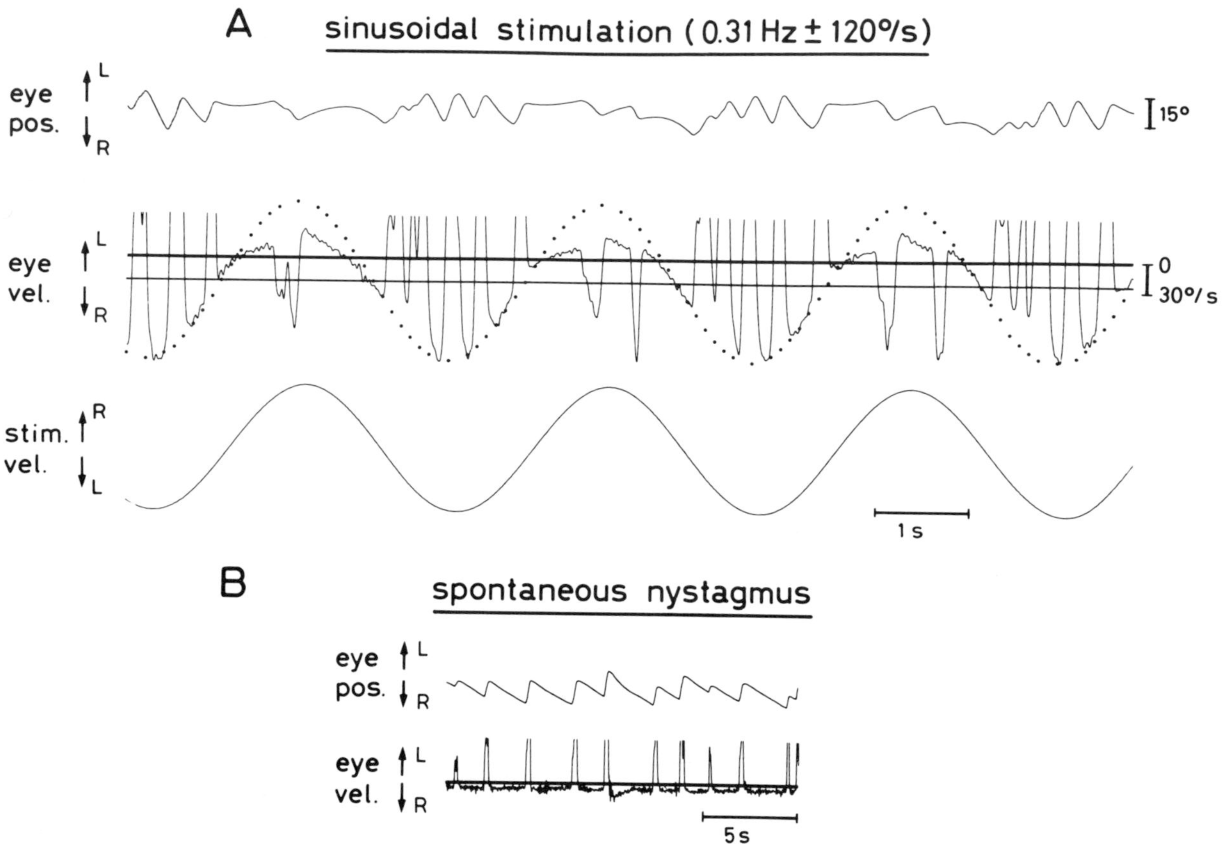

**A** sinusoidal stimulation (0.31 Hz ± 120°/s)

eye pos. ↑L ↓R                                                                    15°

eye vel. ↑L ↓R                                                                    0  30°/s

stim. vel. ↑R ↓L                                                                  1 s

**B** spontaneous nystagmus

eye pos. ↑L ↓R

eye vel. ↑L ↓R                                                                    5 s

*Fig. 2.* Actual eye movements recorded 5 days after right labyrinthectomy. A. Response to sinusoidal oscillation at 0.31 Hz ± 120°/s. In the middle trace eye velocity is plotted together with the sinusoid (dotted line), better fitting the hemicycle of the nystagmic slow phase velocity profile relative to rotation towards the intact side. This sine closely matches the slow phase eye velocity also when the animal is rotated in the opposite direction, but only up to zero crossing level (thick line). Then a flattening of the response is evident. The thin line represents the DC shift computed with the fitting procedure (23°/s). B. Spontaneous nystagmus recorded from the same animal. Note that the slow phase velocity of the spontaneous nystagmus is much lower than the computed DC shift during stimulation (from Maioli et al., 1983).

side remains consistently at 0.4–0.5. Responses to rotation to the *deafferented* side show more variability, but, without exception, the gain is distinctly lower than that for rotation to the intact side, i.e., a clear asymmetry is present. Between 5–10 days p.o. two groups of animals were noted; one group increased the gain on rotation to the intact side to ca. 0.75 (Fig. 3), while it remained low in the other. No consistent improvement of symmetry was observed. In the third period slowly developing changes occur (Fig. 3): symmetry clearly improves so that the values in the chronic state are only slightly lower than those of the controls. While all the above data were obtained from measurements made in the dark, it should be realized

that the VOR in the chronic state is nicely compensatory when measured in the light (Precht et al., 1981). This implies that optokinetic reflexes substitute for partial loss of vestibular functions. Presumably, in the animal with the head free to move, plastically adapted neck proprioceptive influences on the eyes further add to the overall performance of the gaze stabilizing systems (Dichgans et al., 1973a) (see also Chapter 12).

Returning to the long term deficiencies of VOR performance, as revealed by measurements in the dark, it is of great importance to realize the complete lack of any correlation between recovery of gain and balance (see Section 2.1.1). Thus, within the first 3–4 days p.o., the nystagmus at

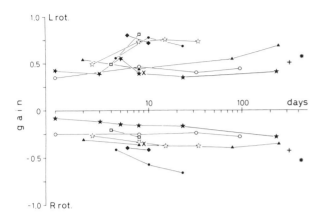

*Fig. 3.* Time course of VOR gain changes following unilateral vestibular nerve section (right side). Responses obtained from ten cats are illustrated. Gain was computed after subtracting from the responses the slow phase velocity of the spontaneous nystagmus (when present). Note the marked VOR asymmetry lasting for many months after the lesion (from Maioli et al. 1983).

rest is almost completely abolished even when measured in the dark, whereas at the same time no appreciable improvement of VOR gain and symmetry occurs. Similar findings were obtained when the phase of the VOR was studied (Maioli et al., 1983). The poor plastic capacity of the VOR gain control in labyrinth damaged animals in the early stage is surprising, since the cat, as well as other species, have been shown to adapt their VOR very quickly and strongly when wearing reversing prisms (Melvill Jones & Davies, 1976; Robinson, 1976; Keller & Precht, 1979a). In the second stage, however, some animals improved their VOR gains (Fig. 3) with a time course similar to that of intact cats wearing prisms. Apparently, when this critical state is missed, possibly by largely passive motor behaviour, only a very slow gain enhancement occurs.

The finding that compensation processes of static and dynamic vestibular symptoms are independent confirms the important distinction made by Haddad et al. (1977) between gain and balance control (see also Section 3). The two systems are functionally and structurally separate, since they are affected differently by lesions. Thus, lesion of the flocculus impairs the gain control (Robinson, 1976) without much affecting balance (Schaefer & Meyer, 1974; Haddad et al., 1977), and section of

the optic chiasm impairs balance and not gain control (Harris & Cynader, 1981b).

The striking difference between the time course of recovery of ocular balance and VOR gain raises another important problem. As mentioned in Section 2.2.2 rebalancing of resting activity in the vestibular nuclei is generally assumed to be responsible for behavioral balance. If neuronal balance had occurred the situation would be very similar to that in which one canal was made non-functional by plugging. However, after acute canal plugging, VOR is symmetrical, although at half gain (Money & Scott, 1962; Zuckerman, 1967; Barmack & Pettorossi, 1981), whereas in hemilabyrinthectomized animals showing ocular balance at rest large asymmetries prevail. This discrepancy will be further discussed in the next section.

Other deficiencies of the VOR system such as abnormalities in response phase, time constants, gaze holding failure in the dark, and also optokinetic abnormalities will not be treated here since no corresponding unit data are available (for details see Courjon et al., 1977; Maioli et al., 1983; Precht et al., 1981).

### 2.1.4. Responses of vestibular neurons to canal stimulation

*Acute stage.* As already mentioned in Section 2.1.2, *acutely* after the unilateral vestibular neurotomy, type I horizontal canal neurons on the *intact* side show an approximately two-fold increase of their resting rates. On the other hand, their mean sensitivities to angular accelerations decrease by about one half (Markham et al., 1977). This drop in sensitivity can be explained by the removal of inhibitory commissural vestibular influences and is in very good agreement with a similar change of VOR gain on rotation to the intact side (see Section 2.1.3). A similar reduction in sensitivity was obtained with vestibular neurons after unilateral canal plugging (Abend, 1978) (Chapter 9), a procedure which does not affect peripheral and central resting discharges but renders one canal non-responsive to rotation.

On the *deafferented* side acutely after the lesion very few type I units are found and they do not at all, or only weakly, respond to very high angular accelerations (Shimazu & Precht, 1966).

For the most part, they had no or very little resting discharge. The silence of type I units presumably is caused by the combined action of increased cross inhibition (two-fold increase in resting rate on the intact side) and ipsilateral disfacilitation.

On the other hand, type II neurons are as frequently found on the deafferented side as in control animals. Since they are inhibitory neurons receiving their input from the contralateral canal system (Shimazu & Precht, 1966), this finding is easily understood.

Rotation to the damaged side reduces the velocity of the spontaneous nystagmus without reversing the direction of eye movement (Section 2.1.3). This behavior is explained by the absence of resting rate of type I neurons on the damaged side. When evoked eye movements reverse their direction their gain is lower (Fig. 3), probably because the excitatory activity arriving from the deafferented type I neurons which have now recovered some resting level is small in amplitude, and inhibitory VORs contribute little to the movement.

The conclusion that VOR slow phase is mainly determined by the increase of sensitivity in the vestibular nuclei is indirectly supported by the fact that both the VOR gain on rotation to the intact side and vestibular neuron activity on the intact side acutely drop to one half, inspite of the complete loss of contribution of the type I neurons on the damaged side at this stage (Maioli et al., 1983). If the inhibitory VOR were to contribute much, the VOR gain should drop by more than one half.

*Chronic stage.* Data are available (Precht et al., 1966; Maioli et al., 1983), on responses beginning one month after the lesion. On the *intact* side type I responses were as frequently found as in control animals, whereas type II responses were extremely rare (practically absent). Since the latter units normally receive their input from the contralateral side only, the disappearance of this response type is readily explained.

On the *deafferented* side the most striking feature was the dearth of type I responses in comparison to the intact side or control animals. The number of type I units per cat in control animals

was at least 3-times as large.

The frequency of occurrence of type II responses was similar to that found in control animals. In addition, the efficacy of contralateral electrical stimulations in evoking responses in type II neurons was not significantly changed (Ried et al., 1984). These findings may indicate that the connections between the intact nucleus and contralateral type II neurons were not changed significantly by plastic processes occurring after the lesion. A similar conclusion was reached in a previous study (Precht et al., 1966).

One possibility to explain the striking reduction in type I responses would be the occurrence of transneuronal degeneration of central vestibular neurons after deafferentation. However, this possibility is very unlikely since no significant reduction in number of cells on the deafferented side was noted when compared to the intact side (Ried et al., 1984). Another possibility might be that lesion-induced sprouting, demonstrated to occur in the vestibular nuclei after vestibular nerve lesion (Korte & Friedrich, 1979), altered the vestibular circuitry. In this context it is important to recall that, in unilaterally canal-plugged animals, type I units occur as frequently on the plugged as on the intact side, although the sensitivity is reduced by half on both sides (Abend, 1978).

The reduction of the size of the type I population on the deafferented side could explain the long term asymmetry (poorer response on rotation to the damaged than to the intact side) observed in the VOR (see Section 2.1.3). Also, the VOR symmetry present in unilaterally canal-plugged animals is in agreement with the above mentioned unit data. Finally, the ca. 50% reduction in VOR gain on rotation to the intact side, or to either side in the canal-plugged preparation, is readily explained by the corresponding reduction in sensitivity of type I vestibular neurons.

Are the sensitivities of the remaining responsive type I units altered, increased or decreased, when compared to controls, i.e., does the commissure change its efficacy? To answer this question responses of vestibular units in control animals have to be likewise studied with only one labyrinth functioning, e.g., in unilaterally canal-plugged animals. Alternatively, one can use

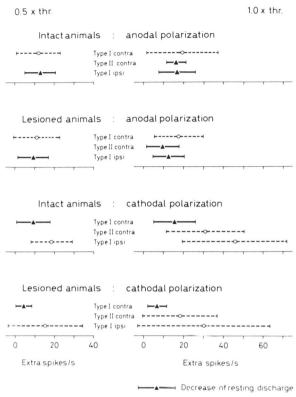

0.5 x thr.                                1.0 x thr.

Intact animals : anodal polarization

├----○----┤    Type I contra    ├-------○--------┤
               Type II contra        ┝━▲━┥
   ┝━━▲━┥     Type I ipsi          ┝━━▲━┥

Lesioned animals : anodal polarization

├----○----┤    Type I contra    ┝-----○-----┤
               Type II contra     ┝━━▲━━┥
  ┝━▲━┥       Type I ipsi         ┝━━▲━┥

Intact animals : cathodal polarization

   ┝━▲━┥      Type I contra       ┝━━▲━┥
               Type II contra    ┝-------○--------┤
├----○----┤    Type I ipsi      ┝----------○-----------┤

Lesioned animals : cathodal polarization

   ┝▲┥        Type I contra       ┝▲┥
               Type II contra    ┝------○-------┤
├------○--------┤ Type I ipsi    ┝------------○-----------┤

0    20    40    0    20    40    60

Extra spikes/s        Extra spikes/s

┝━━▲━━┥ Decrease of resting discharge
┝---○---┤ Increase of resting discharge

*Fig. 4.* Summary diagram showing the results obtained with type I and type II units of control and lesioned cats in response to polarizing stimuli of the ipsi- or contralateral labyrinths. On the left- and right-hand side responses to 0.5 × thr and 1 × thr stimulations are illustrated, respectively. The mean values and standard deviations of response increases and decreases are given in extra spikes/s (difference between firing rate at rest and during stimulation). For details see text (from Ried et al., 1984).

polarizing stimulation of the labyrinth to assess response sensitivities in control and deafferented animals. Ried et al. (1984) have chosen the latter approach and found that, by applying anodal stimuli in *control* animals (Fig. 4), the mean decrease in firing of ipsilateral type I units corresponds to a very similar mean decrease in contralateral type II, and increase in contralateral type I, firing. Similar, but opposite, results were obtained with cathodal stimuli. Thus, the commissure transmits the labyrinthine input in a one-to-one fashion and, therefore, contributes about one half to the total sensitivity of type I neurons. This finding explains the 50% reduction in sensitivities of type I neurons in canal-plugged animals; the symmetrical, but 50% reduced, VOR gain in

the plugged or unilaterally damaged preparations; and the 50% reduction of type I sensitivity following contralateral lesions (see above).

Type I units recorded on the deafferented side in the chronic animals showed no significant changes in response sensitivities (increase or decrease) to galvanic stimuli (Fig. 4), suggesting that the commissural path did not become more effective, i.e., did not compensate for the loss of a significant population of units. In a previous study (Precht et al., 1966) employing repetitive single shock stimulation at the contralateral labyrinth, a lower threshold for commissural inhibition was noted. The differences in results in the two studies may be due to differences in methods of stimulation and/or of measuring effects. Given that the results obtained with polarizing stimuli agree with those obtained in canal-plugging experiments involving natural stimulation, polarizing stimuli may better reveal the overall efficacy of the commissure. Also, the finding that significant changes in commissural efficacy were not present agrees with the persisting deficits in the VOR symmetry in unilaterally deafferented animals.

## 2.2. Recovery of otolith system after lesion

### 2.2.1. Behavioural studies

It is generally assumed that most of the tonic changes in head and eye positions (see Section 2.1.1) and part of the asymmetrical tone of the limbs is caused by macular deafferentation (see Sections 2.1.1 and 3). Neck torque may, via neck-limb reflexes, further enhance asymmetry in tone of limb musculature (Magnus & de Kleijn, 1913). It is of interest to note that those parts of the vestibular nuclear complex (LVN, DVN and caudal MVN) receiving strong otolith inputs are known sources for vestibulo-spinal tracts supplying neck and limb motoneurons (cf., Refs. in Pompeiano, 1975).

Tonic alterations in head and eye position recover to a large extent after unilateral lesions. Thus, tonic ipsilateral head tilt in the cat is greatly reduced within ca. 10 days p.o. (Putkonen et al., 1977) provided cats are kept in the light during the recovery period (see Chapter 12). On the other hand, contrary to nystagmus (Section 2.1.1) tonic head and eye tilt in the rat is strongly reduced within a few hours after the lesion and vision is not required for recovery, at least not in the albino rat (Llinás & Walton, 1979b).

Few studies are available on the recovery of macular reflex behavior in animals following unilateral lesions. Thus, recovery of ocular counter-rolling was studied in the monkey (Krejcova et al., 1971) and guinea pig (Kusakari et al., 1973). In man, ocular counter-rolling has been measured in patients who had one labyrinth removed, and this work was summarized recently by Diamond and Markham (1981). Although the available data are rather conflicting it nevertheless appears that, particularly on rotation to the intact side, significant deficiencies remain for long time periods when the effects of vision are minimized.

Recovery of certain postural reactions to free fall have been observed in unilaterally labyrinthectomized monkeys (Lacour et al., 1979; Lacour & Xerri, 1980): acutely after the lesion vision plays an important role for reflex responses measured in various muscles, whereas in the chronic state the remaining labyrinth appears to be sufficient (see also Chapters 10 & 12).

### 2.2.2. Resting activity of vestibulospinal neurons after lesion

Acutely after unilateral labyrinthine lesions, the resting activity of ipsilateral Deiters' neurons has been measured in the decerebrate, paralyzed cat (Hoshino & Pompeiano, 1977; Xerri et al., 1983). The mean resting rate decreased from $43.6 \pm 54.4$ imp/s in controls to $23.4 \pm 20$ imp/s in acutely deafferented animals. It may be assumed that similar changes occur in other species. Measurements employing the $^{14}$C-labelled 2-deoxy-D-glucose technique in the acutely deafferented rat indirectly support this conclusion by showing asymmetric metabolic activity in the bilateral vestibular nuclei (Llinás & Walton, 1979b).

In a later stage, i.e., when behavioural balance has been re-established, the mean resting rate of Deiters' neurons on the deafferented side remains low (Xerri et al., 1983). This finding is surprising but, since measurements on the intact side are missing, it may well be that resting rate of the intact side has been adjusted to that of the deafferented side. Metabolic activity measured with

the 2-deoxyglucose technique in the rat indicates similar values on either side. Furthermore, when spinal transsections were performed in compensated guinea pigs (Azzena et al., 1977; Jensen, 1979a) resting activity of LVN and DVN (descending VN) units increased on the intact, and decreased on the deafferented, side indicating that resting rates on the intact side have, indeed, been adjusted. The data also suggest an important contribution of ascending inputs to resting rate of vestibular neurons in the chronic state as well as to compensation of behavioral deficits. In fact, animals show a decompensation following spinal lesions (Jensen, 1979b; Azzena, 1969). The compensatory action of spinal influences may also explain most of the decompensatory effects of inferior olive and cerebellar nuclear lesions observed in the rat (Llinás & Walton, 1979b); both structures are mediators of spinal ascending inputs to other brain stem centers including the vestibular nuclei. Decompensation of already compensated guinea pigs was also observed after trigeminal neurotomy (Petrosini & Troiani, 1979).

These lesion studies indicate that rebalancing of resting rate involves many systems which have direct and/or indirect access to the vestibular nuclei. However, it should again be realised that symmetrical tone in other sensorimotor systems and nuclei is likewise important for compensation of balance deficits.

### 2.2.3. Responses of vestibulospinal units to macular stimulation

Are vestibulospinal units — acutely or chronically after the lesion — still capable of responding to macular stimulations?

Xerri et al. (1983) measured the responses of cat Deiters' neurons to slow tilt (0.026 Hz; $\pm 10°$) about the longitudinal body axis in acutely and chronically deafferented as well as in labyrinth intact animals. All recordings were obtained from the deafferented nucleus.

In *control* animals, lateral roll yields about twice as many $\alpha$ as $\beta$ responses ($\alpha$ responses are characterized by increase/decrease in firing on ipsilateral side-down/side-up roll while $\beta$ responses show the reverse pattern). Soon after the lesion (2–3 days p.o.) the number of $\beta$ responses increased so that the $\beta/\alpha$ ratio tended to approach one. The increase in β responses was particularly clear in the dorsocaudal division of Deiters' nucleus which projects to more distal spinal segments. Whereas the proportion of units responding to tilt decreased (from 91 to 72%) in the rostroventral LVN, no significant change was obtained in the dorsocaudal part. The mean sensitivities and gains of Deiters' units increased after the lesion. While in control cats rostroventral units were about twice as sensitive as dorsocaudal ones, those in animals soon after deafferentation no longer showed such a difference due to the remarkable increase in sensitivities of dorsocaudal units. The mean response phase lead (re. position) decreased from + 12.3° in controls to 3.3° in acutely lesioned animals.

From previous electrophysiological studies it is known that Deiters' neurons are excited polysynaptically from the contralateral labyrinth (Shimazu & Smith, 1971; Precht et al., 1967). It may be assumed that the responses found in the deafferented Deiters' nucleus were mediated by these polysynaptic pathways involving also the cerebellum, since cerebellectomy affected the distribution of response patterns as well as response symmetry (Hoshino & Pompeiano, 1977). When decerebrate cats were subjected to cerebellectomy and high spinal transsection, units in the rostroventral Deiters', ipsilateral to the deafferentation, were still affected by tilt; these responses were presumably mediated by vestibulo-reticulo-vestibular crossed connections in the medulla (Hoshino & Pompeiano, 1977). That reticular units, in particular those in the lateral reticular nucleus and surrounding regions, respond to tilt in hemilabyrinthectomized cats has been demonstrated (Pompeiano & Hoshino, 1977; Xerri et al., 1981a). In fact, compared to controls (Kubin et al., 1980), unilateral labyrinthectomy produced only slight asymmetric changes in mean resting rate, gain, sensitivity and distribution of response types of reticular neurons located in both sides of the brain stem. Moreover, cerebellectomy did not much affect the response properties of the units in unilaterally labyrinthectomized cats (Xerri et al., 1981b). It appears from these studies that the brain stem has a balancing system, the reticular formation, which is not severely affected by unilateral deafferentation and may, therefore, redistri-

bute the activity arising from the maculae of the intact side through the brain stem. However, since with acute lesions severe disturbances of postural balance and macular reflexes are observed (Section 2.2.1), close to normal neuronal balance and dynamics in reticular systems are not immediately sufficient to balance posture, reflexes and responses of vestibular units on the deafferented side.

Several months after the lesion the proportion of responsive units was higher in the rostroventral (76.7%) than in the dorsocaudal division of LVN (61.6%), thus approaching control values (Xerri et al., 1983). Gain and sensitivity of units decreased compared to the acute stage and, therefore, also approached control values. However, the ratio of β/α units remained similar as in the acute stage. Finally, response phases tended to be similar to those found in control experiments, i.e., the smaller lead noted acutely was observed to change to larger response leads. The overall response dynamics were also affected by the lesion: whereas in control animals one group of units showed frequency independent phases and sensitivities, others increased their sensitivities and phase lags with higher frequencies. After acute or chronic lesions response phase did not change with frequency; the frequency dependent increase in sensitivity typical of one group of control units was absent in the acute stage but partially recovered in animals in the chronic state. Whereas the initial lack of dynamic vestibular unit properties could explain deficiencies in macular reflex performance in the acute stage, their partial recovery could contribute to improvement of reflexive control.

### 2.2.4. Ascending influences on vestibulospinal neurons

As was the case for recovery of LVN resting discharge, spinal ascending systems probably contribute also to recovery of response properties of macular vestibular neurons. When the spinal cord was transsected in posturally compensated guinea pigs (Tolu et al., 1980) severe disturbances in the relative distribution of α versus β response types, characteristic of compensated animals, were observed. At present it is not known how exactly spinal ascending systems exert their influence on

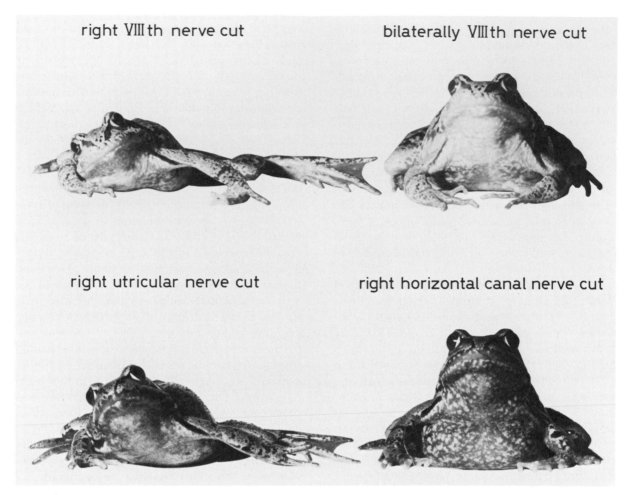

right VIIIth nerve cut

bilaterally VIIIth nerve cut

right utricular nerve cut

right horizontal canal nerve cut

*Fig. 5.* Posture of blinded frogs after acute vestibular lesions as specified above each animal. Note the fairly normal posture of the two animals on the right.

LVN neurons. Candidates are spinoreticular tracts receiving macular and various inputs from limb and neck proprioceptors and projecting via LVN to vestibular neurons both directly and via the cerebellum (cf., Coulter et al., 1976; Pompeiano & Hoshino, 1977). Spino-olivary tracts may likewise be important as suggested above (Section 2.2.1).

## 3. Studies performed in submammalian species

One of the reasons for selecting a lower vertebrate for investigations is its assumed greater simplicity in the central organization of its reflexes. The numerous differences in the central organization of optokinetic and vestibular reflexes for instance between frogs and mammals — some of

which will be described later — support this assumption of greater physiological simplicity. Because of the simpler organization of their gaze stabilizing reflexes, these animals are promising subjects in which some basic problems may be studied more easily and thoroughly than in animals of great physiological complexity.

### 3.1. Lesion-induced behavioural deficits

Unilateral labyrinthectomy results in well-known postural changes and in less well-known deficits in dynamic vestibular reflexes. As will be shown in Sections 3.1.1 and 3.1.2, particular aspects of these deficits can be attributed to the loss of information from particular receptor organs, and recovery of function can occur rather independently for postural and dynamic canal reflex deficiencies. Mainly dynamic reflex behavior and neuronal activity related to the horizontal semicircular canals will be considered here, since only scant information is available about the organization of static and dynamic otolith reflexes and related neuronal activity.

### 3.1.1. Deficiencies in postural reflexes

Unilateral labyrinthectomy in frogs results in a characteristic asymmetric posture of the head, the trunk and the limbs (Fig. 5), as described originally by Goltz (1870) and Ewald (1892). According to the lesion experiments of de Kleijn (1914), the asymmetric limb position can be considered to be predominantly due to the torque of neck and trunk rather than a direct consequence of the asymmetry in the activity of vestibulospinal pathways. As first described by McNally and Tait (1933) and Tait and McNally (1934), it is predominantly the removal of the utricle (Fig. 5), that is responsible for the postural symptoms observed after hemilabyrinthectomy. Lesions of other individual nerve branches, e.g., that of a horizontal semicircular canal (Fig. 5), does not cause obvious postural symptoms in frogs. Eye position is similarly affected, even though much less conspicuously. Owing to the small ocular motor range in frogs, the deviation amounts only to about 3° (Dieringer & Precht, 1981). In the pike, however, lesion of the nerve of a horizontal semicircular canal results in a larger tonic deviation of the eyes towards the side of the lesion without any accompanying body curvature, which is usually present after hemilabyrinthectomy (Lowenstein, 1937). In contrast to mammals, neither in pike (Lowenstein, 1937), frogs (Dieringer et al., 1982) or in several reptilian species (Trendelenburg & Kühn, 1908), was a spontaneous ocular nystagmus observed to occur after hemilabyrinthectomy or after section of the nerve of a horizontal canal. Instead, eye position just deviates tonically towards the side of the lesion.

It may appear from these studies, that posture in frogs crucially depends upon symmetrical activity arising from utriculospinal pathways. However, bilaterally labyrinthectomized, blinded frogs can maintain a fairly normal posture (Fig. 5) as is the case after a high spinalization (Franzisket,

1951), indicating that propriospinal reflexes by themselves have the potential to maintain a normal posture.

In frogs recovery of posture after unilateral lesions follows an exponential time course, and takes at least 2 months (Kolb, 1955). Similar observations were made by a number of investigators in several species of fishes (see Schaefer & Meyer, 1974). The effects of additional lesions, pharmacological treatments and centrifugation of the animal on the time course of postural recovery is discussed in Chapters 12 & 18.

### 3.1.2. Deficiencies in the dynamic reflex behaviour

After a bilateral labyrinthectomy the head of swimming snakes is no longer stabilized in space but swings back and forth in the horizontal plane (Trendelenburg & Kühn, 1908). In the pike, after a section of the nerve of a horizontal canal, pendulations of the head towards the side of the labyrinthine defect occur during forward swimming. These symptoms are striking, since normal pike keep their head perfectly stable during forward swimming (Lowenstein, 1937). These examples emphazise the importance of vestibulocollicular reflexes (VCR), which compensate in intact frogs or turtles for up to 80–90% of an imposed passive gaze displacement (Dieringer et al., 1983).

Soon after hemilabyrinthectomy, velocity steps or sinusoidal oscillations applied to frogs or turtles in the dark evoke only unidirectional VCR responses directed towards the lesioned side (McNally & Tait, 1925; Trendelenburg & Kühn, 1908). In the frog, the same is true acutely after a section of the nerve of a horizontal canal (Gribenski, 1963) (Fig. 6B). Since in the latter preparation head position is normal (Fig. 5), the lack of a VCR response to the intact side cannot be the result of a misalignment of the horizontal canal on the intact side. However, in the frog (Fig. 6) as in pike (Lowenstein, 1937) after a hemilabyrinthectomy, as after a section of a horizontal canal nerve, bidirectional but asymmetrical vestibulo-ocular reflex (VOR) responses can be evoked. Thus, the species differences formerly suggested by reports of unidirectional VCR responses in frog and bidirectional VOR responses in pike (discussed by Gribenski, 1963; and

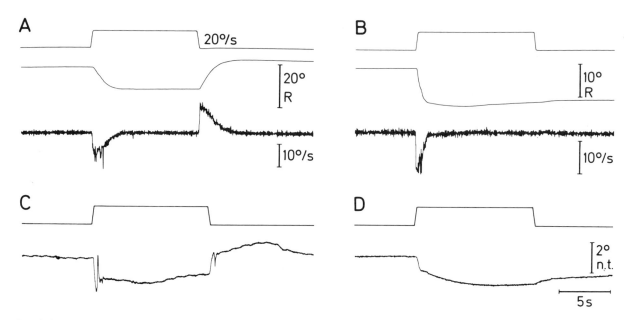

*Fig. 6.* Vestibulo-collicular and vestibulo-ocular reflex responses, of intact and acutely lesioned frogs to velocity steps in the dark. A, C. Head and right eye movements, respectively, of an intact animal in response to anticlockwise table rotation (top traces) recorded with search coils (head fixed in C). B, D. The same stimulus applied to another animal acutely after section of its right horizontal canal nerve. Note absence and presence of a post-rotatory collicular (B) and ocular (D) response and difference in amplifications of head poisiton (middle) and head velocity (bottom) traces between A and B. R, head movements to the right; n.t., movements to the right eye in a naso-temporal direction. (From Dieringer and Precht, unpublished.)

Lowenstein, 1974, pp. 88–90) can now be explained by differences in the thresholds of VCR and VOR responses (Dieringer & Precht, 1982a).

Acutely after the section of a horizontal canal nerve, the frog's VCR responses towards the lesioned side are less reduced (see also Fig. 6) than after hemilabyrinthectomy (Dieringer & Precht, 1981). This difference might be explained by the different head position of both groups of animals (see above). VOR responses directed towards the lesioned side — measured with the head fixed in a normal position — are only little reduced in both groups of frogs, and response thresholds for accelerations are similar to those of intact animals (about $2°/s^2$). These relatively small lesion effects will be further discussed in Section 3.2.2.

Optokinetically evoked compensatory head movements in frogs in the acute stage after labyrinthectomy can be symmetrical and can reach a velocity gain only little reduced with respect to that of intact animals. The occurrence of head saccades superimposed upon compensatory movements directed towards the intact side

(Dieringer & Precht, 1981) will not be further discussed here, since the neurological basis of this symptom is at present unclear (see, however, the hypotheses of Berthoz concerning the role of the saccadic system in compensation in Chapter 12). The effects of hemilabyrinthectomy on optokinetically evoked head movements are relatively small when compared to those in mammals, and can be explained by the differences in the organization of the optokinetic systems. At variance with other vertebrates studied so far, neuronal activity related to slow phase eye or head velocity is not stored centrally in frogs, and the resting discharge of central vestibular neurons is, with very few exceptions, not modulated by optokinetic stimuli (Dieringer et al., 1983). Accordingly, silencing of central vestibular neurons after hemi- or even after bilateral labyrinthectomy affects only slightly the velocity gain of optokinetically evoked head (and probably also eye) movements.

Over time, recovery of deficits in the VOR was observed in the pike (Lowenstein, 1937) and also in the VCR of frogs (Gribenski, 1963) after section of a horizontal canal nerve. However, as far as quantitative studies are concerned, a systematic investigation of the time course and of the degree of recovery of the dynamics of the VOR and the VCR is missing, except for some preliminary observations made in hemilabyrinthectomized frogs by Dieringer and Precht (1981). Only 25% of the frogs developed a symmetrical VCR over the period of 2–3 months. In the remaining animals head movements directed towards the intact side could only be evoked at higher accelerations ($25–100°/s^2$). The gain of these responses was highly variable (Dieringer & Precht, 1981). Since all these animals had recovered a fairly normal posture, the recovery process resulting in a newly balanced head position, and that resulting in a symmetrical gain of VCR responses, can have different time constants, as in the cat (Section 2.1.3). These time constants of recovery of head posture and dynamic VCR responses could be influenced by information signaling deficiencies in posture (at rest) and dynamic reflex performance (only during locomotion). Just how far forced locomotion can improve the recovery of dynamic reflex performance should be tested in future experiments.

## 3.2. Changes in response properties of central vestibular neurons after vestibular lesion

In intact frogs direct horizontal VOR and VCR pathways appear to be similarly organized as in the cat, (for a review see Precht, 1979). However, response properties of central vestibular neurons (VN) to vestibular stimuli differ from those in cat or monkey, in response sensitivity and phase relative to head acceleration (for mammals see Goldberg & Fernandez, 1975a; Precht, 1979 and Baker et al., 1981a).

### 3.2.1. Response properties of horizontal vestibular nucleus neurons in intact frogs

Mean acceleration sensitivity of horizontal primary afferents is several times higher in frog than in cat or squirrel monkey (Blanks & Precht, 1976). VN, however, have similar gains in these different species (Richter, 1974; Dieringer & Precht; unpublished data). With respect to primary afferent fibers the gain of VN is slightly reduced in frogs, but enhanced in mammals. This

last difference is best explained by the absence and presence of a functional commissural inhibition in frogs and mammals, respectively (Ozawa et al., 1974; Dieringer & Precht, 1979a,b; Shimazu & Precht, 1966). Correlated with the lack of a functioning velocity storage element in the brainstem of frogs, time constants of VN are not prolonged with respect to those of primary afferent fibers (Dieringer & Precht, 1982b; Dieringer et al., 1983).

### 3.2.2. Response properties of horizontal vestibular nucleus neurons in hemilabyrinthectomized frogs

No data are available about responses of VN in the acute stage in lesioned frogs. As far as frogs, posturally compensated in the chronic stages, are concerned, only results from a preliminary study, involving 10 animals, are available (Dieringer & Precht, 1981). From these results, the following findings might be of relevance.

(1) As in intact animals, about 50% of the neurons responding to vestibular stimulation were spontaneously inactive on either side of the brain stem. Resting rates of the remaining 50% of neurons did not differ significantly in their range (1–30 Hz) nor in their mean values (12.4 ± 9.7 H on the intact side; 12.1 ± 9.1 Hz on the lesioned side) from those of intact animals (8.2 ± 6.5 Hz). Since in acutely lesioned animals VN (identified by electrical stimulation of the VIIIth nerve) with a resting discharge were only rarely encountered (Dieringer & Precht, 1979a,b), some of the VN in chronic frogs can be assumed to have regained spontaneous activity. This assumption is strongly supported by the results obtained by Flohr et al. (1981) employing $^{14}C$-labelled 2-desoxy-D-glucose as an indicator for metabolic activity (Chapter 18).

(2) In intact animals, out of 123 central vestibular neurons, 78% exhibited type I, 17% type II and 5% type III responses. In frogs in the chronic stages, on the intact side, only neurons (12) with a type I response have been encountered so far. On the lesioned side, out of 20 neurons, three exhibited, at lower levels of acceleration, a type I, and at higher levels, a type III response. The remaining neurons on the lesioned side (85%) showed type II responses. Sensitivity of type I neurons on the intact side and of type II neurons on the

lesioned side (tested at a frequency of 0.25 Hz and amplitudes between ± 5 and 40°) had a range similar to that in intact animals.

From these results, it appears that the response patterns encountered on the lesioned side differ from those observed in intact animals. However, type II neurons on the lesioned side cannot easily be subdivided into those that had this response pattern prior to the lesion and those that acquired it subsequent to the lesion. Compared to intact animals, it is easy to find type II neurons on the lesioned side of animals in the chronic stages, and often multiunit background type II discharge is encountered. Thus, the number of neurons exhibiting type II responses on the lesioned side of frogs in the chronic stages might have increased with respect to intact animals.

The lack of type I responses on the lesioned side of hemilabyrinthectomized frogs could be related to the poor recovery of dynamic VCR (Section 3.1.2) in the majority of animals (75%) tested. Since these single unit recording experiments were carried out in a different group of animals prior to the behavioral studies, it could turn out that VN responses are more appropriate in animals showing better reflex recovery. Accordingly, in future experiments vestibular response patterns of chronically lesioned animals should be correlated with the status of recovery of the dynamic reflexes of each individual.

Alternatively, recovery of dynamic reflexes after hemilabyrinthectomy could be a process, during which the partially missing vestibular input is supplemented by inputs from other sensory modalities. Optokinetic inputs most likely play a minor role in frogs, because in animals, in the acute and chronic stages, optokinetically evoked head movements are not strikingly different in their velocity gain with respect to intact animals. In addition, occasional tests of VN located on the lesioned side of chronically lesioned animals with optokinetic stimuli, failed to modulate their resting activity as in intact animals, indicating that, at least in the vestibular nuclei, the central responsiveness to optokinetic stimuli is not altered. However, proprioceptive spinal inputs could very well be involved in the recovery of static and dynamic reflexes (observed in a minority of animals in the dark), as proposed by many others working with anurans (Kolb, 1955; Trabal et al., 1980; Dieringer & Precht, 1981). These ideas have recently gained strong support due to the results of Amat et al. (1984). After bilateral labyrinthectomy, the number of cerebellar neurons (Purkinje cells and others units) responsive to neck and limb stimulation increased from 5 and 12% (intact) to 61 and 65% (in animals in the chronic stage), respectively. The response characteristics and the distribution of units responsive to optokinetic stimuli, however, remained similar to those described for intact animals. Interestingly, this increase in the number of units responsive to somesthetic input occurs in the area that lost its normal vestibular input, with the result that in animals in the chronic post lesion stages, but not in intact animals, single units can be activated by both optokinetic and somesthetic stimuli.

Part of the dorsal root fibers of amphibians are known to ascend ipsilaterally up to the cerebellum (Joseph & Whitlock, 1968). On its way small side branches leave this tract to terminate in the reticular formation, the trigeminal and vestibular nuclei (Antal et al., 1980). Recently these projections were studied autoradiographically in intact frogs and chronically hemilabyrinthectomized frogs by Dieringer et al. (1984). Comparison of the density of the accumulated silver grains showed a strikingly higher density in the vestibular nuclear complex but not in cerebellum of chronically lesioned animals. These results suggest that already existing dorsal root axons sprouted within the vestibular nuclear complex after the lesion, but that these fibers did not invade areas of the cerebellum (such as auricular lobe or dorsal rim) where in intact animals many vestibular, but no dorsal root, afferents terminate (Antal et al., 1980). Thus, part of the increased responsiveness of cerebellar neurons to somesthetic inputs, described by Amat et al. (1984), might be explained by a synaptic reorganization of dorsal root and other ascending spinal inputs at the level of the partially deafferented vestibular nuclear complex.

Besides defining the systems involved, it is important for the purpose of understanding 'vestibular compensation' to know where and how these changes occur. Even though the behavior of compensated — as of intact — animals results from the distributed properties of all networks involved in balance and gain control, as emphasized by Llinás and Walton (1979b), a redistribution of activity at these various levels can still result from changes in the synaptic efficacy of remaining inputs converging on neurons that are partially deafferented by hemilabyrinthectomy. Thus, an increase in the excitatory and inhibitory synaptic efficacy of converging pathways can alter the output of a nucleus sufficiently to produce a whole chain of effects in various motor- and interneuronal networks. Alterations in synaptic efficacy of pathways terminating within the deafferented vestibular nucleus were studied by Dieringer and Precht (1977; 1979a,b) and will be summarized in the next section.

### 3.2.3. Changes in synaptic efficacy of pathways terminating in the partially deafferented vestibular nucleus

Single electrical stimuli of the anterior branch of the VIIIth nerve evoke field potentials in the vestibular nuclei on both sides. The characteristics of these field potentials were used as a measure of electrode location and for an adjustment of stimulation intensity, to allow a comparison of the results obtained in different animals. Primary afferents exert a powerful excitation upon ipsilateral, central vestibular neurons. Typically, in these neurons a burst of spikes is evoked. This burst arrives in many other structures, including the contralateral vestibular nucleus, which it reaches via the vestibular commissure and where it weakly excites second and higher order vestibular neurons (Ozawa et al., 1974; Dieringer & Precht, 1979a). In chronically lesioned frogs ($\geq$ 60 days) comparable stimuli evoke bursts of almost identical parameters (thresholds, numbers of spikes, interspike intervals) in neurons of the vestibular nucleus on the intact side. However, these bursts are much more potent, and evoke more active responses in a much higher percentage of vestibular neurons on the lesioned side. Therefore, neither the excitability nor the output pattern of vestibular neurons on the intact side changes postoperatively, and the increased efficacy must have developed in the partially deafferented vestibular nucleus somewhere between the commissural terminals and the spike trigger zones of the postsynaptic neurons.

Changes in synaptic efficacy of the commissu-

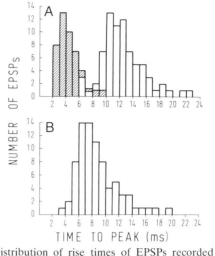

Fig. 7. Distribution of rise times of EPSPs recorded from neurons in the ipsi- and contralateral vestibular nuclei. A. Comparison between the rise times of EPSPs elicited from primary afferents (crosshatched bars) and from commissural fibers in acutely lesioned animals. B. In chronically hemilabyrinthectomized animals the same commissural input induces EPSPs with rise times that are on the average shifted towards shorter values (from Dieringer and Precht, 1977).

ral system were further studied by means of intracellular recordings. As a result, it was found that the improved synaptic transmission is characterized, on average, by a significantly shorter rise time (Fig. 7), and a larger amplitude of the evoked excitatory post synaptic potentials (EPSPs) elicited in chronic animals by stimulation of the contralateral VIIIth nerve. In addition, the potency of inhibitory pathways is also increased on the lesioned side. The onset of some of these inhibitory potentials has latencies too long to be attributed to the vestibular commissure, but occurs at a time when cerebellar Purkinje cells are activated. Removal of the cerebellum reduces the number of inhibited vestibular neurons. Thus, inhibition of partially deafferented vestibular neurons by cerebellar and brain stem neurons increases in parallel with their excitatory commissural input.

The mechanism(s) responsible for the observed alterations in the EPSP parameters is (are) unclear. As the most likely explanation we favor the assumption of reactive synaptogenesis. This assumption should be tested in morphological studies. A reduction of acetylcholinesterase activity on the deafferented side has been proposed as an alternative mechanism by Flohr et al.

(1981). Besides the problem that such a mechanism would fail to account for the decrease of rise times of the evoked EPSPs, the pharmacological evidence for this hypothesis is so far rather circumstantial and cholinergic synapses have until now not been described in the vestibular nuclear complex of the frog.

Whatever the mechanism for the increased synaptic efficacy of commissural terminals on the chronically deafferented side turns out to be, other pathways converging on these partially deafferented vestibular neurons might presumably increase their efficacy as well, and might turn out to be functionally equally, if not more, important. As far as postural recovery is concerned, the Bechterew symptom clearly suggests that resting activity of vestibular neurons on the lesioned side does not entirely depend upon commissural excitation. As far as response patterns to oscillations in the horizontal plane are concerned, a predominance of type II responses on the lesioned side would be in agreement with an increase in commissural efficacy, but would not necessarily be helpful for a recovery of dynamic reflexes. A functional interpretation of these synaptic modifications paralleling behavioral recovery awaits experiments employing natural stimuli in animals with well defined postural and dynamic reflex characteristics.

## 4. Concluding remarks

The review has shown that the question of whether recovery of vestibular functions following VIIIth nerve section occurs cannot be answered in a straightforward way. While it is true that some vestibular functions such as the maintenance of ocular, head and body balance at rest are restored reasonably well, dynamic vestibular reflexes such as VOR and VCR recover less readily. This applies for both mammals and submammalian species. It should also be emphasized again that the time courses of functional recovery differ considerably between species, i.e., submammalian species, in general, require more time to improve vestibular functions than mammals. However, even amongst mammals some deficits, such as head tilt, are rather quickly normalized in some species (rat) and take much longer in others (cat). Also ocular balance is achieved faster than normal head position in the cat while the

converse is true in the rat. Obviously, very different recovery mechanisms are taking place.

In spite of the long term deficiencies in dynamic vestibular reflexes per se, most animals show — in the chronic state — a rather well-coordinated motor performance. This is because other systems such as optokinetic and proprioceptive reflexes supplement for lost vestibular functions. These other systems are probably also important for the acquisition of vestibular recovery.

As for the neuronal mechanisms responsible for recovery of some, and poor recovery of other, vestibular functions, relatively little is known and much more physiological and anatomical studies need to be done. Recovery of balance of eye and head position is most likely achieved by recovery of symmetrical resting rate in the vestibular nuclei *and* related systems. How initially silent neurons regain tonic firing activity is not known although, for the most part, firing may be due to synaptic activation rather than true spontaneous activity in partially deafferented neurons. Potentially, all inputs converging on vestibular neurons and related structures may be involved in regenerating the resting rate. This could be achieved by a change in the synaptic efficacy of remaining terminals, converging upon deafferented vestibular neurons. There is good electrophysiological evidence for such a mechanism in the frog. A similar mechanism might also be present in the cat, since anatomical studies suggest that synaptic reorganization takes place postoperatively.

As for the poor recovery of dynamic vestibular reflexes, recent single unit work performed in the cat and frog suggests that the changes in synaptic organization between the bilateral vestibular nuclei occurring after lesion are not necessarily beneficial for the recovery of dynamic vestibular reflexes. Why, in some individuals, dynamic reflex performance recovers to a higher degree than in others is not known. It could be related to the amount of locomotor activity a given animal engages in after the lesion.

### Acknowledgements
This work was supported by the Swiss National Science Foundation (Grant numbers 3.505.79 and 3.616.80), and by the Dr. Eric Slack-Gyr Foundation.

Adaptive mechanisms in gaze control
Facts and theories
*Eds. Berthoz & Melvill Jones*
© 1985 Elsevier Science Publishers BV (Biomedical Division)

Chapter 18

# Neurotransmitter and neuromodulator systems involved in vestibular compensation

H. Flohr, W. Abeln & U. Lüneburg

*Department of Neurobiology, University of Bremen, NW 2, D 2800 Bremen 33, F.R.G.*

## 1. Introduction

Unilateral labyrinthectomy, or unilateral vestibular neurectomy, causes a characteristic disorganization of posture and movement, as detailed in chapter 17. Following this acute stage a remarkable degree of recovery of most functions usually occurs, with some degree of species dependence (Schaefer & Meyer, 1974).

Despite documentation of many behavioral, anatomical and physiological aspects of this compensation process, our understanding of the central changes underlying functional recovery is still vague. In particular, it is not clear which changes in cellular physiology (e.g., synaptic conductivity, reactive synaptogenesis) are involved, where these are located, by which causal factors (i.e., local or remote trophic influences) modifications are induced, nor which central mechanisms are responsible for the formation of functionally adequate circuits (Flohr et al., 1981).

## 2. Effects of drugs on the compensated state

### 2.1 Drug-induced decompensation and overcompensation

A possible clue to the origin of the central changes may be provided by the observation that the compensated state is labile, being reversibly or irreversibly abolished by certain surgical or pharmacological interventions. Two syndromes can be distinguished. Decompensation consists of a reversal of the compensation and the reappearance of symptoms characteristic of the acute stage (Fig. 1). It can be produced by destruction of various CNS structures, e.g., by hemispherectomy (Di Giorgio, 1939; Menzio, 1949), spinal cord transection (Azzena, 1969), bilateral destruction of the fastigial nuclei (Carpenter et al., 1959), chemically induced lesions of the inferior olive (Llinás et al., 1975; Llinás & Walton, 1979a), and by severance of the intervestibular commissures (Bienhold & Flohr, 1978). Decompensation can also be brought about by various pharmacological agents, in particular by drugs that alter the concentration of central transmitters at their respective receptor sites by affecting their release, disposal at the binding sites or inactivation.

Overcompensation comprises symptoms with postural and locomotor deficiencies opposite to those observed in the precompensated state, e.g., head deviation and circling to the intact side, abduction of the ipsilateral and adduction of the contralateral limbs (Fig. 2). These symptoms can be elicited by various drugs, often antagonists to those which induce decompensation. The first part of this paper will review the current data concerning drug-induced decompensation and overcompensation.

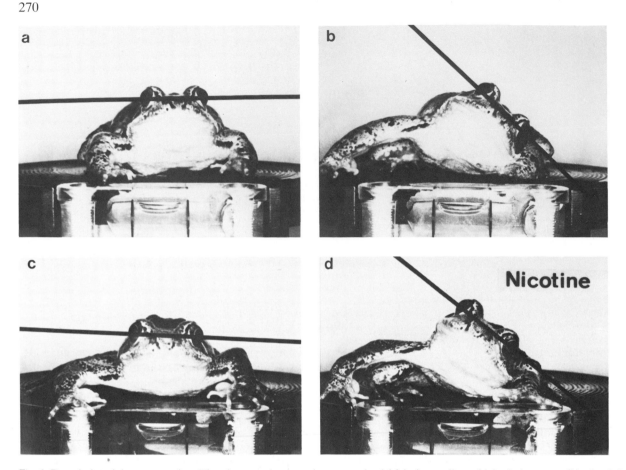

*Fig. 1.* Drug-induced decompensation. The photographs show the same animal (a) before unilateral labyrinthectomy, (b) after left hemilabyrinthectomy, (c) in the compensated state (71 days after hemilabyrinthectomy), and (d) 30 min after intracisternal injection of 2.0 mg/kg nicotine; the drug application causes reappearance of all postural symptoms characteristic of the acute stage.

## 2.2 Cholinergic transmitter systems

Present knowledge on the transmitter systems in afferent and efferent vestibular pathways is rather fragmentary. Steiner and Weber (1964), Yamamoto (1967) and Matsuoka et al. (1973) have shown that acetylcholine-sensitive neurons are present in the Deiters' nucleus of the cat. Summarizing from the above authors, about 50% of the neurons were excited by electrophoretically applied acetylcholine, an effect which could be blocked by atropine. Single unit responses to vestibular nerve stimulation were usually enhanced by physostigmine, given i.v., and this effect could

be counteracted by scopolamine. However, neurons were also found in which the effect of vestibular stimulation was depressed or unaffected by physostigmine (Matsuoka et al., 1973). Afferents from the reticular formation also appear to be mediated by cholinergic neurons since they could be modified by physostigmine. Again the discharge rate evoked by reticular stimulation was increased in some neurons and decreased in others by i.v. administration of physostigmine.

In the frog the compensated state can be strongly influenced by acetylcholine agonists and antagonists. Systemic or intracisternal injection of

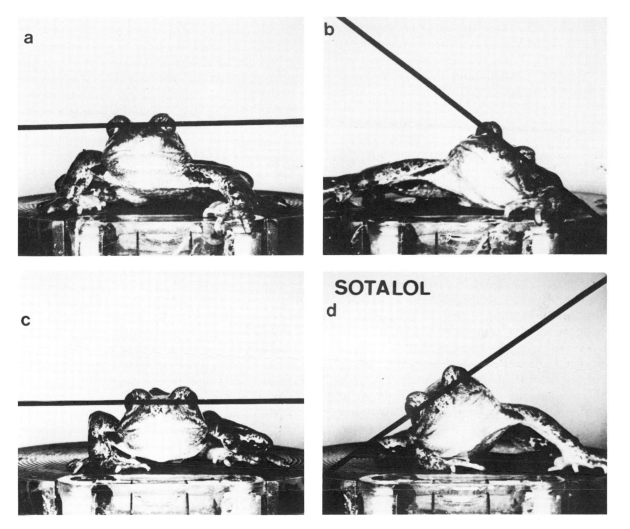

*Fig. 2.* Drug-induced overcompensation. The photographs show the same animal (a) before unilateral labyrinthectomy, (b) after left hemilabyrinthectomy, (c) in the compensated state (75 days after hemilabyrinthectomy), and (d) 30 min after intracisternal injection of 1.0 mg/kg sotalol; the drug application induces postural deficiencies opposite to those in the precompensated state.

cholinesterase inhibitors (physostigmine, paraoxon, parathion, BW 284*) induces an immediate and complete decompensation (Bienhold & Flohr, 1980). The effects are dose dependent, reversible and independent of the time interval between hemilabyrinthectomy and drug treatment, i.e., they are apparent in both partially and completely compensated animals.

Cholinomimetics, such as arecoline, carbachol,

nicotine, muscarine, oxotremorine, methacholine and bethanechol, given intracisternally, have the same decompensatory effect (Abeln et al., 1981). As with cholinesterase inhibitors these effects are dose dependent, reversible and can be elicited in both partially and fully compensated animals.

In contrast, cholinolytics, such as atropine and scopolamine, acting on the previously compensated animal, cause overcompensation with postural and locomotor symptoms contrary to those observed in the acute stage or following decompensation (Abeln et al., 1981).

*1,5-bis-(4-allyldimethyl-ammoniumphenyl)pentan-3-one dibromide.

In species other than the frog, evidence also exists that cholinergic transmitter systems play a comparable role in the maintenance of the compensated state. Epshtein and Shipov (1970) and Schaefer and Meyer (1981), for example, have reported decompensation in the guinea pig following anticholinesterase administration, whilst Ghelarducci (cf., Pompeiano, 1972) has shown that nystagmus reappears in cats treated with physostigmine. It is also interesting that atropine reduces or abolishes the nystagmus in the acute state following unilateral labyrinthectomy in the cat (Yules et al., 1966).

## 2.3. Adrenergic transmitter systems

Investigations of Yamamoto (1967) have established the presence of catecholamine-sensitive neurons in the Deiters' nucleus of the cat. Noradrenaline (NE), administered microelectrophoretically to single units, had a marked direct excitatory effect on about 50% of the neurons in the lateral vestibular nucleus (LVN). Both, spontaneous discharge and response to peripheral stimulation were enhanced. There was no indication of an inhibitory NE action within the LVN.

NE agonists and antagonists have pronounced effects on the compensated state in the frog (Abeln & Flohr, 1982). Noradrenaline, administered intracisternally, causes decompensation. Ephedrine, which facilitates NE release, and clonidine, an $\alpha$-adrenoceptor agonist, act similarly, whereas phentolamine, an $\alpha$-adrenoceptor blocker, leads to overcompensation. All effects are dose dependent, reversible and can be elicited in all phases of the compensation process.

## 2.4 GABA-ergic transmitter systems

There is considerable evidence for the involvement of $\gamma$-aminobutyric acid (GABA) as an inhibitory transmitter in vestibulo-ocular, vestibulo-cervical and vestibulo-vestibular (commissural) pathways (Obata, 1965; Obata et al., 1967; Obata & Highstein, 1970; Ten Bruggencate & Engberg, 1971; Precht et al., 1973a, b; Baker, 1976). In the cat commissural inhibition can be blocked by antagonists of one or other of the two presumed transmitters — GABA or glycine. A combined injection of picrotoxin or bicuculline together with strychnine eliminates all signs of vestibular inhibition, indicating that commissural inhibition is mediated by no more than two types of inhibitory neurons (GABA- and glycinergic) (Precht et al., 1973 a, b; Baker, 1976). Modification of the GABA-ergic commissural pathways seem to play an important role in the compensation process. In the cat the efficacy of commissurally mediated inhibition increases during compensation on the side of the lesion, and the threshold for inhibition of type I neurons in the chronically deafferented vestibular nucleus is significantly lowered (Precht et al., 1966).

The frog, unlike the cat, normally has a poorly developed commissural inhibition (Ozawa et al., 1974). Following unilateral labyrinthectomy, however, an effective crossed inhibition mediated by a vestibulo-cerebello-vestibular loop and by the brain stem commissures develops. These newly formed pathways are GABA-ergic; picrotoxin abolishes all inhibitory responses (Dieringer & Precht, 1979).

Recent findings on the effects of GABA agonists and antagonists on the compensated state in the frog support the assumption that the above mentioned plastic changes are indeed essential for the functional recovery observed at the behavioral level. In the frog, intracisternal administration of the directly acting GABA receptor agonist, muscimol, induces decompensation, whilst the GABA receptor blocker, picrotoxin, acts in the opposite manner to produce overcompensation. Both effects are dose dependent and reversible. (Abeln & Flohr, unpublished) (Table 1).

## 2.5. Conclusions: synaptic changes possibly involved in vestibular compensation

The above effects of various pharmacological agents on the compensated state suggest that different brain stem transmitter systems are implicated in the compensatory reorganization of the vestibular system; this, in turn, is a strong argument for assuming that synaptic changes are involved. However, taken together the reported findings do not yet permit any simple generalization about the specific roles the particular trans-

Table 1

| Drug | Species | Effect | | Effective dose (mg/kg) | Route |
|------|---------|--------------|------------------|------------------------|-------|
| | | Decompensation | Overcompensation | | |
| **AChE-inhibitors** | | | | | |
| BW 284 | frog | + | | 0.5 | i.c. |
| Paraoxon | frog | + | | 6.0 | i.l. |
| | frog | + | | 0.02 | i.c. |
| | guinea pig[a] | + | | 1.0 | i.v. |
| Parathion | frog | + | | 80.0 | i.l. |
| | frog | + | | 0.5 | i.c. |
| Eserine | frog | + | | 120.0 | i.l. |
| | frog | + | | 1.5 | i.c. |
| | cat[b] | + | | | i.v. |
| DFP[c] | frog | + | | 3.0 | i.c. |
| **Cholinomimetics** | | | | | |
| Nicotine | frog | + | | 2.0 | i.c. |
| Oxotremorine | frog | + | | 0.25 | i.c. |
| Arecoline | frog | + | | 3.0 | i.c. |
| Muscarine | frog | + | | 0.25 | i.c. |
| Carbachol | frog | + | | 0.25 | i.c. |
| Bethanechol | frog | + | | 2.0 | i.c. |
| Methacholine | frog | + | | 2.0 | i.c. |
| Bungarotoxin | frog | + | | 0.001 | i.c. |
| **Cholinolytics** | | | | | |
| Atropine | frog | | + | 1.0 | i.c. |
| Scopolamine | frog | | + | 3.0 | i.c. |
| **NE-agonists** | | | | | |
| Ephedrine | frog | + | | 1.5 | i.c. |
| Norepinephrine | frog | + | | 0.075 | i.c. |
| Clonidine | frog | + | | 0.6 | i.c. |
| **NE-antagonists** | | | | | |
| Sotalol | frog | | + | 1.0 | i.c. |
| Phentolamine | frog | | + | 1.7 | i.c. |
| **GABA-agonist** | | | | | |
| Muscimol | frog | + | | 0.0004 | i.c. |
| **GABA-antagonist** | | | | | |
| Picrotoxin | frog | | + | 0.004 | i.c. |

[a] Schaefer & Meyer, 1981
[b] cf. Pompeiano, 1972
[c] Diisopropyl fluorophosphonate

mitter systems might play, and a number of interpretations would currently seem viable.

Decompensation can be obtained not only by pharmacological intervention but also, as mentioned above, by additional lesions of various remote CNS structures. Some authors (Schaefer & Meyer, 1974; Llinás & Walton, 1979b) have therefore postulated that compensation requires

more than localized changes in the vestibular system and is effected by concerted, multilocular changes in different CNS regions. This implies that no single, identifiable 'trace' would be responsible for the process. Incidentally, the finding that various transmitter systems are involved does not contradict this hypothesis.

The arguments on which the above hypothesis

is based are tenable, but not obligatory. It is also conceivable that the wealth of observations apparently documenting the involvement of widely distributed CNS structures merely indicate that, during compensation, a reorganization of afferents from different remote systems has been brought about by localized and identifiable changes within the vestibular complex into which these afferents converge, rather than the remote site itself.

One such attempt to explain the diversity of phenomena characteristic of the compensated state by assuming specific, localized changes within the vestibular complex has recently been undertaken by Galiana et al. (1984) (see also Chapter 22). The essential assumptions of this hypothesis are: (a) that there are pathways interconnecting the bilateral vestibular nuclei which form a positive feedback loop, and (b) that functional adaption is achieved by selective gain changes in the commissural system. The properties of such an arrangement are fundamentally different from those of a feedforward type of commissural interconnection and not intuitively obvious. The predictions arising from an analytical evaluation of this hypothesis are consistent with all behavioral and neurophysiological findings known to date. In particular, this model provides plausible explanations for a number of apparently contradictory observations, e.g., the fact that Bechterew phenomena and decompensation can both be elicited from the compensated state. The model is also fully compatible with the present pharmacological data (Galiana et al., 1984). The outcome indicates that relatively local events could theoretically account for many of the diverse phenomena mentioned above, although it is also important to emphasize that the mathematical statement of this model does not necessarily restrict its modifiable influence to a single commissural location.

### 3. Drug-induced alterations of the compensation process

#### 3.1. Effects of drugs that modify neurotransmission

The compensation process can be accelerated or

delayed by pharmacological agents. Schaefer and Meyer (1973), Schaefer et al. (1978) and Schaefer and Meyer (1981) have shown that drugs with a narcotic or sedative action component (such as barbiturates, alcohol, various neuroleptics and diazepam) slow down vestibular compensation, whilst a marked acceleration is caused by excitants (such as caffeine, pentetrazole, metamphetamine, strychnine and paraoxon). Until now these observations have received surprisingly little attention, but recently Keller and Smith (1983) have directed interest to a hypothesis which might provide a background for interpreting some of the above findings. These authors demonstrated that adaptation of the vestibulo-ocular reflex to altered visual conditions was significantly suppressed in catecholamine-depleted cats. This led them to conclude that brain catecholamines (CA) might be involved in the regulation of plastic processes in the vestibular system just as they appear to be in the visual system (Kasamatsu & Pettigrew, 1976; Kasamatsu & Pettigrew, 1979; Kasamatsu et al., 1979; Daw et al., 1981).

The idea that the widespread CA systems of the brain play a role in controlling adaptive plastic processes was first proposed by Kety (1970, 1972). According to this hypothesis a biogenic amine, released generally throughout the CNS, serves both (a) as a mediator of signals identified as significant for survival, and (b) as a modulator of synapses that are currently in a state of excitation or have recently been active. A nervous system so constructed would not only respond on the basis of a genetically determined input and output response code but would also have the capability of developing new, elaborate and adaptive networks on the basis of its experience.

Some of the above pharmacological observations would suggest that this hypothesis could also be extended to the processes underlying vestibular compensation. The idea that CA systems play a general role in regulating plastic processes would in that case be given substantial support.

#### 3.2. Possible role of neuropeptides

Flohr and Lüneburg (1982) have recently reported in frog that ACTH-like neuropeptides are involved in regulating the plastic processes

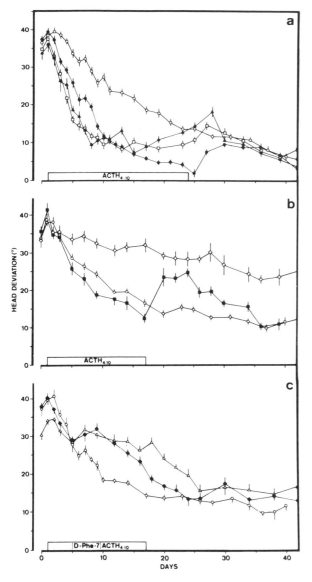

*Fig. 3*. a. Effect of ACTH$_{4-10}$ on compensation following unilateral labyrinthectomy in *Rana temporaria*. ACTH$_{4-10}$ was administered daily from the 1st to the 24th postoperative day. Three different doses were tested: ●, ACTH$_{4-10}$, 250 µg/kg per day ($n=35$); □, ACTH$_{4-10}$, 35 µg/kg per day ($n=20$); ▲, ACTH$_{4-10}$, 5 µg/kg per day ($n=20$); ○, NaCl-treated control group ($n=50$). b. Time course of vestibular compensation in *Rana temporaria* following hypophysectomy with and without ACTH$_{4-10}$ treatment. Hypophysectomy was carried out 8–12 days prior to labyrinthectomy. ◇, hypophysectomy only ($n=10$); ■, hypophysectomy plus ACTH$_{4-10}$ administration from the 1st to the 17th day after hemilabyrinthectomy, 250 µg/kg per day ($n=14$); ○, NaCl-treated control group ($n=30$). c. Effect of [D-Phe-7]ACTH$_{4-10}$ on vestibular compensation. [D-Phe-7]ACTH$_{4-10}$ was given from the 1st to the 17th day following hemilabyrinthectomy. Two different doses were

responsible for vestibular compensation. It was shown: (a) that the compensation process can be considerably accelerated by treatment with ACTH$_{4-10}$, a fragment of the adrenocorticotropic hormone (Fig. 3a); (b) that the compensation process is slowed down significantly by hypophysectomy (Fig. 3b); (c) that the compensation process so impaired can be restored by administration of ACTH$_{4-10}$ (Fig. 3b); (d) that the specific ACTH$_{4-10}$ antagonist [D-Phe-7]ACTH$_{4-10}$, which contains a dextrorotatory amino acid in position 7 of the molecule, inhibits vestibular compensation (Fig. 3c). Investigations by Horn and Rayer (1980) in Xenopus laevis have also demonstrated that hypophysectomy delays compensation.

An increasing number of studies in the last decade have established that the pituitary and hypothalamic petides, ACTH and α- and β-melanocyte stimulating hormone (MSH), are involved in learning and memory processes. This has been confirmed for a range of behavioral tasks, such as active and passive avoidance, visual discrimination and habituation, and for a variety of species including amphibia (De Wied & Gispen, 1977; Horn et al., 1979). Moreover, these effects are independent of the classic endocrine actions of the respective hormones. Apparently, the behaviorally active part of these peptides is the amino acid sequence 4–10 of ACTH (Greven & De Wied, 1973). Some of the effects in complex learning tasks are remarkably similar to those observed in vestibular compensation. As in vestibular compensation the restorative effect of ACTH$_{4-10}$ on acquisition performance in hypophysectomized animals is transitory; when treatment is discontinued, performance gradually declines to control levels (Bohus et al., 1973). These findings might help in understanding the possible mechanism of peptide action. It appears that ACTH-like peptides are not directly involved in the formation of the memory trace (since such effects might be expected to endure beyond the acquisition phase), but produce a brain state that is optimal for storage processes. This has led

tested: △, 1000 µg/kg per day ($n=15$); ◆, 250 µg/kg per day ($n=15$); ○, NaCl-treated control group ($n=30$); ordinates, head deviation in degrees, mean value ± S.E.; abscissas, time in days.

Flohr and Lüneburg (1982) to propose a concept in which neuropeptides are assumed to be part of an intrinsic control system that guides adaptive plastic changes.

### 3.3 Conclusions: neurochemical factors involved in the control of plastic processes

As mentioned above, vestibular compensation does not consist of a repair of the original circuitry because a restoration of the labyrinth and regeneration of the vestibular nerve do not take place. This necessarily implies a reorganization of the remaining structures. Furthermore, this 'rewiring' does not result in a functionally meaningless outcome but rather leads to a new and complex circuitry, the activity of which is appropriate for the restoration of normal function. In other words, it is a goal-directed process induced by some recognized 'error' in the system and directed to its elimination. It would seem highly improbable that the restitution of complex functional circuits and the selective formation of new connections could be a direct consequence of the lesion per se, as in somehow implicit in notions such as locally produced collateral sprouting at, or supersensitivity of, partially deafferented neurons. Changes so induced would not necessarily lead to functionally appropriate connections, but rather to randomly formed synapses which may or may not be mis-matched to functional needs. It must, therefore, be assumed that the elementary plastic changes are 'appropriate' or 'selective', and organized topologically in such manner as to enable an adaptive behavioral response. Consequently, Flohr et al. (1981) have suggested that compensation is effected by specific parametric feedback control mechanisms that guide adaptive changes, including recovery processes, in the adult CNS. A corollary of this suggestion is that neural nets capable of learning and recovery would not only need modifiable elements but also mechanisms for the regulation of these elements. Such mechanisms would provide a feed-back of the system's output to its internal structural elements, enable error signals to be measured and classified, and afford control over the state of the modifiable elements within the net. Flohr et al. (1981) have presented

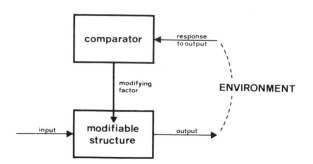

*Fig. 4.* Schematic represenation of a learning (or self-adaptive) system. The adaptive part (lower black box) changes its structure and output depending on the effects of previous outputs. The reactions of the environment are registered, evaluated and transformed into modifying factors controlling the parameters of the adaptive part.

experimental evidence in support of the proposition that the neuronal modifications responsible for vesibular compensation are not a direct consequence of the lesion itself but of an error signal caused by the lesion. If this signal is modified experimentally, the compensation process is markedly influenced — accelerated, delayed or even reversed. Fig. 4 outlines the simplest logistic structure of such a control system. It is common to all adaptive plastic processes and appears to be evidence at the behavioral level, although its physiological representation has yet to be defined.

One concrete idea as to how such feedback control could be realized physiologically is the Marr-Albus-Ito hypothesis concerning adaptive modification of the vestibulo-ocular reflex (Ch. 14). The crucial element in this hypothesis is a heterosynaptic modification at the Purkinje cell level. Two types of synapses are proposed: those transmitting signals and those acting as a 'teaching line' to modify the efficacy of the former. The implications of this concept are such that it appears doubtful whether the hypothesis could be applied to adaptive plasticity in general. Firstly, it implies a pre-existing modifying loop in every modifiable circuit. Secondly, it infers that a program, or several programs, have evolved which, when activated by particular stimuli, guide adaption to specific, and only to specific, situations. This, in turn, would mean that the actual adaptive modifications are selected from a set of genetically predetermined possibilities. Some phenomena, habituation or imprinting, for instance, might well belong to this class of process, but trial and error learning must have a different logistic structure, since new programs and structures, which could hardly be genetically anticipated, have to be sought and confirmed. Such deliberations have led Flohr and Lüneburg (1982) to propose an alternative concept in which humoral factors such as neuropeptides are assumed to participate in the postulated control mechanism, possibly acting as mediators of the error signal to the modifiable elements. The logistic structure of such a 'humoral' system would differ from that implicated by the concept of heterosynaptic modification in that the resultant cellular effects would be anatomically generalized rather than localized. This diffuse broadcast of a 'to-whom-it-may-concern' signal,

however, is exactly what is needed for bringing about concerted, goal-directed modulations in a distributed system. If the modulatory hormone action were coupled with ongoing or shortly terminated cellular activities, it would, in the long term, act preferentially on those structures generating the initiating output. By means of trial and error, the modulatory action would positively reinforce functionally adequate processes or inhibit inadequate processes. Such a mechanism would exert continuous control over the adaptive state of a given network.

An approach focusing on the nature of such neurohumoral control mechanisms would most likely lead to a better understanding of post-lesion adaptive plasticity and, indeed, plastic processes in general.

# Section IIB

## Systematic interpretation of neuronal mechanisms

Adaptive mechanisms in gaze control
Facts and theories
*Eds. Berthoz & Melvill Jones*

# Chapter 19

# Tensorial aspects of the multidimensional approach to the vestibulo-oculomotor reflex and gaze

## A. Pellionisz

*Department of Physiology and Biophysics, New York University Medical Center, 550 First Avenue, New York, NY 10016, USA*

## 1. Introduction

Gaze control has recently been interpreted by tensor network theory of the CNS, which applies to multidimensional natural coordinate systems (Pellionisz & Llinás, 1979a,b, 1980, 1982a; Ostriker et al., 1985). The vestibulo-oculomotor reflex has also been described by a matrix analysis method, which reduces this system to arbitrary frames that are three-dimensional throughout (Schultheis & Robinson, 1981; Robinson, 1982; Ezure & Graf, 1984a,b) (Chapters 1 & 20). While a detailed tensorial computer model of the complex gaze system is offered elsewhere (Ostriker et al., 1985), two specific, yet important and timely tensorial aspects of the VOR and the adaptive gaze are pointed out in this paper, in order to better illuminate the differences and the similarities of these two approaches. First, it is shown mathematically how the problem of motor coordination is treated tensorially as a covariant-contravariant Eigenvector problem in *overcomplete* sensorimotor systems, through the generalized inverse of the covariant metric tensor (Pellionisz, 1983a, 1984a). Second, it is emphasized that there is a need for a hierarchical analysis of *nested sensorimotor networks* underlying gaze control, as dictated by the concept of Metaorganization, which explains the genesis and modification of neuronal networks that implement the functional geometries of the CNS (Pellionisz, 1983b, 1984c).

### 1.1. Multidimensional approaches to the central nervous system and to the vestibulo-ocular reflex

When Sherrington (1906) promulgated the classic concept of reflexes, he warned against its oversimplification. "The main secret of nervous co-ordination lies evidently in the compounding of reflexes. . . . But though the unit reaction in the integration is a reflex, not every reflex is a unit reaction, since some reflexes are compounded of simpler reflexes. A simple reflex is probably a purely abstract conception, because all parts of the nervous system are connected together and no part of it is probably ever capable of reaction without affecting and being affected by various other parts . . ." (Sherrington, 1906).

Indeed, the gaze system has been regarded since Flourens (1826) as an interconnected multivariable system where *all* vestibular canals affect the function of *all* eye muscles (cf. the classical analyses by Helmholtz, 1896, Weiland, 1898 or Lorente de Nó, 1932). However, this complex interpretation of the whole had to be supported by a convergent triad of experimental, formal and conceptual means capable of handling such complexities. Such an experimental approach, in the form of registering the contraction of all extraocular muscles, was pioneered by Szentágothai (1950). A corresponding formal treatment, in the form of conventional vector analysis, was attempted by Krewson (1950). An outstanding conceptual interpretation, in the form of the potent quarternion-theory, was introduced by Westheimer (1957). The complex approach to the gaze system, nevertheless, has only rarely been pursued in recent times (Nakayama, 1974), due perhaps to the lack of cohesion among these difficult experimental, formal and conceptual methods.

Instead, despite the warnings about oversimplification, studies of some 'reflexes', most particularly that of the VOR, had gradually become reduced into a single scalar variable, the 'gain' of the system (for a most recent example, see Miles, 1982). This trend towards simplification was based on the systems' analysis approach, borrowed from engineering, assuming that some simple reflexes can be regarded as single-variable control loops (cf., Robinson, 1968; Stark, 1968; Young, 1969).

It has been claimed that tensor network theory provides new conceptual and formal means to facilitate a unified approach which aims at the true structuro-functional complexity of the CNS (Pellionisz & Llinás, 1979a,b, 1980, 1982a). Since tensor network theory was introduced, there has been a dramatic return of the interest towards multidimensional analysis of CNS, especially those systems, such as the VOR, where such relationships can be quantitatively established (Berthoz et al, 1981a; Schultheis & Robinson, 1981; Robinson, 1982; Goldberg et al. 1982; Simpson, 1983; Ezure and Graf, 1984b) (Chapters 1 and 20).

### 1.2. Problems with a multidimensional approach reduced to three-dimensional matrix analysis

A multidimensional analysis of the CNS presents serious conceptual problems, for instance, how to interpret neuronal function that is expressed in natural coordinates and in hyperspaces with *different* dimensions. Secondly, it also poses the burden of quantitative elaboration of such transformations. Therefore, it was proposed that the tensorial approach, which can state the functional meaning of network transformations in a highly abstract, coordinate system-free manner, should be coupled with computer modeling, which can numerically accomplish such quantitation (Pel-

lionisz & Llinás, 1979b). A tensorial computer model of the gaze system is presently being developed (Ostriker et al., 1985). Some central conceptual problems that appear to be unresolved in the literature, however, can be focused upon in this paper from a purely theoretical viewpoint.

Any multidimensional approach appears more suitable to the VOR than reducing it into a single-variable gain-control mechanism. Nevertheless, some problems of the three-dimensional matrix approach, which may lie in the setting of its goals, call for attention. The issue is *not* that the CNS requires three-dimensional, instead of one-dimensional analysis because it relates to the physical three-dimensional space. CNS functional manifolds are not one or three dimensional, but at times very highly *multidimensional* functional hyperspaces spun over the firings of a large number of neurons. A humble approach is the one that lets the brain be investigated in its own grandeur instead of reducing it into a flat shadow. The reduced approach was designed to elevate the description from one to three dimensions, attainable by no more than matrix-analysis (cf., Chapter 20), and not to tensorially analyze the transformations of natural coordinates in various CNS functional hyperspaces *with differing dimensions*. As a basic simplification in the reduced approach, in order to contain vectorial expressions into three dimensions, artificial systems of coordinates had to be introduced. Some problems that arise from this simplification are as follows.

(1) Enforcing a three-dimensional description entails artificially reducing the six-muscle extraocular motor system into a three-dimensional one by pairing 'agonist and antagonist' muscles, even though their axes of eye rotation, such as that of the superior and inferior recti in human, may lie as far apart as 36° (Robinson, 1975b). In addition to this morphological reality, physiological evidence is also available to show that the activation of so-called 'agonist and antagonist' eye muscles is grossly asymmetrical (Barmack, 1976). Indeed, textbooks warn against the ". . . misleading custom of linking extraocular muscles together, usually into pairs . . . Limited views of this kind may have a mnemonic value, but they ignore the inescapable fact that in any ocular rota-

tion *all* six muscles must change in length. . . . it is impossible to dogmatize as to whether every muscle is contracted precisely in step with the progressive inhibition of an antagonist" (Williams & Warwick, 1975; p. 1125). Beyond the mathematical error that 'averaging of vectors' represents, under these conditions, by changing from intrinsic frames of reference to imaginary ones, the goal of understanding the CNS function in its own terms becomes elusive again.

(2) One of the most significant conceptual problems of sensorimotor integration is the way in which the CNS transforms an expression in a lower dimensional sensory frame into one in a higher dimensional motor frame. This problem underlying motor coordination has been raised, and a tensorial solution was suggested, by Pellionisz and Llinás (1979b, 1980, 1982a), and quantitatively elaborated by Pellionisz (1984a). On the other hand, reducing the system to three-dimensionality throughout, eliminates rather than tackles the very problem of overcompleteness which most warrants a multidimensional approach.

(3) Not analyzing the system in its intrinsic (or natural) coordinates permits only a lumped description of the whole sensorimotor transformation in one single step, by one 'brain stem matrix' of the VOR (Robinson, 1982). However, the VOR has long been known to be based on a 'reflex arc' composed of at least three sequential steps (Lorente de Nó, 1933), from the primary vestibular neurons to secondary vestibular neurons to oculomotor neurons, even if the premotor neurons of the internuclear brain stem apparatus (cf., Baker & Berthoz 1977; Baker et al., 1981a) are ignored. Recently, one of the basic considerations of the reduced approach, requiring that secondary vestibular neurons receive no convergence from various semicircular canals (Robinson, 1982), was found to be conrary, in many instances, to experimental findings of projections to these neurons from up to all six canals (Baker et al., 1983).

To facilitate multidimensional VOR analysis without the need for these simplifying assumptions, a quantitative elaboration of the previously introduced tensorial scheme is presented below.

## 2. Motor coordination as a covariant-contravariant Eigenvector problem in overcomplete sensorimotor frames intrinsic to CNS

### 2.1. Extrinsic and intrinsic systems of coordinates for CNS function

Whenever the function of the CNS is related to physical objects of the world (external to the living organism), the complex multivariable spatial and temporal relationships can conveniently and concisely be given in *systems of coordinates*. The vestibulo-ocular reflex, which turns the eye in a manner that compensates for head movement, thereby allowing a stable field of vision, has been spatially characterized by authors too numerous to mention. In all cases the morphological orientation of the ocular motor system and the vestibular sensory apparatus was established in the frames of reference selected by the *observer* (cf., Fig. 1.).

While, as a matter of course, any arbitrarily chosen system of coordinates can be applied to an extrinsic description of such physical geometries, for reasons of convenience the traditional orthogonal Cartesian XYZ system is utilized by all authors. On the other hand, however, the individual sensors (vestibular semicircular canals) and motor effectors (individual eye muscles) constitute frames of reference of another type. These are *intrinsic* to the CNS, since neuronal firings express physical actions in these natural systems of coordinates. Accordingly, one has to accomplish two different tasks: first, to determine how the actual physical arrangements of natural systems of coordinates relate to the extrinsic, usually Cartesian, frames of the observer; and second, to explain how the CNS expresses its function in its own natural coordinates. For instance, how does the CNS implement a sensorimotor transformation from the three components of the covariant vector that the oblique set of semicircular canals sense, to the six components of the contravariant vector that activate the non-orthogonally arranged extraocular muscles?

The first goal was reached a century ago by Volkmann (1869), who established the rotational

284

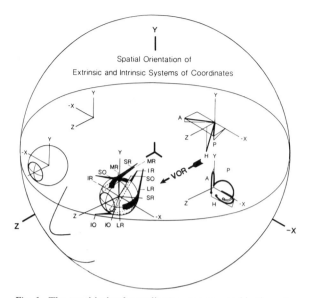

**Spatial Orientation of Extrinsic and Intrinsic Systems of Coordinates**

*Fig. 1.* The two kinds of coordinate systems, used in the external description and in the inner workings of the vestibulo-ocular reflex (VOR). Extrinsic, yet biologically oriented mirror-symmetric XYZ Cartesian frames (for the lateral sides of the body) are used as medial, dorsal and anterior, respectively. As in biological organisms with lateral symmetry, right-hand rule applies to the right side, and left to the left-side. The 'standard' position for visual demonstration presents XYZ with equal axes, 120° apart. Semicircular canals represent the HAP intrinsic system of vestibular coordinates, marked as: H, horizontal; A, anterior; and P, posterior. Eye muscles and their corresponding eye-rotational axes are denoted by: LR, lateral rectus; MR, medial rectus; SR, superior rectus; IR, inferior rectus; SO, superior oblique; IO, inferior oblique. These abbreviations apply throughout the paper. The diagram of the eye muscle orientation is drawn with the utilization of the computer model by Ostriker et al. 1985, and therefore both the paired sensory and unpaired motor systems are shown in a quantitatively exact manner.

axes corresponding to the individual contractions of the human eye muscles. Similar data have been recently provided also for other species (Simpson, 1983; Ezure and Graf, 1984a). Similarly, the excitatory sensitivity axes of each semicircular vestibular canal are also quantitatively known (Blanks et al., 1972, 1975b; Simpson, 1983, Ezure and Graf, 1984a). These data can be given in any extrinsic frame. Consequently, while the Cartesian system is used exclusively, the XYZ conventions vary. Although some yield advantages over the others, the variations may represent a source of confusion. In the approach presented here (see also Ostriker et al., 1985) two mirror-symmetric XYZ systems are used for the two lateral sides of

the body (medial, dorsal and anterior directions, respectively), with a right-hand rule for the right side, and left-hand rule for the left side (Fig. 1.). The XYZ are chosen to correspond to pitch, yaw and roll, no matter which side is referenced. As a result of this natural extrinsic convention, the morphological data are identical numerically and in sign for both sides. For visual demonstration purposes, a 'standard' frontal-lateral view of the head is used throughout the paper (pitched down 45°, and then yawed 45° to the left, so that the XYZ system appears with circular symmetical axes 120° apart).

The geometrical arrangement of the sensory and motor systems shown in Fig. 1. are based on data in Fig. 2 (Volkmann, 1869; Blanks et al., 1975a). Based on an implicit argument that the vestibular apparatus measures the same head acceleration vector, and the misalignment of canal orientations on the two sides is within close limits, it became a practice to average the covariant (cosine) components provided by corresponding semicircular canals of the vestibular systems of the two sides, and thus arrive at a unified vestibular coordinate system as shown in Figs. 1 and 2. (cf., Robinson 1982; Ezure and Graf 1984a,b). This is inevitable to the reduced approach, in order to arrive at a three-variable apparatus. While for the proposed tensorial treatment such averaging is not a requirement at all, this assumption of a combined vestibular system will be maintained temporarily because (a) compared to pairing muscles this pairing yields only a relatively minor error but, more importantly, (b) it facilitates comparison of the approaches, and (c) it shows how the CNS may transform a three-dimensional sensory input into an overcomplete, six-dimensional output. Nevertheless, it is necessary to point out that 'averaging' of vectors is only permissible when the components are of equal magnitude. In contrast to the extraocular apparatus, this assumption is a reasonable one in the case of the vestibular system since, given the maximal deviation in humans of 24° of the canals of the two sides, the maximal deviation of the activation of paired or non-paired canals is 7%. From calculations presented later in this paper it will be evident (see Fig. 3F, IR and SR) that in the case of the extraocular muscles the difference in mag-

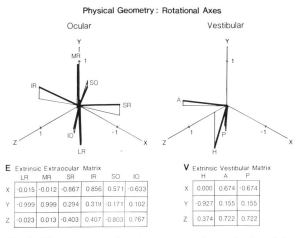

**Physical Geometry : Rotational Axes**

Ocular                                Vestibular

**E** Extrinsic Extraocular Matrix

|   | LR | MR | SR | IR | SO | IO |
|---|-----|-----|-----|-----|-----|-----|
| X | -0.015 | -0.012 | -0.867 | 0.856 | 0.571 | -0.633 |
| Y | -0.999 | 0.999 | 0.294 | 0.319 | -0.171 | 0.102 |
| Z | -0.023 | 0.013 | -0.403 | 0.407 | -0.803 | 0.767 |

**V** Extrinsic Vestibular Matrix

|   | H | A | P |
|---|-----|-----|-----|
| X | 0.000 | 0.674 | -0.674 |
| Y | -0.927 | 0.155 | 0.155 |
| Z | 0.374 | 0.722 | 0.722 |

*Fig. 2.* The sensory and motor systems of coordinates of the VOR, intrinsic to CNS function, as defined by the extrinsic vestibular matrix V and extrinsic eye muscle matrix E. The directions in three-dimensional XYZ space of the unit (normalized) rotational axes, belonging to individual eye muscle contractions, are shown in the left. The excitatory activation-axes of the combined semicircular canals of the two vestibuli are shown on the right. To facilitate visual perception of the three-dimensional directions of the axes, their orthogonal projection to the XZ plane is also indicated. The tables of extrinsic eye muscle matrix E and extrinsic vestibular matrix V represent the data base used throughout the paper (after Volkmann, 1869 and Blanks et al., 1975a,b respectively).

nitude between the activation of a so-called 'agonist-antagonist pair' can be as high as 2670%, and thus pairing of the extraocular muscles is impermissible.

The sensory and motor systems of coordinates, intrinsic to the CNS, are shown in Fig. 2. From the diagram, the differences in the direction and the number of axes of the input and output frames are evident, although the visual perception of the three-dimensional physical arrangement of the rotational axes does require some practice. From the orientation of vestibular directions it is clear that, in human subjects, a 24° down-pitched position would produce the largest excitation of the horizontal canals in case of a horizontal yaw, a position which is used to evoke a 'mostly' horizontal eye rotation (cf., numerical example later in the paper). It is of interest, that this position for maximal horizontal activation is *not* the position for minimal anterior and posterior activation. That position can be calculated from the cross product of A and P canals, yielding a 12° down-pitch. The numerical results for this (and for any)

head-rotation can be calculated using the scheme of Fig. 7, connected to the extrinsic frame (if required) through the extrinsic matrices V and E shown in Fig. 2.

## 2.2. Tensorial scheme of the VOR

The second task, relevant to CNS function, is to reveal how sequential parallel networks of the 'three neuron reflex arc' may transform a head rotation, given by a covariant reception vector, into a contravariant motor execution vector. The tensor approach, which can deal with intrinsic coordinates, suggests a solution to the problem of an increase in dimensionality and shows the interim expressions that are required after each network-transformation. The solution is based on the idea introduced by Pellionisz and Llinás (1979a), shown in the form of a conceptual scheme (Pellionisz & Llinás 1980; Fig. 4), and elaborated into a qualitative neuronal network-implementation (Pellionisz & Llinás 1982a, Fig. 8). The notion that in overcomplete expressions the counterpart of the covariant metric tensor can be obtained by its generalized inverse was introduced by Pellionisz (1983a); a detailed numerical model showing the computed generalized inverse was later given by Pellionisz (1984a,b).

The basic tensorial scheme is shown in Fig. 3. According to the tensor concept, the physical object (invariant) that is extrinsic to the CNS, is expressed in various intrinsic neuronal frames of reference in co- and contravariant forms. In the case of the VOR, the rotation of the head around a physical axis, e.g., as given in Fig. 3, can be represented as a unit-vector with a physical orientation which is, of course, expressible in an extrinsic, e.g., Cartesian frame as (0.000,−0.924, 0.374) in this example 4. This input was chosen for illustration as it is the so-called 'purely' horizontal stimulation. The head-rotation around this axis is the physical invariant, which is represented throughout the VOR in different vectorial expressions, and which finally emerges at the output as an identical physical entity, the movement of the eye. In reality, the compensatory eye movement is opposite to the head movement. However, since it is not presently known at which point of the neuronal 'reflex arc' the sign of the trans-

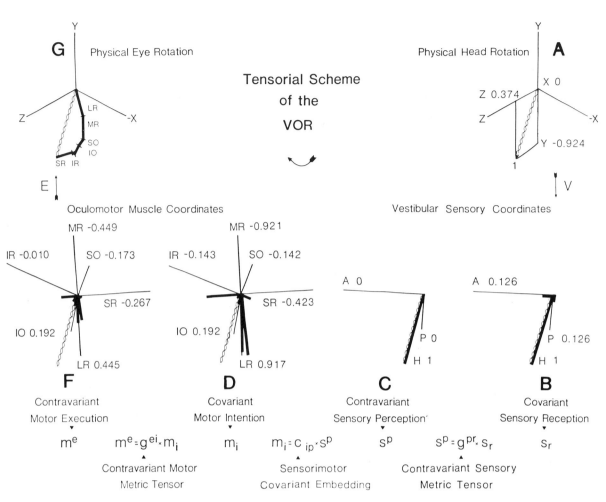

**G** Physical Eye Rotation

Tensorial Scheme
of the
VOR

Physical Head Rotation **A**

Oculomotor Muscle Coordinates

Vestibular Sensory Coordinates

**F**
Contravariant
Motor Execution

**D**
Covariant
Motor Intention

**C**
Contravariant
Sensory Perception'

**B**
Covariant
Sensory Reception

$$m^e \qquad m^e = g^{ei} \times m_i \qquad m_i \qquad m_i = c_{ip} \times s^p \qquad s^p \qquad s^p = g^{pr} \times s_r \qquad s_r$$

Contravariant Motor
Metric Tensor

Sensorimotor
Covariant Embedding

Contravariant Sensory
Metric Tensor

*Fig. 3.* Tensorial scheme of the VOR. A physical entity, a coordinate-system invariant head rotation is vectorially expressed in extrinsic, orthogonal Cartesian frames (A,G), and in intrinsic non-orthogonal vestibular and extraocular muscle-frames, both covariantly and contravariantly in either (B,C,D,F). A, an arbitrarily selected head rotation, corresponding to maximal excitation of the horizontal canals is expressed in an extrinsic, Cartesian XYZ frame. The extrinsic vestibular matrix $V$ (Fig. 2) transforms these XYZ extrinsic coordinates into HAP intrinsic covariant components, as shown in B (for the vestibular HAP, see Fig. 2V). The BCDF three-step sequence is implemented by neuronal networks peforming a sensory metric $g^{pr}$, sensorimotor transfer $c_{ip}$, and motor metric transformations $g^{ie}$. The last intrinsic neuronal expression is the contravariant motor execution vector $m^e$, which generates a physical rotation by activating the eye muscles. The extrinsic eye-muscle matrix $E$ (Fig. 2) can be used to calculate the Cartesian components of this rotation, which emerges as the physical resultant of infinitesimal rotations produced by eye muscle contractions (G). The numerical expressions are provided by the calculations shown in the rest of the Figures. All calculations throughout the paper are given in infinitesimal components so that their summation yields identical result in any permutation.

formation reverses, the VOR is shown throughout this paper as yielding an eye movement identical to the head movement.

The first expression of the external physical invariant in natural coordinates occurs in the vestibular semicircular canals, a physically obvious covariant expression in the non-orthogonal HAP vestibular frame (see Fig. 2, cf., Pellionisz and

Llinás 1980, Robinson 1982). Such an expression of the invariant was called covariant *sensory reception* (Pellionisz & Llinás 1982a), $s_r$ in short, the covariant nature of the vector shown by the subscript. At the other end of the VOR, the compensatory eye movement emerges as the physical resultant, contravariant vectorial expression of the contractions of six extraocular eye muscles (cf., the physical addition of six components in Fig. 3F, yielding the same rotation as in the A input). In Fig. 3E, the *motor expression vector* is symbolized by $m^e$, the superscript denoting the contravariant character of the vector. The vectorial components are shown numerically, as calculated later in the paper. The question of how the CNS arrives from this covariant three-component vector to the contravariant six-vector by a transformation, is first of all a general biological problem, that of *coordination*. However, it can also be looked at as a morphological problem of how 'reflex arcs' implement a *sequence* of network transformations, and it can also be phrased as a mathematical problem of how the tensorial expressions can be obtained in an *overcomplete* space, i.e., in more than three-dimensional spaces for physical movements. All three aspects of this central issue have long been addressed, in the form of (a) analyzing coordination in the CNS and cerebellar reflexes (Sherrington, 1906; Flourens 1826), (b) emphasizing the at least 'three-neuron reflex arc' (Lorente de Nó, 1933; Szentágothai, 1950), and (c) pointing out the overcompleteness through explicit statements such as "it is possible to abduct the eye to the same degree in innumerable ways" (Weiland, 1898). The tensorial scheme in Fig. 3. provides an answer to these classical questions by explaining the sequence of parallel transformations in overcomplete natural frames, and yields a blueprint that not only provides the known function but, as shown elsewhere (Pellionisz, 1984c), can also be generated and modified to perfection by physical CNS procedures.

The two interim vectors are the contravariant expression of the invariant in the sensory frame (*sensory perception* $s^p$; see Fig. 3C), and the covariant expression in the motor frame (motor intention, $m_i$, Fig. 3D). The three transformations necessary to obtain these vectorial versions of the invariant are a contravariant sensory metric $g^{pr}$, to transform a covariant expression into a contravariant one in the same sensory space, a motor metric-type transformation $g^{ei}$ which makes a similar conversion in the motor space, and a sensorimotor transformation $c_{ip}$, a covariant embedding that transforms a contravariant sensory expression into a covariant motor version. The theoretical need of these specific in-

terim versions was pointed out in the original papers by Pellionisz and Llinás (1980, 1982a). The distributed structure of the 'three neuron reflex arc' provides a morphological basis for the existence of interim expressions.

### 2.2.1. Vestibular sensory metric tensors, and their characterization by Eigenvectors

The calculation of the sensory metric is straightforward (cf., Fig. 3. in Pellionisz & Llinás, 1980). Accordingly, the matrix of the *covariant sensory metric* has already been published (Robinson, 1982). A re-calculation of $g_{rp}$ is given by Fig. 4A (note the different conventions, in our case *left*-hand rule for *left*-side). For a triplet of paired canal-axes, which is *not* an overcomplete system (cf., Fig. 4B), the contravariant vestibular metric tensor can be obtained by simple inversion of the covariant vestibular metric tensor. Robinson (1982) did not calculate it since he argued that "the metric tensor . . . need not be specifically recognized" (cf., Chapter 20).

In reality, however, it is not the published *covariant* sensory metric that is relevant to the function of CNS neuronal networks. The vestibulum measures these covariants, which can be calculated from the extrinsic components of the rotation via the covariant metric, for reasons of simple physics. Thus, the CNS needs to construct, through neuronal networks, the other type of metric tensor, the *contravariant* metric in order to obtain the counterpart of the physically measured covariant vectorial version. Then, with both co- and contravariant expressions available, internal sensory judgements on the external invariants (e.g., in this case, directions) can be made (cf., Pellionisz & Llinás, 1982a).

Recognition of the sensory metric tensor yields immediate experimental paradigms that have hitherto escaped attention. It is basic mathematical knowledge, also noted in neuroscience (e.g., by the pioneering work of Anderson et al., 1977), that matrices can most profoundly be characterized by their Eigenvectors. Paraphrased, these are special input vectors to a matrix for which the output will be changed only in 'magnitude' but not in 'direction' (see, e.g., Petrofrezzo, 1966). Such Eigenvectors of the sensory metric can readily be calculated by any of the several com-

288

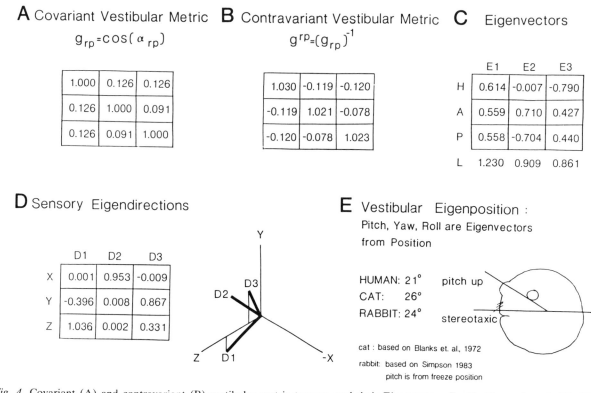

**A** Covariant Vestibular Metric
$$g_{rp} = \cos(\alpha_{rp})$$

| 1.000 | 0.126 | 0.126 |
|-------|-------|-------|
| 0.126 | 1.000 | 0.091 |
| 0.126 | 0.091 | 1.000 |

**B** Contravariant Vestibular Metric
$$g^{rp} = (g_{rp})^{-1}$$

| 1.030 | -0.119 | -0.120 |
|-------|--------|--------|
| -0.119 | 1.021 | -0.078 |
| -0.120 | -0.078 | 1.023 |

**C** Eigenvectors

| | E1 | E2 | E3 |
|---|-------|--------|--------|
| H | 0.614 | -0.007 | -0.790 |
| A | 0.559 | 0.710 | 0.427 |
| P | 0.558 | -0.704 | 0.440 |
| L | 1.230 | 0.909 | 0.861 |

**D** Sensory Eigendirections

| | D1 | D2 | D3 |
|---|--------|-------|--------|
| X | 0.001 | 0.953 | -0.009 |
| Y | -0.396 | 0.008 | 0.867 |
| Z | 1.036 | 0.002 | 0.331 |

**E** Vestibular Eigenposition :
Pitch, Yaw, Roll are Eigenvectors
from Position

HUMAN: 21°   pitch up
CAT:    26°
RABBIT: 24°   stereotaxic

cat : based on Blanks et. al., 1972

rabbit: based on Simpson 1983

pitch is from freeze position

*Fig. 4.* Covariant (A) and contravariant (B) vestibular metric tensors, and their Eigenvectors *E* with Eigenvalues *L* (C). The physical directions in the XYZ three-dimensional space, corresponding to the normalized Eigenvectors (C), are shown in D. These *D* Eigendirections are shown not normalized. E, experimental subject in a pitched-up position aligns the vestibular Eigendirections with the Earth-referenced yaw, pitch and roll directions. Note that such position is in contrast to the usual pitched-*down* orientation that is used for maximal stimulation of the horizontal canals.

monly used methods, and are tabulated in Fig. 4C. Since, for Eigenvector input, the output differs only by the Eigenvalue coefficient, it follows that the Eigenvectors of the covariant and contravariant metric are the same, with reciprocal Eigenvalues. Those physical directions in the XYZ three-dimensional space that yield these vestibular Eigenvectors, are calculated from the data presented in the extrinsic vestibular matrix shown in Fig. 2V, and are shown in Fig. 4 (note, that the vectors are not normalized, in order to provide a measure of the Eigenvalues). From the diagram of Fig. 4D it is evident that there is a position, attainable in the human by pitching the head up from the stereotaxic plane by an angle of $21° = \arctan(0.396/1.036)$, where pitch, yaw and roll around the X, Y, Z axes, respectively, will stimulate the vestibulum by an Eigenvector.

Thus, if one were to test the vestibular apparatus for its special *overall* performance, this simple tilt *up* into an 'Eigenposition' would lend itself easily to an experimental analysis. This is contrary to the not trivially justifiable experimental habit of tilting the head *down* by 24°, in order to align *one* coordinate axis with the rotation. It is noteworthy that in natural tests for the ultimate vestibular performance, such as in free fall or in an ice-skating piroutte, subjects appear to adopt an easily measurable pitched-up head position.

Since all vectorial relationships in this paper can be given in a reference frame-independent tensorial notation (see Fig. 3), different data bases, similar to the one shown for the human in Fig. 2, will be readily applied to model the VOR of various species. Within the scope of this paper, the calculated results on the cat (cf., data from

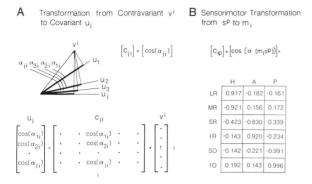

**A** Transformation from Contravariant $v^i$ to Covariant $u_j$

**B** Sensorimotor Transformation from $s^p$ to $m_i$

$$[c_{ji}] = [\cos(\alpha_{ji})]$$

$$[c_{ip}] = [\cos(\alpha(m_i s^p))] =$$

| | H | A | P |
|---|---|---|---|
| LR | 0.917 | -0.182 | -0.161 |
| MR | -0.921 | 0.156 | 0.172 |
| SR | -0.423 | -0.830 | 0.339 |
| IR | -0.143 | 0.920 | -0.234 |
| SO | -0.142 | -0.221 | -0.991 |
| IO | 0.192 | 0.143 | 0.996 |

$$
\begin{bmatrix} \cos(\alpha_{1i}) \\ \cos(\alpha_{2i}) \\ \cos(\alpha_{ji}) \end{bmatrix} =
\begin{bmatrix} \cdot & \cdot & \cos(\alpha_{1i}) & \cdot & \cdot \\ \cdot & \cdot & \cos(\alpha_{2i}) & \cdot & \cdot \\ \cdot & \cdot & \cos(\alpha_{ji}) & \cdot & \cdot \end{bmatrix}
\cdot
\begin{bmatrix} \cdot \\ \cdot \\ 1 \\ \cdot \end{bmatrix}_i
$$

*Fig. 5.* An explanation of the method of covariant embedding in general (A), and in the specific case of sensorimotor vestibulo-extraocular transformation (B). Such transformation may be performed from a contravariant vector to a covariant one. Note, that this direction is opposite to the sensory covariant to motor contravariant sequence. The covariant embedding procedure makes no restrictions regarding the dimensionality of either frame; thus an increase in dimensionality is also possible. The example in A illustrates a five-to-four dimensional transformation, but it applies equally to an $n$ to $k$, where $n$ and $k$ may be any integer. Further explanation is in the text.

Blanks et al., 1972 and Ezure and Graf, 1984a) or on the rabbit (cf., data from Simpson, 1983 and Ezure and Graf, 1984a) are given only for this 'Eigenposition', see Fig. 4E. This yields 26° for the cat, and 24° for the rabbit.

### 2.2.2. Sensorimotor covariant embedding from the vestibular to the oculomotor system of coordinates

In any *sensorimotor* system, by definition, somewhere and at least once, a neuronal network has to be found that executes a transformation through which the external physical invariant is expressed in a *sensory* frame at the input side, and in a *motor* frame at the output side. For an understanding of the nature of sensorimotor integration, it is inevitable that an exact explanation be provided of how such a transformation may occur in the CNS. The covariant embedding procedure suggests such a transfer, implementable by neuronal networks (see Pellionisz & Llinás, 1980, 1982a). However, it assumes the availability of a *contravariant* sensory expression (to be provided by the contravariant sensory metric tensor) and yields a vectorial expression of the invariant in the required motor space, but in a *covariant* form. A

covariant, when physically executed, yields an *improper* invariant. Therefore, the covariant sensorimotor embedding procedure necessitates an additional, contravariant motor metric tensor (Pellionisz & Llinás 1980, 1982a).

Covariant embedding, as demonstrated in Fig. 5., is based on the principle of independence in establishing covariant components along any number of axes. Let a physical invariant be represented by an $i$-dimensional contravariant vector, $v^i$ (with physical components), and let us calculate the covariant components of the same invariant along the $j$ axes of the $u_j$ covariant vector (let $i=5$, and $j=4$, although there will be no restrictions to either $i$ or $j$). Given a physical component of unit-vector of $v^i$ (along an axis), it can be measured along each axes of $u_j$. These cos(alpha) components will yield the $i$-th column in the $c_{ji}$ matrix of the covariant embedding. It is emphasized that either of the $v$ or $u$ vectors can be of any dimensions, and the covariant embedding can still be implemented with unique components. Therefore, a basis for both the sensorimotor transfer and the change of dimensionality (e.g., from a lower to a higher) is conceptually established. Quantitatively speaking, a table of cosines of the angles among sensory and motor axes can be calculated by the inner product of the unit-vectors shown in Fig. 2, yielding $c_{ip}$ in Fig. 5B. The question of how such a sensorimotor covariant embedding network can be generated by the CNS was answered by Pellionisz (1984c).

In summary, starting with any physical invariant, such as head rotation, the vestibular canals will sense its covariant components. Through the contravariant sensory metric, the contravariant sensory expression is made available. This contravariant vectorial version of the physical invariant is amenable to the covariant sensorimotor embedding procedure, which yields a vectorial expression in the motor frame, but in projection-type covariant components. Therefore, to complete the VOR transformations, a last conversion, a covariant to contravariant motor transformation must be made available, as elaborated below.

### 2.2.3. Covariant- to-contravariant motor transformation

Given a motor frame of reference, such as the

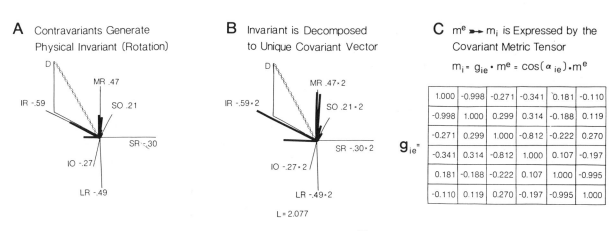

**A** Contravariants Generate Physical Invariant (Rotation)

**B** Invariant is Decomposed to Unique Covariant Vector

**C** $m^e \longrightarrow m_i$ is Expressed by the Covariant Metric Tensor

$$m_i = g_{ie} \cdot m^e = \cos(\alpha_{ie}) \cdot m^e$$

$g_{ie} =$

| 1.000 | -0.998 | -0.271 | -0.341 | 0.181 | -0.110 |
|---|---|---|---|---|---|
| -0.998 | 1.000 | 0.299 | 0.314 | -0.188 | 0.119 |
| -0.271 | 0.299 | 1.000 | -0.812 | -0.222 | 0.270 |
| -0.341 | 0.314 | -0.812 | 1.000 | 0.107 | -0.197 |
| 0.181 | -0.188 | -0.222 | 0.107 | 1.000 | -0.995 |
| -0.110 | 0.119 | 0.270 | -0.197 | -0.995 | 1.000 |

(A) MR .47, IR -.59, SO .21, SR -.30, IO -.27, LR -.49

(B) MR .47·2, IR -.59·2, SO .21·2, SR -.30·2, IO -.27·2, LR -.49·2, L = 2.077

**D** Covariant Metric Tensor is Characterized by its Eigenvectors

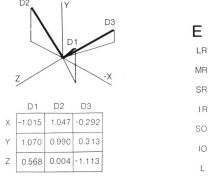

|  | D1 | D2 | D3 |
|---|---|---|---|
| X | -1.015 | 1.047 | -0.292 |
| Y | 1.070 | 0.990 | 0.313 |
| Z | 0.568 | 0.004 | -1.113 |

**E**

|  | E1 | E2 | E3 |
|---|---|---|---|
| LR | -0.427 | -0.484 | -0.199 |
| MR | 0.436 | 0.470 | 0.212 |
| SR | 0.387 | -0.298 | 0.558 |
| IR | -0.119 | 0.585 | -0.424 |
| SO | -0.488 | 0.205 | 0.473 |
| IO | 0.475 | -0.269 | -0.448 |
| L | 2.497 | 2.077 | 1.423 |

**F** Eigenvectors are Identical for Contravariant Metric: Moore-Penrose Generalized Inverse

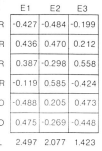

$g^{ie} =$

| 0.214 | -0.214 | -0.075 | -0.057 | -0.030 | 0.044 |
|---|---|---|---|---|---|
| -0.214 | 0.214 | 0.083 | 0.048 | 0.032 | -0.045 |
| -0.075 | 0.083 | 0.321 | -0.268 | 0.081 | -0.063 |
| -0.057 | 0.048 | -0.268 | 0.296 | -0.060 | 0.035 |
| -0.030 | 0.032 | 0.081 | -0.060 | 0.273 | -0.268 |
| 0.044 | -0.045 | -0.063 | 0.035 | -0.268 | 0.266 |

*Fig. 6.* Moore-Penrose generalized inverse acting as a contravariant metric in overcomplete CNS manifolds. A, any given sextuplet of contravariant (physical) components generates a physical resultant. B, the arising physical entity can be measured, using orthogonal projections to the axes, yielding a unique set of covariant components. The numerical data in A and B show an Eigenvector, where each covariant component in B is 2.077 times larger than the contravariant in A. To establish the *reverse* relationship, from a given set of covariants arriving at a unique contravariant (one out of the infinite number of possible expressions), it is required that the Eigenvectors of one expression be transformed to the Eigenvectors of the other. The unique, real-valued and symmetrical covariant metric tensor is given in C, and its Eigenvectors, Eigenvalues and Eigendirections are given in E and D, respectively. F, the Moore-Penrose generalized inverse of the covariant metric tensor, acting as a contravariant metric, transforms covariants into contravariants with the same Eigenvectors and reciprocal Eigenvalues compared to the covariant metric tensor.

six rotational axes corresponding to the contraction of individual eye muscles, the *existence* of both co- and contravariant-type expressions of an invariant can easily be verified (see Fig. 6A,B). Given any six physical components, such as activations of extraocular muscles by motoneurons, the physical entity of an eye movement will emerge. Thus, to any contravariant vectorial expression there exists an invariant (Fig. 6A). Likewise, starting from this invariant, the covariant components can uniquely be established by projections from the invariant onto each axis sepa-

rately; thus a covariant expression of the invariant also exists. As shown in Fig. 6A,B, these components may greatly differ in magnitude.

Thus, since there exists both a covariant and a contravariant expression for an invariant, even if the frame of reference is overcomplete, the question that remains is; how can their relationship be established? The covariant metric tensor can be expressed in a unique manner (since its elements are the cosines of the angles among the axes, cf., Fig. 6C). For the same reason, it is a real-valued, symmetrical matrix. The difficulty arises, however, if one attempts to calculate the contravariant metric by inverting the covariant metric, as could be done if the manifold was Riemannian, and thus Riemannian tensor analysis was applicable. In the multidimensional spaces that govern an overcomplete system of coordinates, however, the covariant metric is singular. Therefore, although there must exist a mathematical device that describes a multitude of possible transformations from a covariant set into a set of contravariant components, a unique solution cannot be identified by inverting this singular covariant metric. This mathematical feature reflects the physical condition, that in an overcomplete frame, the solution is not unique for the covariant-to-contravariant transformation. Given an invariant, the covariants assigned to it are unique, while the invariant itself can physically be assembled in an infinite number of different combinations of contravariant components. While this problem was recognized for eye movements as early as 1898 by Weiland, it has not hitherto been resolved.

It has often been stated that, in tensor theory of the CNS, the most profound questions relate to revealing the geometrical properties of the multidimensional functional manifolds, since it cannot be taken for granted that such spaces are Euclidean, or even Riemannian (cf., Fig. 1. in Pellionisz and Llinás 1982b). While, for didactic purposes two-dimensional diagrams (in the Euclidean space of the paper) have been extensively used to facilitate the understanding of the newly introduced concepts, it has been explicity stated and shown that the metric tensor (which is position independent in Euclidean spaces), is *position dependent* (non-Euclidean) in the overcomplete CNS hyperspaces (cf., Fig. 5. in Pellionisz & Llinás, 1980).

*2.3. Covariant-to-contravariant transformation in special mathematical spaces (overcomplete multidimensional CNS hyperspaces): the Moore-Penrose generalized inverse of the covariant metric tensor acting as a contravariant metric*

There is no a priori reason to assume a Reimannian, let alone Euclidean, geometry for the overcomplete CNS functional hyperspaces. Indeed, since they have never been closely investigated,

they may well turn out to be non-Riemannian in their functional geometry. The gravity of this point is that a rigorous enforcement or a tacit acceptance of axioms that disregard the facts may result in dogmatism or naivete even in scientific research. Thus, the chain of argument in neuroscience, just as in physics or any other natural science, must differ from the one in pure mathematics where there is a respectable place for any solid structure, even one based on imaginary axioms. Accordingly, there the axioms of the geometry of a space are defined first, and the consequences are then explored which follow from the axioms. In neuroscience, the experimentally obtained facts are preeminent. The challenge is to *arrive* at the basic mathematical features of the hyperspaces that lie beneath the rich complexities of findings and to identify and/or *construct* the appropriate abstract structure.

Pursuant to this argument, it is shown below that overcomplete CNS hyperspaces, indeed, appear to be non-Riemannian. This is so at least in the sense that Riemannian tensor analysis must be further generalized following the mathematical groundwork by Moore-Penrose (cf., Albert, 1972; Ben-Israel & Greville, 1980).

The approach presented here is based on the Eigenvectors of the overcomplete covariant-contravariant system. It can be established, both graphically and mathematically, that a particular contravariant physical set of vectorial components may yield an invariant that is uniquely decomposed into a covariant set of projection components, that differ only by a constant coefficient from their contravariant counterparts. Such a numerical example is provided in Fig. 6AB, where each covariant component is 2.077-times larger than its contravariant counterpart. The Eigenvectors and Eigenvalues of a matrix can be calculated by several numerical methods (cf., Petrofrezzo, 1966). The results are presented in tabulated form in Fig. 6E; the directions in physical three-dimensional space that correspond to such Eigenvectors are shown in Fig. 6D. It is noteworthy, but cannot be elaborated here, that such 'Eigendirections' carry physiological significance that are amenable to experimental exploration, similarly to the Eigendirections of the vestibulum. For our present purposes, given that the contra-

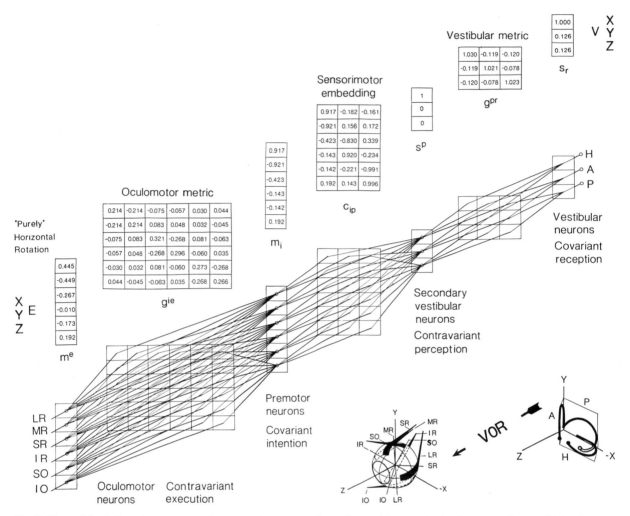

*Fig. 7.* Tensorial solution of an overcomplete sensorimotor transformation and its quantitative (matrix and network) implementation. Combined results of Figs. 4–6, provide a complete set of three intrinsic transformations that convert a three-dimensional covariant vestibular vector $s_r$ into a six-dimensional overcomplete contravariant extraocular vector $m^c$. The intrinsic transformations can be connected (if desired) to any extrinsic frame, e.g., by the extrinsic vestibular- and extraocular matrices of $V$ and $E$ (Fig. 2). The shown numerical example of a particular vestibular input vector $s_r$ is selected since it corresponds to the one in Fig. 3, the case of maximal horizontal stimulation. The scheme can be used for calculation of any eye-muscle activation, emerging from a given vestibular input. In the example shown, note that the activation of 'agonist-antagonist' muscles may yield a grossly asymmetrical contraction of, e.g., the SR and IR muscles, which are activated in a 26.7:1.0 ratio. In addition, *both* muscles are inactivated rather than acting in a push-pull manner. The tensorial scheme requires two interim vectorial expressions of $s^p$ and $m_i$, and thus calls for three separate transformation matrices of vestibular metric tensor $g^{pr}$, sensorimotor embedding $c_{ip}$ and oculomotor metric $g^{ie}$. It is suggested that the interim expression $s^p$ is implemented in the secondary vestibular neurons which receive projections from all canals, and $m_i$ is in the premotor neurons of the internuclear brain stem mechanism.

variant-to-covariant relation is established by the covariant metric tensor, transforming an Eigenvector into an Eigenvector magnified by an Eigenvalue, the contravariant metric-type transformation is expected to change the same covariant Eigenvector into a contravariant one, re-duced by the same Eigenvalue. This conceptual argument leads to the Moore-Penrose generalized inverse of the covariant metric, which yields the required matrix. Indeed, the reader can verify that both $g^{ie}$ (Fig 6F) and $g_{ie}$ (Fig. 6C) share the same Eigenvectors, tabulated in Fig. 6E.

## 2.4. A tensorial blueprint of transformation networks accomplishing an overcomplete VOR function

With the covariant-to-contravariant motor transformation determined, the chain of VOR transformations is now complete, as shown in Fig. 7. The sensorimotor transformation, which utilizes non-orthogonal intrinsic frames of reference, converts a three-dimensional sensory input vector into a unique overcomplete six-dimensional motor output vector. The required interim expressions correspond well to the morphological fact that the VOR pathways do not constitute a single lumped 'brain stem matrix' (Robinson, 1982), but form distinct nuclei with specific structural and functional properties (cf., Lorente de Nó, 1933; Robinson, 1982; Baker et al., 1981a). While XYZ is not part of the VOR per se, for practical purposes it is useful to convert $m^c$, which is expressed in intrinsic coordinates, into XYZ extrinsic coordinates by using the extrinsic eye muscle matrix as shown in Fig. 2E.

Relating the model-explanation shown in Fig. 7. to the exact details of reality calls for substantial further investments at all levels. Nevertheless, a correspondence can be well established on physical grounds for oculomotor neurons performing the contravariant execution function, and primary vestibular neurons acting as covariant receptors. While teleological reasoning postulates no convergence from primary vestibular neurons of various semicircular canals onto single secondary vestibular neurons (Robinson, 1982), evidence was and is available to prove this to be an incorrect assumption. Indeed, labyrinthine convergence on vestibular neurons has been demonstrated both by natural and electrical stimulation (Curthoys & Markham, 1971; Markham & Curthoys, 1972) and it has recently been shown that secondary vestibular neurons may receive input from up to all six vestibular canals (Baker et al., 1983). These findings reasonably correlate to the proposed vestibular metric, which contains nonzero off-diagonal elements. Another point of resonance with ongoing morphological research relates to the premotor neurons, which implement a covariant motor expression in the tensorial scheme. The interstitial, reticular and internuclear premotor-type neurons of the brain stem gaze control apparatus, extensively discussed by Baker and Berthoz (1977), are presently being given thorough attention, furthering the establishment of a correlation of the experimental facts with their model representation. Nevertheless, the significance of the proposed scheme lies in the fact that such increase in dimensionality from sensory to motor apparatus, as explained in Fig. 7, is a ubiquitous feature of the CNS. Indeed, in the gaze control apparatus there exist subsystems, most particularly the neck muscle mechanism, that dramatically deviate from the quasi-orthogonal, non-overcomplete, three-dimensional arrangements that can be adequately described by the reduced matrix analysis. A quantitative example is provided, in a demonstrative diagram (after Pellionisz, 1984b, see Chapter 15), of how the cerebellum may play a covariant-to-contravariant metric-type transformation for neck muscles based on the generalized inverse approach introduced by Pellionisz (1983a, 1984a,b).

The ability to calculate the transformations that are necessary for a sensorimotor integration in an overcomplete system may urge one to seek immediate conclusions regarding the actual morphological implementation of the calculated results. Thus, a word of caution seems appropriate; do not attempt the task unprepared. For instance, the pairing of the vestibular canals is *not* necessary when one utilizes the generalized inverse approach elaborated here. Thus, in the follow-up of this study, it would be important to treat the overcomplete six-canal vestibular system in a non-paired manner, in order to verify whether the error involved in a reduced approximate solution is, indeed, negligible.

A second reason for carefully thinking through a tensorial analysis of the system before arriving at its practical consequence is much more profound, as discussed below.

## 3. The need for a hierarchical analysis of nested sensorimotor systems in a study of the genesis and modification of the gaze control

The above tensorial calculation of an overcomplete sensorimotor transformation can yield the quantitative data for the three basic neuronal connectivities that explain how the VOR may implement its function, *once these matrices are available*. The scheme certainly did not show, however, how the necessary tensor transformation matrices can emerge through the functioning of the CNS. It was shown by Pellionisz (1984c) that the above transformation networks can, indeed, be generated and modified to perfection by the CNS if it follows certain physical procedures in a definite sequence. Such a scheme, where the interim and intrinsic expressions within the VOR are revealed, provides an opportunity to study not just the overall adaptive features of such a system, but actually to identify the sites and means of such genesis and modication. However, while the presented numerical calculation *is* applicable to explain the function of the VOR, the actual physical implementation of the genesis and modification of such sensorimotor geometries (Metageometries) is based on an assumption that the system is a true primary sensorimotor apparatus; but *this assumption does not apply to the VOR*.

### 3.1. Why the VOR is not a primary sensorimotor system: tensorial organization of metageometries through Eigenvectors of the covariants and contravariants belonging to an invariant

The vestibular apparatus is a sensory mechanism that, by means of measuring acceleration, keeps track of the movements of the head. The extraocular muscle system is a motor mechanism that, by means of generating an ideally equal but opposite eye movement, compensates for head movements and thus maintains the direction of the gaze in a moving head. That these sensory and motor systems work with one another, and that they are capable of exhibiting a most intriguing adaptive feature has also been thoroughly studied (see Chapters 2 & 3) (Gonshor and Melvill Jones, 1973, 1976b). Moreover, this modification-phenomenon is not restricted to one dimension only (cf., Berthoz et al., 1981a). Thus, VOR is often regarded as a sensorimotor system which is perhaps the best model for studying 'learning' by the CNS. However, it is asserted here that the VOR is *not*, in the deepest sense, a sensorimotor system, and thus an inadequate model of the genesis and modification of the adaptive sensorimotor function.

The term 'sensorimotor integration', while often utilized, is rarely defined. Tensor network theory, however, provides some means for a desired definition: *sensory function was defined as a covariant vectorial expression by the CNS, of an external physical invariant, while motor function is its contravariant vectorial expression. The transformation from one to the other is based on a metric, comprising a functional geometry* (Pellionisz & Llinás 1980, 1982a,b).

Thus, if the head turn and the eye turn were identical physical objects (in perfect maintenance of gaze they are equal, albeit opposite, movements), the vestibular and the ocular parts of the 'reflex' would be the covariant and corresponding contravariant vectorial expressions of the *same* physical invariant. In a first approximation, the VOR appears to represent both a sensory and a motor vectorial expression of a physical invariant, and thus can be taken for a sensorimotor system. However, a more careful analysis shows this to be an oversimplification.

The vestibulo-ocular reflex is *not*, in itself, a system that closes on the same invariant. It is not a physical necessity that the sensory vestibular reception and extraocular motor action are assigned to the same invariant; one and the same rotation. Indeed, *the vestibular sensory system is incapable of providing any measure of the invariant eye turn that the extraocular muscle system generates*. The adaptive feature of the VOR itself provides a demonstration that achieving such an identity is the *goal* of the VOR and not the *basis* of its operation.

### 3.2. Primary sensorimotor systems of gaze

The above declassification of VOR from a primary sensorimotor system, and from a model suitable in itself for understanding adaptive mechanisms, does not mean that primary sensorimotor systems do not exist in gaze control. In fact, there is more than one such apparatus, but the VOR as a self-contained system is not one of them.

### 3.2.1 Vestibulo-collicular reflex (VCR) as a primary sensorimotor system expressing one invariant, the head-movement

When analyzing gaze control, the most conspicuous physical entity is the movement of the head. It is evident that there exists both a covariant sensory and a contravariant motor mechanism that are directly tied to one and the same object, the head movement. It is physically guaranteed that, in rest, any head movement that is generated by neck muscle action is the same one that is directly observable by the vestibular apparatus. In this sense, both the contravariant generation of the invariant and the covariant vectorial measurement of the same is available in the vestibulo-collicular sensorimotor reflex (cf., the scheme in Pellionisz (1984b) and in Chapter 15).

It is noteworthy that gaze-stabilization in birds occurs predominantly by means of this primary sensorimotor system of head stabilization via neck muscles, in contrast to eye stabilization in primates. Other than the evolutionary argument that primary systems must appear earlier in phylogenesis than secondary hierarchical ones, the explanation for in-flight gaze control by head-stabilization (as opposed to visual stabilization) may be that the vestibular apparatus is very fast in detecting head movements, and thus the neck muscle apparatus can provide a quick response. This is in contrast to the slow retinal apparatus, which would provide the necessary control signals at a time when flying conditions could already be significantly altered. The preference of vestibular control over visual is intuitively obvious to anyone participating in rapid sport activities, such as skiing or skating.

The tensorial scheme presented in this paper could, of course, be quantitatively elaborated for a vestibulo-collicular sensorimotor system (it has already been outlined in Chapter 15), and it may be shown later how such a primary system can be generated and modified by physical CNS processes. However, it is unfortunate that presently no quantitatively precise data base is available for the motor frame of neck (and the limb-trunk) muscle systems, although for the eye comparable data have been available for more than a century (Volkmann, 1869).

### 3.2.2 Retino-ocular reflex (ROR) as a primary sensorimotor system expressing one invariant, the eye movement

There appears to be a second sensorimotor system that expresses both co- and contravariantly the same physical invariant. An eye movement, generated by the extraocular muscle system, could directly be measured by the corresponding retinal displacement of the visual image. In this sense, producing a physical object (eye movement) and detecting the same movement (slip of the retinal image) can serve as a basis on which a sensorimotor system can be generated. Thus, the retino-ocular reflex system is also a self-contained apparatus, that could not only be modeled as shown in this paper, but also physically generated by the CNS (ROR is identical to OKN).

Developing such a system is possible in a stationary head with only the eye moving, and checking, by means of retinal detection of the slip of the visual image on the retina, that the compensation is correct. A major disadvantage of this system over head-stabilization lies in the long-latency visual system. However it also yields some significant advantages over the other. The motor mechanism moves only the eye, in contrast to the much greater mass of the head, and uses only six muscles, in contrast to the more numerous neck muscles. Forthcoming tensorial analysis will quantitate what is already evident at an intuitive level; that this latter system, while slower than the first, yields greater precision.

To elaborate a tensorial scheme for this primary sensorimotor system, the retinal frame of reference must be established. While the persistence through the years of experimentally revealing the natural coordinate systems intrinsic to the neural mechanism of visual-slip detection has already yielded a knowledge of the coordinates for olivo-cerebellar correction (Simpson et al., 1981a), the question of whether the sensory metric utilizes such frames is yet to be answered (cf., tensorial interpretation of tectum by Pellionisz in 1983a).

### 3.3. Hierarchical nesting of the vestibulo-collicular head-stabilization and the retino-ocular eye-stabilization primary systems into the secondary gaze-stabilization system of VOR

The physical process of genesis of Metageometries requires three well-ordered consecutive procedures for each of the two primary sensorimotor systems described above. Once these six procedures are accomplished and the two independent sensorimotor mechanisms perform their function, a relatively simple seventh process, a linkage from one to the other can be established. Thus, a hierarchical hybrid of the VOR will emerge, which has the disadvantage of not being an independently developed sensorimotor system. However, given that its precursory systems are in operation, the hierarchical hybrid has the advantage of combining the speed of one with the precision of the other.

In summary, a quantitative elaboration of overcomplete transformations such as VOR is already possible without resorting to gross oversimplifications of the tensorial approach. Nevertheless, for a thorough analysis, especially of the genesis and modification of the holistic gaze system (cf., Llinás 1974; Llinás et al., 1976) much preparedness seems to be necessary, both in developing the necessary formal techniques, such as the quantitative means of computer models (cf., Ostriker et al., 1985) and in carefully thinking through the rather formidable conceptual implications.

### Acknowledgements

This research was supported by USPHS Grant NS–13742 from NINCDS.

Adaptive mechanisms in gaze control
Facts and theories
*Eds. Berthoz & Melvill Jones*
© 1985 Elsevier Science Publishers BV (Biomedical Division)

# Chapter 20

# The coordinates of neurons in the vestibulo-ocular reflex

## D. A. Robinson

*Departments of Ophthalmology and Biomedical Engineering, The Johns Hopkins University, 355 Woods/Wilmer, 601 N. Broadway, Baltimore, MD 21205, USA*

## 1. Introduction

Most of us have enough trouble measuring eye movements in one dimension, let alone three, and the equipment required to rotate subjects or animals about any axis in space is beyond the means of most of us. So it is not surprising that we mainly study horizontal eye movements and the neurons that create them. Vertical eye movements that are voluntary are also frequently studied, but the vestibulo-ocular reflex less so due to the trouble of oscillating someone in pitch. Torsion eye movements are rarely studied since they are difficult to record, cannot be made voluntarily, and, for the vestibulo-ocular reflex, require oscillating someone in roll. We content ourselves by saying that when we finally work out the neural wiring of the horizontal reflex, the others will follow by a mild application of geometry.

Perhaps so, but interesting questions arise when considering the planes of neurons. (The plane of a neuron may be defined as that plane of eye or head rotation associated with maximum modulation of its discharge rate: e.g., the planes of primary vestibular neurons are those of the canals; the planes of motoneurons are those of the eye muscles.) Consider, for example, a second-order neuron in the vestibular nucleus that relays the signal from the right posterior canal to the left inferior rectus. These neurons carry a head velocity signal (King et al., 1976; Pola and Robinson, 1978) and one would imagine that the plane of this signal is the plane of the right posterior canal. They also carry an eye position signal (ibid.) that is quite independent of head movements and one might imagine that the plane of this signal coincided with that of the muscle (the angle between this canal and that muscle is about 23°). Is it possible that signal components of a single neuron can have different planes or must a neuron have only one plane? As another example, we divide burst neurons into horizontal and vertical for no better reason that those are the only saccade components a monkey can make. But it can make torsional quick phases of vestibular nystagmus so there must exist torsion-related burst neurons. Should the planes of burst neurons be sagittal and coronal or might they lie in the planes of the muscles or canals? These are the types of intriguing questions that arise when one begins to wonder in three dimensions. A step in this direction has already been taken by Simpson and his colleagues (e.g., Simpson et al., 1981a, b) (Chapter 1) who devised a clever scheme to produce optokinetic stimuli in all degrees of freedom (similar to a planetarium projector) and found that the planes of visual neurons in the rabbit's accessory optic system lie close to those of the canals.

There is a practical side to all this; a lesion of

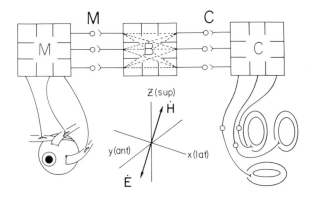

*Fig. 1.* The matrices of the vestibulo-ocular reflex. Eye rotation $\dot{E}$ is a vector driven by a motoneuron vector $M$ through a matrix $[M]$ describing the geometry of the eye muscles. The signal $M$ is driven by the neural output of the canals $C$ through a matrix $[B]$ describing the neural connections between vestibular and oculomotor neurons. $C$ is produced by a head rotation vector $\dot{H}$ through a matrix $[C]$ describing the geometry of the canals. The product of $[M]$, $[B]$ and $[C]$ is the matrix $[VOR]$ that describes the vestibulo-ocular reflex in all three dimensions. Normally $\dot{E}$ equals $-\dot{H}$ in the x (lateral), y (anterior), z (superior) coordinate system shown.

the brain stem might very well disturb eye movements in one plane but not another. Unfortunately, voluntary eye movements are restricted to axes lying in Listing's plane (Alpern 1962, p. 16), so that many axes of rotation are missed. The vestibulo-ocular reflex is not so constrained and in this situation, a misalignment of the eye and head rotation axes could be diagnostic of certain types of lesions. As mentioned, though, the cost and trouble of such measurements currently outweigh the possible benefits. As a result, this review must be content to speculate on the questions that arise and the possible results one might get if and when we can study the planes of central neurons. We will begin by a brief review of how vectors and matrices can be used in such speculations (Robinson, 1982).

## 2. A matrix representation of the vestibulo-ocular reflex

If we are to think of the vestibulo-ocular reflex in all combinations of roll, pitch, and yaw, we must think of a head rotation as a vector $\dot{H}$ with components, in a Cartesian coordinate system

attached to the head (shown in Fig. 1), of $\dot{H}_z$ (yaw), $\dot{H}_x$ (pitch), and $\dot{H}_y$ (roll). Similarly an eye rotation in the head is a vector $\dot{E}$ with coordinates, in the same system, of $\dot{E}_z$ (horizontal — with respect to the head), $\dot{E}_x$ (vertical), and $\dot{E}_y$ (torsional). It is the function of this reflex to make $\dot{E}$ equal to $-\dot{H}$. Since the reflex converts one vector into another, it may be represented as a matrix $[VOR]$,

$$\dot{E} = [VOR]\,\dot{H} \tag{1}$$

If the reflex worked perfectly,

$$
\begin{vmatrix} \dot{E}_z \\ \dot{E}_x \\ \dot{E}_y \end{vmatrix}
=
\begin{vmatrix} -1 & 0 & 0 \\ 0 & -1 & 0 \\ 0 & 0 & -1 \end{vmatrix}
\begin{vmatrix} \dot{H}_z \\ \dot{H}_x \\ \dot{H}_y \end{vmatrix}
\tag{2}
$$

Equation 2 is simply an expanded form of Eqn. 1, in which the components of the vectors are written in a column. Equation 2 expresses three equations obtained by multiplying term by term the $i$th row of the matrix by the $\dot{H}$ column vector to obtain $\dot{E}_i$. Thus,

$$\dot{E}_x = 0\dot{H}_z - 1\dot{H}_x + 0\dot{H}_y \tag{3}$$

etc. The zeros in $[VOR]$ are just as important as the $-1$s since it is just as important that, for example, vertical eye movements ($\dot{E}_x$) be not affected by yaw ($\dot{H}_z$) and roll $\dot{H}_y$) as it is that they compensate ($-1$) for pitch ($\dot{H}_x$).

The reflex may be broken into three parts. On the sensory side the canals transduce $\dot{H}$ into neural modulations of primary vestibular afferents. These signals are combined in pairs through the vestibular commissural system to form three signals: $C_{lrh}$, the modulation of secondary vestibular neurons receiving afferents from the left (lh) and right (rh) horizontal canals; $C_{rpla}$ from the right posterior (rp) and left anterior (la) canal pair; and $C_{ralp}$ from the right anterior (ra) and left posterior (lp) pair. These three signals are components of a vector $C$ that represent the neural encoding of the head velocity vector. The operation of the canals in converting $\dot{H}$ to $C$ is also described by a matrix — the canal matrix $[C]$:

$$C = [C]\,\dot{H} \tag{4}$$

From the measurements of Blanks et al. (1975a) on human canals, the elements of $[C]$ are found to be

$$
\begin{vmatrix} C_{\mathrm{lrh}} \\ C_{\mathrm{rpla}} \\ C_{\mathrm{ralp}} \end{vmatrix} = \begin{vmatrix} 0.927 & 0.0 & -0.374 \\ 0.156 & -0.673 & 0.723 \\ 0.156 & 0.673 & 0.723 \end{vmatrix} \begin{vmatrix} \dot{H}_z \\ \dot{H}_x \\ \dot{H}_y \end{vmatrix} \quad (5)
$$

In a similar fashion, the modulation of motoneurons creates muscle force and rotation of the eye in the plane of that muscle. Again, the muscles operate in pairs through reciprocal innervation. The modulation of the lateral (lr) and medial (mr) rectus pair, $M_{\mathrm{lmr}}$, that of the superior (sr) and inferior (ir) recti, $M_{\mathrm{sir}}$, and that of the superior (so) and inferior (io) obliques, $M_{\mathrm{sio}}$, form the three components of a motor vector $M$. The transformation of $M$ to $\dot{E}$ may be described by a muscle matrix $[M]$,

$$
\dot{E} = [M]\, M \quad (6)
$$

Using numerical values from Robinson (1975b) for the left eye,

$$
\begin{vmatrix} \dot{E}_z \\ \dot{E}_x \\ \dot{E}_y \end{vmatrix} = \begin{vmatrix} 0.999 & 0.016 & 0.14 \\ -0.005 & -0.906 & 0.6 \\ 0.015 & 0.424 & 0.788 \end{vmatrix} \begin{vmatrix} M_{\mathrm{lmr}} \\ M_{\mathrm{sir}} \\ M_{\mathrm{sio}} \end{vmatrix} \quad (7)
$$

The significance of the numbers is discussed elsewhere (Robinson 1982) but they only describe quantitatively what is well known physiologically. For example, from Eqn 7., the action of the vertical recti ($M_{\mathrm{sir}}$) is mainly to move the eye vertically ($\dot{E}_x$) (90.6%), but with some torsion ($\dot{E}_y$) (42.4%), and almost no horizontal movement ($\dot{E}_z$) (1.6%). Similarly, from Eqn. 5, the horizontal canals ($C_{\mathrm{lrh}}$) are very sensitive to yaw ($\dot{H}_z$) (92.7%), insensitive to pitch ($\dot{H}_x$) (0.0) and, because they are tilted backward, moderately sensitive to roll ($\dot{H}_y$) (37.4%).

The purpose of all this quantification is to find the matrix $[B]$ which describes how the connections in the brain stem, between the vestibular nuclei and the motor nuclei, transforms the vector $C$ into $M$,

$$
M = [B]\, C \quad (8)
$$

$[B]$ may be found by combining Eqns. 6, 8, and 4,

$$
\dot{E} = [M]M = [M]\,[B]\,C = [M]\,[B]\,[C]\,\dot{H} \quad (9)
$$

whence, comparing, Eqns. 1 and 9,

$$
[VOR] = [M]\,[B]\,[C] \quad (10)
$$

Solving for $[B]$,

$$
[B] = [M^{-1}]\,[VOR]\,[C^{-1}] \quad (11)
$$

The question now arises as to what $[VOR]$ actually is. Equation 2 assumes ideal performance. The gain of the horizontal reflex is nearly $-1.0$ so long as the subject attempts to fixate an imagined surrounding in the dark during sinusoidal oscillations (as opposed to mental arithmetic when the gain drops to 0.65; Barr et al. 1976) and the vertical gain is probably similar. Closer examination (Collewijn et al., 1981a) shows these gains are about $-0.95$, but we will use $-1.0$ for simplicity in illustrating the method. On the other hand, the gain of the torsion reflex seems to be half that of the others (Berthoz et al., 1981a). Thus, without additional data, and we certainly need more, we estimate $[VOR]$ as

$$
\begin{vmatrix} \dot{E}_z \\ \dot{E}_x \\ \dot{E}_y \end{vmatrix} = \begin{vmatrix} -1 & 0 & 0 \\ 0 & -1 & 0 \\ 0 & 0 & -0.5 \end{vmatrix} \begin{vmatrix} \dot{H}_z \\ \dot{H}_x \\ \dot{H}_y \end{vmatrix} \quad (12)
$$

Substituting this into Eqn. 11 we find $[B]$ to be,

$$
\begin{vmatrix} M_{\mathrm{lmr}} \\ M_{\mathrm{sir}} \\ M_{\mathrm{sio}} \end{vmatrix} - \begin{vmatrix} -1.01 & -0.248 & -0.176 \\ 0.08 & -0.799 & 0.41 \\ 0.112 & 0.031 & -0.621 \end{vmatrix} \begin{vmatrix} C_{\mathrm{lrh}} \\ C_{\mathrm{rpla}} \\ C_{\mathrm{ralp}} \end{vmatrix} \quad (13)
$$

The interpretation of these numbers has been discussed elsewhere (Robinson 1982). Briefly, the main-diagonal terms are large indicating that canal pairs project to the muscle pairs with planes that lie closest to their own. Off-diagonal terms correct for the residual misalignments of those canals and muscle pairs. That none of the numbers in $[B]$ is zero attests to what is often said, without proof, that every canal pair must project

300

to every muscle pair. Note that each number represents four pathways — each of the two canals in a pair excites one muscle and inhibits its angatonist. One cannot interpret the numbers too literally to deduce relative number of fibers in the various projections from canals to motoneurons, because of different neural amplification factors due to synaptic efficacy, different muscle strengths, and so on. Also, there is evidence suggesting that each value in [B] represents the difference between an excitatory and an inhibitory pathway (possibly through the cerebellum) since, during plastic modification of the reflex, the changes in the numbers in [B] can be larger than the numbers themselves. Nevertheless, the numbers do represent the minimum, effective, relative strengths of the necessary projections and their changes in various situations are significant.

## 3. Canal-canal convergence

Convergence of two ipsilateral canals onto a single second-order vestibular neuron would cause the plane of that neuron to lie somewhere between the planes of those two canals. Such convergence does occur between contralateral canal pairs through a commissural inhibitory system, so that when canals in a pair are not coplanar (e.g., the anterior canals and their contralateral posterior partners are misaligned by about 12°) the central neurons adopt the average of the two planes (Robinson 1982). But there is conflicting evidence about convergence from canals lying in very different planes (Wilson & Melvill Jones, 1979, pp. 133, 135). In a previous study (Robinson, 1982) it was argued without proof that such convergence might be undesirable since it could degrade the resolution of the canals.

The argument rests on the observation that the orientation of the vertical canals, about 45° off the sagittal plane, is not something that happened by chance; it is the only position they could assume if they are to be as accurate as possible. This conclusion stems from three constraints: the canal pairs must all be at right angles to each other if they are to resolve the components $\dot{H}$ with the maximum signal-to-noise ratio; the canals must work in push-pull pairs so that one is excited, the other inhibited, regardless of which direction in that

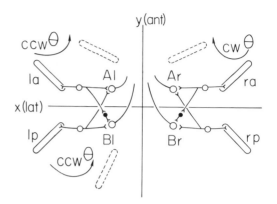

Fig. 2. The problems that would be created by canal-canal convergence. We look down on the vertical canals la, lp, ra, and rp. Al, Bl, Ar, Br, are two pairs of cell groups in the left and right vestibular nuclei that receive convergence from both ipsilateral vertical canals, and their planes are indicated by the equivalent canals drawn in dashed lines. Filled circles are inhibitory neurons. See text for the reason why this scheme would degrade canal resolution.

plane the head moves; and the arrangement must be mirror symmetric around the midsagittal plane (as are all neural structures). If one adds to this the restriction that the canals should not be separated anatomically by long distances to eliminate the case of two canals lying in the midsagittal plane, one in the forehead, the other in the occiput, there is only one configuration left for the vertical canals — 45° off the midsagittal plane. Just about where they are.

A significant amount of canal-canal convergence would destroy the virtue of this arrangement. Fig 2 shows the problem graphically. We will consider only convergence between vertical canals since if that doesn't work neither will other types. Imagine that neuron Al in the left vestibular nucleus receives a projection from the la and lp canals. The projection strengths may be fitted by numbers proportional to cosθ and sinθ respectively where θ is the counter-clockwise (ccw) angle of rotation of the plane of la to Al. If, on the left, we try to maintain orthogonality, then neuron Bl must receive projections from la and lp of strengths −sinθ and cosθ, respectively, to effect, overall, a simple ccw rotation of coordinates by θ. Note that −sinθ requires an inhibitory inter-neuron as shown. We are stuck, however, by the law of mirror symmetry; whatever we do on the left we must also do on the right. In particular, we must set up mirror connections and they will roate the plane of Ar cw by θ compared to ra. But now the plane of Ar is 2θ out of alignment of the plane of Bl and they could no longer constitute a push-pull pair. Thus, the demands of orthogonality on the left are in direct conflict with the demands of mirror symmetry on the right.

If one insists on retaining orthogonality, little or no convergence can be allowed. If one must accommodate significant convergence (not an obvious physiological finding) orthogonality must go. It can be shown that if noise is added to the signals from the canals, a coordinate transformation, into a skewed or orthogonal coordinate system will not increase the noise along the new axes if the original noises were uncorrelated, but if one attempts to reconstruct $\dot{H}$ from signals in skewed coordinates, the noise will create more uncertainty about the size and direction of $\dot{H}$ than if the coordinates were at right angles (see Robinson, 1982, Fig. 3 for a graphical illustration). As the skewed coordinates come closer together the two coordinate signals will contain more redundant information about the projection of $\dot{H}$ in that general direction and extracting the projection of $\dot{H}$ at right angles to this direction necessitates taking the small difference between two large noisy signals. This would still be possible if the system that did the extraction were itself noise-free but this, of course, is not the case. Thus, convergence will degrade the ability to resolve $\dot{H}$. Obviously there is much tolerance in this situation; if coordinates become skewed by only $10 - 20°$ from orthogonality it will have only a negligible effect on the accuracy of resolution. The point is that canal convergence would appear to serve no useful function unless other factors are invoked.

One such factor is that since the eye muscles do not work in the canal planes, one must convert the one to the other (Eqn. 13) sooner or later, and there is no reason not to start at once, with second-order vestibular neurons by using canal-canal convergence. This immediately raises the question of whether second-order neurons are dedicated to a particular motor system or are still general purpose. For the latter case — and this may well pertain to those neurons that carry a pure vestibular signal — it would be best to avoid

convergence and retain orthogonality for best accuracy. In the former case, despite many somatic signals ascending in the spinal cord to the vestibular nuclei, the only clear example to date of dedicated vestibular neurons is the group that carries eye position as well as vestibular signals. For this group, the possibility of convergence is enhanced by the very fact that the eye position signal is likely to represent a plane closer to that of a motoneuron signal than of a canal signal; if the eye position signal and head velocity signal lie in the same plane then the latter has presumably been shifted by canal convergence. To what extent the transformation in Eqn. 13 is performed by such convergence, and how much occurs in central pathways, is not known.

Consequently, the argument that significant canal-canal convergence destroys orthogonality, and hence accuracy, applies only to general-purpose vestibular neurons that are not yet committed to a particular motor system. That such neurons exist is made likely by the complexity of spinal righting reflexes. Unlike the vestibulo-ocular reflex where the transformation required is quite modest, the signal processing involved in using multi-articulated limbs in the control of posture is extremely complex and it seems unlikely that the majority of second-order vestibular neurons are already caught up in such processing.

## 4. Effect of eye position

It is well known that the action of the extra-ocular muscles depends on eye position. For example, when the eye abducts by about 25°, the line of sight lies in the plane of action of the vertical recti (see Fig. 3). These muscles would then purely elevate or depress the eye. If the eye could adduct 65°, these muscles would then roll the eye about the line of sight — pure torsion. Thus, the actions of these muscles might be thought to change rather drastically as the eye assumes various positions, but these observations pertain to muscle actions in the coordinate system of the eye, not the head, because most people, in thinking about such things, are interested in the visual consequences of muscle action. This way of thinking is not at all applicable to the vestibulo-ocular reflex which is only concerned with the rotations of the

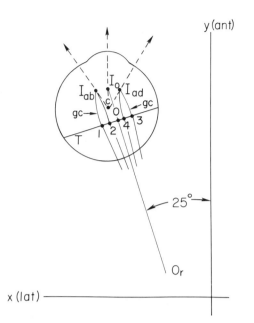

*Fig. 3.* The influence of eye position on muscle action. We are looking down on the left human eye. In primary position the superior rectus runs from its insertion $I_0$ to its origin $0_r$, leaving the globe at point 0 on the circle of tangency $T$ formed by the locus of all points on the globe, from which a line to $0_r$ is tangent to the globe. If the eye abducts or adducts, $I_0$ moves to $I_{ab}$ or $I_{ad}$. If the muscles took the shortest, or great circle path, over the globe (gc), the muscle would leave the globe at point 1 or 3, but lateral restraints allow less side slipping and constrain departure points to loci such as 2 and 4. Since these are the points where the muscle effectively acts on the globe, that action changes only slightly with different eye positions when viewed in a head coordinate system.

eye with respect to the head. It must rotate the eye with respect to the head about the same axis as the head rotates, regardless of which way the eye is looking, if image slip on the retina is to be reduced. The problem of thinking in retinal rather than head coordinates is well illustrated by noting that in the former, the rabbit makes 'torsional' eye movements in response to pitch while humans make 'vertical' eye movements, yet in both cases the eyes are rotating about the x-axis in Fig. 1 (see also Chapter 1).

Consequently we must see to what extent the pulling directions of the muscles change in a head coordinate system as the eye changes position. Fig. 3 shows that we should not expect a large change. The insertion point of the sr in the primary position is shown by $I_0$. From here the muscle

runs over the globe and leaves it at point 0 on the circle of tangency $T$ to run straight to its origin $0_r$. From a mechanical standpoint the muscle acts as though it exerted all its force at the point 0 and it will rotate the globe in a plane containing 0, $0_r$, and the center of the globe C. On abduction the insertion moves to $I_{ab}$ and we are now faced with an unresolved problem. If the muscle were completely free to slip sideways, it would take a great circle path (gc) over the globe. The plane of the circle would contain points $0_r$, C, and $I_{ab}$ and it defines the shortest path for the muscle to take from $I_{ab}$ to $0_r$. The muscle would act on the globe at point 1 and rotate the eye in the plane of the great circle.

Muscles, however, are not free to slideslip arbitrarily and it is easy to show that in certain eye positions, the shortest path would require tendons to slip half or all the way around the globe! (Robinson 1975b). Muscles are restrained by Tenon's capsule and other fascia so that they cannot deviate too far from the path on the globe that they take in the primary position. Thus, the path that leaves the globe at point 2 is more realistic. Similarly in adduction the muscle would not take a great circle path (gc) and depart at point 3 but would be restrained to a point of action such as point 4. Since the paths of these muscles have never been measured one can only guess at the stiffness of the elastic restraints to side-slipping. As this stiffness increases, the point of action of the muscle will move away from points 1 and 3, through points 2 and 4, toward point 0. If the stiffness were large enough the point would even cross through 0 to points on the other side. Thus, it is possible that the stiffness is such that the point of action would remain at 0 for different eye positions in which case the action of the muscle in orbital coordinates would not depend at all on eye position. Consequently, the claim that the pulling directions of muscles depends on eye position is not to be taken for granted, it may not be true, and certainly must be demonstrated, if one measures pulling direction with respect to the head. In any event, Fig. 3 shows that the plane of action of a muscle varies very little, if at all, with eye position and certainly by amounts far less than one would be led to suppose thinking in terms of eye coordinates.

A very crude method has been proposed for estimating a muscle's path and simulating permitted side slipping (Robinson 1975b). Since then, J. M. Miller and I have improved this estimation by a more physiological simulation involving a distributed fascial spring that restrains side slipping (unpublished research). These calculations are part of a mathematical model of the mechanics of how six muscles hold the globe in any position; the model is used to diagnose squint and simulate the results of strabismus surgery. We have adjusted the stiffness of these fascial springs until the overall model gives reasonable simulations of responses to interventions such as palsies and surgery. From this model we can find the unit action vectors (a vector of unit length pointed along the axis about which the eye would turn if acted upon by that muscle alone) of all six muscles in any position of gaze. It is the components of these vectors, combined in pairs, that are the numbers in the $[M]$ matrix (Eqn. 7). That matrix refers to the primary position. When the eye abducts by 30°, these vectors change because of the mechanism illustrated in Fig. 3 so that for small perturbations around that position we must use a new motor matrix $[M_{ab}]$,

$$
\begin{vmatrix} \dot{E}_z \\ \dot{E}_x \\ \dot{E}_y \end{vmatrix} = \begin{vmatrix} 0.998 & 0.002 & 0.056 \\ 0.008 & -0.899 & 0.754 \\ 0.014 & 0.438 & 0.655 \end{vmatrix} \begin{vmatrix} M_{lmr} \\ M_{sir} \\ M_{sio} \end{vmatrix} \quad (14)
$$

The elements of this matrix should be compared to Eqn. 7 to see the changes that occurred as a consequence of the new eye position. The numbers in the first two columns have changed by 1% or less (% of total vector length which is 1.0) which is insignificant. The elements in the third column demonstrate that the changes are greater for short muscles, the obliques in this case, than for long; a point that should be obvious from Fig 3. In abduction the sio have lost the ability to move the eye horizontally by 11%, to tort the eye by 11%, and have gained the ability to move the eye vertically by 14%. (Note that viewed in the coordinates of the eye just the opposite would occur; the obliques become better at torsion in abduction.) These changes in the action of the obliques are still modest but what is most impor-

tant to note is that the horizontal and vertical recti were hardly affected at all by the 30° abduction.

What changes would be required if the brain stem pathways compensated for the changes that did occur in the muscle actions? We can find out by using Eqn. 11, in which we use $[M_{ab}]$ rather than $[M]$. Performing these operations (using Eqn. 12) we find the new brain stem matrix $[B_{ab}]$ to be,

$$
\begin{vmatrix} M_{lmr} \\ M_{sir} \\ M_{sio} \end{vmatrix} = \begin{vmatrix} -1.001 & -0.259 & -0.220 \\ 0.094 & -0.789 & 0.270 \\ 0.123 & 0.047 & -0.662 \end{vmatrix} \begin{vmatrix} C_{lrh} \\ C_{rpla} \\ C_{ralp} \end{vmatrix} \quad (15)
$$

which should be compared to Eqn. 13. The largest change in the first two columns, indicating adjustments of signals from $C_{lrh}$ and $C_{rpla}$, is 1.6% or less. Since the sio are most altered and they lie near the planes of ralp, the connections from $C_{ralp}$ are most affected. In particular, the projection to sir has been decreased by 14% to compensate for the 14% increased participation of sio in vertical movements. The other elements in column three changed by only 4%. As one would suppose, given the modest changes in $[M_{ab}]$, the required changes in $[B_{ab}]$ are also modest. It is not known to what extent some of these gain changes come about automatically through system nonlinearities. As the eye moves eccentrically, recruitment of motor units may create larger changes in force for a given change in neural activity, for example, and that would effectively alter the elements in $[B]$, whether for better or worse is not known. How the oculomotor system compensates for large signal, static nonlinearities in the plant is not yet understood. All we can say is that the nonlinearity introduced by position-dependent muscle geometry (Eqn. 14) is small.

If the position-dependent changes are as small as this analysis suggests, one might wonder if the central nervous system even bothers to correct for them. In goldfish, rabbit and cat, the oculomotor range is only about ± 20° and it is unusual for the eye to spend much time deviated even 15°. For rotatory nystagmus in the cat, for example, quick phases take the eyes about 12° into the direction of turning, slow phases bring them back to 0° (Chun & Robinson, 1978). In this moderate range, the system may be nearly linear although one could not be certain without knowing more about the geometry of cat eye muscles. On the other hand, during a large eye-head reorientation, humans make a large saccade, putting the eye in a very eccentric position, and then, if vision is to remain clear, the vestibulo-ocular reflex must work reasonably well as the head begins to catch up with the eye.

To see what would happen if there were no central compensation we use Eqn. 10, in which $[M]$ is replaced by $[M_{ab}]$. This gives $[VOR_{ab}]$,

$$
\begin{vmatrix} \dot{E}_z \\ \dot{E}_x \\ \dot{E}_y \end{vmatrix} = \begin{vmatrix} -0.999 & 0.025 & 0.044 \\ -0.011 & -1.062 & -0.073 \\ -0.001 & 0.07 & -0.442 \end{vmatrix} \begin{vmatrix} \dot{H}_z \\ \dot{H}_x \\ \dot{H}_y \end{vmatrix} \qquad (16)
$$

which should be compared to Eqn. 12 which we are assuming as normal. Most of the changes occur in the four lower right elements which compensate for the misalignment between the vertical canals and the cyclovertical muscles (sir, sio). Because the plane of action of sio shifted, all these terms went up or down by about 7%. Thus, for example, roll ($\dot{H}_y$) will now create a 7.3% vertical eye movement ($\dot{E}_x$). We should, however, note that the usual situation is that the head is rotating in the direction of the eye displacement. This occurs during either active eye-head reorientation or passive rotations in the dark (Melvill Jones, 1964). It is less usual, for example, to be looking up while rotating to the left. In Eqn. 16 a yaw head movement ($\dot{H}_z$) produces negligible eye movements around the x- and y-axes (second and third elements in the first column). If one made a 30°, left eye-head reorientation and the post-saccadic head velocity were 100°, in addition to the normal, horizontal, compensatory movement, the eye would make an unwanted, simultaneous vertical movement at 1.1°/s. Collewijn et al. (1981a) showed, by precise eye movement recordings in humans, that the gain of the vestibulo-ocular reflex is seldom better than 0.95, even with vision, (we have used gains of 1.0 here (Eqn. 12) only for simplicity) so that a horizontal retinal slip of about 5°/s may be expected at this time. The vertical retinal slip is so much less than the horizontal that, at least in this case, it would seem

unnecessary for the nervous system to take steps to compensate for the small position dependency of muscle action.

This same point is illustrated by vertical movements. When the eye looks up 30°, the motor matrix becomes $[M_{up}]$,

$$
\begin{vmatrix} \dot{E}_z \\ \dot{E}_x \\ E_y \end{vmatrix} = \begin{vmatrix} 0.999 & 0.25 & 0.414 \\ 0.05 & -0.874 & 0.625 \\ -0.008 & 0.416 & 0.662 \end{vmatrix} \begin{vmatrix} M_{lmr} \\ M_{sir} \\ M_{sio} \end{vmatrix} \qquad (17)
$$

The biggest changes compared to Eqn. 7 are the 23 and 27% increases in the ability of sir and sio to contribute to horizontal eye movements. Except for a 12% decrease in the contribution of sio to $\dot{E}_y$ all the other terms change by 5% or less. Note especially that the horizontal recti continue to rotate the eye about an axis vertical with respect to the head; the last two terms in the first column are still negligible. If these muscles had rotated the eye about an axis tilted back 30°, the last element in the first column would have been sin 30° or 0.5. To see the consequences of these changes, assuming that the brain stem took no steps to compensate them, we find that $[VOR_{up}]$ is

$$
\begin{vmatrix} \dot{E}_z \\ \dot{E}_x \\ \dot{E}_y \end{vmatrix} = \begin{vmatrix} -0.993 & 0.071 & -0.201 \\ -0.054 & -0.983 & -0.017 \\ 0.022 & 0.048 & -0.44 \end{vmatrix} \begin{vmatrix} \dot{H}_z \\ \dot{H}_x \\ \dot{H}_y \end{vmatrix} \qquad (18)
$$

The biggest change is a 20% dependence of $\dot{E}_z$ on roll ($\dot{H}_y$). The rest of the terms have changed by 7% or less. In particular, if the head moves in the direction of the eye position (pitch, $\dot{H}_x$), the movement is compensated by 98.3%, and unwanted horizontal and torsion components appear, of 7.1% and 4.8%, respectively. The latter produces no retinal slip near the fovea, the former would produce slip comparable to that normally produced by the inadequacy of the vertical reflex itself.

While this study has not attempted to examine all possible eye positions and directions of head movements, it suggests that the pulling directions of eye muscles, in the coordinate system of the head, change so little with eye position that the visual sequelae are not worth correcting. Note that these effects are so small that it would require great care just to measure them in the laboratory. It is not certain if this applies to other animals. A shorter orbital cone compared to the size of the eye would make $[M]$ more susceptible to eye position (as illustrated by the obliques in Eqn. 14) but a smaller oculomotor range would make it less so. In addition, sub-primates tend to have their eye muscles inserted closer to the equator (a terminology that regards the front of the eye as the north pole) and this can make $[M]$ quite insensitive to eye position. If, in Fig. 3, $I_0$ were directly above C (on the equator) the effective point of action of the muscle, if free to side slip, would depend not at all on eye position. In summary, these considerations suggest that the eye muscles are so designed as to make their planes of action relatively independent of eye position, and that no special effort is taken by the central nervous system to compensate for the small nonlinearities that do exist. I suggest that, until proven otherwise, this is the most reasonable hypothesis to adopt.

## 5. Plasticity

One of the most intriguing applications of the matrix approach is to observe the changes required in $[B]$ when plastic deformations of the vestibulo-ocular reflex occur, usually in response to dissociation of head motion and retinal image motion by magnifying lenses (e.g., Miles & Fuller, 1974) or reversing prisms (e.g. Gonshor & Melvill Jones, 1976). Many of these studies caused plastic changes in the gain of the horizontal reflex, which not only requires similar changes in the upper left element of $[B]$, but also significant changes in the other two elements in the first row of $[B]$ to prevent roll from creating unwanted horizontal eye movements (Robinson, 1982). Three studies have demonstrated plasticity in more than one dimension. Berthoz et al. (1981a) showed that reversing prisms cause a decrease in the gain of the torsion reflex as well as the horizontal reflex without affecting vertical gain. These changes required significant alterations in all nine elements of the $[B]$ matrix (Robinson, 1982). Callan and Ebenholtz (1982) produced op-

tical tilt with spectacles and showed that horizontal head movements can be made to produce vertical eye movements. Schultheis and Robinson (1981) did the opposite in the cat by associating horizontal retinal slip with pitch head movements.

Following a previous analysis (Robinson, 1982), let us illustrate the use of matrices in displaying such results. These authors showed that after several hours of such visual-vestibular experience, pitch, in the dark, created a horizontal eye velocity that was 25% of the vertical head velocity. The vertical component of eye movement was normal as was the horizontal reflex. Consequently the reflex matrix $[VOR']$ would be,

$$
\begin{vmatrix} \dot{E}_z \\ \dot{E}_x \\ \dot{E}_y \end{vmatrix} = \begin{vmatrix} -1 & -0.25 & 0 \\ 0 & -1 & 0 \\ 0 & 0 & -0.5 \end{vmatrix} \begin{vmatrix} \dot{H}_z \\ \dot{H}_x \\ \dot{H}_y \end{vmatrix} \quad (19)
$$

Assuming this would also happen in humans, the brain-stem matrix $[B']$ required, using Eqn. 11 with $[VOR']$, is

$$
\begin{vmatrix} M_{lmr} \\ M_{sir} \\ M_{sio} \end{vmatrix} = \begin{vmatrix} -1.009 & -0.062 & -0.362 \\ 0.08 & -0.801 & 0.412 \\ 0.112 & 0.029 & -0.619 \end{vmatrix} \begin{vmatrix} C_{lrh} \\ C_{rpla} \\ C_{ralp} \end{vmatrix} \quad (20)
$$

As might be expected the only significant changes in $[B']$ from Eqn. 13 occur in the last two elements of the first row; those elements that express the coupling between the vertical canals and the horizontal muscles. The magnitude of one element increased while the other decreased by the same amount (0.186). The reason is easy to see. In roll, $C_{rpla}$ and $C_{ralp}$ have the same magnitude and sign. Consequently, when the first row of $[B']$ is multiplied by these canal components the changes cancel so the effect on $M_{lmr}$ is not changed. In pitch, however $C_{rpla}$ and $C_{ralp}$ have opposite signs so that the changes add. The result is that pitch now creates horizontal eye movements without producing any other effect.

This example illustrates what by now is obvious — all nine elements in the matrix $[B]$ must be under adaptive parametric control. The job to be done by this control system might at first seem to be a very complicated one. If one replaced the elements of $[B]$ with nine terms of form $b_{ij}$ (the term in the $i$th row and $j$th column) and performed the multiplications indicated in Eqn. 10, each element in $[VOR]$ would contain all nine of the $b_{ij}$. If the elements of $[VOR]$ are to be set to nine given values, as in Eqn. 12, it would seem necessary for the central nervous system (CNS) to solve nine simultaneous equations in nine unknowns. Put another way, a change in any one of the elements in $[B]$ will change every element in $[VOR]$. If the CNS tried to vary another element of $[B]$ to correct just one of the incorrect terms in $[VOR]$, it may make other terms in $[VOR]$ even worse. Thus, it would appear that the CNS must take into account all these interactions at once, which is equivalent to solving nine equations simultaneously. The CNS, however, has solved this problem very simply.

First, it should be noted that there is general agreement that each element in $[B]$ consists of a direct, brain stem pathway in parallel with a cerebellar pathway. It is not important whether the cerebellum contains (Ito, 1982a; Robinson, 1976), or does not contain (Llinás & Walton, 1979a), the requisite modifiable synapses (see Chapters 14 & 15); it is certain, however, that a lesion of the latter path abolishes plasticity, indicating that each element of $[B]$ should be written as $b_{ij} + \beta_{ij}$, where $b_{ij}$ is a fixed gain associated with the brain-stem pathways and $\beta_{ij}$ is a modifiable gain associated with a cerebellar pathway. In cat and monkey, at least, the gains of the vestibulo-ocular reflex are not far from normal after flocculectomy, so that we will assume values for $b_{ij}$ equal to those in Eqn. 13, and that the $\beta_{ij}$ are normally all zero; other choices would not conflict with the following analysis. Presumably when some disorder changes the elements of $[VOR]$, the resulting dysmetria causes the $\beta_{ij}$ to change and return $[VOR]$ to normal. How does the CNS know which $\beta_{ij}$ to change and by how much?

It is generally agreed that in animals without pursuit (e.g. rabbit; the cat has such poor pursuit (Evinger & Fuchs, 1978) that it could be included), retinal image motion is the error signal for the plastic control of the vestibulo-ocular reflex. The gain of the reflex will go up, down or twist (Eqn. 19), always in an attempt to decrease any retinal image slip that is coincident with head rotation. For primates where pursuit can create en bloc slip of the visual surround on the retina during head movements, image slip of the background per se is no longer a perfect indicator of inadequate vestibulo-ocular corrections (Miles & Lisberger, 1981a). Nevertheless, the point is moot and we will continue our analysis on the assumption that retinal slip is still the main source of error detection in controlling the reflex. Simpson and his colleagues (e.g., Simpson et al., 1981a,b) have found that direction-selective cells in the accessory optic system and flocculi of the rabbit can be grouped in three categories, cells responding to horizontal retinal slip and cells responding to retinal slip caused by visual motion in vertical planes lying about 45° from the midsagittal. These are planes lying near those of the canals and eye muscles. Thus, the retina appears to transduce retinal slip in coordinates close to those of the canals or muscles. Retinal slip, of course, is itself a vector $\dot{e}$ with components $\dot{e}_x$, $\dot{e}_y$, and $\dot{e}_z$ in the coordinates of Fig. 1 and the collected neural outputs of the direction-selective cells may be expressed as components $R_1$, $R_2$, and $R_3$, of a vector $R$ produced by the retinal matrix $[R]$,

$$R = [R]\,\dot{e} \qquad (21)$$

These cells are very nonlinear but we will consider their behaviour for small $\dot{e}$ and continue using linear analysis. We will assume a similar arrangement in humans. This is a highly speculative point that needs investigation but this analysis is speculative by nature and the conclusions we will draw are valid whatever the findings are in primates.

The simplest hypothesis for deciding which $\beta_{ij}$ to change, and by how much, given dysmetria, is shown in Fig. 4. It suggests that the central nervous system examines $R$ and $C$ and when there is coincident activity of $R_i$ and $C_j$, it adjusts $\beta_{ij}$ up or down until $R_i$ is driven suitably close to zero. Let us see how well this scheme works by an example.

Since $C$ is in canal coordinates, it would, at first, seem reasonable to put $R$ in the same coordinates so they may be compared directly. In that case the matrix $[R]$ would be identical to $[C]$. One can fine $\dot{e}$ as the difference between the rotation of the visual world with respect to the head, $\dot{W}_h$,

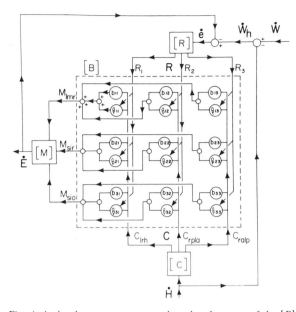

*Fig. 4.* A simple arrangement to alter the elements of the [B] matrix (in dashed lines) to eliminate dysmetria. The visual system is assumed to convert the retinal slip vector $\dot{e}$ into a neural vector $R$ in coordinates close to those of the canals or muscles. $\dot{H}$, as in Fig. 1, passes through [C] to produce $C$. The three components of $R$ and $C$ distribute into the nine elements of [B] as shown. Dysmetria is signaled by retinal slip $R_i$ that is coincidental with canal activity $C_j$. When this happens, $\beta_{ij}$ is turned up or down until $R_i$ goes to zero and orthometria is restored. Some arrows and + signs have been omitted to avoid clutter but all elements in [B] are similar to the arrangement for $b_{11}$. $\dot{W}$ is the velocity of the visual world and is normally zero.

and eye velocity in the head, $\dot{E}$ (Fig. 4). In a stationary visual environment, $\dot{W}_h$ equals $-\dot{H}$ so that

$$\dot{e} = -\dot{H} - \dot{E} \qquad (22)$$

or

$$\dot{e} = -(\dot{H} + [VOR]\dot{H}) = ([-I] \quad [VOR]) \dot{H} \qquad (23)$$

The more [VOR] departs from the ideal (Eqn. (2) or $-1$ times the identity matrix [I]) the greater the retinal slip. We can find $R$ from Eqn. 21 with [R] replaced by [C], Eqn. 22, and the inverse of Eqn. 4,

$$R = [C]\dot{e} = [C]([-I] - [VOR])\dot{H} =$$
$$[C]([-I] - [VOR])[C^{-1}]C = [VV]C \qquad (24)$$

The matrix [VV], for visual-vestibular interaction, gives the amount of retinal slip $R_i$ that will occur during a head rotation that excites canal $C_j$. Thus, $VV_{ij}$ should tell one how much to change $\beta_{ij}$.

Suppose, for example, we change $b_{22}$, in Eqn. 13, from $-0.799$ to $-0.6$ to simulate a lesion. Call this matrix [B']. We can find [VOR'] in the usual manner (Eqn. 10),

$$\begin{vmatrix} \dot{E}_z \\ \dot{E}_x \\ \dot{E}_y \end{vmatrix} = \begin{vmatrix} -1.0 & -0.002 & 0.002 \\ -0.028 & -0.879 & -0.13 \\ -0.013 & -0.057 & -0.439 \end{vmatrix} \begin{vmatrix} \dot{H}_z \\ \dot{H}_x \\ \dot{H}_y \end{vmatrix} \qquad (25)$$

Comparison with Eqn. 12 shows the extent of the dysmetria. Most off diagonal terms are less than 3%. The main problem is 12–13% shifts in the last two terms of the second row. We use Eqn. 23 to find the relationship between $\dot{e}$ and $\dot{H}$, which is $[-I] - [VOR]$,

$$\begin{vmatrix} \dot{e}_z \\ \dot{e}_x \\ \dot{e}_y \end{vmatrix} - \begin{vmatrix} 0.00 & 0.002 & -0.002 \\ 0.028 & -0.121 & 0.13 \\ 0.013 & 0.057 & -0.561 \end{vmatrix} \begin{vmatrix} \dot{H}_z \\ \dot{H}_x \\ \dot{H}_y \end{vmatrix} \qquad (26)$$

The large image slip in roll ($-0.561$) is to be expected since the gain of that reflex is half normal. The 12–13% in the last two terms of the second row are a direct consequence of the dysmetrias of Eqn. 25. Finally, from Eqn. 24 we find [VV],

$$\begin{vmatrix} R_1 \\ R_2 \\ R_3 \end{vmatrix} \cdot = \begin{vmatrix} -0.04 & 0.148 & 0.119 \\ 0.077 & -0.413 & -0.23 \\ 0.077 & -0.170 & -0.23 \end{vmatrix} \begin{vmatrix} C_{lrh} \\ C_{rpla} \\ C_{ralp} \end{vmatrix} \qquad (27)$$

This matrix gives the retinal slip $R$ that will always accompany the canal stimulation $C_j$. There is, however, a problem in interpreting [VV] because the low gain (0.5) of the torsional reflex (Eqn. 12) causes a lot of retinal slip that is normally tolerated. To see this, one can put the normal reflex (Eqn. 12) into Eqn. 24 and derive its visual-vestibular interaction matrix, call it $[VV_0]$,

$$[VV_0] = \begin{vmatrix} -0.04 & 0.119 & 0.119 \\ 0.077 & -0.23 & -0.23 \\ 0.077 & -0.23 & -0.23 \end{vmatrix} \qquad (28)$$

Note that there is little retinal slip in yaw (first column) or in pitch, because in pitch $C_{rpla}$ equals $-C_{ralp}$ so the terms in the second and third columns cancel out. It is only in roll, when $C_{rpla}$ equals $C_{ralp}$, that slip is large. This pattern of retinal slip is no doubt tolerated by the human CNS because it interferes only slightly with vision. Torsion of the eye about the line of sight does not displace images on the fovea, causes only mild retinal slip in the parafovea and largely affects only the far periphery. Because the visual cells that are probably most effective in inducing plastic changes are densely packed around the fovea, and are not well excited by torsional image slip, the transformation $[R]$ could be made nonlinear to reflect such a retinal geometry. Alternately, the pattern could be suppressed centrally. We shall assume the latter and represent the acceptance of torsional image slip by the CNS by subtracting $[VV_0]$ from $[VV]$ to observe only the changes in $[VV]$ from normal. We can call the result $[\Delta VV]$. Then,

$$[\Delta VV] = [VV] - [VV_0] = [C] \, ([-I] - [VOR']) \, [C^{-1}]$$
$$- [C] \, ([-I] - [VOR]) \, [C^{-1}] \quad (29)$$

or, collecting terms

$$[\Delta VV] = [C] \, ([VOR] - [VOR']) \, [C^{-1}] \quad (30)$$

If we define $[\Delta VOR]$ as the difference between the normal $[VOR]$ and the dysmetric $[VOR']$, Eqn. 30 becomes just,

$$[\Delta VV] = [C] \, [\Delta VOR] \, [C^{-1}] \quad (31)$$

Subtracting Eqn. 25 from Eqn 12 to get $[\Delta VOR]$ and performing the indicated multiplications gives the same result as subtracting Eqn. 28, term by term, from Eqn. 27. The result is

$$[\Delta VV] = \begin{vmatrix} 0 & 0.029 & 0 \\ 0 & -0.183 & 0 \\ 0 & 0.06 & 0 \end{vmatrix} \quad (32)$$

The term $\Delta VV_{22}$ indicates that $\beta_{22}$ should be changed by $-0.183$ which will very nearly correct for the lesion ($b_{22}$ was changed by 0.199). The

other two non-zero terms (0.029, 0.06) are small errors suggesting, incorrectly, changes in $\beta_{12}$ and $\beta_{32}$. They are, however, quite small. Thus, the scheme in Fig. 4 will work very well when the visual system transduces retinal slip in canal coordinates. If it had used a very different coordinate system, without correction, the misalignment between $R$ and $C$ would have caused the change in $b_{22}$ to create incorrect terms throughout $[\Delta VV]$ thus degrading the ability of the simple scheme in Fig. 4 to specify the needed changes in $\beta$. Of course the retina is free to use any coordinate system so long as $R$ was subsequently transformed into canal-like coordinates but that would, of course, entail additional neural wiring.

It might be supposed that the canal coordinates are the optimal ones for that part of the visual system that detects relative, world motion but that is not the case, at least from the standpoint of plasticity. A lesion in $[B]$ can cause eye movements that create retinal slip in several components of $R$ for a given canal excitation. The small numbers 0.029 and 0.06 in Eqn. 32 are an example. Larger lesions would make this cross talk worse. Put another way, a lesion in $[B]$ does not lie in canal coordinates; it lies between the canal and muscle coordinates. Thus, the detection of this lesion should not be confined entirely to the canal system as in Eqn. 31. We can show that the ideal coordinates for the retinal slip system are those of the muscles. Since $[M]$ converts neural signals to eye movements we would want the repercussions of eye movements (retinal slip) to be translated back into neural signals by $[M^{-1}]$. Thus, let $[R]$ equal $[M_r^{-1}]$. The subscript r reminds us that this is a retinal matrix that could differ from $[M^{-1}]$ if lesions occurred. This, in effect, replaces $[C]$ in Eqn. 30 with $[M_r^{-1}]$ whence,

$$[\Delta VV] = [M_r^{-1}] \, [VOR] \, [C^{-1}]$$
$$- [M_r^{-1}] \, [VOR'] \, [C^{-1}] \quad (33)$$

From Eqn. 11, the first term on the left is $[B]$, the normal brain stem connections. These are the desired connections. By the same token, the second term is the $[B']$ for the dysmetric connections. They are the undesired connections. Consequently, the difference in Eqn. 33 gives the needed changes in $b_{ij}$ directly and tells exactly which $\beta_{ij}$ to change and by how much. Operationally, Eqn. 33 reduces to

$$[\Delta VV] = [M_r^{-1}] [\Delta VOR] [C^{-1}] \quad (34)$$

If one applies this in our example, one gets

$$[\Delta VV] = \begin{vmatrix} 0 & 0 & 0 \\ 0 & -0.199 & 0 \\ 0 & 0 & 0 \end{vmatrix} \quad (35)$$

which exactly describes the change in $\beta_{22}$ for the lesion we created. Consequently, for a brain stem lesion, the scheme in Fig. 4 will work most accurately if the retina transduces retinal slip in the planes of the eye muscles rather than the canals. In humans, these planes are not very different: the mean plane for larp is 22° away from that of sir while that for ralp is only 6° from that of sio so that it might be hard experimentally to distinguish between the two hypotheses. Any coordinate system lying between that of the muscles and canals would obviously work quite well; the theoretical analysis merely shows that, given a choice, the former is better than any other for purposes of detecting the source of brain stem dysmetria.

What happens if the lesion affects $[M]$ and $[C]$ as well as $[B]$? Returning to Eqn. 29 but using $[M_r^{-1}]$ for $[R]$,

$$[\Delta VV] = [M_r^{-1}] [C^{-1}] ([I] - [C] [C'^{-1}]) + [B] - [M_r^{-1}] [M'] [B'] \quad (36)$$

where the primes denote matrices affected by a lesion. If the lesion were confined only to $[B']$ ($[M']$ and $[C']$ equal to [M] and [C], respectively), this equation reduces to

$$[\Delta VV] = [B] - [B'] \quad (37)$$

which is the correct diagnosis, but if lesions occur in the canals or muscles, Eqn. 36 does not give the correct answer. The latter may be found by letting $[B'']$ be the brain stem matrix that has repaired all lesions;

$$[\Delta B] = [B''] - [B'] = [M'^{-1}] [VOR] [C'^{-1}] - [B'] = [M'^{-1}] [M] [B] [C] [C'^{-1}] - [B'] \quad (38)$$

This equation agrees with Eqn. 36 only in the case when the lesion is confined to the brain stem.

If the lesion is confined to the canals Eqn. 36 becomes

$$[\Delta VV] = [M_r^{-1}] [C^{-1}] ([I] - [C] [C'^{-1}]) \quad (39)$$

while, from Eqn. 38,

$$[\Delta B] = [B] ([C] [C'^{-1}] - [I]) \quad (40)$$

These equations are similar but not equal. Note that if the retina worked in canal coordinates ($[R]$ equal to $[C]$), Eqn. 39 would still not equal Eqn. 40. To give some idea of the error, a canal lesion was simulated by assuming that $C_{rpla}$ decreased to half its normal value. Thus, $[C']$ was taken from Eqn. 5 with the 2nd row multiplied by 0.5 and used in Eqns. 39 and 40,

$$[\Delta B] = \begin{vmatrix} 0 & -0.248 & 0 \\ 0 & 0.798 & 0 \\ 0 & -0.031 & 0 \end{vmatrix}$$

$$[\Delta VV] = \begin{vmatrix} 0 & -0.203 & 0 \\ 0 & -0.997 & 0 \\ 0 & -0.267 & 0 \end{vmatrix} \quad (41)$$

The estimate of the needed correction by $[\Delta VV]$ is not bad but it is far from perfect.

If the lesion is confined to the muscle,

$$[\Delta VV] = ([I] - [M_r^{-1}] [M']) [R] \quad (42)$$

while

$$[\Delta B] = ([M'^{-1}] [M] - [I]) [B] \quad (43)$$

again similar but not identical. To assess the error, a lesion was simulated in $[M]$ by reducing the strength of the sir. That is, Eqn. 7 was modified by multiplying all elements in the 2nd column by 0.5. The results from Eqns. 39 and 40 are,

$$[\Delta B] = \begin{vmatrix} 0 & 0 & 0 \\ 0.08 & -0.799 & 0.41 \\ 0 & 0 & 0 \end{vmatrix}$$

$$[\Delta VV] = \begin{vmatrix} 0 & 0 & 0 \\ 0.073 & -0.498 & 0.106 \\ 0 & 0 & 0 \end{vmatrix} \qquad (44)$$

This time the visual-vestibular scheme in Fig. 4 underestimates rather than overestimates the required changes in the $b_{ij}$.

It should be stressed that these errors do not require us to throw out the hypothesis in Fig. 4. As a negative feedback scheme it will continue, hour by hour, altering the $\beta_{ij}$ in small increments until dysmetria is eliminated. It will not stop until $[VOR]$ is back to normal and the pattern of retinal slip, $\dot{e}$ or $R$, is back to the tolerated level. The only question is how long it takes the system to converge. The worse the estimate for $[\Delta B]$, as in Eqns. 41 and 44, the longer the process will take. The only danger is that for certain combinations of lesions the estimate could be bad enough to cause the system to go around in circles and fail to converge. Given the sorts of miscalculations in Eqns 41 and 44, this is unlikely to happen, and given the duration of observed gain changes (2 — 3 days), the failure of the system in Fig. 4 to make the most accurate estimate of dysmetria in certain cases is not sufficient grounds to reject this simple model.

Nevertheless, several issues are raised by these considerations. It can be shown that $[\Delta VV]$ calculates the needed corrections with even more error when multiple lesions accumulate over the years. One cause is that $[M_r^{-1}]$ fails more and more to reflect the true value of $[M^{-1}]$ as $[M]$ undergoes successive lesions. It raises the interesting question of whether the CNS can recalibrate $[R]$ if $[M]$ should suffer a lesion. By observing the retinal motion $\dot{e}$ for any given command $M$, the CNS can easily calculate what $[R]$ should be to equal the current $[M^{-1}]$, and that would remove one source of error in Eqn. 36. Whether this happens is not known. A second issue is that from Eqn. 29 it can be seen that $[VV_0]$ will change if $[C^{-1}]$ changes. Since $\dot{e}$ determines what is tolerated, not $[VV_0]$,

the latter must be adapted during recovery since, if the $\beta$'s change until $[\Delta VV]$ is zero, $[VOR]$ will not return to normal. This is tantamount to the recognition by the CNS that $[C]$ has changed. These problems raise a much deeper issue: if one regards $C$ as an efference copy and $\dot{e}$ as reafference, and tries to detect dysmetria by matching efference copy to expected reafference, one ends up proposing internal models of the sensory and motor systems involved, and this raises the problem that if peripheral dysmetria is discovered, one should modify the internal models. On the other hand, the scheme in Fig. 4 does not explicitly propose such models which would make it far more complicated. If the system works without them, as this analysis suggests, then the simpler system is to be preferred although that may depend on the sophistication of the species. These questions are beyond the scope of this report but it is interesting that the vestibuloocular reflex is a system more mathematically tractable than most and allows one to address these issues in a very specific way.

The conclusion that the visual signals $R$ should be in muscle rather than canal coordinates is confounded by the problems that arise when the lesion is in $[C]$ or $[M]$. One gets into the argument of which system is most often damaged. Evidently no choice of coordinates for $R$ will cover all three cases and the choice of canal coordinates does not give a correct answer for any of the three cases. Since the choice of muscle coordinates for $R$ gives a correct answer for at least one of the three cases it would seem reasonable to choose this hypothesis until contrary evidence or theories are found.

It should be noted that retinal slip detection depends on eye position. The vector $\dot{e}$ is in a head-coordinate system and the pattern of activity it creates in the retina will vary with eye position. This parametric adaptive system, however, only responds to consistent pairing of $R_i$ and $C_j$ that persists over minutes or hours. Since the average eye position over such time intervals is the primary position, it would appear that variation due to changes in eye position will average out.

## 6. Conclusions

The theoretical considerations in this chapter, using vectors and matrices to describe the vestibulo-ocular reflex, have led to three predictions.

1. Significant convergence of fibers from orthogonal canals onto second-order vestibular neurons is unlikely since such an arrangement would degrade the accuracy with which the canals can resolve head velocity. This consideration, however, applies only to neurons that supply the canal signal for use by a large number of complex spinal reflexes. It need not apply to vestibular neurons that are dedicated to a single reflex, such as the vestibulo-ocular reflex, where transformations for specific muscles could begin at once on second-order neurons by such convergence.

2. The pulling directions of the eye muscles vary so little in the head coordinate system with different eye positions, especially when the eye is deviated in the direction of the head movement, that it is probably unnecessary for the nervous system to compensate for the small errors so created.

3. The nervous system can easily detect which of the nine brain stem connections needs to be changed to eliminate vestibulo-ocular dysmetria by observing coincidental activity between retinal slip in the $i$th direction and that of the $j$th canal pair, and adjusting the connections between the $j$th canal pair and the $i$th muscle pair. This process is most accurate when retinal image slip is transduced in the coordinates of the eye muscles.

These observations are interesting and constitute hypotheses to be tested by experimental results. They also continue to show the usefulness of matrix analysis, at least for some purposes, in dealing with coordinate systems in the vestibulo-ocular reflex.

**Acknowledgements**

This work was supported by EY00598 from the National Eye Institute, U. S. Department of Health and Human Services. Computer facilities were supported by EY01765 of the same Institute. I thank A. McCracken for preparing the manuscript and C. Bridges for the illustration.

Adaptive mechanisms in gaze control
Facts and theories
Eds. Berthoz & Melvill Jones

# Chapter 21

# An adaptive equalizer model of the primate vestibulo-ocular reflex

F. A. Miles[a], L. M. Optican[a] & S. G. Lisberger[b]

[a]Laboratory of Sensorimotor Research, National Eye Institute, National Institutes of Health, Bethesda, MD 20205 and [b]Department of Physiology, University of California, San Francisco, CA 94143, U.S.A.

## 1. The adaptive interface between the labyrinth and the eyeball

The vestibulo-ocular reflex (VOR) performs the function of stabilizing the gaze in space during head movements. The reflex senses head rotations through the semicircular canals, whose afferent discharges enter the brain stem and ultimately result in the activation of the motoneurons innervating the eye muscles. If the reflex were perfect, it would generate compensatory eye movements exactly equal in magnitude (unity gain) and opposite in direction (180° phase shift) to the head movements. Over the biologically important frequency range, 0.05–5 Hz, the reflex comes close to achieving this, at least in the monkey: deviations from perfect antiphase behavior are very minor except towards the extremes of the frequency range, when slight phase lead is evident at low frequencies and slight phase lag at high; gain is usually within 10% of unity except at the uppermost limit of the frequency range where it tends to exceed unity by 30–40% (Keller, 1978; Lisberger et al., 1983; Miles & Eighmy, 1980).

The canal afferents that provide the reflex with all of its information about head turns display somewhat complicated dynamic behavior: while to a first approximation the canals can be regarded as accelerometers that perform a single integration so that primary afferent discharges effectively encode head velocity, individual afferents display a wide range of phase lags (Miles & Braitman, 1980), and all become increasingly phase advanced on head velocity below 0.1 Hz and above 1 Hz (Fernandez & Goldberg, 1971). Furthermore, the oculomotor plant that transforms the motoneuron discharges into compensatory eye movements acts as a lowpass filter whose gain is constant only at frequencies below about 0.1 Hz, and above this shows progressively decreasing gain and increasing phase lag. Clearly, the physical input and output elements of the VOR exhibit frequency dependent behavior over the range 0.05–5 Hz that is not seen in the overall reflex. Thus, as Skavenski and Robinson (1973) pointed out, the central nervous system must provide an interface whose dynamics compensate almost exactly for the dynamics of the labyrinth and the oculomotor plant, introducing different amounts of gain and phase lag at different frequencies. In a pioneering paper, Skavenski and Robinson (1973) treated the reflex as a lumped system and derived transfer functions for the labyrinth and oculomotor plant from the discharge characteristics of the 'average' canal primary afferent and eye muscle montoneuron, respectively. These workers drew attention to the fact that, while the discharges of the canal primary afferents effectively encode head velocity, the motoneurons discharge in relation to the position as well as the velocity of the eyes; from this they inferred that the brain introduces considerable phase lag into the vestibular head velocity signal in order to produce the antiphase eye position signals and must, therefore, perform the mathematical function of an integrator. Since that time, Robinson has gone on to derive a detailed transfer function for the central nervous link of the VOR, treating it as a lumped system (Robinson, 1981a,b).

It has often been noted that the VOR is an open-loop system, and its gain has been shown to be regulated by a visually mediated, long term learning process. When the visual inputs associated with head turns are magnified or minified with optical devices such as telescopic spectacles, the gain of the VOR gradually undergoes appropriate (adaptive) changes (for recent reviews see Collewijn, 1981a; Ito, 1975; Melvill Jones, 1977; Miles & Lisberger, 1981b). However, while adaptive gain control has been the subject of many studies, little attention has been directed at the problem of fine tuning the system's phase: it seems reasonable to assume that an adaptive mechanism is needed to ensure that the brain introduces appropriate, differing phase lags at each frequency. Robinson's transfer functions provide a precise, elegant mathematical description of the signal processing that must be done by the nervous system. However, a lumped structure is only one way to perform this processing. Recent studies have begun to provide some new insights into the long term regulation of the phase of the VOR and to point out some limitations in the structure of present models of the basic reflex.

## 2. Frequency selective adaptation and phase crossover

A number of studies on a variety of species have revealed that when animals are adapted to telescopic spectacles — or equivalent optical conditions — using restricted frequencies of sinusoidal oscillation, the associated changes in VOR gain are always greatest at the frequencies used for adaptation (rabbit: Collewijn & Grootendorst, 1979; monkey: Lisberger et al., 1983; cat: Robin-

son, 1976 and Godaux et al., 1983b; fish: Schairer & Bennett, 1981; birds: Wallman et al., 1982) (see Ch. 2). In the rabbit, this frequency selective adaptation is very sharply tuned, and only very minor gain changes are evident a mere octave above or below the adapting frequency (Collewijn & Grootendorst, 1979). Furthermore, the rabbit shows occasional after effects in the dark, when its eyes continue to oscillate spontaneously at the adapting frequency even after the platform used to oscillate the animal has been stopped. These observations led Collewijn and Grootendorst (1979) to postulate that the adaptive mechanism in the rabbit involves a storage system for patterns of motion, which registers eye movements and retinal slip; normal compensatory eye movements are then assumed to result from visual and vestibular inputs, plus any previously stored patterns whose retrieval is now triggered by sensory-motor interactions matching those that originally led to the storage (Collewijn, 1981a) (see Ch. 3). This interesting hypothesis is reminiscent of the 'pattern center' invoked to explain motion sickness and particularly the after effects of prolonged irregular motions (Groen, 1957). Along these same lines, Melvill Jones and Gonshor (1982) have also recently suggested that "the central generation of a predicted periodic function" might account for the frequency dependent phase shifts seen in the ocular response to active head oscillations following adaptation to left-right reversed vision in humans.

However, the pattern storage idea provides a less satisfactory explanation for the frequency selective adaptation that we have recently described in the monkey: in this species, after effects appear to be lacking, frequency selectivity is much less sharply tuned, and orderly phase shifts are evident at adjacent frequencies (Lisberger et al., 1983). These phase shifts were particularly intriguing: frequency selective increases in VOR gain were associated with phase lead below the adapting frequency and phase lag above, while frequency selective decreases in gain showed the converse — phase lag below the adapting frequency and phase lead above. For convenience we referred to this seemingly complex pattern of phase shifts around the adapting frequency as 'phase crossover'. Similar phase shifts are evident in the data of Godaux et al. (1983b), who studied frequency selective decreases in gain in the cat. Current lumped models cannot explain such findings and, arguing by analogy with the spatial-frequency channel hypothesis that has been invoked to explain frequency selective elevation of visual detection thresholds for spatial-frequency gratings (Campbell & Robson, 1968), we have suggested that the central pathways in the VOR are organized into parallel, overlapping temporal-frequency channels. Since we envisage broadly tuned channels, we are not suggesting that they perform a Fourier transform, but rather that they act as bandpass filters.

## 3. The channels hypothesis

While the gain changes in frequency dependent adaptation studies first led us to consider a channeled type of organization, it was the associated phase shifts which suggested that the channels must differ in their dynamics. Indeed, it seemed to us that such a channel model could offer a surprisingly simple explanation for what otherwise seemed to be a perplexing pattern of phase shifts. The increased lag at frequencies above the adapting frequency following an increase in gain was taken to indicate that, of the channels contributing to the VOR in that frequency range, the modified channel(s) must be contributing more lag than the average; likewise, the decreased lag at frequencies below the adapting frequency was taken to indicate that, of the channels contributing in that frequency range, the modified channel(s) must be contributing less lag than the average. If we assume that all channels have essentially the same complement of dynamic elements, and differ only in the time constants of those elements, then we might infer that a given channel shows progressively increasing phase lag with increasing frequency, and that at any given test frequency, low frequency channels would show more phase lag than high frequency channels. If adaptation at a particular frequency is assumed to selectively alter the gains of the individual channels in proportion to the magnitude of their contributions to the responses at that frequency, then a gain change with no phase shift would be expected at that frequency. However, such adapta-

tion would disrupt the usual balance among the channels contributing to responses at adjacent frequencies: above the adapting frequency, the modified channels would be those contributing more lag than the average, and below the adapting frequency they would be those contributing less lag than the average. It follows then that increases in gain would result in excessive lag above the adapting frequency and inadequate lag below and so forth.

The establishment and maintenance of an appropriate gain and phase for the VOR over the full range of functional frequencies would be a matter of adjusting the relative contributions of the different temporal-frequency channels that subscribe to the performance at each frequency. Thus, each channel is assumed to have an independently adjustable gain element that is the basis for an adaptive tuning mechanism operating to offset the frequency dependent dynamics seen in the primary afferents and the plant. Conceptually, this is equivalent to the spectrum equalizer in a high-fidelity sound reproduction system, which emphasizes or de-emphasizes portions of the audio spectrum to match the listening room's acoustics.

Our initial attempt to show the validity of the temporal-frequency channels hypothesis was able to demonstrate that such models could display frequency selectivity and phase crossover (Lisberger et al., 1983). We did not wish to employ any dynamic elements not already invoked by Skavenski and Robinson (1973) and, in effect, we merely produced a distributed version of their lumped model. Instead of lumping the labyrinthine inputs and central pathways, we segregated them into three channels according to their dynamic response properties; three channels (high-, middle- and low-frequency) were deemed the minimum necessary to demonstrate the basic phenomena. Work by Goldberg et al. (1981), Shimazu and Precht (1965) and ourselves (Lisberger & Miles, 1980; Miles & Braitman, 1980), had already suggested that vestibular primary afferents with differing dynamics project to different cells in the vestibular nuclei, and we assumed that this separation was preserved up to the level of the motoneurons, at which point everything became lumped through the common muscle ten-

316

don. Thus, the neural part of our model was configured as three channels, each consisting of a subpopulation of primary afferents, a modifiable gain element and a lag element representing Skavenski and Robinson's direct and integrated inputs to motoneurons. The transfer functions for the primary afferents were taken from Fernandez and Goldberg (1971) and were distributed in an orderly fashion such that those with least lag provided the inputs to the high frequency channel and so forth. The relative weighting of the direct and integrated inputs to motoneurons was varied systematically across channels so that the direct path was emphasized most in the high frequency channel. With this arrangement, these weightings determined the motoneurons' relative sensitivities to eye velocity ($r$) and eye position ($k$), hence the weightings used in the model were selected to concur with the range of $r/k$ values recorded in motoneurons by Skavenski and Robinson (1973) and Robinson (1970). However, it was found that frequency selectivity could only be obtained if the integrators were assumed to be 'leaky' and the degree of leakiness of the integrators was distributed systematically across the channels, being least in the low frequency channel and greatest in the high: it was not sufficient to merely distribute the differing dynamics seen in primary afferents across channels. Since all of the elements had simple linear transfer functions, it was possible to obtain Bode plots describing phase and gain at any frequency analytically. Selectively altering the gain of the middle channel resulted in frequency selective gain changes peaking at 0.25 Hz with appropriately directed changes in phase shift above and below this frequency.

While this simple three-channel model establishes the feasibility of using channels to explain frequency selectivity and phase crossover, in its original form it has serious deficiencies that limit its utility. Firstly, the overall transfer function always exhibits less phase lag than is actually observed. Secondly, while increases in gain following selective adjustments of the middle channel are always greatest at the particular frequency of 0.25 Hz, gain fails to decrement appropriately at higher frequencies. This deficiency results from the poor delineation of the high frequency limits of the channels. Increasing the number of chan-

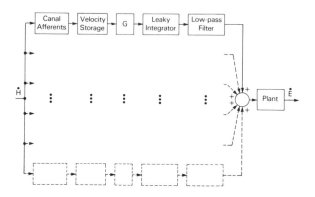

*Fig. 1.* A block diagram showing the layout of the basic components in a six channel version of our equalizer model of the VOR. Individual channels are assumed to converge on the lumped plant at the level of the motoneuron. $\dot{H}$ represents head velocity and $\dot{E}$ represents eye velocity.

nels could provide some improvement but these shortcomings can only be completely eliminated by introducing an additional lag element into each of the channels so that they acquire the transfer characteristics of true bandpass filters. Accordingly, we now propose a more complete channels hypothesis that incorporates these additional lag elements and can reproduce our observations on the gain and phase of the normal and adapted VOR quite faithfully.

## 4. An equalizer model of the VOR

Fig. 1 shows the basic structure of our revised channels model of the VOR. We shall first consider the transfer functions of the individual elements of the system together with the salient features of their frequency response characteristics, and then proceed to consider the performance of the whole system, especially its ability to simulate a normal VOR and show frequency selective adaptive gain changes with appropriate phase crossover. As far as possible, all parameters are based on data taken from the monkey.

An important feature of our model of the VOR is that it is linear, so that its behaviour can be described entirely by linear differential equations. These equations are usually represented by transfer functions in the Laplace domain, which are rational polynomial functions of a complex frequency ($s$) and describe mathematically how the system transforms its input to produce the output.

When a system, such as the VOR, is described by subsystems in series or cascade, the overall transfer function can be determined by simply multiplying together the transfer functions of each of the subsystems.

One simple way to visualize the functional operation of such systems is to construct asymptotic Bode diagrams, which are straight line approximations to the gain and phase of the transfer function. As a rational polynomial, the transfer function can be completely described by the roots of its numerator (its 'zeros') and its denominator (its 'poles'). The poles and zeros are at the frequencies corresponding to the time constants of the system. In an asymptotic Bode plot, these are the frequencies at which the line segments intersect (the 'corner' frequencies). Log-log scales are used in Bode diagrams so that products of transfer functions can be derived by simple addition.

### 4.1. The vestibular primary afferent input

The transfer function describing the gain and phase of semicircular canal primary afferent discharge modulation ($\dot{H}'_c$) in relation to head velocity ($\dot{H}$) was taken from Fernandez and Goldberg (1971), and in Laplace transform notation is given by

$$\frac{\dot{H}'_c(s)}{\dot{H}(s)} = \frac{s}{(sT_1 + 1)(sT_2 + 1)} \frac{sT_A}{(sT_A + 1)}(sT_L + 1) \qquad (1)$$

where $s$ is the Laplace complex frequency. The first factor on the right hand side represents the physics of the torsion-pendulum model of the cupula, where $T_1$ is 5.7 s and $T_2$ is 0.003 s, and is assumed to be the same for all channels. However, at low frequencies the phase lag of the primary afferent discharge was less than that expected from the torsion-pendulum model and the second factor, an adaptation element, was introduced to account for this. Based on the phase lag discrepancy at 0.0125 Hz, $T_A$ was estimated to range from 30 s to values so high as to be indistinguishable from infinity. A further important deviation from the torsion-pendulum model was seen in the behavior of primary afferents at high frequencies, where they showed increased gain and diminished phase lag; the third factor, a simple lead element, was incorporated to account for this. The phase lag discrepancies above 1 Hz provided estimates for $T_L$ ranging from 0.013 to 0.094 s. Fernandez and Goldberg also found that $T_A$ and $T_L$ tended to co-vary, such that a high degree of adaptation tended to be associated with pronounced high frequency lead. We have therefore distributed values of $T_A$ and $T_L$ systematically across the various channels, such that afferents with the most adaptation (low $T_A$) and high frequency lead (high $T_L$) are assumed to innervate the highest frequency channel (see Table 1). The frequency dependence of the canal afferent modulations ($\dot{H}'_c$) relative to head velocity ($\dot{H}$) for a representative channel (number 3) is summarized in the Bode diagram in Fig. 2B (dashed line).

Table 1

Parameters used to define channels.

The following parameters were common to all channels: $T_{ok}$ and $T_1 = 5.7$ s; $T_i$ and $T_{e1} = 0.24$ s; $T_2 = 0.003$ s; $T_{e2} = 0.016$ s; $b = 0.928$ s.

| Chan | 1 | 2 | 3 | 4 | 5 | 6 |
|------|------|------|------|------|------|------|
| $T_A$ | 1000 | 420 | 215 | 114 | 56.8 | 31.8 |
| $T_L$ | 0.015 | 0.020 | 0.027 | 0.035 | 0.047 | 0.063 |
| $T_{B1}$ | 420 | 17.7 | 3.98 | 0.88 | 0.19 | 0.04 |
| $T_{B2}$ | 20 | 4.42 | 1 | 0.22 | 0.047 | 0.01 |
| $G$ | 2 | 4 | 4 | 4 | 4.75 | 1.25 |

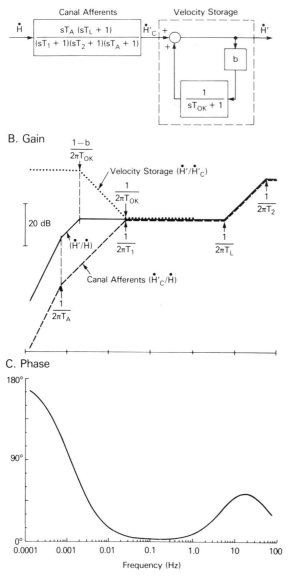

A. Transfer Functions

B. Gain

C. Phase

## 4.2. The velocity storage mechanism

The low frequency performance of the VOR is much better than that expected from the time constant of the cupula ($T_1$, 5.7 s), and it has become usual to invoke a central velocity storage mechanism to increase the time constant of the VOR to about 16 s in the case of the monkey (Waespe & Henn, 1977a; Buettner et al., 1978; Raphan et al., 1979; Robinson, 1977b, 1981a,b). In effect, the velocity storage mechanism operates to improve the vestibular system's estimate of head velocity at low frequencies. Since the increased time constant is evident at the level of the secondary vestibular neurons (Waespe & Henn, 1977a), the storage mechanism is assumed to receive its inputs directly from canal primary afferents. We have used Robinson's model of the velocity storage mechanism, which incorporates a lag element, $(sT_{ok} + 1)^{-1}$, in a positive feedback loop with a gain element $b$ (see Fig. 2A). The transfer function for this arrangement, which relates the improved estimate of head velocity ($\dot{H}'$) to the canal afferent's estimate ($\dot{H}'_c$), is given by

$$\frac{\dot{H}'(s)}{\dot{H}'_c(s)} = \frac{1}{1-b} \left[ \frac{sT_{ok} + 1}{s(\frac{T_{ok}}{1-b}) + 1} \right] \qquad (2)$$

This lag element has a zero at frequency $(2\pi T_{ok})^{-1}$ Hz and a pole at frequency $[2\pi T_{ok}/(1-b)]^{-1}$ Hz. By arranging for this zero to exactly cancel the pole due to the cupula time constant at $(2\pi T_1)^{-1}$ Hz, a new pole is created for the labyrinthine signal at $[2\pi T_{ok}/(1-b)]^{-1}$ Hz. Accordingly, $T_{ok}$ was set at 5.7 s and $b$ at 0.928 s for every channel, effectively moving the pole for the labyrinthine signal from 0.028 to 0.002 Hz; this can be seen in the Bode diagram of Fig. 2B.

### 4.3. The neural channels

In the central portion of our original three channel model, we employed Skavenski and Robin-

*Fig. 2.* Frequency dependence of the semicircular canal primary afferents and the central velocity storage mechanism. A. Transfer functions for canal afferents (Fernandez & Goldberg, 1971) and Robinson's (1981a,b) positive feedback model of the velocity storage mechanism. $\dot{H}$, head velocity; $\dot{H}'_c$, the canal primary afferent's estimate of head velocity; $\dot{H}'$, the vestibular system's estimate of head velocity. B. Asymptotic Bode diagram showing frequency dependence of the gains of the canal afferents (dashed line), the velocity storage mechanism (dotted line) and their combination (continuous line). $T_A$ and $T_L$ are assumed to vary across channels (see Table 1) and the values seen in this Figure were those used in channel 3. C. Phase shift of the final vestibular output signal in channel 3

($\dot{H}'$) relative to head velocity ($\dot{H}$). Note that, for this channel, the gain of the vestibular signal is flat and its phase only slightly advanced on head velocity over the physiologically important frequency range 0.05–5 Hz.

son's scheme involving direct and indirect (integrated) pathways whose relative weightings, we assumed, varied across channels, thereby contributing to the separation of the channels at high frequencies and also accounting for the range of $r/k$ values among the motoneurons (Lisberger et al., 1983). In order to achieve adequate separation of the channels at low frequencies we assumed that the integrator pathways functioned imperfectly (leaked), and that the time constant of the leakiness ($T_{B1}$) was shortest in the high frequency integrator and longest in the low frequency integrator. However, the upper frequency limits of the channels in our initial model were so poorly differentiated that the narrow bandpass characteristic implicit in any channel hypothesis was missing. Such broad 'channels', regardless of their number, could never faithfully reproduce the details of our data on frequency selective adaptation, e.g., the roll off in gain characteristically seen above the adapting frequency following frequency selective increases in gain (except to a very small degree below a frequency of $(2\pi T_{e1})^{-1}$, i.e. 0.66 Hz). If frequency selectivity and phase crossover are to be adequately explained by a linear channels hypothesis, then it is imperative that the channels act as a series of relatively narrow, albeit overlapping, bandpass filters covering the full range of biologically important frequencies (0.05–5 Hz). Operationally, this is most easily achieved by introducing one additional lag element into the central neuronal portion of each channel and distributing their time constants ($T_{B2}$) so as to impose different high frequency limits on the different channels. Clearly, this new time constant should be shortest in the high frequency channels and longest in the low frequency channels.

The complete transfer function for these central channels, describing each channel's output modulation ($R'_L$) in relation to its input, is given by

$$\frac{R'_L(s)}{\dot{H}'(s)} = \frac{T_{B1}}{(sT_{B1}+1)}(sT_i + 1)\frac{1}{(sT_{B2} + 1)} \qquad (3)$$

Note that the input to these channels ($\dot{H}'$) represents the vestibular system's estimate of head velocity. The first factor on the right hand side of Eqn. 3 is a lag element representing the leaky

integrator that sets the low frequency cut-off in each channel at $(2\pi T_{B1})^{-1}$ Hz (except in channel 1, where $1/T_{B1} < (1-b)/T_{ok}$, hence the low frequency cut-off for this channel is due to the pole created by the velocity storage mechanism at $(1-b)/2\pi T_{ok}$ Hz. The second factor is Skavenski and Robinson's velocity feed-forward signal that operates as a lead element to cancel the major lag factor in the plant (see later). The third factor is our newly introduced lag element that operates as a lowpass filter and sets the high frequency cut-off in each channel at $(2\pi T_{B2})^{-1}$Hz*. The frequency dependence of a representative channel (number 3) is shown in a Bode diagram in Fig. 3B (dotted line). It should be noted that if $b$ were to vary across channels it could further accentuate the low frequency separation between channels, but only below $(2\pi T_1)^{-1}$ Hz.

### 4.4 The oculomotor plant

We have assumed that the dynamics of the plant (eye muscles, globe and orbital tissues) are lumped because in a given muscle all fibers pull on a common tendon, which in turn operates on the common globe, etc. The transfer function of the plant, describing eye velocity ($\dot{E}$) in relation to average motoneuron discharge rate modulation ($R$), was taken from Robinson (1981a), and is given by

$$\frac{\dot{E}(s)}{R(s)} = \frac{s\ e^{-sT}}{(sT_{e1} + 1)(sT_{e2} + 1)} \qquad (4)$$

where $R$ is the sum of the outputs, ($R'_L$), from all of the channels. The time constant, $T_{e1}$, is determined by the ratio of the slopes of the curves relating motoneuron discharge rates to eye velocity ($r$) and eye position ($k$), and averages 0.24 s. The time constant $T_{e2}$ is determined by the ratio of the slopes of the curves relating motoneuron discharge rate to eye acceleration ($m$) and eye velocity ($r$), and averages 0.016 s. The exponen

---

*Actually, this is only strictly true for channels 1–4; in channel 5, $T_{B2}$ is exactly cancelled by the zero due to $T_L$, so that the high frequency pole for this channel is due to $T_{e2}$; for channel 6, $T_{B2} < T_L$, hence the gain in this channel breaks up at $(2\pi T_L)^{-1}$ Hz and, once again, the high frequency cut-off is due to $T_{e2}$.

320

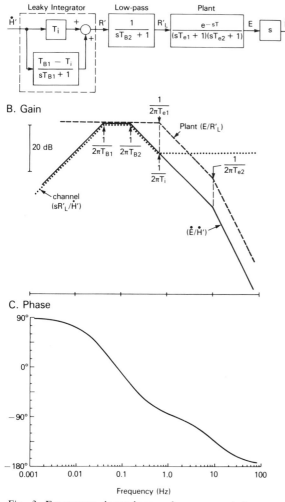

**A. Transfer Functions**

Leaky Integrator    Low-pass    Plant

$\dot{H}'$ → $T_i$ → (+) → $R'$ → $\dfrac{1}{sT_{B2}+1}$ → $R'_L$ → $\dfrac{e^{-sT}}{(sT_{e1}+1)(sT_{e2}+1)}$ → $E$ → $s$ → $\dot{E}$

$\dfrac{T_{B1}-T_i}{sT_{B1}+1}$

**B. Gain**

$\dfrac{1}{2\pi T_{e1}}$

Plant $(E/R'_L)$

20 dB

$\dfrac{1}{2\pi T_{B1}}$  $\dfrac{1}{2\pi T_{B2}}$

$\dfrac{1}{2\pi T_i}$

$\dfrac{1}{2\pi T_{e2}}$

channel $(sR'_L/\dot{H}')$

$(\dot{E}/\dot{H}')$

**C. Phase**

90°

0°

−90°

−180°

0.001    0.01    0.1    1.0    10    100

Frequency (Hz)

*Fig. 3.* Frequency dependence of a representative neural channel (number 3) and the oculomotor plant. A. Transfer functions for Skavenski and Robinson's neural integrator (with leakiness as per Lisberger et al., 1983) and velocity feedforward path, together with our proposed new lag element and Robinson's (1981a,b) model of the plant. $\dot{H}'$, the vestibular system's estimate of head velocity; $R'$, the output of the feedforward and leaky integrator networks, and $R'_L$, this same signal after passage through the lowpass lag element; $\dot{E}$, eye velocity. B. Asymptotic Bode diagrams showing the frequency dependence of the gains of a neural channel (due to the combined effects of the leaky integrator, the velocity feedforward, and the lag elements: dotted line), the plant (dashed line) and their combination (continuous line). Note that the time constants $T_{B1}$ and $T_{B2}$ vary across channels and play a major role in defining the low and high frequency limits, respectively: the values seen here were those used for channel number 3. C. Phase lag introduced by channel number 3 and the plant (combined). Note that there is increasing lag with increasing frequency.

tial function incorporates the effects of a finite delay of about 8 ms ($T$) between motoneuron discharge and eye movement. The Bode diagram in Fig. 3B (dashed line) illustrates the frequency dependence of the plant, expressing eye position relative to average motoneuron discharge modulation. (Note that for simplicity the major pole in the plant at $(2\pi T_{e1})^{-1}$ Hz has been exactly offset by the zero due to Skavenski and Robinson's highpass element in the brain stem $(2\pi T_i)^{-1}$ Hz.)

### 4.5. Parameters defining channels

Each channel in our equalizer model has the overall transfer characteristics of a bandpass filter (see Fig. 4 and 5). At low frequencies, channels are distinguished by the degree of adaptation evident in their primary afferents (determined by the value of $T_A$) and the leakiness of the central integrators (determined by the value of $T_{B1}$). At high frequencies, channels are distinguished largely by the time constants of the new central lag elements ($T_{B2}$) and to a lesser extent by the time constants of the lead elements in their primary afferents ($T_L$). However, of the four parameters that are varied systematically from one channel to another — $T_A$, $T_L$, $T_{B1}$, $T_{B2}$ — only two are absolutely essential to preserve channel-like qualities: the lag elements in the brain governed by $T_{B1}$ and $T_{B2}$.

With such an arrangement, allowing the relative weights of the direct and integrated pathways in the brain stem to vary across channels has little consequence and, as mentioned above, we arranged for the zero due to $T_i$ to exactly cancel the pole due to $T_{e1}$ in the plant (see Fig. 3B). The range of $r/k$ values found in motoneurons would then arise from small imbalances in the strengths of their various channel inputs. This does not necessarily mean that the range of $r/k$ values displayed by motoneurons is of no physiological significance. Others have suggested that the range of dynamics seen in motoneuron discharges results from the selective distribution of vestibular afferents, and may in turn be matched to the mechanical dynamics of the muscle fibers that they innervate (e.g., Baker et al., 1981). Our channels model is not incompatible with the latter idea. However, the range of dynamics evident in these

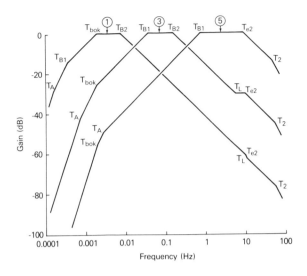

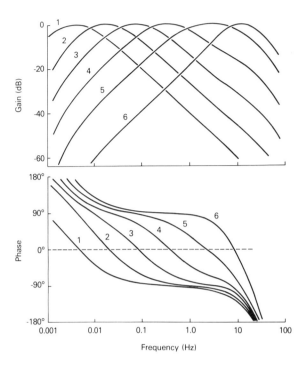

*Fig. 4.* Channels as bandpass filters. Asymptotic Bode diagrams indicate how the various proposed lead and lag elements operate to define the frequency selectivity of the individual channels. The three curves show the frequency dependence of the VOR gain ($\dot{E}/\dot{H}$) that would result from the independent operation of each of the channels 1, 3, and 5 in a six channel version of our equalizer model.

*Fig. 5.* Bode plots indicating the overall transfer characteristics of each channel in a six channel version of the adaptive equalizer model. Each curve indicates the amplitude or phase relations between eye velocity and head velocity, and was computed by adjusting the simple gain elements, $G$, to zero for all of the channels except that one to be characterized. Note that the channels have the gain profiles of bandpass filters.

$r/k$ values is much smaller than that which must be displayed by the channels in our model: new dynamic elements must be invoked to adequately define channels.

## 4.6. The performance of the equalizer model

The Bode plots in Fig. 6 show the performance of a six channel version of our model. No special biological significance attaches to this number of channels: it was sufficient to generate smooth Bode plots of the VOR, relatively free from obtrusive edge effects, yet allowing frequency selective changes over the full, biologically important, frequency range with a magnitude and resolution close to that which we actually observed. While a more realistic representation might involve an extensive continuum of numerous overlapping channels, we do not feel that such numbers are critical for any of the concepts that we wish to explore here. The parameters selected for each channel are listed in Table 1. In most instances, the upper and lower corner frequencies for each channel are determined by the values of $T_{B1}$ and $T_{B2}$, respectively. Increasing the separation

of these two poles in each of the channels undermines the sharpness of the frequency selective gain changes, while conversely, decreasing the separation undermines the smoothness of the combined VOR Bode plot; that only six channels are employed is clearly an important factor here and an aesthetically acceptable compromise was achieved with separations of about 1/2 decade. The selected ranges of values for $T_{B1}$ and $T_{B2}$ produced channels with center frequencies extending from 0.004 to 12 Hz. The individual contributions of the channels to the overall response are each assumed to be regulated by an adaptive mechanism that operates entirely through the simple gain element, $G$. We have made no attempt to characterize this adaptive mechanism. Initial values for $G$ were selected manually by successive approximations to achieve a normal VOR: gain close to unity and phase lag close to

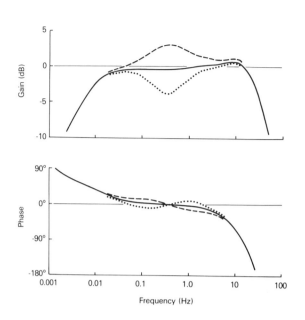

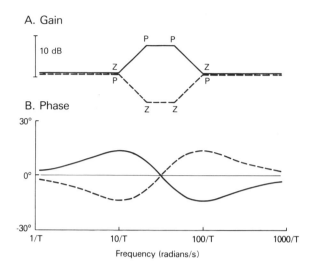

Fig. 7. Frequency selective gain changes and phase crossover. A. Asymptotic Bode plots for a lead-lag element (continuous line) that shows a frequency selective increase in gain with two adjacent poles (p) and a lag-lead element (dashed line) that shows a frequency selective decrease in gain with two adjacent zeros (z). B. Shows the associated phase shifts, with phase crossover occurring at the mid-point frequencies.

Fig. 6. Bode plots indicating the frequency dependence of the normal VOR gain and phase (eye velocity relative to head velocity) produced by the six channel equalizer model after individual channel gains had been suitably adjusted (continuous line): see Table 1 for the actual values used. Also shown are the frequency selective gain changes and phase crossover following selective increases (dashed lines) or decreases (dotted lines) in the gain of channel 4.

ideal (i.e., 180°) in the frequency range 0.1–1 Hz, with inadequate lag and diminishing gain at low frequencies, and increasing gain with further increasing phase lag at higher frequencies.

The proposed equalizer model contains a dynamic element (pole) not needed in the original lumped model proposed by Skavenski and Robinson, yet the frequency responses of the VORs produced by the two models are virtually identical. One reason for this is that these poles are spread over a wide frequency range and are added in parallel, so that their 90° of phase lag is spread over a wide range. In addition, part of the extra phase lag compensates for the extra phase lead introduced in the channeled model by unlumping the canal afferents. These two factors make the net lag of the whole reflex less than would have been expected from the addition of an extra pole to the lumped model.

If the gain of any one of the channels 2 to 5 is selectively altered, the model shows frequency selective gain changes, together with appropriate

phase crossovers, centering around frequencies ranging from 0.01 to 3 Hz. Fig. 6 shows the effect of increasing the gain of channel 4 by 75% or decreasing it by 50%: the changes in gain are clearly maximal at 0.36 Hz — which in effect represents the 'adapting frequency' — and decrement with frequency at a rate which approximates that which we observed in the monkey; appropriate phase crossover is also evident at 0.36 Hz, e.g., increases in gain result in phase lead below this frequency and phase lag above it.

An appreciation of the mechanisms underlying phase crossover comes from the realization that in a linear system a frequency selective increase in gain must involve two adjacent poles, while a frequency selective decrease in gain must involve two adjacent zeros (see Fig. 7). Poles are always associated with progressively increasing phase lag with increasing frequency, and zeros with the converse. Thus, it follows that a peak in the gain profile must be associated with increasing lag with increasing frequency, while a trough must be accompanied by decreasing lag with increasing frequency: phase crossover.

## 5. Adaptive mechanisms

### 5.1. An adaptive equalizer model

The equalizer model in Fig. 1 has the virtue of being a simple, linear representation that reproduces all of the essential data from the monkey. It is basically a channeled version of Skavenski and Robinson's original model of the VOR with one important addition: a simple lag element. However, to form a complete adaptive model, a specific mechanism, organized into frequency selective channels to identify those VOR channels whose gains need adjustment, is still needed.

The neural correlate of temporal-frequency channels would be the phase shift of the signals that they transmit. In our view, phase shift could play a key role in identifying the sites (i.e., the channels) that are in need of gain adjustment. If the channels model is to be invoked to explain frequency selective changes in VOR gain, then it must be assumed that the adaptive mechanism is able to identify the channels that contribute to the VOR at the adapting frequency, and we feel that the phase of the impulse traffic in the channel could provide the basis for this recognition. This hypothesis assumes that adaptation depends upon a precise phase coherence between the vestibular and error inputs to the site of changes. In the time domain, this phase relationship would be manifested as a precise timing alignment of the vestibular and error inputs; such temporal coincidence is an implicit feature of most models of the adaptive mechanism (Ito, 1972; Davies & Melvill Jones, 1976; Miles & Lisberger, 1981b; Robinson, 1976) (see Chs. 3 & 14).

### 5.2. An adaptive lumped model

Since the equalizer model is linear, it is possible to formulate a lumped model with the same overall transfer function. An equivalent lumped model could be formulated by simply adding more poles and zeros to the Skavenski and Robinson model to provide for the frequency selective behavior of the VOR. In the normal state, all of the 'extra' zeros would have to exactly cancel all of the 'extra' poles, since by definition they are not seen in the overall transfer function. Frequency

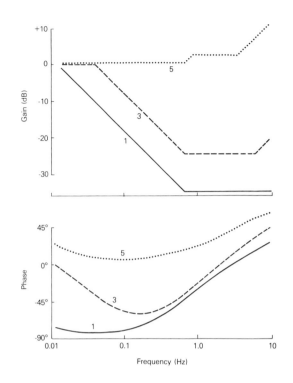

Fig. 8. Bode diagrams showing the frequency responses of sample vestibular signals in the equalizer model. The gain and phase of the signal, $R'$, representing the output of the leaky integrator combined with its vestibular input (see Fig. 3A), are plotted relative to head velocity for the channels 1, 3 and 5.

selective adaptation would be achieved by causing the pole-zero pairs to separate, thereby revealing their existence to the external observer, in accord with the simple rules seen in Fig. 7. For example, a gain increase with phase crossover would require two pole-zero pairs to split: one pair, at a frequency below the adapting frequency, would have to separate with the zero going to a lower frequency than the pole; the other pair, at a frequency above the adapting frequency, would have to separate with the zero going to a higher frequency than the pole. To lower the gain, the reverse would have to happen (see Fig. 7). A mechanism for achieving pole-zero separation was seen in the velocity storage mechanism discussed earlier (Fig. 2A,B); in this case, the separation between the zero (at $(2\pi T_{ok})^{-1}$ Hz) and the pole (at $[2\pi T_{ok}/(1-b)]^{-1}$ Hz) is determined by $b$, a simple gain element.

The lumped and channeled adaptive models are similar in that they both extend Skavenski and

Robinson's model with extra poles, and they can both be adjusted by changing simple gain elements. (The lumped model also requires extra zeros, but this is not a critical consideration.) The channeled VOR pathways in the equalizer model are regulated by a channeled adaptive controller. However, even if the VOR pathways are all lumped, the adaptive controller must still be channeled, since those gain elements controlling the separation of poles and zeros must be independently adjustable.

In the equalizer model, the gain elements control the contributions of channels whose dynamics are fixed. Conceptually, it is relatively simple to imagine how the system might derive error signals by comparing the outputs of the channels with a central correlate of retinal slip (or gaze velocity: Miles & Lisberger, 1981b). This would indicate the extent to which any particular channel's contribution was affecting the overall system error. The problem of determining error is much more difficult in the lumped adaptive model: errors occurring early in the VOR pathway would be present at all subsequent points in the system, rendering it difficult to identify the offending element(s); a simple mechanism for achieving this has so far eluded us.

## 6. Neural correlates of channels

The bandpass characteristic determined by the two poles, $T_{B1}$ and $T_{B2}$, would be expected to show up in the transfer functions of central neurons in the vestibulo-ocular pathway(s). Why have single-unit studies of the VOR not reported evidence suggesting the existence of bandpass filters? To answer this question we must consider the expected discharge properties of neurons encoding signals such as $R'$ and $R'_L$ in Fig. 3A. This requires that we derive the transfer functions relating these signals to head movements or compensatory eye movements. The Bode plots in Figs. 8 and 9 show the frequency responses for $R'$ and $R'_L$, respectively, relative to head velocity, in the physiological range 0.05–5 Hz for channels 1, 3 and 5. (Head velocity can be regarded as an intended eye velocity signal, with an appropriate sign change.)

The signal $R'$ is the output of each channel's leaky integrator combined with its vestibular input. As shown in Fig. 8, at this stage of signal processing the high-frequency channels (e.g., number 5) would still have the major dynamic characteristics of primary afferent vestibular signals, their activity modulating nearly in phase with head velocity. At the other extreme, activity in the low frequency channels (e.g., number 1) would modulate almost 90° phase lagged behind head velocity and would seem more related to intended eye position. Intermediate channels (e.g., number 3) would have phase lags around 45° and might appear to be carrying both position and velocity signals. None of this is inconsistent with currently available recordings from putative vestibulo-ocular relay neurons (Buettner et al., 1978; Fuchs & Kimm, 1975; Keller & Daniels, 1975; Keller & Kamath, 1975; King et al., 1976; Lisberger & Miles, 1980; Miles, 1974; Pola & Robinson, 1978; Waespe & Henn, 1977a).

The signal $R'_L$ is the final output of each channel. As shown in Fig. 9, high frequency channels (e.g., number 5) would still effectively encode head velocity. The effect of the lowpass filter, $T_{B2}$, would become very evident in the low frequency channels over the physiological range: signals here would show more phase lag than has ever been reported in the literature. However, if the lag elements responsible for $T_{B2}$ were in the synaptic coupling at the motoneuron membrane, and the motoneurons were each assumed to receive inputs from many channels, then single unit recording techniques would not sample these individual channel outputs. It is this point which leads us to assume that the system becomes lumped at the level of the motoneuron (in contrast to Baker et al., 1981). Unfortunately, this creates a problem for the adaptive mechanism: how would the system derive a channel-specific error signal? This would require channel output collaterals whose synapses within the adaptive mechanism show the same lowpass filter dynamics as those on to motoneurons.

Experimental evidence for a channelled structure may be obtainable with correlation techniques. Spike triggered averaging between vestibular premotor neurons and ocular motoneurons should reveal the lag element $T_{B2}$. Intracellular stimulation of these premotor neurons could also

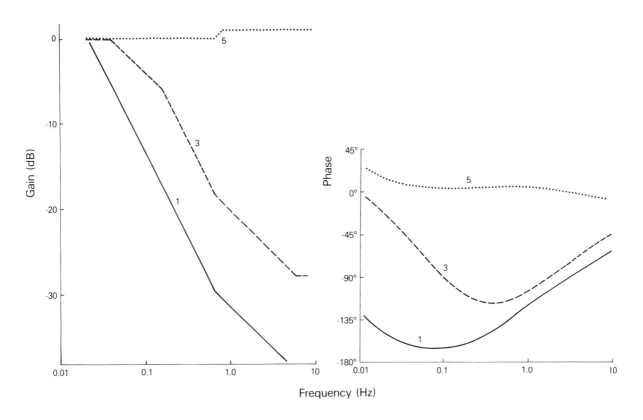

*Fig. 9.* Bode diagrams showing the frequency responses of the individual channel output signals that converge on motoneurons. The gain and phase of the signal $R'_L$ (see Fig. 3A) are plotted relative to head velocity for the channels 1, 3 and 5.

be employed. There should be a wide range of coupling time constants and, to support our channels hypothesis, they should be selectively distributed such that the longest time constants are associated with premotor neurons whose vestibular modulations show the greatest phase lag relative to head velocity.

## 7. Conclusions

This chapter has presented a new linear model of the vestibulo-ocular reflex that extends the lumped, linear model of Robinson (1981a,b). By introducing frequency bandpass channels, the new model can reproduce not only the normal VOR, but also frequency selective gain changes (with phase crossover). The model contains a new dynamic element, a lowpass filter, and has the transfer characteristics of an equalizer. Comparison with an equivalent lumped model shows that the channel structure of the equalizer model sim-

plifies the task of the adaptive mechanism. It is conjectured that the error signal used by the adaptive controller might be obtained by comparing the output of each channel with a central correlate of retinal slip or some other co-varying parameter (e.g., gaze velocity).

Although developed to explain experimental data concerning frequency selective adaptation, the adaptive equalizer model is mainly of interest because it can explain how the nervous system might compensate for the frequency dependent dynamics of the labyrinth and oculomotor plant. Thus, we envisage a highly versatile adaptive mechanism capable of tuning the developing reflex and then maintaining its performance despite the inevitable deterioration of its components. Rigorous tests of hypotheses about brain function require precise, mathematical formulations rarely achievable in practice. Happily, oculomotor function seems to be one of the exceptions. By its explicit nature the structure of the equalizer model raises new issues in thinking about the vestibu-lo-ocular reflex and may allow further progress in both theoretical and experimental studies of this fundamental brain function.

**Acknowledgements**

S.G.L. is supported by NIH grant EY03878, by the Alfred P. Sloan Foundation and the McKnight Foundation.

Adaptive mechanisms in gaze control
Facts and theories
*Eds. Berthoz & Melvill Jones*
© 1985 Elsevier Science Publishers BV (Biomedical Division)

# Chapter 22

# Commissural vestibular nuclear coupling: a powerful putative site for producing adaptive change

## H.L. Galiana

*Aerospace Medical Research Unit, Department of Physiology, McGill University, 3655 Drummond Street, Montréal, Québec, Canada H3G 1Y6*

## 1. Introduction

Parts I and II of this book demonstrate an abundance of recent advances in our understanding of the neurophysiology and neuroanatomy of central neural networks, responsible for the control of gaze and its adaptive modulation. Indeed, the many interactive elements have today become too complex for reliable intuitive interpretation of their functional significance. As a result, powerful analytical tools are now being introduced to properly evaluate the operation of the whole system. For example, we have seen the application of matrix theory in expanding our understanding of VOR operation to multiple degrees of freedom (Chapters 15, 19 and 20). The potential variety of central responses in multiple parallel pathways has been explored by Miles et al. (Chapter 21) as a possible mechanism for frequency selective adaptation of the VOR. In the saccadic system too, Optican (Chapter 4) has proposed analytically viable models to account for identified adaptive characteristics in the related pulse and step generating mechanisms of this system (see also Ch. 12).

However, a notable feature common to all these studies is that they envisage the system under question as a linear model in which bilateral connectivity between the two sides of the brain serves only to improve the reliability, and perhaps the sensitivity, of central processes. In other words, the lumped linear model is presumed to represent equally well the dynamic properties of pathways on one side of the brain stem, or of push-pull interactions between the two sides. In particular, consideration does not appear to have been given previously to the possibility that the bilateral aspect of these central processes may have an important role to play in defining the *dynamics*, as well as the sensitivity, of observed reflexes.

This chapter aims to show that commissural pathways interconnecting the two sides of the brain stem represent a powerful putative site for adaptative modulation of *both* the static (gain, resting rates) and dynamic (time constants) characteristics of vestibular responses. This postulate relies on the probability that some commissural pathways form closed positive feedback loops between the bilateral vestibular nuclei (VN). Admittedly, such a structural property remains to be proven experimentally. Nevertheless, as detailed elsewhere (Galiana & Outerbridge, 1984; Galiana et al., 1984), it is highly compatible with currently available experimental observations.

First, the experiments of Shimazu and Precht (1966) suggested that type I vestibular cells in the medial VN excite contralateral type II cells, and that these in turn inhibit type I cells on the same side. Recently, Nakao et al. (1982) used spike triggered averaging to prove that type II cells can inhibit monosynaptically 2° tonic type I cells projecting to the abducens nuclei, concurring with the findings of McCrea et al. (1980) using horseradish peroxidase (HRP). Hence some commissural pathways passing through type II cells in the cat act on *efferent* secondary vestibular neurons (viz., $V_L$ projecting to $O_R$ via $a_R$ or $g_R$ in Fig. 1).

Second, some secondary type I vestibular cells, projecting to the contralateral abducens nuclei, also project to the contralateral medial VN, an area symmetrically contralateral to that of their soma (McCrea et al., 1980, 1981). Furthermore, many type II cells in these same areas exhibit, albeit in mirror fashion, all of the known characteristics of efferent type I cells: for example, modulation with saccades or quick phases, a long time constant reflecting integration of the canal signal during normal VOR responses, and a deterioration in the integration time constant after cerebellectomy (Nakao et al., 1982; Keller & Precht, 1979b). Taken together, these results imply that at least some commissural type II cells are excited by contralateral *efferent* vestibular fibers, thereby closing the loop between the VN (in Fig. 1, only commissural projections via the gains $g_R$ and $g_L$ satisfy these conditions).

Given the known susceptibility of commissural pathways for plastic change (Dieringer & Precht, 1979a,b; Ott, 1982; Korte & Friedrich 1979) (Chapter 17), and the observed parallel improvement in both static and dynamic reflexes during recovery from unilateral vestibular lesions (Schaefer & Meyer, 1981; Dieringer & Precht, 1981; Maioli et al., 1983), the commissural system should be explored as a potential target for adaptive modulation of reflexes, in the healthy or lesioned brain. As will be shown below, the commissural system is considered as a prime candidate here, because small parametric changes in closed loops at this level could have unexpectedly powerful repercussions on reflex response characteristics.

Before proceeding with the analytic treatment, it should be emphasized that the following study concentrates specifically on the effects of parametric (e.g., gain) changes at various possible sites, relying on analysis of simple models of the coupled VN to draw conclusions about the functional consequences. That is, the effects of possible 'memory traces' are to be compared, without delving into the more complicated issue of the nature of any local plastic mechanism or the 'teaching line' which would force the plastic change. Also, cross-midline pathways in this study are not restricted conceptually to the brain stem commissure, but could include a general trans-midline system through reticular and/or cerebellar pathways.

## 2. Static properties of commissural coupling

### 2.1. Analytic statement

This study will make use of simplified representations of coupling between the bilateral VN, in order to develop a feeling for the particular properties of feedback coupling between neural pools. In this section, dynamics will be omitted for the moment (see Section 3), and the system will be assumed linear. Thus, here, only the resting rates and sensitivities of central cells, namely the secondary VN cells of Fig. 1, will be related to the strength of cross-midline pathways. In Fig. 1, both feedback commissural pathways (with gains $g_R$ and $g_L$) and more classical feed-forward commissural pathways (with gains $a_R$ and $a_L$) have been included for generality. The effect of each type on the characteristics of central responses ($O_R$ and $O_L$) to primary afferent activity can be quite different (refer to Galiana et al., 1984, for a more detailed comparison). The simple static model in Fig. 1 could represent elements of the system in cat, for example, with disynaptic mutual inhibition via the brain stem commissure, and more indirect, multisynaptic excitation across the midline via vestibulo-reticulo-cerebellar pathways (Shimazu & Precht, 1966; Furuya et al., 1976); (Chapter 17). Here and elsewhere in this study, the subscripts R and L always refer to elements or activities on the right and left side of the brain stem, respectively.

In Fig. 1, activities on vestibular afferents are represented by the variables $V_R$ and $V_L$, while non-vestibular inputs are indicated with $r_R$ and $r_L$. Simple summation of the four inputs on each side gives

$$O_R = V_R + r_R + a_R V_L - g_R O_L$$
$$O_L = V_L + r_L + a_L V_R - g_L O_R$$

By recombining like terms, it can be shown that

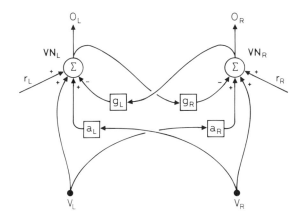

*Fig. 1.* A simple model of cross-midline coupling between the vestibular nuclei (VN). The subscripts $R$ and $L$ refer to the right and left side, respectively, of the brainstem. $V$, activity on primary vestibular afferents; $r$, activity on non-vestibular afferents; $O$, responses of VN efferent cells, projecting to motor nuclei; $g$, gain of inhibitory commissural pathways, linking the VN in feedback, closed-loop fashion; $a$, gain of excitatory cross-midline pathways, projecting multisynaptically from primaries to VN cells in feed-forward, push-pull fashion.

the efferent responses will be given by,

$$O_R = \frac{r_R + V_R(1-a_L g_R) - g_R(r_L + V_L) + a_R V_L}{1 - g_R g_L}$$

(1)

$$O_L = \frac{r_L + V_L(1-a_R g_L) - g_L(r_R + V_R) + a_L V_R}{1 - g_R g_L}$$

Note that because of the closed loop which links the two efferent responses (via *g*'s), commissural gains on *both* sides affect responses on *both* sides. On the other hand, purely feed-forward commissural connections would never have this property. This can be seen by setting all *g*'s to zero in Eqn. 1: then a feed-forward commissural gain (e.g., $a_R$) can only affect responses on one side (e.g., $O_R$).

The expressions in Eqn. 1 can be greatly simplified under certain conditions, as will be shown below. However, the general equations are worth noting here, as they are useful in the following arguments on compensation after lesions.

Assuming that vestibular primaries are mod-

ulated reciprocally about a constant resting level so that,

$$V_R = v + \Delta V$$
$$V_L = v - \Delta V$$

(2)

(where $v$ is primary resting rate) and allowing for bilateral symmetry in central gains and activities in the healthy system ($g_R = g_L = g$; $r_R = r_L = r$; $a_R = a_L = a$), then substituting Eqn. 2 into Eqn. 1 results in

$$O_R = \frac{r + v(1+a)}{1 + g} + \frac{\Delta V (1-a)}{1 - g}$$

(3)

$$O_L = \frac{r + v(1+a)}{1 + g} - \frac{\Delta V (1-a)}{1 - g}$$

(Note use of $1 - g^2 = (1-g)(1+g)$).

In Eqn. 3, the first terms represent resting efferent activity, whilst the second terms show the central modulations produced by changes in primary vestibular activity ($\Delta V$). Thus, it can be seen that the resting rates on the two sides will remain balanced for any level of commissural gains in the symmetrical model. On the other hand, the sensitivity of efferent response to peripheral stimulation is related to $(1-a)/(1-g)$. Several useful conclusions can be drawn: (i) the efferent cells will be excited by ipsilateral peripheral nerve stimulation (type I) for any combination of inhibitory and excitatory gains less than one ($a,g<1$); (ii) the sensitivity on efferent fibers will be greater than that of the primary sensor if net commissural inhibition is larger than the overall commissural excitation ($(1-a)/(1-g)>1$ implies $g>a$); (iii) the gain of efferent fibers (e.g., $O_R/\Delta V$) will be very sensitive to the level of commissural inhibition in closed loops, since as $g$ approaches one, the factor $1/(1-g)$ can become ver large.

Conditions (i) and (ii) above will be assumed as true in the normal system, for compatibility with observations in mammals. In turn, vestibular reflexes such as the VOR should be related to the central sensitivities, since VN efferent fibers generally project in push-pull fashion to the ocular motor nuclei. Considering eye movements to the right as positive, and bearing in mind the sign inversion due to the connectivity from central to ocular motor nuclei, Eqn. 3 yields

$$VOR \propto O_L - O_R = -2\,\Delta V\,(1-a)/(1-g) \qquad (4)$$

It is therefore clear that both the static characteristics of central responses and the VOR gain could vary greatly with commissural efficacy. The question now is what happens to VOR gain and central responses in the model of Fig. 1, after unilateral loss of primary modulation on one side? It will be shown that model responses after such a lesion are compatible with reported observations, assuming that compensation relies on known commissural changes (Dieringer & Precht, 1979; Ott, 1982).

## 2.2. After unilateral labyrinthectomy

A labyrinthectomy on the left side in Fig. 1 is equivalent to setting $V_L = v - \Delta V = 0$, with intact $V_R = v + \Delta V$ in Eqn. 1. Hence in the *acute* stage when central symmetry can still be assumed,

$$O_R = \frac{r(1-g) + v(1-ag)}{1-g^2} + \frac{\Delta V(1-ag)}{1-g^2}$$

$$(5)$$

$$O_L = \frac{r(1-g) - v(g-a)}{1-g^2} - \frac{\Delta V(g-a)}{1-g^2}$$

Comparing this equation with the normal conditions in Eqn. 3, the central responses in the acute case now show an increased resting activity (first term) and decreased sensitivity to the primary modulation $\Delta V$ (second term), when measured on the healthy side ($O_R$). On the lesioned side (left) however, *both* the resting activity, if present, and the sensitivity to primary modulation are decreased from normal levels. This can be verified by comparing Eqn. 5 to Eqn. 3 under the conditions $a<g<1$. All of these results are compatible with experimental observations in the acute stage after a labyrinthectomy, for example, head tilt and spontaneous nystagmus (slow phase) towards the lesioned side.

The VOR gain in this condition is reduced to

half of normal since in Eqn. 5,

$$(O_L-O_R) = -\Delta V(1-ag+g-a)/(1-g^2) = -\Delta V\,(1-a)/(1-g)$$

Note that Eqn. 5 only holds if the nucleus on the lesioned side remains spontaneously active or, more generally, if its spontaneous resting activity is positive, i.e.

$$r(1-g) - v(g-a) > 0$$

However in reality VN cells on the lesioned side are often silent in the acute condition, implying $v(g-a) > r(1-g)$, as would be expected with large primary resting rates ($v$) and a normal system with dominating inhibitory commissures ($g>a$). In this case, the central responses would initially be

$$O_L = 0$$
$$O_R = (r+v) + \Delta V \qquad (6)$$

which also indicates an increase in resting rate and a decrease in central sensitivity on the healthy side.

Restoration of resting activity on the lesioned side ($O_L$) during compensation could be achieved by forcing asymmetry in the commissural gains, thereby correcting for the asymmetry in afferent firing levels. In this case, Eqn. 5 must be restated in its more general form, allowing for such structural asymmetry. This is done by substituting $V_L = 0$ in the more general form of Eqn. 1;

$$O_R = \frac{r(1-g_R) + v(1-a_Lg_R)}{1-g_Rg_L} + \frac{\Delta V(1-a_Lg_R)}{1-g_Rg_L}$$

$$(7)$$

$$O_L = \frac{r(1-g_L) - v(g_L-a_L)}{1-g_Rg_L} - \frac{\Delta V(g_L-a_L)}{1-g_Rg_L}$$

Thus, after a left loss, balance of central resting rates (when $\Delta V=0$) requires equal numerators in the first terms of Eqn. 7, or

$$r(1-g_R) + v(1-a_Lg_R) = r(1-g_L) - v(g_L-a_L)$$

By recombining, the following condition results,

$$\frac{(1 + g_L)}{(1 + g_R)} = \frac{r + a_L v}{r + v} \qquad (8)$$

Eqn. 8 sets a general condition on valid relative weights of inhibitory and excitatory commissural pathways, but does not define a unique set.

However, assuming for the moment that balance has been achieved, the new VOR gain will be defined (from Eqn. 7) by the relation

$$VOR \propto O_L - O_R = \frac{-\Delta V[1 + g_L - a_L(1+g_R)]}{1 - g_R g_L}$$

which, by substituting Eqn. 8, can be reduced to

$$VOR \propto \frac{-\Delta V (1+g_R)(1-a_L) r}{(1-g_R g_L)(r+v)} \qquad (9)$$

Thus, in order to preserve the compensatory nature of the VOR, the new commissural gains are restricted to $a_L < 1$, and $g_R g_L < 1$. Referring to Eqn. 8, this implies that balance recovery must be achieved with $g_R > g_L$, that is, stronger inhibition on the healthy than on the lesioned side. Several strategies could satisfy this condition, such as only decreasing the inhibition on the lesioned side, or only increasing it on the healthy side.....etc. Referring to Eqn. 9, the first strategy would decrease the VOR gain even further below acute deficient levels; the second strategy could improve it. However the most efficient way to simultaneously balance central activities and increase the VOR gain above acute levels, would be *bilateral* increases in the commissural inhibition, albeit to asymmetric levels.

It is worth noting that the parameter conditions derived above would guarantee Type I responses on the healthy side, but not necessarily on the lesioned side, and this despite an improved and appropriate VOR. Though commissural excitation on the lesioned side was restricted to less than one, it may have been forced to values greater than the ipsilateral commissural inhibition in the initial process of restoring spontaneous activity in acutely silenced cells (i.e., with $a_L > g_L$ in Eqn. 7). As a result, Type II responses would be observed with greater frequency on the lesioned side (see $O_L$, first and second terms in Eqn. 7).

## 2.3. After unilateral canal plugging

If only primary *modulation* is blocked on the left side, as achieved for example by canal plugging (see Chapter 9), this is equivalent to setting only $\Delta V_L = 0$ in Fig. 1 (Eqns. 1 and 2). No net change in resting symmetry at either input or output levels would result acutely, and central responses would now be expressed as

$$O_R = \frac{r + v(1+a)}{1 + g} + \frac{\Delta V(1-ag)}{1 - g^2}$$
$$\qquad (10)$$
$$O_L = \frac{r + v(1+a)}{1 + g} - \frac{\Delta V(g-a)}{1 - g^2}$$

In the acute condition, resting activities are balanced and equal to the normal condition (compare Eqn. 3). However the VOR gain is reduced by half (viz., $O_L - O_R$), as in the case of a unilateral labyrinthectomy. Central sensitivities are also less than normal, though still of Type I bilaterally since $g > a$ is assumed in the healthy system.

As in the case of unilateral labyrinthectomy, the VOR gain could be increased by bilaterally increasing the commissural inhibition ($g$), though here at *equal* rates since symmetry in resting rates is already satisfied. This would be associated with a bilateral decrease in the new central resting rates, since the first terms in Eqn. 10 decrease with increases in $g$. This could be corrected by increasing commissural excitation ($a$ in Fig. 1) in a parallel fashion though not necessarily at the same rate.

Since the primary resting rates are already adequate on both sides and, since initially $a < g$ in the normal system, it can be shown that the required change in excitatory gain ($a$) to maintain near normal resting activity would be much smaller than any change in inhibitory gain ($g$). Hence, inhibitory commissures would continue to dominate during VOR adaptation ($g > a$) and central responses on *both* sides would remain throughout Type I. This would be in contrast to the case of unilateral labyrinthectomy, where loss of primary resting activity may require predominance of commissural excitation on the lesioned side in order to restore spontaneous activity (previous section), thereby resulting in Type II sensitivities on the lesioned side.

## 2.4. Summary of static properties

The above analytic study illustrates how both the balance of central resting rates in the bilateral brain stem, and the gain of push-pull reflexes such as the VOR, could be manipulated by organized control over neural pathways in a generalized commissural system. It is only required that at least some of the commissural connections provide closed feedback loops across the midline.

The analytic predictions are compatible with experimental observations. For example, Dieringer & Precht (1979) reported increases in the efficacy of both excitatory and inhibitory commissural pathways in the frog, after unilateral labyrinthectomy. Similarly, observations confirm a higher incidence of Type II responses on the lesioned side after unilateral labyrinthectomy, but a normal distribution of Type I responses after adaptation of the VOR following unilateral canal plugging (Chapter 17). Thus, increased inhibition from the remaining labyrinth to the VN on the lesioned side is fully compatible with Type II responses on that side. The first represents short delay effects, which may dominate during testing of evoked potentials with artificial stimulation; while the second may only appear in integrated responses to more natural stimuli, reflecting the combination of both short (disynaptic inhibition) and longer (multisynaptic excitation) pathways.

If a second labyrinthectomy were performed in a *fully compensated animal*, the resulting Bechterew phenomenon (Chapters 9, 18 and 20) would follow directly from asymmetric commissural gains in feedback loops, now distributing unevenly the currently symmetrical inputs remaining to the VN ($r_R = r_L$ in Fig. 1; see Galiana et al., 1984, for more details). In fact, any intervention which disturbs the bias in resting rates for which the system has compensated (whether surgical or pharmacological) will cause a decompensation or overcompensation in the model. This is because the asymmetry in commissural gains which affects responses on both sides would no longer be appropriate for the new conditions. This particular property could never follow from plasticity in

a system of purely feed-forward commissures: other processes would have to be included.

The implication of non-cerebellar pathways in vestibular compensation seems clear, since cerebellar lesions may retard but never completely block recovery of postural balance, or elimination of spontaneous nystagmus (Llinás et al., 1975; Haddad et al., 1977). However, adaptive gain control of the balanced VOR can be completely lost following such lesions (Haddad et al., 1977; Ito et al., 1974b), and it is interesting that cerebellar lesions involving trans-midline connections seem the most detrimental to oculomotor adaptive function (Eckmiller & Westheimer, 1983; Schaefer & Meyer, 1981). The results to date cannot tell us whether the cerebellum forms part of the pathways serving as a 'teaching line' and/or is required as part of a larger commissural network. It is worth noting here that only one intervention so far apparently completely blocks vestibular compensation, and that is section of the vestibular commissure as shown in frog by Bienhold and Flohr (1978).

Vestibular compensation most likely relies on neural plasticity integrated over several sites (Llinás & Walton, 1979b). However, the fact that recovery of central symmetry and VOR adaptation often proceed at different rates (Chapter 17) (Schaefer & Meyer, 1981; Paige, 1983a,b) is not sufficient in itself to require different 'memory traces' or sites of plasticity for each process. This remains an open question. For example, one could argue that both systems rely on commissural plasticity, but that the 'teaching line' signalling VOR deficiencies cannot influence commissural VN pathways until these have recovered sufficient spontaneous activity to allow plastic modulation by the error signal.

## 3. Dynamic properties of commissural coupling

So far, the significance of commissural feedback loops has only been investigated in terms of their influence on central resting rates and steady state reflex gains, with no regard as to possible repercussions on reflex dynamics. This aspect will now be investigated, using a simple extension of the model in Fig. 1. As in the previous section, the analysis will first study the healthy, normal VOR,

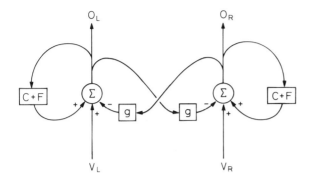

*Fig. 2.* A bilateral representation of VOR central pathways, during slow phase compensatory responses. The VN are linked across the midline by mutual inhibition of gain, *g* (refer to Fig. 1), and receive ipsilateral signals via feedback from cerebellar and brainstem pathways, respectively represented by *C* and *F* (see text; figure simplified from Fig. 2 of Galiana & Outerbridge, 1984).

so that structural symmetry can be assumed. Possible mechanisms for adaptation of the normal VOR will then be explored and compared. Changes in VOR dynamics following unilateral canal plugging, and their subsequent recovery in the model will then be discussed.

### 3.1. The VOR model

A simplified version of the VOR model presented by Galiana & Outerbridge (1984) will be used here to illustrate the following arguments. Thus, in Fig. 2, The bilateral VN, denoted by the summing symbol, $\Sigma$, are interconnected by inhibitory commissural pathways of gain $g$, as in Fig. 1. Each VN also receives feedback signals through ipsilateral cerebellar pathways of gain $C$, and brain stem pathways with gain $F$.

For reasons previously discussed (Galiana & Outerbridge, 1984), the gain $F$ is presumed to represent a filtering process in the brain stem, whose response resembles that of a first-order filter with a time constant near that of the eye plant ($\sim0.3$ s). Hence, though the ipsilateral feedback loops can be lumped in one element of gain '$C+F$', each remains expressed separately. This is because $F$ is envisioned as a model of the eye plant, and is therefore not expected to vary during plas-

tic adaptation of the VOR with normal eye plant dynamics. Thus, only the relative effects of parametric changes in cerebellar ($C$) or commissural ($g$) pathways will be compared in the following analysis. Because $F$ is assumed to play the role of an eye plant model, the VN responses will be shown to incorporate not only an integration function on primary signals, but also will have the required frequency characteristics to compensate for the eye plant dynamics, as suggested by Skavensky and Robinson (1973) for premotor neurons.

The VN responses, $O_R$ and $O_L$, in Fig. 2 can be considered as representing 2° vestibular cells projecting to the ocular motor nuclei. Since here we are dealing with dynamic responses, the Laplace transform of variables will be used so that equations can be manipulated algebraically. Thus, VN responses to the primary signals, $V_R$ and $V_L$, can be expressed as

$$O_R = V_R - gO_L + (C+F)\,O_R$$
$$O_L = V_L - gO_R + (C+F)\,O_L$$

Recombining to solve for each VN output,

$$O_R = \frac{V_R\,(1-C-F) - gV_L}{(1-C-F+g)\,(1-C-F-g)} \tag{11}$$

$$O_L = \frac{V_L\,(1-C-F) - gV_R}{(1-C-F+g)\,(1-C-F-g)}$$

where boldface type is used to represent the Laplace transform of variables. The filter, $F$, is assumed to have a gain, $K$, and time constant, $T$, so that in Laplace transforms it is expressed as

$$F = K\,/\,(Ts+1) \tag{12}$$

where $s$ is the Laplace variable. As in the previous section, one can assume $V_R = v/s + \Delta V$, $V_L = v/s - \Delta V$ during normal modulation of canal primary afferents. Substituting this and Eqn. 12 into Eqn.

11, and assuming zero initial conditions, we find that,

$$O_R = \frac{v\,(Ts+1)}{(1-C-K+g)\,(T_cs+1)\,s}$$

$$+ \frac{\Delta V\,(Ts+1)}{(1-C-K-g)\,(T_ds+1)}$$

$$O_L = \frac{v\,(Ts+1)}{(1-C-K+g)\,(T_cs+1)\,s}$$

$$- \frac{\Delta V\,(Ts+1)}{(1-C-K-g)\,(T_ds+1)}$$

(13)

where

$$T_c = T\,(1-C+g)\,/\,(1-C-K+g)$$

$$T_d = T\,(1-C-g)\,/\,(1-C-K-g)$$

(14)

As before, the first terms in the VN responses refer to resting activity, while the second terms now include the dynamics of responses to reciprocal modulation on the primaries. Thus a special dynamic property of feedback coupling across the midline is already clear: namely, despite the presence of a single time constant ($T$) in the processes on each side of the brain stem, bilateral coupled responses will exhibit *two* time constants widely separated in amplitude ($T_c$ and $T_d$ in Eqn. 14). Neither of these two time constants is equal to that of the original brain stem filter ($F$). In Eqn. 13, the first terms will be referred to as the 'common mode' responses, with time constant $T_c$, because they represent central responses to those components which are *common* to the bilateral afferent activity. The second terms will be referred to as the 'difference mode' responses, with time constant $T_d$, caused by those components of primary modulation on the two sides which are reciprocal or *differential* ($\Delta V$ in this case).

In the case of inhibitory commissural connections ($g>0$ in Fig. 2), Eqns. 13 and 14 indicate that the central responses to *reciprocal* modulation on the primaries will also be reciprocal (opposite sensitivities to $\Delta V$) and have a time constant ($T_d$) which can be (from Eqn. 14) much larger than the time constant ($T$) of the brain stem

filter. In fact, the difference mode responses can approach the 'integral' of primary modulation ($\Delta V$), so that $T_d$ represents the VOR time constant.

On the other hand, the common mode responses (first terms in Eqn. 13) to equal bilateral primary resting rates will have a much shorter time constant ($T_c \ll T_d$, when $g>0$ in Eqn. 14), and will not even be observed if central activity is already at its normal resting level. That is, if the filter initial conditions are at the normal resting level of $R = Kv/(1-C+g)$, rather than the assumed zero level, then the first terms in Eqn. 13 would be reduced to $R/s$, a simple D.C. bias.

Interestingly, should excitatory mutual coupling dominate between two neural pools ($g<0$ in Fig. 2), then the dynamics of common and difference modes in Eqn. 13 will be reversed: i.e., responses to equal bilateral inputs will now reflect a long integrating time constant, while responses to opposite or reciprocal inputs will have short time constants and opposite sensitivities in the two pools. Thus, feedback coupling between neural pools may play a significant role in postural or limb control as well, since multi-modal responses are known to occur during muscle agonist-antagonist interactions (Humphrey et al., 1983).

Here, mutual inhibition is assumed to dominate in the brain stem VOR, so that a large time constant ($T_d$) and stability in the system can be guaranteed for all parameters satisfying $(1-C-K-g)>0$. Also, because of the assumption that the brain stem filter time constant is near that of the eye plant, the lead term ($Ts+1$) in the VN responses will compensate for the eye plant dynamics. Hence these VN responses are suitable premotor ocular signals.

### 3.2. Controlling dynamics in the normal VOR

Fig. 2 represents the bilateral VOR in the normal system, in the slow phase mode. Insofar as conjugate ocular responses are concerned, an equivalent linear model of the VOR can be derived from Fig. 2. By neglecting the effects of initial conditions (see Galiana & Outerbridge, 1984, for a discussion on this point), the difference between $O_R$ and $O_L$ in Fig. 2 can be represented by the lumped VN response, $O$, in the linear model of

Fig. 3. VN responses in turn drive the eye plant whose time constant $T_e$ is presumed near that of the filter $F$ $(=T)$. Note that contrary to most linear models of the VOR, the effects of both commissural $(g)$ and ipsilateral feedback $(C+F)$ loops on response dynamics have been preserved, as indicated. However, in moving to this linear equivalent, all information on central resting rates and the rapid common mode of responses has been lost.

For the purposes of this article, the primary modulation in response to head rotation will be modelled as a simple overdamped angular accelerometer, with a normalized gain of one. Thus, if $\dot{H}$ represents horizontal head velocity, the Laplace transform of the primary modulation is given by

$$\Delta V = \dot{H}\, sT_1/(sT_1+1) \tag{15}$$

with $T_1$ representing the slow canal time constant of approximately 4 s in cat.

The overall responses to head rotation in Fig. 3 can then be found by substituting Eqn. 15 for $\Delta V$ in Eqn. 13 and solving for $O = O_R - O_L$, so that

$$O\,/\,\dot{H} = G\,s\,T_1\,(Ts+1)\,/\,(T_1s+1)(T_ds+1)$$
$$\dot{E}\,/\,\dot{H} \propto -\,G\,s^2\,T_1\,T\,/\,(T_1s+1)(T_ds+1) \tag{16}$$

where $G = 2\,/\,(1-C-K-g)$ and, as before, $T_d = T(1-C-g)/(1-C-K-g)$. Remember that model parameters are assumed to be set at levels which provide for a large $T_d$, and that $T_e$ is assumed equal to the central filter time constant $T$. From Eqn. 16, the gain of the VOR in the canal passband is therefore proportional to $G \cdot T/T_d$, which reduces to $2/(1-C-g)$. Hence it is clear that both the VOR gain and its time constant $(T_d)$ will vary with the parameters $C$ and $g$. In fact, at least in this case of the VOR in the dark where visual effects have not been included, it would not be possible to differentiate between parametric changes at cerebellar or commissural levels, because they affect the conjugate VOR responses in exactly the same way.

These comments are illustrated in Fig. 4, showing the frequency characteristics of central and ocular response gains to head velocity, as deter-

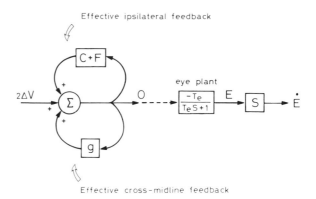

Effective ipsilateral feedback

eye plant

Effective cross-midline feedback

Fig. 3. An equivalent linear representation of the bilateral model presented in Fig. 2. VN efferent signals, $O$, project directly to the eye plant, controlling eye position, $E$. Note that the original effect of commissural feedback loops on VOR dynamics has been preserved, as indicated by the loop gain, $g$. The eye plant is represented by a first-order filter with time constant $T_e$. $2\Delta V$ represents the push-pull modulation on vestibular afferents during head angular rotation.

mined from Eqn. 16. The vertical scale is only to be used for reference in determining *relative* gain changes over the frequency range: actual gain levels could be shifted up or down by varying primary and oculomotor synaptic sensitivities.

The gain of central VN responses with respect to head velocity is presented in Fig. 4A (solid lines). Above the canal break frequency $(1/2\pi T_1)$, these central responses would resemble tonic vestibular cells, modulating with head position during sustained slow phase compensation in the dark. Below this canal break frequency, the VN cells have a much larger gain and appear to be 'tuned' to head velocity over a bandwidth which is very sensitive to the level of cerebellar or commissural gain. An example of decreasing the model loop gains is depicted by the dashed line, and predicts decreased central gain, and increased phase lead at the lower frequencies. Because of the premotor nature of these modelled VN cells, their gain levels off at the frequency corresponding to the eye plant time constant.

The corresponding gain of the VOR in the dark ($\dot{E}/\dot{H}$ is presented in Fig. 4B. Again, it is clear that decreases in VOR gain, achieved by decreasing cerebellar or commissural loop gains, will be associated with deterioration in the VOR

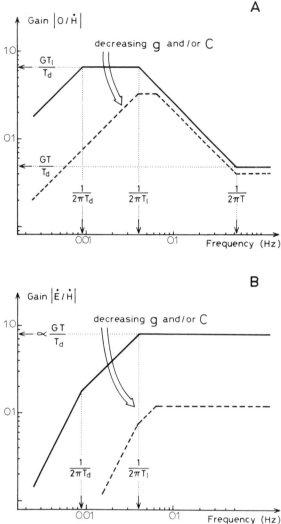

Fig. 4. The gain characteristics of VN (A) and ocular (B) responses in Fig. 3, are described with respect to head velocity ($H$) at different sinusoidal frequencies. The solid lines are an example of the VOR characteristics with $T_e = T = 0.3$ s; $T_d = 15$ s; and a canal time constant $T_1 = 4$ s. The dashed lines describe changes in response dynamics as commissural and/or cerebellar loops decrease in gain (see text).

time constant. This can be seen as a shift of the VOR towards the right.

These analytic predictions are compatible with experimental observations. For example, Keller and Precht (1979a) reported such decreases in the VOR time constant, when forcing reductions in the VOR gain with reversing prisms. More re-

cently, Maioli et al. (1983), and Paige (1983a,b) reported that unilateral vestibular interventions caused reductions in the acute VOR gain, associated with deterioration in the time constant of central integration. Neural plasticity in VOR feedback loops could account for the fact that dynamic modifications often accompany any gain changes.

Cerebellar and commissural loop changes would theoretically be equally effective, and may well proceed in parallel, though not necessarily at the same rate. This is deduced from the fact that vestibular compensation which is known to be associated with commissural changes proceeds very slowly (days or weeks) and continues even in the absence of cerebellar pathways (Haddad et al., 1977). On the other hand, the synaptic efficacy of Purkinje cells in VOR cerebellar pathways has been shown to be modifiable at very short latencies (Ito et al., 1982c).

### 3.3. VOR dynamics after unilateral canal plugging

VOR dynamics after unilateral plugging of the horizontal canal would be expected to have characteristics different from the normal case, because primary inputs to the VN would no longer have their purely complementary nature. This is better illustrated by returning to a bilateral representation of the reflex (see Fig. 2 and Eqn. 11). If one substitutes

$$V_R = v/s + \Delta V; \; V_L = v/s,$$

into Eqn. 11, remembering that $F = K/(Ts+1)$, then if the system is initially at its normal resting rate when rotational stimulation begins, the responses can be expressed as

$$O_R = \frac{v}{s(1-C+g)}$$

$$+ \frac{\Delta V \,(Ts+1)}{2(1-C-K-g)(T_d s+1)}$$

$$+ \frac{\Delta V \,(Ts+1)}{2(1-C-K+g)(T_e s+1)}$$

$$\tag{19}$$

$$O_L = \frac{v}{s(1-C+g)}$$

$$- \frac{\Delta V\,(Ts+1)}{2(1-C-K-g)(T_d s+1)}$$

$$+ \frac{\Delta V(Ts+1)}{2(1-C-K+g)(T_c s+1)}$$

The time constants $T_d$ and $T_c$ are as defined previously in Eqn. 14.

Thus, at the central level, there are two important effects of restricting primary modulation to one side. First, there is the expected halving of central difference mode responses (2nd terms in Eqn. 19, compare to Eqn. 13), which provide the reciprocal long time constant modulations driving the VOR. Second, there now appears another component in central responses, the common-mode (3rd terms in Eqn. 19), which is modulated in equal fashion on both sides by primary modulation, and reflects a much shorter time constant ($T_c < T_d$). This second component does not appear in normal responses to reciprocal, bilateral primary modulations (see text related to Eqn. 13). This characteristic of bilateral coupled networks should be kept in mind, when attempting to compare the properties of central responses during any form of one-sided stimulation, whether by rotation or electrical stimulation.

As before, the gain of the VOR in the canal passband would be related to the difference between $O_R$ and $O_L$ in Eqn. 19, i.e., to $1/(1-C-g)$ in this case. This acute gain level could be gradually restored to near normal levels by increasing the cerebellar and/or commissural pathway gains. However, note that in the case of the now observable common mode responses (3rd terms in Eqn. 19), parametric changes along commissural and cerebellar loops are *not* equivalent. In fact, increases in cerebellar efficacy would increase the amplitude of central common mode responses, while increases in commissural gain would decrease the common mode response.

Thus, the observations of Paige (1983b) (see also Chapter 9) would tend to support a commissural role in VOR adaptation after unilateral plugging of the horizontal canal in squirrel monkey. He reported the occurrence of a bias in the VOR, which was dependent on stimulus intensity under two conditions: (i) during rotation at peak head velocities greater than 360°/s in the normal animal, and (ii) at lower head velocities (>120°/s) in the acutely plugged animal. This bias was subsequently reduced as VOR gain and time constant improved, so that it could only be observed at the larger stimulus levels. Only commissural gain changes in the model would be compatible with the observations.

Since these results were obtained with monocular measurements, they may reflect a VOR component in vergence control of eye movements. The analytic results here indicate that the common mode component of central vestibular responses could cause such biases, given bilateral excitatory projections to, say, the oculomotor (III) nuclei (Furuya & Markham, 1981; Uchino et al., 1982). This component would appear whenever reciprocity in bilateral input levels was lost, e.g., (i) when the primary on one side is cut off by high intensity contralateral rotation, or (ii) when reciprocity is eliminated by total loss of modulation on one side.

### 3.4. Summary of dynamic properties

It would appear that commissural pathways should be investigated as a powerful putative site for adaptive control of VOR gain and dynamics, not only in the lesioned subject, but also in normals. The deteriorated VOR time constant which is observed acutely after unilateral labyrinthectomy or unilateral canal plugging (Chapter 9) (Maioli, 1983) would be compatible with the postulate that commissural pathways contribute to the realization of the VOR integrator. In the first case, the commissural feedback loop would become ineffective due to silencing or very low resting rates on VN cells in the lesioned side. In the second case, there would be less recruitment of commissural fibers (i.e., effectively a smaller 'g') because of the reduced central modulation with head rotation. This could represent another factor in the often noted observation that VOR gain and time constant can improve with the intensity of vestibular stimulation, though this is more usually ascribed to a general increase in alertness. As shown analytically, the same arguments could apply in the case of cerebellar plasticity during adaptation of the normal VOR. However, only commissural changes seem compatible here with the pattern of observations during adaptation to unilateral canal plugging.

It is worth noting that the frequency characteristics described in Fig. 4 are remarkably similar to those presented by Miles et al. (Chapter 21) in an equivalent frequency range. Perhaps commissural coupling between many pools of VN cells, each tuned to the desired bandpass range, would be one mechanism of realizing the parallel channels they propose for selective frequency tuning of the VOR. After all, the firing patterns of secondary VN cells projecting to the motor nuclei in the cat can range all the way from near-primary characteristics, to purely tonic activity modulated by eye position (Baker & Berthoz, 1974; Hikosaka et al., 1977; Berthoz et al., 1981b; Nakao et al., 1982). One example to achieve various cell populations in the VN has been presented elsewhere (Galiana & Outerbridge, 1984). It is also likely that commissural pathways play a role in defining the matrix elements used to represent three-dimensional VOR transformations from sensory to oculomotor planes of operation (see Chapter 20).

Should vestibular adaptation rely on plasticity at commissural levels, then the new VOR characteristics would affect any visual reflexes which share these pathways. Second-order VN cells are known to respond equally well during vestibular nystagmus, or optokinetic nystagmus in the appropriate directions, within the range of stimulus amplitudes allowing linear responses (Waespe & Henn, 1979a). Many behavioural observations during VOR adaptation are consistent with sharing of adapted pathways by these reflexes (Paige, 1983a,b; Lisberger et al., 1981; Keller and Precht, 1979a), and so support the plausibility of a commissural role.

In this context, it is sometimes stated that decreases in the OKN gain, which may accompany adaptive decreases in the VOR gain, are 'maladaptive', on the grounds that high gains in visual pathways would always be useful (Lisberger et al., 1981). However, in all cases the new VOR in the light is always appropriate for the adapted conditions. Furthermore, VOR adaptation cannot be achieved without access to visual errors (Chapter 2), and a purely optokinetic stimulus is not natural to our environment. It might therefore be more pertinent to consider the performance of the VOR in the light, when evaluating the 'adaptive' quality of any change. Incidentally, one could argue that with a reduced VOR gain, visual pathways need no longer be so strong in order to permit occasional suppression of the VOR, whereas they would have to be more powerful to effectively suppress a VOR of increased gain.

## 4. Conclusions

Because of the known highly plastic synaptic efficacy in Purkinje cells, it is often argued that cerebellar pathways are the sole contributor to VOR adaptation, especially when the new VOR characteristics are within normal reflex operation and easily achieved (Chapters 3 and 14). However, one cannot ignore the fact that commissural changes are known to occur during long term vestibular compensation, and that such changes could theoretically equally contribute to adaptation of VOR dynamics. Hence, commissural pathways should be further explored as a powerful putative site for vestibular reflex plasticity.

Clearly, cerebellar pathways can contribute to rapid modifications of the VOR (Waespe et al., 1983; Ito, 1982; Ito et al., 1982a,b,c; Lisberger & Fuchs, 1978a,b; Dufosse et al., 1978a,b; Robinson, 1976), and might even initially suffice for small adaptive changes. However, there is no reason to presuppose that the contributing plastic site should remain at the cerebellar level. Despite constant reflex characteristics at the ocular level, neural plasticity could be progressively transferred to another site, in the long term, such as the commissural connections. Eventually the new VOR dynamics could depend fully on modifications in this alternate site, just as proposed by Miles and Lisberger (1981b). This would explain the presence of both rapid (minutes or hours) and slow (days) components reported in the time courses of VOR adaptation, when faced with difficult visual or lesion-induced adjustments (Gonshor & Melvill Jones, 1976b; Miles & Eighmy, 1980; Mandl et al., 1981; Maioli et al, 1983). When a required change is within the reach of the rapid component, only the short time constant would be observed, despite possible long term transference of the adaptive load to alternate neural pathways. In essence, the presence of a long term component in such cases may be masked by the maintained adequate performance at the ocular level.

Much more information on the characteristics of central vestibular responses throughout long term adaptation of the VOR is needed. Preliminary studies indicate that measurements during the VOR in the dark would not suffice to resolve present controversies (Galiana, 1983). This would require additional protocols to manipulate and observe associated visual-vestibular interactions at cerebellar and brainstem levels.

Adaptive mechanisms in gaze control
Facts and theories
Eds. Berthoz & Melvill Jones
© 1985 Elsevier Science Publishers BV (Biomedical Division)

Epilogue

# A compendium of questions concerning adaptive mechanisms

## G. Melvill Jones & A. Berthoz

After travelling with us thus far the reader may well be left wondering where the boundaries lie between established fact and imaginative speculation. Indeed, in the Introduction we were at pains to point out that one of our prime objectives was to focus on unanswered, rather than settled, questions. It is afterall curiosity for the approachable unknown which activates the valid scientific quest.

## 1. The fact of behavioural adaptation

There is, however, a single factual base on which all our contributors seem to agree: that is, the definition of a new class of behaviourally induced adaptive changes which can be realised in adult reflexes without invasive interference of the nervous system. Thus, we have seen that alteration of optic gain, whether augmentation, diminution or sign inversion, always produces more or less appropriate changes in the VOR. Again, maintained visual suppression of the reflex by a head-fixed target rapidly reduces VOR output towards a new 'ideal' gain of zero (Chapters 2 and 3). Halving the reflex input by surgical obstruction of fluid circulation in the lumen of one semicircular canal leads to vision-dependent gain recovery towards the 'ideal' value of unity (Chapter 9). Not only scalar gain, but also geometric relations between sensory input and motor output vectors prove readily malleable (Chapters 2 and 20).

Such findings are not restricted to the vestibulo-oculomotor system alone. In the saccadic system both gain and system dynamics are suscepti-ble to controlled remodelling (Chapter 4). The integrative mechanisms responsible for head-eye coordination can be adaptively changed according to a variety of different strategies (Chapter 12). Adaptive coupling between the separate neural mechanisms responsible for accommodation and vergence has been demonstrated (Chapter 5). Evidence suggests an adaptive potential in visuo-postural pathways (Chapter 2). Even the 'inviolate' monosynaptic spinal stretch reflex is no longer exempt from behavioural induction of 'adaptive' change (Wolpaw et al., 1983a,b).

Evidently, externally imposed behavioural influences can and do penetrate the CNS to produce functionally advantageous rearrangement of internal parameters such as neural gain, network dynamics (e.g., time constants) and even vectorial transforms between related sensory-motor functions: and all this in 'involuntary' reflex pathways previously thought to be relatively 'hard wired' in the mature nervous system.

## 2. Underlying cellular processes

So much for established fact. But reaching beyond the behavioural phenomena themselves towards their underlying central mechanisms we find ourselves teetering on the brink of controversy and speculation. First of all, can we even hope to lump these various behavioural phenomena into a single class of adaptive mechanisms? Almost certainly not. We have seen for example in Chapter 2 that, at one extreme, small changes incurred by prescription spectacles can be induced very rapidly whilst, at the other extreme, much longer term effects have been found in experiments extending over weeks and months. Again, while simple magnifying or diminishing lenses produce almost machine-like 'single state' system changes, reversing optics eventually induce puzzling, more complex, phenomena superimposed on the 'simple' ones (Chapter 2). In the saccadic system (Chapter 4), at least three different kinds of adaptive response, obeying quite different rules, have been described: and, as already noted, with free head movement the human subject can apparently choose from a variety of different available adaptive strategies, presumably based on quite different cellular mechanisms (Chapter 12).

In vestibular compensation for unilateral 8th nerve lesion (Chapters 17 and 18) the problem is further complicated by calling simultaneously for adjustment of differential bias as well as gain. The physiological resolution of this difficulty brings us face to face with one of the most fascinating questions of all: do the behaviourally induced adaptive phenomena described in Part I of the book depend in any way upon central plastic cellular processes akin to those known to be induced by neural lesions? It now seems certain that the bilateral imbalance induced in central vestibular nuclei by unilateral nerve ablation does indeed activate such processes; at least at the level of the intervestibular commissures (Chapter 17). But are these processes restricted to the influence of the peripheral nerve lesion per se? Or can they also be invoked by external 'behavioural' stimuli, such as retinal image slippage, produced for example by persistent unidirectional nystagmus or inadequate vestibular input to the VOR? Despite the rather 'heretical' implications of this possibility, it is not out of line with findings of Tsukahara (1981) and colleagues, noted in Chapter 3. Recall that, after crossing the peripheral innervation of the hind limb, synaptic changes occurred at the remote central level of the red nucleus which were akin to those resulting from direct central neural lesions.

If these implications prove valid we may ask what kind of 'trophic' influences would be at play in generating a plastic central response to a behaviourally induced 'command'? Further than

this, we may ask whether such processes, if they occur, would be confined to adjustments of transmission efficacy within genetically predetermined pathways; or, on the other hand, might even extend to growth of new pathways, as seems to occur during metamorphosis of the flatfish (Chapter 1)? At the time of writing, answers simply are not available to questions such as these. Nevertheless, bearing in mind the factual nature of the behaviourally defined phenomena, we can at least be certain that there must be some kind of relevant central change; which raises the problem of the adaptive cellular response to a level of feasible exploratory investigation.

## 3. Significance of network design in the remodelling process

Turning from the cellular processes themselves to the part they might play in modifying the input-output characteristics of a cohesive reflex neural network, we have seen a variety of postulates emerge from different research teams (Chapters 3–5, 8, 12, 19–22). Historically the first working hypothesis, conceived by Ito and his colleagues (Chapter 14), focused on the concept of a special neural mechanism for adaptive control in a given reflex network. Specifically, for the VOR a transcerebellar side path comes under the influence of climbing fibre signals keyed to retinal image slippage. In turn these latter signals modulate the parameter of neural gain in the side path so as to readjust the overall VOR in such a way as to reduce the image slippage and thus restore automatic image stabilization during head movement.

It has been argued that this kind of 'personalized' or 'special' adaptive control might be too extravagant in neural tissue to cater for the full extent of known modifiability, including for example the broad range of conditioned reflexes (e.g., Flohr, 1983). Thus, at the opposite end of the spectrum of possibilities, a generalized scheme could be envisaged as operating through the medium of what might be termed a 'broadcast' system. Briefly an adverse behavioural situation would release a neuromodulator agent(s) which plays specifically upon those network pathways exhibiting abnormal activity, eventually to readjust their active state in such a way as to achieve a functionally advantageous alteration of behavioural performance and so in turn reduce the agent's release.

The 'diffuse' concept envisaged by Llinás and Pellionisz (Chapter 15) would seem to lie somewhere between these two extremes. They argue against the specific 'motor learning' role of cerebellar cortex in favour of a distributed process, acting at multiple sites within a given network. In the broader framework of their general tensor theory of sensory-motor signal processing (Chapter 19), the adaptive phenomenon is envisaged as an ubiquitous mechanism which essentially establishes and maintains proper signal transformations throughout all stages in the sequential moulding of a neural message on its way from the sensory periphery, through the CNS, to the final executive motor outflow.

As we have seen, a number of alternate hypotheses have been offered. There has for example been recurrent reference to the neurophysiological findings of Miles, Lisberger and colleagues (reviewed by Miles & Lisberger, 1981b), which also argue against the location of an adaptive 'learning' element of the VOR in cerebellar cortex. Rather, it is proposed that a derived signal of gaze velocity error is fed out from cerebellar cortex, to produce a suitable error-nulling gain change at some hypothetical site in the brain stem. Galiana (Chapter 22) suggests a site in the inter-vestibular commissural pathways which could theoretically serve this role. A particular feature here is the potentially powerful utilization of putative positive feedback loops linking the two sides of the bilateral system. In that chapter, emphasis is further placed on the potential for controlled alterations of efficacy in such pathways to produce dramatic (adaptive?) changes of system dynamics as well as gain; even to account for the concept of frequency selective channels proposed in Chapter 21.

Clearly, as at the cellular level, there is as yet no concensus on the question of where, or how, central processes act upon the system as a whole to bring about the behaviourally defined adaptive phenomena. Section IIB does, however, show that the very diversity of contemporary approaches offers a wide scope for further development in this intriguing field. The section also demonstrates the important fact that understanding cellular mechanisms per se is not enough; the part they play in the whole neural network must also be understood before the behavioural effect of a given change in synaptic efficacy can be rationalised.

## 4. Perceptual and reflex correlates

The modern introduction of 'alert behaving animals' to the neurophysiologist's laboratory is bringing the normally functioning nervous system within reach of the invasive microelectrode. The development is proving more significant than it might at first appear since, in conjunction with human experiments, it promises to yield insightful links between identified neural 'messages' in the CNS and related 'messages' formulated in the mind as perceptual impressions.

Let us be more specific to illustrate the point. Recent neurophysiological studies of vestibular neural signals in the brainstem of alert behaving animals (Chapter 16) have demonstrated a form of central neural message, (reflecting head movement relative to space), which may be quite different from, but more valid than, either of the two major primary afferent signals (vestibular and visual) from which it, (the central signal) is derived. Technically, the 'lead' transfer function of the semicircular canal becomes complemented by a centrally derived 'lag' function driven by vision, to form a 'symbiotic' whole (Robinson, 1977a,b), which constitutes a new central 'best estimate' of the real physical event. It is this new emergent central signal (rather than either of the two primary ones), which best correlates with reflexly induced slow phase eye movement.

The key issue here is that, in corresponding human experiments, perceptual impressions tend to follow the induced eye movement and hence, presumably, the 'reflexly' emergent central message, rather than the simple sum of peripheral, but individually *in*appropriate primary afferent signals. Does this indicate that common (brain stem?) processing may be at play in generating meaningfully related perceptual and reflex events. Seen in this light it is not altogether surprising to find that adaptive phenomena also demonstrate strong correlates between perceived and reflex events: recall the close relation between perceived self rotation and the adaptively augmented VOR reported by Gauthier & Robinson (1975) and reviewed in Chapter 2.

## 5. Matters of the mind

Even more provocative is the fact that a similar conclusion has recently been drawn for adaptive alterations induced by maintained mental effort alone, that is, in the absence of any visual input at all (Chapter 13). Simply 'thinking' of looking at a head-fixed target during head rotation produced 'adaptive' attenuation of the dark-tested VOR: and this attenuation also correlated well with a correspondingly attenuated perception of vestibularly sensed body movement in the dark. It seems that mental effort per se is capable of 'adaptively' altering fundamental neural parameters in the central symbiotic system. Does this imply that without meaningful contact between the internal world of the CNS and the external physical world, there will be drifting of controlling neural parameters according to the prevailing mental state? And bearing in mind the correlated relations between reflex performance and perceptual sensations, does this imply that without adaptive 'homeostasis' through contact with the real physical world, the veridical nature of its mental perception stands to be jeopardized? (Melvill Jones, 1983a).

Of course at this point we are trespassing somewhat recklessly in the fanciful fields of wild speculation. But should there be any truth in the matter, perhaps we have here new clues to mechanisms which underly disorganization of the mind. On the one hand we have seen, in Chapter 13, that normal human subjects exposed to prolonged periods of sensory deprivation become peculiarly susceptible to strong illusory perceptions. Could these be attributable to effective opening of the parametric feedback loop, normally essential for maintaining both proper reflex function and the veracity of perception? On the other hand we have also seen, in Chapter 11 that certain clinical conditions seem to arise from abnormal function of the adaptive mechanisms themselves. Presumably these, like all other body functions, are not except from pathological interference. In which case perhaps a new class of neurological syndromes will emerge, linked by a common type of failure which might be termed 'maladaptive disease'.

In the long term, and bearing in mind the perceptual and reflex correlates discussed above, we may even ask whether this conceptual approach could be extended to diseases of the mind? Is it possible, for example, that some psychotic conditions associated with illusory perceptions might also be attributable to pathological interference with those 'adaptive' processes which normally establish and maintain an acceptable level of veracity between the mentally perceived event and its physical reality?

### Enfin!

This brings us to the close of our 'review'. We have seen a fair spectrum of experimental findings which together define a somewhat novel aspect of homeostatic control within the central nervous system. Yet, as in any lively field of research, experimental and theoretical findings are opening up more questions than they resolve. However, as emphasised above, it was not our intent merely to recount, without question, the new knowledge which has emerged thus far. Rather, our main purpose has been to encourage the scientific quest in an emergent area where viable questions are currently unfolding in extravagant abundance. Our objective will indeed be fulfilled if the tales we have told stimulate interest and active research in this challenging new speciality of neuroscientific research.

# Bibliography

Abel, L.A., Schmidt, D., Dell'Oso, L.F. & Daroff, R.B. (1978) Saccadic system plasticity in humans. Ann. Neurol. 4, 313–318.

Abeln, W. & Flohr, H. (1982) Adrenergic synaptic changes in vestibular compensation. Verh. Dtsch. Zool. Ges. Fischer Verlag, 213.

Abeln, W., Bienhold, H. & Flohr, H. (1981) Influence of cholinomimetics and cholinolytics on vestibular compensation. Brain Res. 222, 458–462.

Abend, W.K. (1978) Response to constant angular accelerations of neurons in the monkey superior vestibular nucleus. Exp. Brain Res. 31, 459–473.

Albert, A. (1972) Regression & the Moore-Penrose Pseudoinverse. Academic Press, New York.

Albus, J.S. (1971) A theory of cerebellar function. Math. Biosci. 10, 25–61.

Allen, D.C. (1974) Vertical prism adaptation in anisometropes. Am. J. Opt. Physiol. Optics 51, 252–259.

Alley, K.E., Baker, R. & Simpson, J.I. (1975) Afferents to the vestibulo-cerebellum and the origin of the visual climbing fibers in the rabbit. Brain Res. 98, 582–589.

Allum, J.H.J. & Graf, W. (1977) Time constants of vestibular nuclei neurons in the goldfish: A model with ocular pro-prioception. Biol. Cybern. 28, 95–99.

Allum, J.H.J., Graf, W., Dichgans, J. & Schmidt, C.L. (1976) Visual vestibular interactions in the vestibular nuclei of the goldfish. Exp. Brain Res. 26, 463–485.

Alpern, M. (1946) The after-effect of lateral duction testing on subsequent phoria measurement. Am. J. Optom. Arch. Am. Acad. Optom. 23, 442–447.

Alpern, M. (1962) Part I: Movements of the eyes. In: II. Davson (Ed.) The Eye, Vol. 3. Academic Press, New York, pp. 3–187.

Alpern, M. (1969) Movements of the eyes. In: H. Davson (Ed.) The Eye, Vol. 3, 2nd Edn. Academic Press, New York, pp. 1–214.

Alpern, M. & David, H. (1958) Effects of illuminance quantity on accommodation of the eyes. Ind. Med. 27, 551–555.

Alpern, M. & Ellen, P. (1956a) A quantitative analysis of the horizontal movements of the eyes in the experiments of Johannes Mueller. I. Methods and results. Am. J. Ophthalmol. 42, 289–296.

Alpern, M. & Ellen, P. (1956b) A quantitative analysis of the horizontal movements of the eyes in the experiments of Johannes Mueller. II. Effect of variation in target separation. Am. J. Ophthalmol. 42, 296–303.

Alpern, M. & Larson, B.F. (1960) Vergence and accommodation: IV. Effect of luminance quantity on the AC/A. Am. J. Ophthalmol. 49, 1140–1149.

Alpern, M., Kincaid, W.M. & Lubeck, M.J. (1959) Vergence and accommodation: III. Proposed definitions of the AC/A ratios. Am. J. Ophthalmol. 48, 143–148.

Amat, J., Matus-Amat, P. & Vanegas, H. (1984) Visual (optokinetic) and somesthetic inputs to the cerebellum of bilaterally labyrinthectomized frogs. Neuroscience 11, 835–891.

Anderson, J.A., Silverstein, J.W., Ritz, S.A. & Randall, S.J. (1977) Distinctive features, categorical perception, and probability learning: Some applications of a neural model. Psychol. Rev. 84, 413–451.

Antal M., Tornai I., Székely G. (1980) Longitudinal extent of dorsal root fibres in the spinal cord and brain stem of the frog. Neuroscience 5, 1311–1322.

Arrott, A.P. (1982) Torsional eye movements in man during linear accelerations. S.M. Thesis, M.I.T., Cambridge, MA.

Arshavsky, Y.I., Gelfand, I.M. and Orlovsky, G.N. (1983) The cerebellum and control of rythmical movements. Trends Neurosci. 6, 417–422.

Atkin, A. & Bender, B. (1968) Ocular stabilization during oscillatory head movements. Arch. Neurol. (Chicago) 19, 559–566.

Atkinson, J. (1979) Development of optokinetic nystagmus in the human infant and monkey infant. An analogue to development in kittens. In: Freeman R. (Ed.) Developmental Neurobiology of Vision. Plenum Press, New York, pp. 277–287.

Autrum, H. (1959) Das Fehlen unwillkürlicher Augenbewegungen beim Frosch. Naturwiss. 46, 435.

Azzena, G.B. (1969) Role of the spinal cord in compensating the effects of hemilabyrinthectomy. Arch. Ital. Biol. 107, 43–53.

Azzena, G.B., Mameli, O. & Tolu, E. (1977) Vestibular units during decompensation. Experientia 33, 234–236.

Baarsma, E.A. & Collewijn H. (1974) Vestibulo-ocular and optokinetic reactions to rotation and their interaction in the rabbit. J. Physiol. (London) 238, 603–625.

Baarsma, E.A. & Collewijn, H. (1975) Changes in compensatory eye movements after unilateral labyrinthectomy in the rabbit. Arch. Oto-Rhino-Laryngol. 211, 219–230.

Bahill, T., Adler, D. & Stark, L. (1975a) Most naturally occurring human saccades have magnitudes of 15 degrees or less. Invest. Ophthalmol. 14, 468–469.

Bahill, T., Clark, M. & Stark, L. (1975b) Glissades-eye movements generated by mismatched components of the saccadic motoneural control signal. Math. Biosci. 26, 203–218.

Bahill, T., Hsu F.K. & Stark, L (1978) Glissadic overshoots are due to pulse width errors. Arch. Neurol. 35, 138–142.

Baird, I.L. (1974) Some aspects of the comparative anatomy and evolution of the inner ear in submammalian vertebrates. Brain Behav. Evol. 10, 11–36.

Baker, C.L. & Braddick, O.J. (1985) Temporal properties of the short range process in apparent motion. Perception.

Baker, J., Goldberg, J., Peterson, B. & Schor, R. (1982) Oculomotor reflexes after semicircular canal plugging in cats. Brain Res. 252, 151–155.

Baker, R., Goldberg, J., Hermann, G. & Peterson, B. (1983) Convergence of canal inputs to secondary neurons in cat vestibular nuclei. Soc. Neurosci. Abstr. 9, 315.

Baker, R. (1976) Pharmacological profile of inhibition in the

346

vestibular and ocular nuclei. In: P.B. Bradley & B.N. Dhawan (Eds.) Drugs and Central Synaptic Transmission. MacMillan, London and Basingstoke, pp. 227–234.

Baker, R. & Berthoz, A. (1974) Organisation of vestibular nystagmus in the oblique oculomotor system. J. Neurophysiol. 37, 195–217.

Baker, R. & Berthoz, A. (1977) Control of Gaze by Brain Stem Neurons, Developments in Neuroscience, Vol. 1. Elsevier, Amsterdam.

Baker, R. & Highstein, S.M. (1978) Vestibular projections to medial rectus subdivision of oculomotor nucleus. J. Neurophysiol. 41, 1629–1646.

Baker, R., Precht, W. & Llinás, R. (1972) Cerebellar modulatory action on the vestibulo-trochlear pathway in the cat. Exp. Brain Res. 15, 364–385.

Baker, R., Evinger, C. & McCrea, R.A. (1981a) Some thoughts about the three neurons in the vestibular ocular reflex. In: B. Cohen (Ed.) Vestibular and Oculomotor Physiology. Ann. N.Y. Acad. Sci. 374, 171–188.

Baker, R., Delgado-Garcia, J.M. & McCrea, R. (1981b) Morphological and physiological effects of axotomy on cat abducens motoneurons. In : H.Flohr & W.Precht (eds) Lesion-induced neuronal plasticity in sensorimotor systems. Springer Verl. Berlin, pp. 51–63.

Baker, R., Graf, W. & Spencer, R.F. (1982) The vertical vestibulo-ocular reflex. In: A. Roucoux & M. Crommelinck (Eds.) Physiological and Pathological Aspects of Eye Movements. Dr. W. Junk, The Hague, pp. 101–116.

Balaban, C.D., Ito, M. & Watanabe, E. (1981) Demonstration of zonal projections from the cerebellar flocculus to vestibular nuclei in monkeys (*Macaca fuscata*). Neurosci. Lett. 27, 101–105.

Baloh, W.R., Honrubia, V. & Konrad, H.R. (1977) Ewald's second law reevaluated. Acta Oto-Laryngol. 83, 475–479.

Baloh, R.W., Yee, R.D. & Honrubia, V. (1978) Internuclear ophthalmoplegia. Arch. Neurol. 35, 484–489.

Baloh, R.W., Yee, R.D. & Honrubia, V. (1980) Optokinetic asymmetry in patients with maldeveloped foveas. Brain Res. 186, 211–216.

Baloh, W.R., Henn, V. & Jäger, J. (1982) Habituation of the human vestibulo-ocular reflex with low frequency harmonic acceleration. Am. J. Otolaryng. 3, 235–241.

Baloh, R.W., Kimm, J. & Hassul, M. (1983) A comparison of the dynamics of the rabbit and human vestibulo-ocular reflex. Exp. Neurol. 81, 245–256.

Baloh, R.W., Lyerly, K., Yee, R.D. and Honrubia, V. (1984) Voluntary control of the human vestibulo-ocular reflex. Acta Oto-Laryngol 97, 1–6.

Bard, C., Paillard, J. & Fleury, M. (1982) Contribution of head movement to the projective aiming accuracy in adults. Soc. Neurosci. Abstr. 8, 289.

Barlow, H.B. & Gaze, R.M. (1977) A discussion on the structural and functional aspects of plasticity in the nervous system. Phil. Trans. R. Soc. London. Ser. B 278, 243–244.

Barmack, N.H. (1976) Measurement of stiffness of extraocular muscles of the rabbit. J. Neurophysiol. 39, 1009–1019.

Barmack, N.H. (1979) Immediate and sustained influence of visual olivo-cerebellar activity on eye movement. In: R.E.

Talbot & D.R. Humphrey (Eds.) Posture and Movement: Perspective for Integrating Sensory and Motor Research on the Mammalian Nervous System. Raven Press, New York, pp. 123–168.

Barmack, N.H. (1981) A comparison of the horizontal and vertical vestibulo-ocular reflexes of the rabbit. J. Physiol. (London) 314, 547–564.

Barmack, N.H. (1982) Influence of bilateral plugs of pairs of semicircular canals on optokinetic and vestibular ocular reflexes. In: A. Roucoux & M. Crommelink (Eds.) Physiological and Pathological Aspects of Eye Movements. D.W. Junk, The Hague, pp. 193–200.

Barmack, N.H. & Erickson, R.G. (1981) Optokinetic and vestibulo-ocular reflexes in rabbits with bilateral plugs of the horizontal or anterior semicircular canals. Soc. Neurosci. Abstr. 7, 483.

Barmack, N.H. & Nelson, B.J. (1982) Influence of long-term optokinetic stimulation on eye movements of the rabbit. Soc. Neurosci. Abstr. 8, 292.

Barmack, N.H. & Pettorossi, V.E. (1981) The influence of unilateral horizontal canal plugs on the horizontal vestibulo-ocular reflex of the rabbit. In: H. Flohr & W. Precht (Eds.) Lesion-induced Neuronal Plasticity in Sensorimotor Systems. Springer Verlag, Berlin, Heidelberg, New York, pp. 231–239.

Barmack, N.H. & Simpson, J.I. (1980) Effects of microlesions of dorsal cap of inferior olive of rabbits on optokinetic and vestibulo-ocular reflexes. J. Neurophysiol. 43, 182–206.

Barnes, G.R. (1979a) Vestibulo-ocular function during coordinated head and eye movements to acquire visual targets. J. Physiol. (London) 287, 127–147.

Barnes, G.R. (1979b) Head-eye coordination in normals and in patients with vestibular disorders. Adv. Oto-Rhino-Laryngol. 25, 197–201.

Barnes, G.R. & Edge, A. (1983) The effects of strobe rate of head-fixed visual targets on suppression of vestibular nystagmus. Exp. Brain Res. 50, 228–236.

Barnes, G.R. & Forbat, L.N. (1979) Cervical and vestibular afferent control of oculomotor response in man. Acta Oto-Laryngol. 88, 79–87.

Barnes, G.R. & Smith, R. (1981) The effects on visual discrimination of image movement across the stationary retina. Aviat. Space Environ. Med. 52, 466–472.

Barnes, G.R. & Sommerville, G.P. (1978) Visual target acquisition and tracking performance using a helmet-mounted sight. Aviat. Space Environ. Med. 49, 565–572.

Barnes, W.J.P. & Horridge, G.A. (1969) Interactions of the movements of the two eyecups in the crab (*Carcinus*). J. Exp. Biol. 50, 651–671.

Barr, C.C., Schultheis, L.W. & Robinson, D.A. (1976) Voluntary, non-visual control of the human vestibulo-ocular reflex. Acta Oto-Laryngol. 81, 365–375.

Bast, T.H., Anson, B.J. & Gardner, W.D. (1947) The developmental course of the human auditory vesicle. Anat. Rec. 99, 55–74.

Baumgarten, R. von, Benson, A., Berthoz, A., Brandt, T., Brand, U., Bruzek, W., Dichgans, J., Kass, J., Probst, T., Scherer, H., Vieville, T., Vogel, H. & Wetzig, J. (1984) Effects of rectilinear acceleration and optokinetic and caloric stimulations in space. Science 225, 208–211.

Bechterew, W., von (1883) Ergebnisse der Durchschneidung des N. Acusticus, nebst Erörterung der Bedeutung der semicirculären Kanäle für das Körpergleichgewicht. Pflügers Arch. Gesamte Physiol. Menschen Tiere 30, 312–347.

Becker, W. & Fuchs, A.F. (1969) Further properties of the human saccadic system: eye movements and correction saccades with and without visual fixation points. Vision Res. 9, 1247–1258.

Becker, W. & Jürgens, R. (1975) Saccadic reactions to double step stimuli: evidence for model feedback and continuous information uptake. In: G. Lennerstrand & P. Bach-y-Rita (Eds.) Basic Mechanisms of Ocular Motility and their Clinical Implications. Pergamon, Oxford, pp. 519–524.

de Beer, G.R. (1947) How animals hold their heads. Proc. Linn. Soc. (London) 159, 125–139.

Bender, M.B. (1965) Oscillopsia. Arch. Neurol. 13, 204–213.

Ben-Israel, A. & Greville, T.N. (1980) Generalized Inverses: Theory and Applications. Robert E. Krieger, England.

Benjamins, C.E. & Huizinga, E. (1928) Untersuchungen über die Funktion des Vestibularapparates bei der Taube. Pfluegers Arch. Gesamte Physiol. 217, 105–123.

Bennet, H. & Savill, Th. (1889) A case of permanent conjugate deviation of the eyes and head, the result of a lesion limited to the VIth nucleus with remarks on associated lateral movements of the eyeballs and rotation of the head and neck. Brain 12, 102–116.

Benson, A.J. (1970) Interactions between semicircular canals and graviceptors. In: D.E. Busby (Ed.) Recent Advances in Aerospace Medicine. Reidel, Dordrecht, pp. 249–261.

Benson, A.J. (1977) Possible mechanisms of motion and space sickness. In: Life Sciences Research in Space, ESA SP-130, Proceedings of a Symposium held at Cologne/Porz Wahn, Germany, May 1977, p. 101–108.

Benson, A.J. & Barnes, G.R. (1978) Vision during angular oscillation: the dynamic interaction of visual and vestibular mechanisms. Aviat. Space Environ. Med. 49, 340–345.

Benson A.J. & Bodin M.A. (1966) Interaction of linear and angular accelerations on vestibular receptors in man. Aerospace Med. 37, 144–154.

Berlin, E. (1871) Beitrag zur Mechanik der Augenbewegungen. Albrecht v. Graefes Arch. Ophthalmol. 17/2, 154–203.

Berman, N. & Cynader, M. (1972) Comparison of receptive-field organization of the superior colliculus of Siamese and normal cats. J. Physiol. (London) 224, 363–389.

Berman, N & Daw, N.W. (1977) Comparison of the critical period for monocular and directional deprivation in cats. J. Physiol. (London) 265, 249–259.

Bernstein, N.A. (1947) O Postroyenii Dvizheniy (On the Construction of Movements), Moscow, Medgiz.

Bernstein, N.A. (1967) The coordination and regulation of movements. Pergamon Press, New York.

Berthoz, A. & Anderson, A. (1971a) Frequency analysis of vestibular influence on extensor motoneurons. I. Response to tilt in forelimb extensors. Brain Res. 34, 370–375.

Berthoz, A. & Anderson, A. (1971b) Frequency analysis of vestibular influence on extensor motoneurons. II. Relationship between neck and forelimb extensors. Brain Res. 34, 376–380.

Berthoz, A. & Anderson, A. (1972) Frequency analysis of vestibular influence on extensor motoneurons. III. Neck and forelimb motor unit activity after hemilabyrinthectomy. Brain Res. 45, 236–240.

Berthoz, A. & Droulez, J. (1982) Linear self motion perception. In: Wertheim, Wagenaar & Leibowitz (Eds) Tutorials in Motion Perception. Plenum Press, London, pp. 157–199.

Berthoz, A., Melville Jones, G. & Bégué, A. (1981c) Long-term effects of dove prism vision on torsional VOR and head-eye coordination. In: H. Flohr & W. Precht (Eds) Lesion-induced Neuronal Plasticity in Sensorimotor Systems. Springer Verlag, Berlin, pp. 277–283.

Berthoz, A. & Llinás, R. (1974) Afferent neck projection to the cat cerebellar cortex. Exp. Brain Res. 20, 385–401.

Berthoz, A. & Melvill Jones, G. (1981) Modifications of head-eye coordination during reversing prism adaptation. Neurosci. Lett. Suppl. 7, 111.

Berthoz, A., Jeannerod, M., Vital-Durand, F. & Oliveras, J.L. (1975a) Development of vestibulo-ocular responses in visually deprived kittens. Exp. Brain Res. 23, 425–442.

Berthoz, A., Pavard, B. & Young, L.R. (1975b) Perception of linear horizontal self motion induced by peripheral vision (linear vection). Exp. Brain Res. 23, 471–489.

Berthoz, A., Lacour, M., Soechting, J. & Vidal, P.P. (1979). The role of vision in the control of posture during linear motion. In: O. Pompeiano & R. Granit (Eds.) Reflex Control of Movement and Posture. Elsevier, Amsterdam, 197–209.

Berthoz, A., Melvill Jones, G. & Bégué, A.E. (1981a) Differential visual adaptation of vertical canal-dependent vestibulo-ocular reflexes. Exp. Brain Res. 44, 19–26.

Berthoz, A., Yoshida, K. & Vidal, P.P. (1981b) Horizontal eye movement signals in second-order vestibular nuclei neurons in the cat. In: B. Cohen (Ed.) Vestibular and Oculomotor Physiology. Ann. N.Y. Acad. Sci. 374, 144–156.

Berthoz A., Melvill Jones G. & Bégué A. (1981c) Long term effects of dove prism vision on torsional VOR and head-eye coordination. In: H. Flohr & W. Precht (Eds.) Lesion Induced Neuronal Plasticity in Sensorimotor Systems. Springer Verlag, Berlin, 277–283.

Berthoz, A., Vidal, P.P. & Corvisier, J. (1982) Brain stem neurons mediating horizontal eye position signals to dorsal neck muscles of the alert cat. In: A. Roucoux & M. Crommelinck (Eds.), Physiological and Pathological Aspects of Eye Movements. Dr W. Junk, The Hague, pp. 385–398.

Bexton, W.H., Heron, W. & Scott, T.H. (1954) Effects of decreased variation in the sensory environment. Can. J. Psychol. 8, 70–76.

Bienhold, H. & Flohr, H. (1978) Role of commissural connections between vestibular nuclei in compensation following unilateral labyrinthectomy. J. Physiol. (London) 284, 178 P.

Bienhold, H. & Flohr, H. (1980) Role of cholinergic synapses in vestibular compensation. Brain Res. 195, 476–478.

Biguer, B. & Prablanc, C. (1981) Modulation of the vestibulo-ocular reflex in eye-head coordination as a function of target distance in man. In: A. Fuchs & W. Becker (Eds) Progress in Oculomotor Research. Elsevier, Amsterdam, New York, pp. 525–530.

Bilotto, G., Goldberg, J., Peterson, B.W. & Wilson, V.J.

348

(1982) Dynamic properties of vestibular reflexes in the decerebrate cat. Exp. Brain Res. 47, 343–352.

Birukow, G. (1937) Untersuchungen über den optischen Drehnystagmus und über die Sehshärfe beim Grasfrosch (*Rana temporaria*). Z. Vgl. Physiol. 25, 92–142.

Bizzi, E. (1981) Eye-head coordination. In: V.B. Brooks (Ed.) Handbook of Physiology: The nervous system. Am. Physiol. Soc., Bethesda, pp. 1321–1336.

Bizzi, E., Kalil, R.E. & Tagliasco, V. (1971) Eye-head coordination in monkeys: evidence for centrally patterned organization. Science 173, 452–454.

Bizzi, E., Kalil, R.E., Morasso, P. & Tagliasco, V. (1972a) Central programming and peripheral feedback during eye-head coordination in monkeys. In: J. Dichgans & E. Bizzi (Eds.), Cerebral Control of Eye Movements and Motion Perception. Karger, Basel, pp. 220–232.

Bizzi, E., Kalil, R.E. & Morasso, P. (1972b) Two modes of active eye-head coordination in monkeys. Brain Res. 40, 45–48.

Bizzi, E., Polit, A. & Morasso, P. (1976) Mechanisms underlying achievement of final head position. J. Neurophysiol. 39, 435–444.

Blair, S. & Gavin, M. (1979) Response of the vestibulo-ocular reflex to differing programs of acceleration. Invest. Ophthalmol. 18, 1086–1090.

Blakemore, C. & Cooper, G.F. (1970) Development of the brain depends on the visual environment. Nature 228, 477–478.

Blakemore, C. & Donaghy M. (1980) Coordination of head and eyes in the gaze changing behaviour of cats. J. Physiol. (London) 300, 317–335.

Blanks, R.H.I. & Precht, W. (1976) Functional characterization of primary vestibular afferents in the frog. Exp. Brain Res. 25, 369–390.

Blanks, R.H.I. & Precht, W. (1978) Response properties of vestibular afferents in alert cats during optokinetic and vestibular stimulation. Neurosci. Lett. 10, 225–229.

Blanks, R.H.I., Curthoys, I.S. & Markham, C.H. (1972) Planar relationships of semicircular canals in the cat. Am. J. Physiol. 223, 55–62.

Blanks, R.H.I., Curthoys, I.S. & Markham, C.H. (1975a) Planar relationships of the semicircular canals in man. Acta Oto-Laryngol. 80, 185–196.

Blanks, R.H.I., Estes, M.S. & Markham, C.H. (1975b) Physiological characteristics of vestibular first order canal neurons in the cat. II. Response to constant angular acceleration. J. Neurophysiol. 38, 1250–1268.

Blanks, R.H.I., Giolli, R.A. & Torigoe, Y. (1982) Descending projections of the medial terminal nucleus of the accessory optic systems: A light autoradiographic study in rat and rabbit. Soc. Neurosci. Abstr. 8, 204.

Bles, W. & Vianney de Jong, J.M.B. (1982) Cervico-vestibular and visuo-vestibular interaction. Acta Oto-Laryngol. 94, 61–72.

Boeder, P. (1962) Co-operative action of extraocular muscles. Br. J. Ophthalmol. 46, 397–403.

Boehmer, A., Henn, V. & Suzuki, J.I. (1982) Compensatory eye movements in the monkey during high frequency sinusoidal rotations. In: A. Roucoux & M. Crommelinck (Eds.) Physiological and Pathological Aspects of Eye Movements. Dr. W. Junk, The Hague, pp. 127–130.

Bohus, B., Gispen, W.H. & De Wied, D. (1973) Effect of lysine vasopressin and ACTH$_{4-10}$ on conditioned avoidance behaviour of hypophysectomized rats. Neuroendocrinology 11, 137–142.

Botros, G. (1979) The tonic oculomotor function of the cervical joint and muscle receptors. Adv. Oto-Rhino-Laryngol. 25, 214–220.

Boylls, C.C., Jr. (1978) Prolonged alterations of muscle activity induced in locomoting premammillary cats by microstimulation of the inferior olive. Brain Res. 159, 445–450.

Bower, J. & Llinás, R. (1982) Simultaneous sampling and analysis of the activity of multiple, closely adjacent, cerebellar Purkinje cells. Soc. Neurosci. Abstr. 8, 830.

Bower, J. & Llinás, R. (1983) Simultaneous sampling of the responses of multiple, closely adjacent, Purkinje cells responding to climbing fiber activation. Soc. Neurosci. Abstr. 9, 607.

Bracchi, F., Gualtierotti, T., Morabito, A. & Rocca, E. (1975) Multi day recordings from the primary neurons of the statoreceptors of the labyrinth of the bull frog, Acta Oto-Laryngol. 334, 1–27.

Braddick, O.J. (1980) Low level and high level processes in apparent motion. Phil. Trans. R. Soc. London Ser. B, 137–151.

Braitenberg, V. & Onesto, N. (1961) The cerebellum as a timing organ. Discussion of an hypothesis. Proc. 1st. Int. Conf. Med. Cybernet., Giannini, Naples, pp. 1–19.

Brandt, T., Dichgans, J. & Buechele, W. (1974) Motion habituation: Inverted self-motion perception and optokinetic after-nystagmus. Exp. Brain Res. 21, 337–352.

Brecha, N., Karten, H.J. & Hunt, S.P. (1980) Projections of the nucleus of the basal optic root in the pigeon: An autoradiographic and horseradish peroxidase study. J. Comp. Neurol. 189, 615–670.

Breinin, G.M. & Chin, N.B. (1973) Accommodation, convergence, and aging. Doc. Ophthalmol. 34, 109–121.

Breuer, J. (1874) Über die Funktion der Bogengänge des Ohrlabyrinthes. Med. Jahrbücher, Wien, Heft 1, 72–124.

Breuer, J., (1891) Über die Funktion der Otolithen-Apparate. Pfluegers Arch. Gesamte Physiol. Menschen Tiere 48, 195–306.

Brindley, G.S. (1964) The use made by the cerebellum of the information that it receives from sense organs. IBRO Bull., 3,80.

Brodal, A. & Høivik, B. (1964) Site and mode of termination of primary vestibulocerebellar fibers in the cat. Arch. Ital. Biol. 102, 1–21.

Budelmann, B.U. (1977) Structure and function of the angular acceleration receptor systems in the statocysts of cephalopods. Symp. Zool. Soc. London 38, 309–324.

Budelmann, B.U. & Wolff, H.G. (1973) Gravity response from angular acceleration receptors in *Octopus vulgaris*. J. Comp. Physiol. 85, 283–290.

Budelmann, B.U. & Young, J.Z. (1982) Untersuchungen zum okulomotorischen System von *Octopus vulgaris*. Verh. Dtsch. Zool. Ges. 75, 266.

Buettner, U.W. & Büttner, U. (1979) Vestibular nuclei activity in the alert monkey during suppression of vestibular and optokinetic nystagmus. Exp. Brain Res. 37, 581–593.

Buettner, U.W., Büttner, U. & Henn, V. (1978) Transfer characteristics of neurons in vestibular nuclei of the alert monkey. J. Neurophysiol. 41, 1614–1628.

Buettner, U.W., Henn, V. & Young, L.R. (1981) Frequency response of the vestibulo-ocular reflex (VOR) in the monkey. Aviat. Space Environ. Med. 52, 73–77.

Buizza, A. & Schmid, R. (1982) Visual vestibular interaction in the control of eye movement: mathematical modelling and computer simulation. Biol. Cybern. 43, 209–223.

Buizza, A., Leger, A., Berthoz, A. & Schmid, R. (1979) Otolithic acoustic interactions in the control of eye movements. Exp. Brain Res. 36, 509–522.

Buizza, A., Leger, A., Droulez, J., Berthoz, A. & Schmid, R. (1980) Influence of otolithic stimulation by horizontal linear acceleration on optokinetic nystagmus and visual motion perception. Exp. Brain Res. 39, 165–176.

Bullock, T.H. & Horridge, G.A. (1965) Structure and Function in the Nervous System of Invertebrates, Vol. I/II. W.H. Freeman, San Francisco and London.

Burlet, de, H.M. & Versteegh, C. (1930) Über Bau und Funktion des Petromyzonlabyrinthes. Acta Oto-Laryngol. Suppl. 13, 5–58.

Burlet, de, H.M. & Koster, J.J. (1916) Zur Bestimmung des Standes der Bogengänge un der Maculae acusticae in Kaninchenschädel. Arch. Anat. Physiol. Anat. Abstr., 59–100.

Burrows, M. & Horridge, G.A. (1968) The action of the eyecup muscles of the crab (*Carcinus*) during optokinetic movements. J. Exp. Biol. 49, 223–250.

Büttner, U. & Henn, V. (1976) Thalamic unit activity in the alert monkey during natural vestibular stimulation. Brain Res. 103, 127–132.

Büttner, U. & Waespe, W. (1981) Vestibular nerve activity in the alert monkey during vestibular and optokinetic nystagmus. Exp. Brain Res. 41, 310–315.

Büttner, U. & Waespe, W. (1984) Purkinje cell activity in the primate flocculus during optokinetic stimulation, smooth pursuit eye movements and VOR-suppression. Exp. Brain Res. 55, 97–104.

Büttner, U., Waespe, W. & Henn, V. (1976) Duration and direction of optokinetic afternystagmus as a function of stimulus exposure time in the monkey. Arch. Psychiatr. Nervenkr. 222, 281–291.

Callan, J.W. & Ebenholtz, S.M. (1982) Directional changes in the vestibulo-ocular response as a result of adaptation to optical tilt. Vision Res. 22, 37–42.

Camis, M. (1912) Contributi alla fisiologia del labirinto. III. effetti della labirintectomia nel cane particolarmente sulla innervatione vaso-motoria. Folia Neurobiol. 6, 138–165.

Camis, M. (1930) The Physiology of the Vestibular Apparatus. (trans. R.S. Creed) Oxford University Press, London.

Campbell, F.W. (1954) Accommodation reflex. Br. Orthopt. J. 11, 13–17.

Campbell, F.W. (1957) The depth of field in the human eye. Opt. Acta 4, 157–164.

Campbell, F.W. & Robson, J.G. (1968) Application of Fourier analysis to the visibility of gratings. J. Physiol. (London) 197, 551–566.

Campbell, F.W. & Westheimer, G. (1959) Factors influencing accommodation responses of the human eye. J. Opt. Soc. Am. 49, 568–571.

Campbell, F.W. & Westheimer, G. (1960) Dynamics of accommodation responses of the human eye. J. Physiol. (London) 151, 285–295.

Campbell, F.W., Robson, J.G., & Westheimer, G. (1959) Fluctuations of accommodation under steady viewing conditions. J. Physiol. (London) 145, 579–594.

Carpenter, M.B., Fabrega, H. & Glinsmann, W. (1959) Physiological deficits occurring with lesions of labyrinth and fastigial nuclei. J. Neurophysiol. 22, 222–234.

Carpenter, M.B., Stein, B.M. & Peter, P. (1972) Primary vestibulo-cerebellar fibers in the monkey: distribution of fibers arising from distinctive cell groups of the vestibular ganglia. Am. J. Anat. 135, 221–250.

Carpenter, R.H.S. (1972) Cerebellectomy and transfer function of the vestibulo-ocular reflex in the decerebrate cat. Proc. R. Soc. London Ser. B 181, 353–374.

Carpenter, R.H.S. (1977) Movements of the Eyes. Pion, London, 420 pp.

Carter, D.B. (1963) Effects of prolonged wearing of prism. Am. J. Optom. Arch. Am. Acad. Optom. 40, 265–273.

Carter, D.B. (1965) Fixation disparity and heterophoria following prolonged wearing of prisms. Am. J. Optom. Arch. Am. Acad. Optom. 42, 141–152.

Chalupa, L.M. & Rhoades, R.W. (1978) Modification of visual response properties in the superior colliculus of the golden hamster following stroboscopic rearing. J. Physiol. (London) 274, 571–592.

Cheng, M. & Outerbridge, J.S. (1975) Optokinetic nystagmus during selective retinal stimulation. Exp. Brain Res. 23, 129–139.

Chun, K.-S. & Robinson, D.A. (1978) A model of quick phase generation in the vestibuloocular reflex. Biol. Cybern. 28, 209–221.

Ciuffreda, K.J. & Kenyon, R.V. (1983) Accommodative vergence and accommodation in normals, amblyopes, and strabismics. In: C.M. Schor & K.J. Ciuffreda (Eds.) Vergence Eye Movements: Basic and Clinical Aspects. Butterworths, Boston, pp. 101–173.

Ciuffreda, K.J., Kenyon, R.V. & Stark, L. (1979) Abnormal saccadic substitution during small amplitude pursuit tracking in amblyopis eyes. Invest. Ophthalmol 18, 506–516.

Clément G., Courjon, J.H, Jeannerod, M. & Schmid, R. (1981) Unidirectional habituation of vestibulo-ocular responses by repeated rotational or optokinetic stimulations in the cat. Exp. Brain Res. 42, 34–42.

Cohen B., (1981) Vestibular and oculomotor physiology. Int. Meet. Baramy Soc., Ann. N.Y. Acad. Sci. 374, 892 pp.

Cohen, B. & Suzuki, J.-I. (1963) Eye movements induced by ampullary nerve stimulation. Am. J. Physiol. 204, 347–351.

Cohen, B., Suzuki, J.-I. & Bender, M. (1964) Eye movements from semicircular canal nerve stimulation in the cat. Ann. Oto-Rhino-Laryngol. 73, 153–165.

Cohen, B., Goto, K., Shanzer, S. & Weiss, A.H. (1965) Eye

movements induced by electric stimulation of the cerebellum in the alert cat. Exp. Neurol. 13, 145–165.

Cohen, B., Krejcova, H. & Highstein, S. (1970) Ocular counterrolling induced by static head tilt in the monkey. Fed. Proc. Abstr. 29, 454.

Cohen, B., Uemura, T. & Takemori, S. (1973) Effects of labyrinthectomy on optokinetic nystagmus (OKN) and optokinetic afternystagmus (OKAN). Equilibrium Res. 3, 88–93.

Cohen, B., Matsuo, V. & Raphan, T. (1977) Quantitative analysis of the velocity characteristics of optokinetic nystagmus and optokinetic after-nystagmus. J. Physiol. (London) 270, 321–344.

Cohen, B., Henn, V., Raphan, T. & Dennett, D. (1981) Velocity storage, nystagmus and visual-vestibular interactions in humans. In: B. Cohen (Ed.) Vestibular and Oculomotor Physiology. Ann. N.Y. Acad. Sci. 374, 421–433.

Cohen, B., Suzuki, J., Raphan, T., Matsuo, V. & deJong, V. (1982) Selective labyrinthine lesions and nystagmus induced by rotation about off-vertical axis. In: G. Lennerstrand, E. Keller & D.S. Zee (Eds.) Functional Basis of Ocular Motility Disorders, Pergamon, Oxford, pp. 337–346.

Cohen, B., Suzuki, J. & Raphan, T., (1983) Role of the otolith organs in generation of horizontal nystagmus; effects of selective labyrinthine lesions. Brain Res. 276, 159–164.

Collewijn, H. (1969) Optokinetic eye movements in the rabbit: input-output relations. Vision Res. 9, 117–132.

Collewijn, H. (1970a) Dysmetria of fast phase of optokinetic nystagmus in cerebellectomized rabbits. Exp. Neurol. 28, 144–154.

Collewijn, H. (1970b) Oculomotor reactions in the cuttlefish (Sepia officinalis). J. Exp. Biol. 52, 369–384.

Collewijn, H. (1972) An analog model of the rabbit's optokinetic system. Brain Res. 36, 71–88.

Collewijn, H. (1975a) Oculomotor areas in the rabbit's midbrain and pretectum. J. Neurobiol. 6, 3–22.

Collewijn, H. (1975b) Direction-selective units in the rabbit's nucleus of the optic tract. Brain Res. 100, 489–508.

Collewijn, H. (1976) Impairment of optokinetic (after-)nystagmus by labyrinthectomy in the rabbit. Exp. Neurol. 52, 146–156.

Collewijn, H. (1977a) Eye and head movements in freely moving rabbits. J. Physiol. (London) 266, 471–498.

Collewijn, H. (1977b) Gaze in freely moving subjects. In: R. Baker & A. Berthoz (Eds.) Control of Gaze by Brain Stem Neurons. Elsevier, Amsterdam, pp. 13–22.

Collewijn, H. (1977c) Optokinetic and vestibulo-ocular reflexes in dark-reared rabbits. Exp. Brain Res. 27, 287–300.

Collewijn, H. (1981a) The Oculomotor System of the Rabbit and its Plasticity. In: V. Braitenberg (Ed.) Studies of Brain Function, Vol. 5, Springer-Verlag, Berlin, 240 pp.

Collewijn, H. (1981b) The optokinetic system. In: B.L. Zuber (Ed.) Models of Oculomotor Behavior and Control. CRC Press, Boca Raton (F1), pp. 111–137.

Collewijn, H. & Grootendorst, A.F. (1979) Adaptation of optokinetic and vestibulo-ocular reflexes to modified visual input in the rabbit. In: R. Granit & O. Pompeiano (Eds.) Reflex control of Posture and Movement. Progress in Brain Research, Vol. 50. Elsevier, Amsterdam, pp. 772–781.

Collewijn, H. & Kleinschmidt, H.J. (1975) Vestibulo-ocular and optokinetic reactions in the rabbit: changes during 24 hours of normal and abnormal interaction. In: G. Lennerstrand & P. Bach-y-Rita (Eds.) Basic Mechanisms of Ocular Motility and their Clinical Implications. Pergamon Press, Oxford, pp. 477–483.

Collewijn, H. & Tamminga, E. (1984) Human smooth and saccadic eye movements during voluntary pursuit of different motions on different backgrounds. J. Physiol. (London) 351, 217–250.

Collewijn, H., Winterson B.J. & Dubois, M.F.W. (1978) Optokinetic eye movements in albino rabbits: inversion in anterior visual field. Science 199, 1351–1353.

Collewijn, H., Winterson, B.J. & Van der Steen, J. (1980a) Postrotatory nystagmus and optokinetic after-nystagmus in the rabbit: linear rather than exponential decay. Exp. Brain Res. 40, 330–338.

Collewijn, H., Verhagen, A.M. & Grootendorst, A.F. (1980b) Adaptation of the vestibulo-ocular reflex in albino rabbits by selective exposure of the anterior sector of the visual field. Brain Res. 192, 305–312.

Collewijn, H., Martins, A.J. & Steinman, R.M. (1981a) Natural retinal image motion: origin and change. In: B. Cohen (Ed.) Vestibular and Oculomotor Physiology. Ann. N.Y. Acad. Sci. 374, 312–329.

Collewijn, H., Martins, A.J. & Steinman, R.M. (1981b) The time course of adaptation of human compensatory eye movements. Doc. Ophthalmol. Proc. Ser. 30, 123–133.

Collewijn, H., Curio, G. & Grüsser, O.J. (1982a) Spatially selective visual attention and generation of eye pursuit movements. Human Neurobiol. 1, 129–139.

Collewijn, H., Conijn, P. & Tamminga, E.P. (1982b) Eye-head coordination in man during the pursuit of moving targets. In: G. Lennerstrand, D.S. Zee & E.L. Keller (Eds.) Functional Basis of Ocular Motility Disorders. Pergamon Press, Oxford, pp. 369–378.

Collewijn, H., Conijn, P., Martins, L. & A.J., Tamminga, E.P. & Van Die, G.C. (1982c) Control of gaze in man: synthesis of pursuit, optokinetic and vestibulo-ocular systems. In: A. Roucoux & M. Crommelinck (Eds.) Physiological and Pathological Aspects of Eye Movements. Dr. W. Junk, The Hague, 3–22.

Collewijn, H., Martins, A.J. & Steinman, R.M. (1983) Compensatory eye movements during active and passive head movements: Fast adaptation to changes in visual magnification. J. Physiol. (London) 340, 259–286.

Collins, W.E. (1962) Effects of mental set upon vestibular nystagmus. J. Exp. Psychol. 63, 191–197.

Collins, W.E. (1964a) Primary, secondary and caloric nystagmus of the cat following habituation to rotation. J. Comp. Physiol. Psychol. 57, 417–421.

Collins, W.E. (1964b) Task-control of arousal and the effects of repeated unidirectional angular acceleration on human vestibular responses. Acta Oto-Laryngol., Suppl. 190, 1–34.

Collins, W.E. (1974) Habituation of vestibular responses with and without visual stimulation. In: H.H. Kornhuber (Ed.) Handbook of Sensory Physiology, Vol. 6/2. Springer Verlag, Berlin, Heidelberg, New York, pp. 369–388.

Collins, W.E., Schroeder, D.J., Rice, N., Mertens, R.A. & Kranz, G. (1970) Some characteristics of optokinetic eye-movement patterns: a comparative study. Aerosp. Med. 41, 1251–1262.

Comer, C. & Grobstein, P. (1981) Tactually elicited prey acquisition behaviour in the frog, *Rana pipiens*, and a comparison with visually elicited behaviour. J. Comp. Physiol. 142, 141–150.

Conway, J.L., Timberlake, G.T. & Skavenski, A.A. (1981) Oculomotor changes in cats reared without experiencing continuous retinal image motion. Exp. Brain Res. 43, 229–232.

Coriolis, G., (1844) Traité de la Mécanique des Corps Solides et du calcul de l'Effet des machines, 2nd Edn., Paris, 367 pp.

Correia, M.J. & Money, K.E. (1970) The effect of blockage of all six semicircular canal ducts on nystagmus produced by linear acceleration in the cat. Acta Oto-Laryngol. 69, 7–16.

Correia, M.J. Nixson, W.C. & Niven, J.I. (1965) Otolith shear and the visual perception of force directions, discrepancies, and a proposed resolution. NAMI 951. Naval Aerospace Medicine Institute, Pensacola, FL.

Coulter, J.D., Mergner, T. & Pompeiano, O. (1976) Effects of static tilt on cervical spinoreticular tract neurons. J. Neurophysiol. 39, 45–62.

Courjon, J.H., Jeannerod, M., Ossuzio, I. & Schmid, R. (1977) The role of vision in compensation of vestibulo-ocular reflex after hemilabyrinthectomy in the cat. Exp. Brain Res. 28, 235–248.

Courjon, J.H., Flandrin, J.M., Jeannerod, M. & Schmid, R. (1982) The role of flocculus in vestibular compensation after hemilabyrinthectomy. Brain Res. 239, 251–257.

Crampton, G.H. (1962) Directional imbalance of vestibular nystagmus in cat following repeated unidirectional angular acceleration. Acta Oto-Laryngol. 55, 41–48.

Crampton, G.H. (1964) Habituation of ocular nystagmus of vestibular origin. In: M.B. Bender (Ed.) The Oculomotor System. Harper & Row, New York, pp. 332–346.

Crampton, G.H. & Schwam, W.J. (1961) Effects of arousal reaction on nystagmus habituation in the cat. Am. J. Physiol. 200, 29–33.

Crommelinck, M., Roucoux, A. & Veraart, C. (1982) The relation of neck muscles activity to horizontal eye position in the alert cat. II. Head free. In: A. Roucoux & M. Crommelinck (Eds.) Physiological and Pathological Aspects of Eye Movements. Dr. W. Junk, The Hague, pp. 379–384.

Cross, S.A., Smith, J.L. & Norton, E.W.D. (1982) Periodic alternating nystagmus clearing after vitrectomy. J. Clin. Neuro-ophthalmol. 2, 5–11.

Crum Brown, A. (1874) On the sense of rotation and the anatomy and physiology of the semicircular canals of the internal ear. J. Anat. Physiol. 8, 327–331.

Curthoys, I.S. & Markham, C.H. (1971) Convergence of labyrinthine influences on units in the vestibular nuclei of the cat. I. Natural stimulation. Brain Res. 35, 469–490.

Curthoys, I.S., Blanks, R.H. & Markham, C.H. (1975) The orientation of the semicircular canals in the guinea pig. Acta Oto-Laryngo. 80, 197–205.

Curthoys, I.S., Blanks, R.H.I. & Markham, C.H. (1977) Semicircular canal functional anatomy in cat, guinea pig and man.

Acta Oto-Laryngol. 83, 258–265.

Cynader, M. (1976) The effects of visual deprivation on the cat superior colliculus. Soc. Neurosci. Abstr. 111, 1584.

Cynader, M. (1979) Competitive interactions in postnatal development. In: R. Freeman (Ed.) Developmental Neurobiology of Vision. Plenum Press, New York, pp. 109–120.

Cynader, M. & Chernenko, G. (1976) Abolition of direction selectivity in the visual cortex of the cat. Science 193, 504–505.

Cynader, M. & Hoffmann, K.P. (1981) Strabismus disrupts binocular convergence in cat nucleus of the optic tract. Dev. Brain Res. 1, 132–136.

Cynader, M. & Mitchell, D.E. (1977) Monocular astigmatism effects on kitten visual cortex development. Nature 270, 177–178.

Cynader, M., Berman, N. & Hein, A. (1973) Cats reared in stroboscopic illumination: effects on receptive fields in visual cortex. Proc. Natl. Acad. Sci. U.S.A. 10, 1353–1354.

Cynader, M., Berman, N. & Hein, A. (1975) Cat raised in a one-directional world: effects on receptive fields in visual cortex and superior colliculus. Exp. Brain Res. 22, 267–280.

Cynader, M., Berman, N. & Hein, A. (1976) Recovery of function in cat visual cortex following prolonged deprivation. Exp. Brain Res. 25, 139–156.

Dallos, P.J. & Jones, R.W. (1963) Learning behavior of the eye fixation control system. IEEE, Trans. Autom. Control AC–8, 218–227.

Daniel, J.F. (1928) The Elasmobranch Fishes. University of California Press, Berkeley.

Daniels, P.D., Hassul, M. & Kimm, J. (1978) Dynamic analysis of the vestibulo-ocular reflex in the normal and flocculectomised chinchilla. Exp. Neurol. 58, 32–45.

Darlot, C., Denise, P. & Droulez, J. (1985) Modulation by horizontal eye position of the vestibulo-colic reflex induced by tilting in the frontal plane in alert cat. Exp. Brain Res. (in press).

Davies, P. (1979) Neural adaptation in humans and cats subjected to long-term optical reversal of vision: An experimental and analytical study of plasticity. Ph.D. Thesis, McGill University, Montreal.

Davies, P. & Melvill Jones, G. (1976) An adaptive neural model compatible with plastic changes induced in the human vestibulo-ocular reflex by prolonged optical reversal of vision. Brain Res. 103, 546–550.

Daw, M. & Wyatt, H.J. (1976) Raising rabbits in a moving visual environment: an attempt to modify direction selectivity in the retina. J. Physiol. (London) 240, 309–330.

Daw, N.W., Roder, R.K. & Robertson, T.W. (1981) Effect of 6-hydroxydopamine on plasticity of direction selective cells in visual cortex. Soc. Neurosci. Abstr. 7, 673.

Demer, J.L. (1981) The variable gain element of the vestibulo-ocular reflex is common to the optokinetic system of the cat. Brain Res. 229, 1–13.

Demer, J.L. & Robinson, D.A. (1982) Effects of reversible lesions and stimulation of olivocerebellar system on vestibuloocular reflex plasticity. J. Neurophysiol. 47, 1084–1107.

Demer, J.L. & Robinson, D.A. (1983) Different time constants for optokinetic and vestibular nystagmus with a single

352

velocity-storage element. Brain Res. 276, 173–177.

Denieul, P. (1982) Effects of stimulus vergence on mean accommodation response, microfluctuations of accommodation and optical quality of the human eye. Vision Res. 22, 561–569.

Desclin, J.C. & Escubi, J. (1974) Effects of 3-Acetylpyridine on the central nervous system of the rat, as demonstrated by silver methods. Brain Res. 77, 349–364.

Diamond, S.G. & Markham, C.H. (1981) Binocular counterrolling in humans with unilateral labyrinthectomy and in normal controls. In: B. Cohen (Ed.) Vestibular and Oculomotor Physiology. Ann. N.Y. Acad. Sci. 374, 69–79.

Diamond, S.G., Markham, C.H., Simpson, N.E. & Curthoys, I.S. (1979) Binocular counterrolling in humans during dynamic rotation. Acta Oto-Laryngol. 87, 490–498.

Dichgans, J. (1977) Optokinetic nystagmus as dependent on the retinal periphery via the vestibular nucleus. In: R. Baker & A. Berthoz (Eds.) Control of Gaze by Brain Stem Neurons. Elsevier, Amsterdam, pp. 261–267.

Dichgans, J. & Brandt, T. (1972) Visual-vestibular interaction and motion perception. Bibl. Ophthalmol. 82, 327–338.

Dichgans, J. & Brandt, Th. (1978) Visual-vestibular interactions: Effects on self-motion perception and postural control. In: R. Held, H. Leibowitz & H.-L. Teuber (Eds.) Handbook of Sensory Physiology. Perception, Vol. VIII. Springer Verlag, Berlin, pp. 755–804.

Dichgans, J., Held, R., Young L.R. & Brandt, T. (1972) Moving visual scenes influence the apparent direction of gravity. Science 178, 1217–1219.

Dichgans, J., Bizzi, E., Morasso, P. & Tagliasco, V. (1973a) Mechanisms underlying recovery of eye-head coordination following bilateral labyrinthectomy in monkeys. Exp. Brain Res. 18, 548–562.

Dichgans, J., Schmidt, C.L. & Graf, W. (1973b) Visual input improves the speedometer function of the vestibular nuclei in the goldfish. Exp. Brain Res. 18, 319–322.

Dichgans, J., Von Reutern, G.M. & Römmelt, U. (1978) Impaired suppression of vestibular nystagmus by fixation in cerebellar and non-cerebellar patients. Arch. Psychiatr. Nervenkr. 226, 183–199.

Die, Van, G.C. & Collewijn, H. (1982) Optokinetic nystagmus in man. Role of central and peripheral retina and occurrence of asymmetries. Human Neurobiol. 1, 111–119.

Dieringer, N. & Precht, W. (1977) Modification of synaptic input following unilateral labyrinthectomy. Nature (London) 269, 431–433.

Dieringer, N. & Precht, W. (1979a) Mechanism of compensation for vestibular deficits in the frog. I. Modification of the excitatory commissural system. Exp. Brain Res. 36, 311–328.

Dieringer, N. & Precht, W. (1979b) Mechanism of compensation for vestibular deficits in the frog. II. Modifications of the inhibitory pathways. Exp. Brain Res. 36, 329–341.

Dieringer, N. & Precht, W. (1981) Functional restitution of static and dynamic reflexes in the frog after hemilabyrinthectomy. In: H. Flohr & W. Precht (Eds.) Lesion-induced Neuronal Plasticity in Sensorimotor Systems. Springer Verlag, Berlin, Heidelberg, pp. 185–196.

Dieringer, N. & Precht, W. (1982a) Compensatory head and eye movements in the frog and their contribution to stabilization of gaze. Exp. Brain Res. 47, 394–406.

Dieringer, N. & Precht, W. (1982b) Dynamics of compensatory vestibular reflexes in the grass frog, Rana temporaria. In: A. Roucoux & M. Crommelinck (Eds.) Physiological and Pathological Aspects of Eye Movements. Dr. W. Junk, The Hague, pp. 418–423.

Dieringer, N., Precht, W. & Blight, A.R. (1982) Resetting fast phases of head and eye and their linkage in the frog. Exp. Brain Res. 47, 407–416.

Dieringer, N., Cochran, S.L. & Precht, W. (1983) Differences in the central organization of gaze stabilizing reflexes between frog and turtle. J. Comp. Physiol. 153, 495–508.

Dieringer, N., Künzle, H. & Precht, W. (1984) Increased projection of ascending dorsal root fibers to vestibular nuclei after hemilabyrinthectomy in the frog. Exp. Brain Res. 55, 574–578.

Di Giorgio, A.M. (1939) Effetti di lesioni unilaterali della corteccia sui fenomeni di compenso da emislabirintazione. Atti Accad. Fisiol. Fac. Med. Siena, Ser. XI/2, 382–384.

Dijkgraaf, S. (1959) Kompensatorische Kopfbewegungen bei Aktivdrehung eines Tintenfisches. Naturwissenschaften 46, 611.

Dijkgraaf, S. (1961) The statocyst of Octopus vulgaris as a rotation receptor. Pubbl. Stn. Zool. (Napoli) 32, 64–87.

Dijkgraaf, S. (1963) Nystagmus and related phenomena in Sepia officinalis. Experientia 19, 29–30.

Ditchburn, R.W. & Ginsborg, B.L. (1952) Vision with stabilized retinal image. Nature 170, 36–37.

Dodge, R. (1923) Habituation to rotation. J. Exp. Psychol. 6, 1–35.

Dohlman, G. (1929) Experimentelle Untersuchungen über die galvanische Vestibularisreaktion. Acta Oto-Laryngol. Suppl. 8, 1–48.

Donaghy, M. (1978) The cat's vestibulo-ocular reflex. J. Physiol. (London) 300, 337–351.

Donaghy, M. (1980) The contrast sensitivity, spatial resolution and velocity tuning of the cat's optokinetic reflex. J. Physiol. (London) 300, 353–365.

Doslak, M.J., Kline, L.B., Dell'Osso, L.F. & Daroff, R.B. (1980) Internuclear ophthalmoplegia: recovery and plasticity. Invest. Ophthalmol. 19, 1506–1512.

Douglas, R.M., Flohr, H., Feran, M.T. & Melvill Jones, G. (1982) Improved visual modulation of VOR in the cat. Soc. Neurosci. Abstr., 8, 939.

Dow, R.S. (1938) The effects of unilateral and bilateral labyrinthectomy in monkey, baboon and chimpanzee. Am. J. Physiol. 121, 393–399.

Droulez, J., Berthoz, A. & Vidal, P.P. (1984) Use and limits of visuovestibular interaction in the control of posture. Are there two modes of sensorimotor control? In: M. Igarashi (Ed.) Proc. Int. Symp. Posture and Equilibrium. Karger (in press).

Dubois, M.F. & Collewijn, H. (1979a) The optokinetic reactions of the rabbit: relation to the visual streak. Vision Res. 19, 9–17.

Dubois, M.F.W. & Collewijn, H. (1979b) Optokinetic reactions in man elicited by localized retinal motion stimuli. Vision

Res. 19, 1105–1115.

Duensing, F. & Schaefer, K.P. (1958) Die Aktivität einzelner Neurone im Bereich der Vestibulariskerne bei Horizontalbeschleunigung unter besonderer Berücksichtigung des vestibulären Nystagmus. Arch. Psychiatr. Nervenkr. 198, 225–252.

Duensing, F. & Schaefer, K.P. (1959) Über die Konvergenz labyrinthärer Afferenzen auf einzelne Neurone des Vestibularis Kerngebietes. Arch. Psychiatr. Nervenkr. 199, 345–371.

Dufossé, M., Ito, M. & Miyashita, Y. (1977) Functional localization in the rabbit's cerebellar flocculus determined in relationship with eye movements. Neurosci. Lett. 5, 273–277.

Dufossé, M., Ito, M., Jastreboff, P.J. & Miyashita, Y. (1978a) A neuronal correlate in rabbit's cerebellum to adaptive modification of the vestibulo-ocular reflex. Brain Res. 150, 611–616.

Dufossé, M., Ito, M. & Miyashita, Y. (1978b) Diminution and reversal of eye movements induced by local stimulation of rabbit cerebellar flocculus after partial destruction of the inferior olive. Exp. Brain Res. 33, 139–141.

Duke-Elder, S. & Wybar, K. (1973) Ocular motility and strabismus. In: System of Ophthalmology, Vol. 6. C.V. Mosby, St. Louis.

Easter, S.S., Johns, P.R. & Heckenlively, D. (1975) Horizontal compensatory eye movements in goldfish (Carassius auratus) I. The normal animal. J. Comp. Physiol. 92, 23–35.

Eccles, J.C., Llinás, R. & Sasaki, K. (1966) The excitatory synaptic action of climbing fibres on the Purkinje cells of the cerebellum. J. Physiol. (London) 182, 268–296.

Eccles, J.C., Ito, M. & Szentágothai, J. (1967) The Cerebellum as a Neuronal Machine. Springer Verlag, Berlin, Heidelberg New York.

Eckmiller, R. & Mackeben, M. (1978) Pursuit eye movements and their neural control in the monkey. Pfluegers Arch. 377, 15–23.

Eckmiller, R. & Westheimer, G. (1983) Compensation of oculomotor deficits in monkeys with neonatal cerebellar ablations. Exp. Brain Res. 49, 315–326.

Edgeworth, F.H. (1935) The Cranial Muscles of Vertebrates. University Press, Cambridge.

Ekerot, C.-F. & Kano, M. (1984) Effects of cerebellar cortical inhibition on the long-term depression of parallel fibre-Purkinje cell transmission. Neurosci. Lett. Suppl. 17, 569.

Ekerot, C.-F. & Oscarsson, O. (1981) Prolonged depolarization elicited in Purkinje cell dendrites by climbing fiber impulses in the cat. J. Physiol. (London) 318, 207–221.

Ekerot, C.-F., Ito, M. & Kano, M. (1983) Long-lasting depression of parallel fiber-Purkinje cell transmission caused by conjunctive stimulation of parallel fibers and climbing fibers. Neurosci. Lett. Suppl. 3, 525.

Ellerbrock, V.J. (1948) Further study of effects induced by anisometropic corrections. Am. J. Optom. Arch. Am. Acad. Optom. 25, 430–437.

Ellerbrock, V.J. (1950) Tonicity induced by fusional movements. Am. J. Optom. Arch. Am. Acad. Optom. 27, 8–20.

Ellerbrock, V.J. & Fry, G.A. (1942) Effects induced by anisometropic corrections. Am. J. Optom. Arch. Am. Acad. Optom. 19, 444–459.

Ephstein, E.L. & Shipov, A.A. (1970) Unilateral labyrinthectomy as a model for assessing effect of drugs on vestibular function. Environ. Space Sci. 4, 339–341.

Evinger, C. & Fuchs, A.F. (1978) Saccadic, smooth pursuit, and optokinetic eye movements of the trained cat. J. Physiol. (London) 285, 209–229.

Ewald, J.R. (1892) Physiologische Untersuchungen über das Endorgan des Nervus Octavus. Bergmann, Wiesbaden.

Ewert, J.P. (1967) Elektrische Reizung des retinalen Projection Feldes in Mittelhirn der Erdkröte (Bufo Bufo L.). Pfluegers Arch. 295, 90–98.

Ezure, K. & Graf, W. (1984a) A quantitative analysis of the spatial organization of the vestibulo-ocular reflexes in lateral- and frontal-eyed animals. I. Orientation of semicircular canals and extraocular muscles. Neuroscience 12, 85–93.

Ezure, K. & Graf, W. (1984b) A quantitative analysis of the spatial organization of the vestibulo-ocular reflexes in lateral- and frontal-eyed animals. II. Neuronal networks underlying vestibulo-oculomotor coordination. Neuroscience 12, 95–109.

Ezure, K. & Sasaki, S. (1978) Frequency-response analysis of vestibular-induced neck reflex in cat. I. Characteristics of neural transmissions from the horizontal semicircular canal to neck motoneurons. J. Neurophysiol. 41, 445–458.

Feldon, S.E., Hoyt, W.F. & Stark, L. (1980) Disordered inhibition in internuclear ophthalmoplegia. Analysis of eye movement recordings with computer simulations. Brain 102, 113–137.

Ferin, M., Grigorian, R.A. & Strata, P. (1971) Mossy and climbing fiber activation in the cat cerebellum by stimulation of the labyrinth. Exp. Brain Res. 12, 1–17.

Fernandez, C. & Goldberg, J.M. (1971) Physiology of the peripheral neurons innervating semicircular canals of the squirrel monkey. II. Response to sinusoidal stimulation and dynamics of peripheral vestibular system. J. Neurophysiol. 34, 661–675.

Fernandez, C. & Goldberg, J.M. (1976a) Physiology of peripheral neurons innervating otolith organs of the squirrel monkey. I. Response to the static tilts and to long-duration centrifugal force. J. Neurophysiol. 39, 970–984.

Fernandez, C. & Goldberg, J.M. (1976b) Physiology of peripheral neurons innervating otolith organs of the squirrel monkey. II. Directional selectivity and force-response relations. J. Neurophysiol. 39, 985–995.

Fernandez, C. & Goldberg, J.M. (1976c) Physiology of peripheral neurons innervating otolith organs of the squirrel monkey. III. Response dynamics. J. Neurophysiol. 39, 996–1008.

Ferran, M.T., Douglas, R.M. & Melvill Jones, G. (1984) Adaptation of visual vestibular interaction without alteration of VOR or visuo-motor performance. Soc. Neurosci. Abstr. 9, 910.

Fincham, E.F. (1951) The accommodation reflex and its stimulus. Br. J. Ophthalmol. 35, 381–393.

Fincham, E.F. (1955) The proportion of ciliary muscle force required for accommodation. J. Physiol. (London) 128, 99–112.

Fincham, E.F. & Walton, J. (1957) The reciprocal actions of accommodation and convergence. J. Physiol. (London) 137, 488–508.

Fisch, U. (1973) The vestibular response following unilateral vestibular neurectomy. Acta Oto-Laryngol. 76, 229–238.

Flandrin, J.M. & Jeannerod, M. (1977) Lack of recovery in collicular neurons from the effects of early deprivation or neonatal cortical lesions in kitten. Brain Res. 120, 362–366.

Flandrin, J.M., Kennedy, H. & Amblard, B. (1976) Effects of stroboscopic rearing on the binocularity and directionality of cat superior colliculus neurons. Brain Res. 101, 576–581.

Flandrin, J.M., Courjon, J.H., Jeannerod, M. & Schmid, R. (1979a) Vestibulo-ocular responses during the states of sleep in the cat. Electroencephalogr. Clin. Neurophysiol. 46, 521–530.

Flandrin, J.M., Courjon, J.H. & Jeannerod, M. (1979b) Development of vestibulo-ocular response in the kitten. Neurosci. Lett. 12, 295–299.

Fleming, D.G., Vossius, W., Bowman, G. & Johnson, E.L. (1969) Adaptive properties of the eye tracking system as revealed by moving head and open loop studies. Ann. N.Y. Acad. Sci. 156, 825–850.

Flohr, H. (1983) Control of plastic processes. In: E. Basar, H. Flohr, H. Haken & A.J. Mandell (Eds.). Synergetics of the Brain. Springer Verlag, Berlin, New York, Tokyo, pp. 60–74.

Flohr, H. & Lüneburg, U. (1982) Effects of ACTH$_{4-10}$ on vestibular compensation. Brain Res. 248, 169–173.

Flohr, H. & Precht, W. (1981) Lesion-induced neuronal plasticity in sensorimotor systems. Springer Verlag, Berlin, 400 pp.

Flohr, H., Bienhold, H., Abeln, W. & Macskovics, I. (1981) Concepts of vestibular compensation. In: H. Flohr & W. Precht (Eds.) Lesion-induced Neuronal Plasticity in Sensorimotor Systems. Springer Verlag, Berlin, pp. 153–172.

Flom, M.C. (1960a) On the relationship between accommodation and accommodative convergence. I. Linearity. Am. J. Optom. Arch. Am. Acad. Optom. 37, 474–482.

Flom, M.C. (1960b) On the relationship between accommodation and accommodative convergence. III. Effects of orthoptics. Am. J. Optom. Arch. Am. Acad. Optom. 37, 619–632.

Flourens, P. (1826) Experiences sur les canaux semi-circulaires de l'oreille, dans les mammifères. Mem. Acad. R. Sci. Inst. France 9, 467–477.

Flourens, P. (1842) Recherches expérimentales sur les propriétés et les fonctions du système nerveux dans les animaux vertébrés. Edn. 2. Baillière, Paris.

Fluur, E. (1959) Influence of semicircular ducts on extraocular muscles. Acta Oto-Laryngol. Suppl. 149, 1–46.

Fonda, G. (1981) Spectacle correction for aphakia. The prismatic effect. Surv. Ophthalmol. 26, 154–156.

Franzisket, L. (1951) Gewohnheitsbildung und bedingte Reflexe bei Rückenmarksfröschen. Z. Vgl. Physiol. 33, 142–178.

Fraser, P.J. (1981) Semicircular canal morphology and function in crabs. In: T. Gualtierotti (Ed.) The Vestibular System: Function and Morphology, Springer Verlag, New York, Heidelberg, Berlin.

Fraser, P.J. & Sandeman, D.C. (1975) Effects of angular and linear accelerations on semicircular canal interneurons of the crab Scylla serrata.J. Comp. Physiol. 96, 205–221.

Freeman, J.A. (1969) The cerebellum as a timing device: An experimental study in the frog. In: R. Llinás (Ed.) Neurobiology of Cerebellar Evolution and Development. Am. Med. Assoc., Chicago, pp. 397–420.

Fregly, A.R. & Graybiel, A. (1970). Labyrinthine defects as shown by ataxia and caloric tests. Acta Oto-Laryngol. 69, 216–222.

Fuchs, A.F. & Becker, W. (Eds.) (1981) Progress in Oculomotor Research, Developments in Neuroscience, Vol 12. Elsevier, Amsterdam.

Fuchs, A.F. & Kimm, P. (1975) Unit activity in vestibular nucleus of the alert monkey during horizontal angular acceleration and eye movement. J. Neurophysiol. 38, 1140–1161.

Fujita, M. (1982a) Adaptive filter model of the cerebellum. Biol. Cybern. 45, 195–206.

Fujita, M. (1982b) Simulation of adaptive modification of the vestibulo-ocular reflex with an adaptive filter model of the cerebellum. Biol. Cybern. 45, 207–214.

Fuller, J.H. (1980a) The dynamic neck-eye reflex in mammals. Exp. Brain Res. 41, 29–35.

Fuller, J.H. (1980b) Linkage of eye and head movements in the alert rabbit. Brain Res. 194, 219–222.

Fuller, J.H., Maldonado, H. & Schlag, J. (1983) Vestibular-oculomotor interaction in cat eye-head movements. Brain Res. 271, 241–250.

Funk, C. & Anderson, M.E. (1977) Saccadic eye movements and eye-head coordination in children. Percept. Motor Skills. 44, 599–610.

Furuya, N. & Markham, C.H. (1981) Arborization of axons in oculomotor nucleus identified by vestibular stimulation and intra-axonal injection of horseradish peroxidase. Exp. Brain Res. 43, 289–303.

Furuya, N., Kawano, K. & Shimazu, H. (1976) Transcerebellar inhibitory interaction between bilateral vestibular nuclei and its modulation by cerebellocortical activity. Exp. Brain Res. 25, 447–463.

Gacek, R. (1974) Transection of the posterior ampullary nerve for the relief of benign paroxysmal vertigo. Ann. Oto-Laryngol. 83, 590–605.

Galiana, H.L. (1983) A model reconciling central observations during plasticity of the vestibulo-ocular reflex. Soc. Neurosci. Abstr. 9, 523.

Galiana, H.L. & Outerbridge, J.S. (1984) A bilateral model for central neural pathways in the vestibuloocular reflex. J. Neurophysiol (London) 51, 226–257.

Galiana, H.L., Flohr, H. & Melvill Jones, G. (1984) A reevaluation of intervestibular nuclear coupling: its role in vestibular compensation. J. Neurophysiol. 51, 258–275.

Gans, C. & Northcutt, R.G. (1983) Neural crest and the origin of vertebrates: a new head. Science 220, 268–274.

Gauthier, G.M. (1974) Plongée profonde simulée Sagittaire IV à 610 mètres sous Heliox, Rapp. prelim, pp. 1–7.

Gauthier, G.M. & Robinson, D.A. (1975) Adaptation of the human vestibulo-ocular reflex to magnifying lenses. Brain Res. 92, 331–335.

Gernandt, B.E. & Thulin, C.A. (1952) Vestibular connections of the brain stem. Am. J. Physiol. 171, 121–127.

Ghelarducci, B., Ito, M. & Yagi, N. (1975) Impulse discharges from flocculus Purkinje cells of alert rabbits during visual stimulation combined with horizontal head rotation. Brain. Res. 8, 66–72.

Godaux, E., Gobert, C. & Halleux, J. (1983a) Vestibulo-ocular reflex, optokinetic response, and their interactions in the alert cat. Exp. Neurol. 80, 42–54.

Godaux, E., Halleux, J. & Gobert, C. (1983b) Adaptive change of the vestibulo-ocular reflex in the cat: the effects of a long-term frequency-selective procedure. Exp. Brain Res. 49, 28–34.

Goldberg, J.M. & Fernandez, C. (1971) Physiology of peripheral neurons innervating semicircular canals of the squirrel monkey. I. Resting discharge and response to constant angular accelerations. J. Neurophysiol. 34, 635–660.

Goldberg, J.M. & Fernandez, C. (1975a) Vestibular mechanisms. Annu. Rev. Physiol. 37, 129–162.

Goldberg, J.M. & Fernandez, C. (1975b) Responses of peripheral vestibular neurons to angular and linear accelerations in the squirrel monkey. Acta Oto-Laryngol. 80, 101–110.

Goldberg, J.M. & Fernández, C. (1980) Efferent vestibular system in the squirrel monkey: Anatomical location and influence on afferent activity. J. Neurophysiol. 43, 986–1025.

Goldberg, J.M. & Fernandez, C. (1981) Physiological mechanisms of the nystagmus produced by rotations about an earth-horizontal axis. In: B. Cohen (Ed.) Vestibular and Oculomotor Physiology. Ann. N.Y. Acad. Sci. 374, 40–43.

Goldberg, J.M. & Fernandez, C. (1982) Eye Movements and vestibular nerve responses produced in the squirrel monkey by rotations about an earth-horizontal axis. Exp. Brain Res. 46, 393–402.

Goldberg, J.M., Fernandez, C. & Highstein, S.M. (1981) Differential projections of regularly and irregularly discharging vestibular-nerve afferents onto individual secondary neurons of the superior vestibular nucleus in the barbiturate-anesthetised squirrel monkey. Soc. Neurosci. Abstr. 7, 39.

Goldberg, J., Baker, J., Schor, R. & Peterson, B. (1982) Vertical canal contribution to horizontal eye movements. Soc. Neurosci. Abstr. 8, 419.

Goltz, F. (1870) Über die physiologische Bedeutung der Bogengänge des Ohrlabyrinthes. Pfluegers Arch. Gesamte Physiol. Menschen Tiere 3, 172–192.

Gonshor, A. & Melvill Jones, G. (1969) Investigations of habituation to rotational stimulation within the range of natural movement. Proc. Aerosp. Med. Assoc. Meet., San Francisco, pp. 94–95.

Gonshor, A. & Melvill Jones, G. (1971) Plasticity in the adult human vestibulo-ocular reflex arc. Proc. Can. Fed. Biol. Soc. 14, 11.

Gonshor, A. & Melvill Jones, G. (1973) Changes of human vestibulo-ocular response induced by vision-reversal during head rotation. J. Physiol. (London) 234, 102–103.

Gonshor, A. & Melvill Jones, G. (1976a) Short-term adaptive changes in the human vestibulo-ocular reflex arc. J. Physiol. (London) 256, 361–379.

Gonshor, A. & Melvill Jones, G. (1976b) Extreme vestibulo-ocular adaptation by prolonged optical reversal of vision. J. Physiol. (London) 256, 381–414.

Gonshor, A. & Melvill Jones, G. (1980) Postural adaptation

to prolonged optical reversal of vision in man. Brain Res. 192, 239–248.

Graf, W. (1981) Flatfish vestibulo-ocular reflex (VOR): Physiological and anatomical aspects. Biol. Bull. 161, 313.

Graf, W. & Baker, R. (1983) Adaptive changes of the vestibulo-ocular reflex in flatfish are achieved by reorganization of central nervous pathways. Science 221, 777–779.

Graf, W. & Ezure, K. (1983) The validity of matrix analysis for the description of spatial vestibulo-ocular coordination in cat and rabbit. Soc. Neurosci. Abstr. 9, 314.

Graf, W. & Meyer, D.L. (1978) Eye positions in fishes suggest different modes of interaction between commands and reflexes. J. Comp. Physiol. 128, 241–250.

Graf, W. & Meyer, D.L. (1983) Central mechanisms counteract visually induced tonus asymmetries. A study of ocular responses to unilateral illumination in goldfish. J. Comp. Physiol. 150, 473–481.

Graf, W. & Simpson, J.I. (1981) The relations between the semicircular canals, the optic axis, and the extraocular muscles in lateral-eyed and frontal eyed animals. In: A. Fuchs & W. Becker (Eds.) Progress in Oculomotor Research, Developments in Neuroscience Vol. 12, Elsevier, New York pp. 411–420.

Graf, W., McCrea, R.A. & Baker, R. (1981) Morphology of secondary vestibular neurons linked to the posterior canal in rabbit and cat. Soc. Neurosci. Abstr. 7, 40.

Graf, W., McCrea, R.A. & Baker, R. (1983) Morphology of posterior canal related secondary vestibular neurons in rabbit and cat. Exp. Brain Res. 52, 125–138.

Grantyn, A. & Berthoz, A. (1983) Discharge patterns of tecto-bulbo-spinal neurons during visuo-motor reactions in the alert cat. Soc. Neurosci. Abstr. 9, 751.

Grantyn, A. & Berthoz, A. (1985) Burst activity of identified tecto-reticulo-spinal neurons in the alert cat. Exp. Brain Res. 57, 417–421.

Gray, A.A. (1908) The Labyrinth of Animals, Including Mammals, Birds, Reptiles and Amphibians, Vol. I, II. Churchill, London.

Graybiel, A. (1974) Measurement of otolith function. In: H.H. Kornhuber (Ed.) Vestibular System. Handbook of Sensory Physiology. Vol. VI. Springer-Verlag, New York, pp. 233–266.

Graybiel, A. & Fregly, A.R. (1966) A new quantitative ataxia test battery. Acta Oto-Laryngol. 61, 293–312.

Graybiel, A., Miller, E.F., Newsom, B.D. & Kennedy, R.S. (1967) The effect of water immersion on perception of the oculographic illusion in normal and labyrinthine-defective subjects. NAMI-1016. Naval Aerospace Medicine Institute, Pensacola, FL.

Graybiel, A., Stockwell, C.W. & Guedry, F.E. (1972) Evidence for a test of dynamic otolith function considered in relation to responses from a patient with idiopathic progressive vestibular degeneration. Acta Oto-Laryngol. 73, 1–3.

Graybiel, A., Miller, E.F. & Homick, J.L. (1974) Experiment M-131. Human vestibular function. Proc. Skylab Life Sci. Symp., Vol. 1, NASA TM X- 58154, pp. 169–198.

Green, D.G., Powers, M.K. & Banks, M.S. (1980) Depth of focus, eye size and visual acuity. Vision Res. 20, 827–835.

356

Gresty, M.A. (1974) Coordination of head and eye movements to fixate continuous and intermittent targets. Vision Res. 14, 395–403.

Gresty, M.A. (1976) A reexamination of "neck reflex" eye movements in the rabbit. Acta Oto-Laryngol. 81, 386–394.

Gresty, M.A. & Ell, J.J. (1982) Normal modes of head and eye coordination. In: G. Lennerstrand, D.S. Zee & E.L. Keller (Eds.) Functional Basis of Ocular Motility Disorders. Pergamon, Oxford.

Gresty, M.A. & Halmagyi, G.M. (1979) Abnormal head movements. J. Neurol. Neurosurg. Psychiatr. 42, 705–714.

Gresty, M.A. & Leech, J. (1977) Coordination of the head and eyes in pursuit of predictable and random target motion. Aviat. Space Environ. Med. 48, 741–744.

Gresty, M.A., Hess, K. & Leech, J. (1977) Disorders of the vestibulo-ocular reflex producing oscillopsia and mechanisms compensating for loss of labyrinthine function. Brain 100, 693–716.

Greven, H.M. & De Wied, D. (1973) The influence of peptides derived from corticotropin (ACTH) on performance. Structure-activity studies. In: E. Zimmermann, W.H. Gispen, B.H. Marks & D. De Wied (Eds.) Drug Effects on Neuroendocrine Regulation, Progress in Brain Research, 39. Elsevier, Amsterdam, pp. 429–442.

Gribenski, A. (1963) Contribution à l'étude fonctionelle des canaux semi-circulaires chez la grenouille (Rana esculenta). J. Physiol. (Paris) 55, Suppl. VII, 1–95.

Groen, J.J. (1957) Adaptation. Pract. Oto-Rhino-Laryngol. 19, 524–530.

Groen, J.J., Lowenstein, O. & Vendrik, A.J. (1952) The mechanical analysis of responses from the end-organs of the horizontal semicircular canal in the isolated elasmobranch labyrinth. J. Physiol. (London) 117, 329–346.

Grossberg, S. (1964) The theory of embedding fields with applications to psychology and neurophysiology. Studies from Rockefeller Institute for Medical Research.

Guedry, F.E. (1965) Orientation of the rotation axis relative to gravity: its influence on nystagmus and the sense of rotation. Acta Oto-Laryngol. 60, 30–48.

Guitton, D. & Douglas, R.M. (1981) Une comparaison entre les mouvements rapides d'orientation de l'oeil accompagnant les mouvements actifs ou passifs de la tête chez le chat. Rev. Can. Biol. 40, 1, 69–75.

Guitton, D., & Douglas, R.M. & Vollé, M. (1984) Eye-head coordination in cats. J.Neurophysiol. 52, 1030–1050.

Guitton, D., Crommelink, M. & Roucoux, A. (1980) Stimulation of the superior colliculus in the alert cat. I. Eye movements and neck EMG activity evoked when the head is restrained. Exp. Brain Res. 39, 63–73.

Hacket, J.T., Hou, S.-M. & Cochran, S.L. (1979) Glutamate and synaptic depolarization of Purkinje cells evoked by parallel fibers and by climbing fibers. Brain Res. 170, 377–380.

Haddad, G.M. & Robinson, D.A. (1977) Cancellation of the vestibulo-ocular reflex during active and passive head movements in the cat. Soc. Neurosci. Abstr. 3, 155.

Haddad, G.M., Friendlich, A.R. & Robinson, D.A. (1977) Compensation of nystagmus after VIIIth nerve lesions in vestibulo-cerebellectomized cats. Brain Res. 135, 192–196.

Haddad, G.M., Demer, J.L. & Robinson, D.A. (1980) The effect of lesions of the dorsal cap of the inferior olive on the vestibulo-ocular and optokinetic systems of the cat. Brain Res. 185, 265–275.

Haines, D.E. (1977) Cerebellar corticonuclear and cortico-vestibular fibers of the flocculonodular lobe in a prosimian primate (Galago senegalensis). J. Comp. Neurol. 174, 607–630.

Hale, E.G. & Strachan, I.M. (1981) Non-surgical factors in the correction of aphakia. Trans. Ophthalmol. Soc. U.K. 101, 62–64.

Hallett, P.E. (1978) Primary and secondary saccades to goals defined by instruction. Vision Res. 18, 1279–1296.

Hallett, P.E. & Lightstone, A.D. (1976) Saccadic eye movements towards stimuli triggered during prior saccades. Vision Res. 16, 88–106.

Hannen, R.A., Kabrisky, M., Replogle, C.R., Hartzler, V.L. & Roccaforte, P.A. (1966) Experimental determination of a portion of the human vestibular response through measurement of eyeball counterroll. IEEE Trans. Bio-Med. Electron 13, 65–70.

Harris, A.J. (1965) Eye movements in the dogfish Squalus acanthias L. J. Exp. Biol. 43, 107–130.

Harris, L.R. (1980) The superior colliculus and movements of the head and eyes in cats. J. Physiol. (London) 300, 367–391.

Harris, L.R. & Cynader, M. (1981a) The eye movements of the dark-reared cat. Exp. Brain Res. 44, 41–56.

Harris, L.R. & Cynader, M. (1981b) Modification of the balance and gain of the vestibulo-ocular reflex in the cat. Exp. Brain Res. 44, 57–70.

Harris, L.R., Lepore, F., Guillemot, J.P. & Cynader, M. (1980) Abolition of optokinetic nystagmus in the cat. Science 210, 91–92.

Hasegawa, T. (1931) Die Veränderung der labyrinthaeren Reflexe bei zentrifugierten Meerschweinchen. Pfluegers Arch. Gesamte Physiol. Menschen Tiere 229, 205–225.

Hassler, R. & Hess, W.R. (1954) Experimentelle und anatomische Befunde über die Drehbewegungen und ihre nervösen Apparate. Arch. Psychiatr. Neurol. 192, 488–526.

Hassul, M., Daniels, P.D. & Kimm, J. (1976) Effects of bilateral flocullectomy on the vestibulo-ocular reflex in the Chinchilla. Brain Res. 118, 339–343.

Hay, J.C. (1968) Visual adaptation to an altered correlation between eye movement and head movement. Science 160, 429–430.

Heath, G.G. (1956a) The influence of visual acuity on accomodative responses of the eye. Am. J. Optom. Arch. Am. Acad. Optom. 33, 513–524.

Heath, G.G. (1956b) Components of accommodation. Am. J. Optom. Arch. Am. Acad. Optom. 33, 569–579.

Hebb, O. (1949) The Organization of Behavior. Wiley, New York.

Heiligenberg, W. (1977) Principles of Electrolocation and Jamming Avoidance in Electric Fish. A Neuroethological Approach. Studies on Brain Function, Vol. 1. Springer Verlag, Berlin, Heidelberg.

Helmholtz, H. von, (1896) Handbuch der physiologischen Optik. Zweite Auflage. Voss, Leipzig.

Helmholtz, H. von, (1910) Handbuch der physiologischen Optik. Dritte Auflage, Band 3. Voss, Hamburg, Leipzig. Engl. Translation: Helmholtz' Treatise on Physiological Optics. Vol. 3 Dover Press, New York, 1925.

Henn, V., Young, L.R. & Finley, C. (1974) Vestibular nucleus units in alert monkeys are also influenced by moving visual fields. Brain Res. 71, 144–149.

Henn, V., Cohen, B. & Young, L.R. (1980) Visual-vestibular interaction in motion perception and the generation of nystagmus. Neurosci. Res. Bull. 459–651.

Henn, V., Reisine, H., Waespe, W. & Böhmer, A. (1983) Pathophysiology of the vestibular system and its clinical implications. In : J.I. Suzuki (Ed) Clinical Examinations on Vertigo and Loss of Balance, pp. 366–378.

Hennessy, R.T. & Leibowitz, H.W. (1971) The effect of a peripheral stimulus on accommodation. Percept. Psychophys. 10, 129–132.

Henriksson, N.G., Kohut, R. & Fernandez, C. (1961) Studies on habituation of vestibular reflexes. I. Effect of repetitive caloric test. Acta Oto-Laryngol. 53, 333–349.

Henriksson, N.G., Novotny, M. & Tjerstrom, O. (1974) Eye movements as a function of active head turning. Acta Oto-Laryngol. 77, 86–91.

Henson, D.B. (1978) Corrective saccades: Effects of altering visual feedback. Vision Res. 18, 63–67.

Henson, D.B. & Dharamshi, B.G. (1982) Oculomotor adaptation to induced heterophoria and anisometropia. Invest. Ophthalmol. 22, 234–240.

Henson, D.B. & North, R. (1980) Adaptation to prism-induced heterophoria. Am. J. Opt. Physiol. Optics 57, 129–137.

Hering, E. (1868) Die Lehre vom binocularen Sehen. Engelmann, Leipzig.

Highstein, S.M. (1971) Organization of the inhibitory and excitatory vestibulo-ocular reflex pathways to the third and fourth nuclei in rabbit. Brain Res. 32, 218–224.

Highstein, S.M. (1973a) The organization of the vestibulo-oculomotor and trochlear reflex pathways in the rabbit. Exp. Brain Res. 17, 285–300.

Highstein, S.M. (1973b) Synaptic linkage in the vestibulo-ocular and cerebello-vestibular pathways to the VIth nucleus in the rabbit. Exp. Brain Res. 17, 301–314.

Hikosaka, O., Maeda, M., Nakao, S., Shimazu, H. and Shinoda, Y. (1977) Presynaptic impulses in the abducens nucleus and their relation to postsynaptic potentials in motoneurons during vestibular nystagmus. Exp. Brain Res. 27, 355–376.

Hillman, D.E. (1969) Neuronal organization of the cerebellar cortex in amphibia and reptilia. In: R. Llinás (Ed.) Neurobiology of Cerebellar Evolution and Development. Am. Med. Assoc., Chicago, pp. 279–325.

Hirsch, H.V. & Spinelli, D.N. (1970) Visual experience modifies distribution of horizontally and vertically oriented receptive fields in cats. Science 168, 869–871.

van Hoff-van Duin, J. (1978) Direction preference of optokinetic responses in monocularly tested normal kittens and light deprived cats. Arch. Ital. Biol. 166, 471–477.

Hoffmann, K.P. (1979) Optokinetic nystagmus and single cell responses in the nucleus tractus opticus after early monocular deprivation in the cat. In R.D. Freeman (Ed.) Developmental Neurobiology of Vision. Plenum Press, New York, pp. 63–73.

Hoffmann, K.-P. (1981) Neuronal responses related to optokinetic nystagmus in the cat's nucleus of the optic tract. In: A. Fuchs & W. Becker (Eds) Progress in Oculomotor Research. Elsevier, Amsterdam, New York, pp 443–454.

Hoffmann, K.-P. (1982) Cortical versus subcortical contributions to the optokinetic reflex in the cat. In: G. Lennerstrand, D.S. Zee & E. Keller (Eds.) Functional Basis of Ocular Motility Disorders. Pergamon Press, Oxford, New York, pp. 303–310.

Hoffmann, K.-P. & Schoppmann, A. (1975) Retinal input to direction selective cells in the nucleus tractus opticus of the cat. Brain Res. 99, 359–366.

Hoffmann, K.-P. & Schoppmann, A. (1981) A quantitative analysis of the direction-specific response of neurons in the cat's nucleus of the optic tract. Exp. Brain Res. 42, 146–157.

Högyes, E., (1880) On the nervous mechanisms of involuntary associated movements of the eyes. Orvosi Hetilap. 17, (Hungarian) (Ref. in Camis and Creed, 1930).

Högyes, E. (1880–1884) Az associált szemmozgások idegmechanismusáról. Értekezések a természéttudományok köréből. X, 18, 1–62 (1880); XI, 1–100 (1881); XIV, 9, 1–84 (1884). German translation: Högyes, A. (1912) Über den Nervenmechanismus der assoziierten Augenbewegungen. Monatsschr. f. Ohrenheilk. u. Laryngo-Rhinol. 46, 685–740; 809–841; 1027–1083; 1353–1413; 1554–1571.

Holmes, G. (1939) The cerebellum in man. Brain 63, 1

v. Holst, E. (1935) Über den Lichtrückenreflex bei Fischen. Pubbl. Stn. Zool. (Napoli) 15, 143–158.

Holstege, G. & Collewijn, H. (1982) The efferent connections of the nucleus of the optic tract and the superior colliculus in the rabbit. J. Comp. Neurol. 209, 139–175.

Honrubia, V., Scott, B.J. & Ward, P.H. (1967) Experimental studies on optokinetic nystagmus I. Normal cats. Acta Oto-Laryngol. 64, 388–402.

Honrubia, V., Koehn, W.W., Jenkins, H.A. and Fenton, W.H. (1982) Visual-vestibular interaction: effect of prolonged stimulation on the vestibulo-oculomotor reflex responses. Exp. Neurol. 76, 347–360.

Hood, J.D. (1981) Further observations on the phenomenon of rebound nystagmus. In: B. Cohen (Ed.) Vestibular and Oculomotor Physiology. Ann. N.Y. Acad. Sci. 374, 532–539.

Hood, J.D. & Pfalz, C.R. (1954) Observations upon the effects of repeated stimulation upon rotational and caloric nystagmus. J. Physiol. (London) 124, 130–144.

Horn, E. & Rayer, B. (1980) A hormonal component in central vestibular compensation. Z. Naturforsch. 35c, 1120–1121.

Horn, E., Greiner, B. & Horn, I. (1979) The effect of ACTH on habituation of the turning reaction in the toad Bufo bufo. J. Comp. Physiol. 131, 129–135.

Horridge, G.A. and Burrows, M. (1968) The onset of the fast phase in the optokinetic response of the crab (Carcinus). J. Exp. Biol. 49, 299–313.

Hoshino, K. and Pompeiano, O. (1977) Responses of lateral vestibular neurons to stimulation of contralateral macular labyrinthine receptors. Arch. Ital. Biol. 115, 237–261.

Hubel, D.H., & Wiesel, T.N. (1962) Receptive fields, binocular interaction and functional architecture in the cat's visual cortex. J. Physiol. (London) 160, 106–154.

Humphrey, D.R., Smith, A.M., Lamarre, Y., Nichols, T.R., Shinoda, Y. & Bizzi, E. (1983) Reciprocal inhibition and coactivation of antagonist muscles: Two fundamental modes of motor control. Soc. Neurosci. Abstr. 9, 1.

Igarashi, M., Alford, B.R., Kato, Y. & Levy, J.K. (1975) Effect of physical exercise upon nystagmus and locomotor equilibrium after labyrinthectomy in experimental primates. Acta Oto-Laryngol. 79, 214–220.

Igarashi, M., Takahashi, M. & Homick, J.L. (1978a) Optokinetic afternystagmus and postrotatory nystagmus in squirrel monkey. Acta Oto-Laryngol. 85, 387–396.

Igarashi, M., Takahashi, M., Kubo, T., Levy, J.K. & Homick, J.L. (1978b) Effect of macular ablation on vertical optokinetic nystagmus in the squirrel monkey. ORL 40, 312–318.

Igarashi, M., Levy, J.K., Takahashi, M., Alford, B.R. & Homick, J.L. (1979) Effect of exercise upon locomotor balance modification after peripheral vestibular lesions (unilateral utricular neurotomy) in squirrel monkey. Adv. Oto-Rhino-Laryngol. 25, 82–87.

Igarashi, M., Takahashi, M., Kubo, T., Alford, B.R. & Wright, W.K. (1980) Effect of off-vertical tilt and macular ablation on postrotatory nystagmus in the squirrel monkey. Acta Oto-Laryngol. 90, 93–99.

Igarashi, M.H., Isago, T., O-Uchi, W., Kulecz, J., Homick, J. & Reschke, M. (1983a) Visual-vestibular conflict sickness in the squirrel monkey. Acta Oto-Laryngol. 95, 193–198.

Igarashi, M., Isago, H. & Alford, B.R. (1983b) Effects of prolonged optokinetic stimulation on oculomotor and locomotor balance function. Acta Oto-Laryngol. 95, 560–567.

Igarashi, M., Isago, H. O-Uchi, T. & Kubo, T. (1983c) Uvulonodular lesions and eye-head coordination in squirrel monkey. In : C.R. Pflatz (Ed) Advances in Oto-Rhino-Laryngology,

Imbert, M. & Buisseret, P. (1975) Receptive field characteristics and plastic properties of visual cortical cells in kittens reared with or without visual experience. Exp. Brain Res. 22, 25–36.

Ishizuka, N., Mannen, H., Sasaki, S.-I. & Shimazu, H. (1980) Axonal branches and terminations in the cat abducens nucleus of secondary vestibular neurons in the horizontal canal system. Neurosci. Lett. 16, 143–148.

Isu, N. & Yokota, J. (1983) Morphological study on the divergent projection of axon collaterals of medial vestibular nucleus neurons in the cat. Exp. Brain Res. 53, 151–162.

Ito, M. (1970) Neurophysiological aspects of the cerebellar motor control system. Int. J. Neurol. 7, 162–176.

Ito, M. (1972) Neural design of the cerebellar motor control system. Brain Res. 40, 81–84.

Ito, M. (1974) The control mechanism of cerebellar motor system. In: F.O. Schmitt & F.G. Worden (Eds.) The Neurosciences, Third Study Program. MIT Press, pp. 293–303.

Ito, M. (1975) Learning control mechanisms by the cerebellum investigated in the flocculo-vestibulo-ocular system. In: D.B. Tower (Ed.) Basic Neurosciences. The Nervous System, Vol. I. Raven Press, New York, pp. 245–252.

Ito, M. (1976) Cerebellar learning control of vestibulo-ocular mechanisms. In: T. Desiraju (Ed.) Mechanisms in Transmission of Signals for Conscious Behavior. Elsevier, Amsterdam, New York, pp. 1–22.

Ito, M. (1977) Neuronal events in the cerebellar flocculus associated with an adaptive modification of the vestibulo-ocular reflex of the rabbit. In: R. Baker & A. Berthoz (Eds.) Control of Gaze by Brain Stem Neurons. Elsevier, Amsterdam, pp. 391–398.

Ito, M. (1980) Experimental tests of constructive models of the cerebellum. In: Gy. Székely, E. Lábos & S. Damjanovich (Eds.) Advances in Physiological Sciences vol. 30, Neural Communication and Control. Pergamon Press & Akadémiai Kiadó.

Ito, M. (1982a) Cerebellar control of the vestibulo-ocular reflex around the flocculus hypothesis. Annu. Rev. Neurosci. 5, 275–296.

Ito, M. (1982b) Questions in modeling the cerebellum. J. Theor. Biol. 99, 81–86.

Ito, M. (1982c) Experimental verification of Marr-Albus' plasticity: Assumption for the cerebellum. Acta Biol. Acad. Sci. Hung. 33, 189–199.

Ito, M. (1984) The cerebellum and neural control. Raven Press, New York, 580 pp.

Ito, M. & Kano, M. (1982) Long-lasting depression of parallel fiber-Purkinje cell transmission by conjunctive stimulation of parallel fibers and climbing fibers in the cerebellar cortex. Neurosci. Lett. 33, 253–258.

Ito, M. & Miyashita, Y. (1975) The effects of chronic destruction of inferior olive upon visual modification of the horizontal vestibulo-ocular reflex of rabbits. Proc. Jpn. Acad. 51, 716–760.

Ito, M., Nisimaru, N. & Yamamoto, M. (1973a) The neural pathways mediating reflex contraction of extraocular muscles during semicircular canal stimulation in rabbits. Brain Res. 55, 183–188.

Ito, M., Nisimaru, N. & Yamamoto, M. (1973b) The neural pathways relaying reflex inhibition from semicircular canals to extraocular muscles of rabbits. Brain Res. 55, 189–193.

Ito, M., Shiida, T., Yagi, N. & Yamamoto, M. (1974a) Visual influence on rabbit horizontal vestibulo-ocular reflex presumably effected via the cerebellar flocculus. Brain Res. 65, 170–174.

Ito, M., Shiida, T., Yagi, N. & Yamamoto, M. (1974b) The cerebellar modification of rabbit's horizontal vestibulo-ocular reflex induced by sustained head rotation combined with visual stimulation. Proc. Jpn. Acad. 50, 85–89.

Ito, M., Nisimaru, N. & Yamamoto, M. (1976a) Pathways for the vestibulo-ocular reflex excitation arising from semicircular canals of rabbits. Exp. Brain Res. 24, 257–271.

Ito, M., Nisimaru, N. & Yamamoto, M. (1976b) Postsynaptic inhibition of oculomotor neurons involved in vestibulo-ocular reflexes arising from semicircular canals of rabbits. Exp. Brain Res. 24, 273–283.

Ito, M., Nisimaru, N. & Yamamoto, M. (1977) Specific patterns of neuronal connections involved in the control of rabbit's vestibulo-ocular reflexes by the cerebellar flocculus. J. Physiol. (London) 265, 833–854.

Ito, M., Jastreboff, P.J. & Miyashita, Y. (1979a) Adaptive modification of the rabbit's horizontal vestibulo-ocular reflex during sustained vestibular and optokinetic stimulation. Exp. Brain Res. 37, 17–30.

Ito, M., Nisimaru, N. & Shibuki, K. (1979b) Destruction of inferior olive induces rapid depression in synaptic action of cerebellar Purkinje cells. Nature 277, 568–569.

Ito, M., Jastreboff, P.J. & Miyashita, Y. (1980) Retrograde influence of surgical and chemical flocculectomy upon dorsal cap neurons of the inferior olive. Neurosci. Lett. 20, 45–48.

Ito, M., Jastreboff, P.J. & Miyashita, Y. (1982a) Specific effects of unilateral lesions in the flocculus upon eye movement of rabbits. Exp. Brain Res. 45, 233–242.

Ito, M., Orlov, O. & Yamamoto, M. (1982b) Topographical representation of vestibulo-ocular reflexes in rabbit cerebellar flocculus. Neuroscience 7, 1657–1664.

Ito, M., Sakurai, M. & Tongroach, P. (1982c) Climbing fiber induced depression of both mossy fiber responsiveness and glutamate sensitivity of cerebellar Purkinje cells. J. Physiol. (London) 324, 113–134.

Jacob, W. (1928) Über das Labyrinth der Pleuronectiden. Zool. Jahrb., Allg. Zool. 44, 523–574.

Janeke, J.B., Jongkees, L.B. and Oosterveld, W.J. (1970) Relationship between otoliths and nystagmus. Acta Oto-Laryngol. 69, 1–6.

Jäger, J. & Henn, V. (1981a) Habituation of the vestibulo-ocular reflex (VOR) in the monkey during sinusoidal rotation in the dark. Exp. Brain Res. 41, 108–114.

Jäger, J. & Henn, V. (1981b) Vestibular habituation in man and monkey during sinusoïdal rotation. In: B. Cohen (Ed.) Vestibular and Oculomotor Physiology. Ann. N.Y. Acad. Sci. 374, 330–339.

Jäger, J., Henn, V., Lang, W., Miles, T.S. & Waespe, W. (1981) Vestibular unit activity in monkeys with horizontal gaze palsy. In: A.F. Fuchs & W. Becker (Eds.) Progress in Oculomotor Research. Elsevier, Amsterdam, pp. 89–95.

Jeannerod, M. & Hecaen, H. (1979) Adaptation et restauration des fonctions nerveuses. Simep. Ed. Lyon, Fr. 392 pp.

Jeannerod, M., Magnin, M., Schmid, R. & Stefanelli, M. (1976) Vestibular habituation to angular velocity steps in the cat. Biol. Cybern. 22, 39–48.

Jeannerod, M., Clément, G. & Courjon, J.H. (1981) Unilateral habituation of vestibulo-ocular responses in the cat. In: B. Cohen (Ed.) Vestibular and Oculomotor Physiology. Ann. N.Y. Acad. Sci. 374, 340–351.

Jell, R.M., Guedry, F.E. & Hixson, W.C. (1982) The vestibulo-ocular reflex in man during voluntary head oscillation under three visual conditions. Aviat. Space Environ. Med. 53,6, 541–548.

Jensen, D.W. (1979a) Reflex control of acute postural asymmetry and compensatory symmetry after a unilateral vestibular lesion. Neuroscience 4, 1059–1073.

Jensen, D.W. (1979b) Vestibular compensation: Tonic spinal influence upon spontaneous descending vestibular nuclear activity. Neuroscience 4, 1075–1084.

Jensen, D.W. (1983) Survival of function of the deafferentated vestibular nerve. Brain Res. 273, 175–178.

Johnston, R.S. & Dietlein, L.F. (Eds.) (1977) Biomedical Results from Skylab NASA SP-377. Washington, DC: NASA Scientific and Technical Information Office.

Jones, G.M. & Milsum, J. H. (1965) Spatial and dynamic aspects of visual fixation. IEEE Trans. Biomed. Engin. Vol. BME 12, No. 2, pp. 54–62.

Jones, G.M. & Spells, K.E. (1963) A theoretical and comparative study of the functional dependence of the semicircular canal upon its physical dimensions. Proc. R. Soc. London B. 157, 403–419.

Jones, R. (1977) Anomalies of disparity detection in the human visual system. J. Physiol. (London) 264, 621–640.

Jones, R. & Kerr, K.E. (1971) Motor responses to conflicting asymmetrical vergence stimulus information. Am. J. Optom, Arch. Am. Acad. Optom. 48, 989–1000.

Jones, R. & Kerr, K.E. (1972) Vergence eye movements to pairs of disparate stimuli with shape selection cues. Vision Res. 12, 1425–1430.

Joseph, B.A. & Whitlock, D.G. (1968) Central projections of selected spinal dorsal roots in anuran amphibians. Anat. Rec. 160, 297–288.

Jung, R. (1948) Die Registrierung des post-rotatorischen und optokinetischen Nystagmus und die optisch-vestibuläre Integration beim Menschen. Acta Oto-Laryngol. 36, 199–202.

Kalmijn, A.J. (1974) The detection of electric fields from inanimate and animate sources other than electric organs. In : A. Fessard (Ed.) Handbook of Sensory Physiology, Vol. III/3, Springer Verlag, New York, pp. 147–200.

Kalmijn, A.J. (1974) Electro-orientation in sharks and rays: theory and experimental evidence. Scripps Institution of Oceanography Reference Series, Contr. No. 73–39 1–22.

Kasahara, M. & Uchino, Y. (1974). Bilateral semicircular canal inputs to neurons in cat vestibular nuclei. Exp. Brain Res. 20, 285–296.

Kasai, T. & Zee, D.S. (1978) Eye-head coordination in labyrinthine-defective human beings. Brain Res. 144, 123–141.

Kasamatsu, T. & Pettigrew, J.D. (1976) Depletion of brain catecholamines: failure of ocular dominance shift after monocular occlusion in kittens. Science 194, 206–209.

Kasamatsu, T. & Pettigrew, J.D. (1979) Preservation of binocularity after monocular deprivation in the striate cortex of kittens treated with 6-hydroxydopamine. J. Comp. Neurol. 185. 139–162.

Kasamatsu, T., Pettigrew, J.D. & Ary, M. (1979) Restoration of visual cortical plasticity by local microperfusion of norepinephrine. J. Comp. Neurol. 185, 163–182.

Kawano, K. & Miles, F.A. (1983) Adaptive plasticity in short-latency ocular following responses of monkey. Soc. Neurosci. Abstr. 9, 868.

Keller, E.L. (1974) Participation of medial pontine reticular formation in eye movement generation in monkey. J. Neurophysiol. 37, 316–332.

Keller, E.L. (1976) Behavior of horizontal semicircular canal afferents in alert monkey during vestibular and optokinetic stimulation. Exp. Brain Res. 24, 459–471.

Keller, E.L. (1978) Gain of the vestibulo-ocular reflex in monkey at high rotational frequencies. Vision Res. 18, 311–315.

Keller, E.L. (1981) Oculomotor neuron behavior. In: B.L. Zuber (Ed.) Models of Oculomotor Behavior and Control. CRC Press, Boca Raton, pp. 1–19.

Keller, E.L. & Daniels, P.D. (1975) Oculomotor related interaction of vestibular and visual stimulation in vestibular nucleus cells in alert monkey. Exp. Neurol. 46, 187–198.

Keller, E.L. & Kamath, B.Y. (1975) Characteristics of head rotation and eye movement related neurons in alert monkey vestibular nucleus. Brain Res. 100, 182–187.

Keller, E.L. & Precht, W. (1978) Persistence of visual response in vestibular nucleus neurons in cerebellectomized cat. Exp. Brain Res. 32, 591–594.

Keller, E.L. & Precht, W. (1979a) Adaptive modification of central vestibular neurons in response to visual stimulation through reversing prisms. J. Neurophysiol. 42, 896–911.

Keller, E.L. & Precht, W. (1979b) Visual-vestibular responses in vestibular nuclear neurons in the intact and cerebellectomized alert cat. Neuroscience 4, 1599–1613.

Keller, E.L. & Precht, W. (1981) Adaptive modification of brain stem pathways during vestibulo-ocular recalibration. In: H. Flohr & W. Precht (Eds.) Lesion-Induced Neuronal Plasticity in Sensorimotor Systems. Springer Verlag, Berlin, pp. 284–294.

Keller, E.L. & Robinson, D.A. (1972) Abducens unit behavior in the monkey during vergence movements. Vision Res. 12, 369–382.

Keller, E.L. & Smith, M.J. (1983) Suppressed visual adaptation of the vestibuloocular reflex in catecholamine-depleted cats. Brain Res. 258, 323–327.

Kelly, D.A. (1979) Motion and vision. II. Stabilized spatiotemporal threshold surfaces. J. Opt. Soc. Am. 69, 1340–1349.

Kennedy, H., Flandrin, J.M. & Amblard, B. (1980) Afferent visual pathways and receptive field properties of superior colliculus neurons in stroboscopically reared cats. Neurosci. Lett. 19, 283–288.

Kennedy, H., Courjon, J.H. & Flandrin, J.M. (1982) Vestibulo-ocular reflex and optokinetic nystagmus in adult cats reared in stroboscopic illumination. Exp. Brain Res. 48, 279–287.

Kent, P.R. (1958) Convergence accommodation Am. J. Optom. Arch. Am. Acad. Optom. 35, 393–406.

Kenyon, R.V., Ciuffreda, K.J. & Stark, L. (1978) Binocular eye movements during accommodative vergence. Vision Res. 18, 545–555.

Kety, S.S. (1970) The biogenic amines in the central nervous system: their possible roles in arousal, emotion, and learning. In: F.O. Schmitt (Ed.) The Neurosciences, Second Study Program. Rockefeller University Press, New York, pp. 324–336.

Kety, S.S. (1972) Brain catecholamines, affective states and memory. In: J.L. McGaugh (Ed.) The Chemistry of Mood, Motivation, and Memory. Plenum Press, New York, London, pp. 65–80.

Kim, J.H. (1974) Studies on the functional interrelation between the vestibular canals and the extraocular muscles. Korean J. Physiol. 8, 87–103.

King, W.M., Lisberger, S.G. & Fuchs, A.F. (1976) Responses of fibers in medial longitudinal fasciculus (mlf) of alert monkeys during horizontal and vertical conjugate eye movements evoked by vestibular or visual stimuli. J. Neurophysiol. 39, 1135–1149.

Kleijn, de, A. (1914) Zur Analyse der Folgezustände einseitiger Labyrinthextirpation beim Frosch. Pfluegers Arch. Gesamte Physiol. Menschen Tiere 159, 218–223.

Kleinschmidt, H.J. & Collewijn, H. (1975) A search for habituation of vestibulo-ocular reactions to rotary and linear sinusoidal accelerations in the rabbit. Exp. Neurol. 47, 257–267.

Kleyn, de, A. & Versteegh, C. (1933) Labyrinthreflex nach Abscheuderung der Otolithenmembrane bei Meerschweinchen. Pfluegers Arch. Gesamte Physiol. Menschen Tiere 233, 454–465.

Koch, C. & Poggio, T. (1983) A theoretical analysis of electrical properties of spines. Proc. R. Soc. London Ser. B 218, 455–477.

Koenig, E. & Dichgans, J. (1981) Aftereffects of vestibular and optokinetic stimulation and their interaction. In: B. Cohen (Ed.) Vestibular and Oculomotor Physiology. Ann. N.Y. Acad. Sci. 374, 434–445.

Koenig, E., Allum, J.H.J. & Dichgans, J. (1978) Visual-vestibular interaction upon nystagmus slow phase velocity in man. Acta Oto-Laryngol. 85, 397–410.

Koerner, F. & Schiller, P.H. (1972) The optokinetic response under open and closed loop conditions in the monkey. Exp. Brain Res. 14, 318–330.

Kohler, I. (1956). Die Methode des Brillenversuches in der Wahrenhmungspyschologie: Mit Bemerkungen zur Lehre der Adaptation. Z. Exp. Angew. Psychol., 3, 381–417.

Kohler, I. (1962) Experiments with goggles. Sci. Am. 206, 62–86.

Kolb, E. (1955) Untersuchungen über zentrale Kompensation und Kompensationsbewegungen einseitig entstateter Frösche. Z. Vergl. Physiol. 37, 136–160.

Kommerell, G., Olivier, D. & Theopold, H. (1976) Adaptive programming of phasic and tonic components in saccadic eye movements. Investigations in patients with abducens palsy. Invest. Ophthalmol. 15, 657–660.

Kompanejetz, S. (1928) Investigation on the counterrolling of the eyes in optimum head positions. Acta Oto-Laryngol. 12, 332–350.

Kornhuber, H.H. (1959) Der periodisch alternierende Nystagmus (Nystagmus alternans) und die Enthemmung des vestibulären Systems. Arch. Ohren-Nasen-Kehlkopfheilkd. 174, 182–209.

Kornhuber, H.H. (1974) Vestibular System. Handbook of Sensory Physiology. Vol. VI/1,2. Springer Verlag, Berlin.

Korte, G.E. & Friedrich, V.L. (1979) The fine structure of the feline superior vestibular nucleus: identification and synaptology of the primary vestibular afferents. Brain Res. 176, 3–32.

Korte, G.E. & Mugnaini, E. (1979) The cerebellar projection of the vestibular nerve in the cat. J. Comp. Neurol. 184, 265–278.

Kowler, E., Murphy, B.J. & Steinman, R.M. (1978) Velocity matching during smooth pursuit of different targets on different backgrounds. Vision Res. 18, 603–605.

Kreidl, A. (1906) Die Funktion des Vestibularapparates. Ergeb. Physiol. 5, 572.

Krejcova, H., Highstein, S. & Cohen, B. (1971) Labyrinthine and extra-labyrinthine effects on ocular counter-rolling. Acta Oto-Laryngol. 72, 165–171.

Krewson, W.E. (1950) The action of the extraocular muscles.

A method of vector-analysis with computations. Trans. Am. Opthalmol. Soc. 48, 443–486.

Krishnan, V.V., Shirachi, D. & Stark, L. (1977) Dynamic measures of vergence accommodation. Am. J. Optom. Physiol. Optics 54, 470–473.

Kubin, L., Magherini, P.C., Manzoni, D. & Pompeiano, O. (1980) Responses of lateral recticular neurons to sinusoidal stimulation of labyrinth receptors in decerebrate cat. J. Neurophysiol. 44, 922–936.

Kubo, T., Igarashi, M., Jensen, D.W. & Homick, J.L. (1981a) Eye-head coordination during optokinetic stimulation in squirrel monkeys. Ann. Oto-Rhino-Laryngol. 90, 85-88.

Kubo, T., Igarashi, M., Jensen, D.W. & Wright, W.K. (1981b) Head and eye movements following vestibular stimulus in squirrel monkeys. ORL 43, 26–38.

Kubo, T., Igarashi, M., Jensen, D.W. & Wright, W.K. (1981c) Effects of lateral semi-circular canals block on eye-head coordination in squirrel monkeys. Ann. Oto-Rhino-Laryngol. 90, 154–157.

Kusakari, J., Kaneko, Y., Kakizaki, J. (1973) Labyrinthine compensatory eye position of the guinea pig. Laryngoscope 83, 388–396.

Lacour, M. & Xerri, C. (1980) Compensation of postural reactions to free-fall in the vestibular neurotomized monkey. Role of the visual motions cues. Exp. Brain Res. 40, 103–110.

Lacour, M., Roll, J.P. & Appaix, M. (1976) Modifications and development of spinal reflexes in the alert baboon (*Papio Papio*) following an unilateral vestibular neurotomy. Brain Res. 113, 255–269.

Lacour, M., Xerri, C. & Hugon, M. (1979) Compensation of postural reactions to fall in the vestibular neurectomized monkey. Role of the remaining labyrinthine afferences. Exp. Brain Res. 37, 563–580.

Landers, P.H., Taylor, A. (1975) Transfer function analysis of the vestibulo-ocular reflex in the conscious cat. In: G. Lennerstrand & P. Bach-y-Rita (Eds.) Basic mechanisms of ocular motility and their clinical implications. Pergamon Press, Oxford, pp. 505–508.

Langer, T., Fuchs, A.F., Chubb, M.C. Scudder, C.A. & Lisberger, S.G. (1985) Floccular efferents in the rhesus macaque as revealed by autoradiography and horseradish peroxydase. J.Comp. Neurol., in press.

Lanman, J., Bizzi, E. & Allum, J. (1978) The coordination of eye and head movement during smooth pursuit. Brain Res. 153, 39–53.

Lashley, K.S. (1942) The problem of cerebral organization in vision. In: H. Kluever (Ed.) Visual Mechanisms, Biological Symposia, Vol. VII. Jacques Cattel Press, Lancaster, pp. 301–322.

Lebedkin, S. (1924) Über die Lage des Canalis Semicircularis bei Sängern. Anat. Anz. 58, 449–460.

Leigh, R.J. & Zee, D.S. (1980) Eye movements of the blind. Invest. Ophthalmol. 19, 328–331.

Leigh, R.J., Robinson, D.A. & Zee, D.S. (1981) A hypothetical explanation for periodic alternating nystagmus: instability in the optokinetic-vestibular system. In: B. Cohen (Ed.) Vestibular and Oculomotor Physiology. Ann. N.Y. Acad. Sci. 374, 619–635.

Leigh, R.J., Newman, S.A., Zee, D.S. & Miller, N.R. (1982) Visual following during stimulation of an immobile eye (the open loop condition). Vision Res. 22, 1193–1197.

Lennerstrand, G. & Bach-Y-Rita, P. (Eds.) (1975) Basic Mechanisms of Ocular Motility and their Clinical Implications. Pergamon press, Oxford, 584 p.

Lennerstrand, G., Zee, D.S. & Keller, E.L. (Eds.) (1982) Functional Basis of Ocular Motility Disorders. Pergamon press, Oxford, 603 p.

Lestienne, F., Whittington, D. & Bizzi, E. (1981) Single cell recording from the brain stem in monkey: behaviour of preoculomotor neurons during eye-head coordination. In: A. Fuchs & W. Becker (Eds.) Progress in Oculomotor Research. Elsevier, Amsterdam, pp. 325–333.

Lestienne, F., Vidal, P.P. & Berthoz, A. (1984) Gaze changing behaviour in head restrained monkey. Exp. Brain Res. 53, 349–356.

Lichtenberg, B.K., Young, L.R., and Arrott, A.P. (1982) Human ocular counter-rolling induced by varying linear accelerations. Vision Res. 48, 127–136.

Lincoln, J.S., McCormick, D.A. & Thompson, R.F. (1982) Ipsilateral cerebellar lesions prevent learning of the classically conditioned nictitating membrane/eyelid response. Brain Res. 242, 190–193.

Lisberger, S.G. & Fuchs, A. (1974) Responses of flocculus Purkinje cells to adequate vestibular stimulation in the alert monkey: Fixation vs. compensatory eye movements. Brain Res. 69, 347–353.

Lisberger, S.G. & Fuchs, A.F. (1978a) Role of primate flocculus during rapid behavioral modification of vestibuloocular reflex. I. Purkinje cell activity during visually guided horizontal smooth-pursuit eye movements and passive head rotation. J. Neurophysiol. 41, 733-763.

Lisberger, S.G. & Fuchs, A.F. (1978b) Role of primate flocculus during rapid behavioral modification of vestibuloocular reflex. II. Mossy fiber firing patterns during horizontal head rotation and eye movement. J. Neurophysiol. 41, 764–777.

Lisberger, S.G. & Miles, F.A. (1980) Role of primate medial vestibular nucleus in long-term adaptive plasticity of vestibuloocular reflex. J. Neurophysiol. 43, 1725–1745.

Lisberger, S.G. & Miles, F.A. (1981) Channels in the vestibulo-ocular reflex (VOR). Soc. Neurosci. Abstr. 7, 297.

Lisberger, S.G., Miles, F.A. Optican, L.M. & Eighmy, B.B. (1981) Optokinetic response in the monkey: underlying mechanisms and their sensitivity to long-term adaptive changes in vestibuloocular reflex. J. Neurophysiol. 45, 869–890.

Lisberger, S.G., Miles, F.A. & Optican, L.M. (1983) Frequency selective adaptation: Evidence for channels in the vestibulo-ocular reflex? J. Neurosci. 3(6), 1234–1244.

Lisberger, S.G., Miles, F.A. & Zee, D.S. (1984) Signals used to compute errors in monkey vestibulo-ocular reflex: possible role of flocculus. J. Neurophysiol. 52, 1140–1153.

Llinás, R. (Ed.) (1969) Neurobiology of Cerebellar Evolution and Development. Am. Med. Assoc., Chicago, 893 pp.

Llinás, R. (1974) Eighteenth Bowditch Lecture: Motor aspects of cerebellar control. Physiologist 17, 19–46.

Llinás, R. (1984) Rebound excitation as the physiological basis for tremor: A biophysical study of the oscillatory properties of mammalian central neurons in vitro. In: Findlay and Capildeo (Eds.) Movement Disorders: Tremor. MacMillan, London, pp. 165–182.

Llinás, R. & Simpson, J.I. (1981) Cerebellar control of movement. In: A. L. Towe & E.S. Luschei (Eds.) Motor Coordination. Handbook of Behavioral Neurobiology, Vol. 5. Plenum Press, New York, pp. 231–302.

Llinás, R. & Sugimori, M. (1980) Electrophysiological properties of in vitro Purkinje cell dendrites in mammalian cerebellar slices. J. Physiol. (London) 305, 197–213.

Llinás, R. & Volkind, R. (1973) The olivo-cerebellar system: Functional properties as revealed by harmaline-induced tremor. Exp. Brain Res. 18, 69–87.

Llinás, R. and Walton, K. (1979a) Place of the cerebellum in motor learning. In: M.A.B. Brazier (Ed.) Brain Mechanisms in Memory and Learning: From the Single Neuron to Man, IBRO Monograph Series 4. Raven Press, New York, pp. 17–36.

Llinás, R. & Walton, K. (1979b) Vestibular compensation: A distributed property of the central nervous system. In: H. Asanuma & V.J. Wilson (Eds.) Integration in the Nervous System. Igaku-Shoin, Tokyo, New York, pp. 145–166.

Llinás, R. & Yarom, Y. (1981a) Electrophysiology of mammalian inferior olivary neurones in vitro. Different types of voltage-dependent ionic conductances. J. Physiol. (London) 315, 549–567.

Llinás, R. & Yarom, Y. (1981b) Properties and distribution of ionic conductances generating electroresponsiveness of mammalian inferior olivary neurones in vitro. J. Physiol. (London) 315, 569–584.

Llinás, R., Precht, W. & Clarke, M. (1971) Cerebellar Purkinje cell responses to physiological stimulation of the vestibular system in the frog. Exp. Brain Res. 13, 408–431.

Llinás, R., Walton, K., Hillman, D.E. & Sotelo, C. (1975) Inferior olive: its role in motor learning. Science 190, 1230–1231.

Llinás, R., Simpson, J.I. & W. Precht (1976) Nystagmic modulation of neuronal activity in rabbit cerebellar flocculus. Pfluegers Arch. 367, 7–13.

Llinás, R., Yarom, Y. & Sugimori, M. (1981) The isolated mammalian brain in vitro: A new technique for the analysis of the electrical activity of neuronal circuit function. Fed. Proc. 40, 2240–2245.

Loe, D.R., Tomko, D.L. & Werner, G. (1973) The neural signal of angular head position in primary vestibular axons. J. Physiol. (London) 230, 29–50.

Lorente de Nó, R. (1932) The regulations of eye positions and movements induced by the labyrinth. The Laryngoscope 42, 233–332.

Lorente de Nó, R. (1933) Vestibulo-ocular reflex arc. Arch. Neurol. Psychiatr. 30, 245–291.

Löwenstein, O. (1937) The tonic function of the horizontal semicircular canals in fishes. J. Exp. Biol. 14, 473–482.

Löwenstein, O.E. (1974) Comparative morphology and physiology. In: H.H. Kornhuber (Ed.) Handbook of Sensory Physiology, Vol. VI/1, Springer, Berlin, Heidelberg, New York, pp. 75–120.

Löwenstein, O. & Sand, A. (1940) The mechanism of the semicircular canal. A study of responses of single-fibre preparations to angular accelerations and to rotation at constant speed. Proc. R. Soc. London Ser. B. 129, 256–275.

Löwenstein, O. & Thornhill, R.A. (1970) The labyrinth of Myxine: Anatomy, ultrastructure and electrophysiology. Proc. R. Soc. London Ser. B. 176, 21–42.

Löwenstein, O., Osborne, M.P. & Thornhill, R.A. (1968) The anatomy and ultrastructure of the labyrinth of the lamprey (Lampetra fluviatilis L.). Proc. R. Soc. London Ser. B. 170, 113–134.

Ludvigh, E., McKinnon, P. & Zartzeff, L. (1964) Temporal course of the relaxation of binocular duction (fusion) movements. Arch. Ophthalmol. 71, 389–399.

Luschei, E.S. & Fuchs, A.F. (1972) Activity of brainstem neurons during eye movements of alert monkeys. J. Neurophysiol. 35, 445–461.

McCabe, B.F., Ryu, J.H. & Sekitani, T. (1972) Further experiments on vestibular compensation. Laryngoscope 82, 381–396.

McClure, J.A., Copp, J.C. & Lycett, P. (1981) Recovery nystagmus in Meniere's disease. Laryngoscope 91, 1727–1737.

McCormick, D.A., Clark, G.A., Lavond, D.G. & Thompson, R.F. (1982) Initial localization of the memory trace for a basic form of learning. Proc. Natl. Acad. Sci. U.S.A. 79, 2731–2735.

McCrea, R.A., Yoshida, K., Berthoz, A. & Baker, R. (1980) Eye movement related activity and morphology of second order vestibular neurons terminating in the cat abducens nucleus. Exp. Brain Res. 40, 468–473.

McCrea, R.A., Yoshida, K., Evinger, C. & Berthoz, A. (1981) The location, axonal arborization, and termination sites of eye-movement related secondary vestibular neurons demonstrated by intra-axonal HRP injection in the alert cat. In: A. Fuchs & W. Becker (Eds.) Progress in Oculomotor Research. Developments in Neuroscience, Vol. 12. Elsevier, New York, Amsterdam, Oxford, pp. 379–386.

McCrea, R.A., Strassman, A. & Highstein, S.M. (1982) The location and collateral projection of squirrel monkey vestibular neurons with vertical eye position sensitivity. Soc. Neurosci. Abstr. 8, 157.

McNally, W.J. & Tait, J. (1925) Ablation experiments on the labyrinth of the frog. Am. J. Physiol. 75, 155–179.

McNally W.J., & Tait, J. (1933) Some results of section of particular nerve branches to the ampullae of the four vertical semicircular canals of the frog. Q.J. Exp. Physiol. 23, 147–196.

Mach, E. (1875) Grundlinien der Lehre von den Bewegungsempfindungen. Engelmann, Leipzig, Reprint Bonset, Amsterdam, 1967.

Mach, E. (1886) Beiträge zur Analyse der Empfindungen. Jena: Fisher. English translation by C.M. Williams, revised and supplemented by Sydney Waterlow, 1959, Dover, New York.

Mackworth, N.H. & Kaplan, I.T. (1962) Visual acuity when eyes are pursuing moving targets. Science 136, 387–388.

Maddox, E.E. (1886) Investigations on the relationship between convergence and accommodation of the eyes. J. Anat. 20, 475–508, 565–584.

Maekawa, K.E. & Simpson, J.I. (1972) Climbing fiber activation of Purkinje cells in the flocculus by impulses transferred through the visual pathways. Brain Res. 39, 245–251.

Maekawa, K. & Simpson, J.I. (1973) Climbing fiber responses evoked in the vestibulo-cerebellum of rabbit from visual system. J. Neurophysiol. 36, 649–666.

Maekawa, K. & Takeda, T. (1976) Electrophysiological identification of the climbing and mossy fibre pathways from the rabbit's retina to the contralateral cerebellar flocculus. Brain Res. 109, 169–174.

Maekawa, K. & Takeda, T. (1979) Origin of descending afferents to the rostral part of dorsal cap of inferior olive which transfers contralateral optic activities to the flocculus. An HRP study. Brain Res. 172, 393–405.

Magnus, R. (1924) Körperstellung. Springer, Berlin.

Magnus, R. & De Kleijn, A. (1913) Analyse der Folgezustände einseitiger Labyrinthextirpation mit besonderer Berücksichtigung der Rolle der tonischen Halsreflexe. Pfluegers Arch. Gesamte Physiol. Menschen Tiere 154, 178–306.

Maioli, C., Precht, W., & Ried, S. (1982) Vestibuloocular and optokinetic reflex compensation following hemilabyrinthectomy in the cat. In: A. Roucoux & M. Crommelinck (Eds.) Physiological and Pathological Aspects of Eye Movements D.W. Junk, The Hague, pp. 200–208.

Maioli, C., Precht, W. & Ried, S. (1983) Short- and long-term modification of vestibulo-ocular response dynamics following unilateral vestibular nerve lesions in the cat. Exp. Brain Res. 50, 259–274.

Mair, J.W.S. & Fernandez, C. (1966) Pathological and functional changes following hemisection of the lateral ampullary nerve. Acta Oto-Laryngol. 62, 513–531.

Malach, R., Strong, N.P. & Van Sluyters, R.C. (1981) Optokinetic nystagmus in long-term monocularly deprived cats. Soc. Neurosci. Abstr. 7, 733.

Malach, R., Strong, N.P., Olavarria, J. & Van Sluyters, R.C. (1984) Horizontal optokinetic nystagmus in the cat: effects of long term monocular deprivation. Dev. Brain Res. 13, 193–206.

Malcolm, R. & Melvill Jones, G. (1970) A quantitative study of vestibular adaptation in human. Acta Oto-Laryngol. 70, 126–135.

Mandl, G. & Melvill Jones, G. (1979) Rapid visual vestibular interaction during visual tracking in strobe light. Brain Res. 165, 133–138.

Mandl, G., Melvill Jones, G. & Cynader, M. (1981) Adaptability of the vestibulo-ocular reflex to vision reversal in strobe-reared cats. Brain Res. 209, 35–45.

Markham, C.H. & Curthoys, I.S. (1972) Convergence of labyrinthine influences on units in the vestibular nuclei of the cat. II. Electrical stimulation. Brain Res. 43, 383–396.

Markham, C.H., Yagi, T. & Curthoys, I.S. (1977) The contribution of the contralateral labyrinth to second order vestibular neuronal activity in the cat. Brain Res. 138, 99–109.

Marlow, F.W. (1921) Prolonged monocular occlusion as a test for the muscle balance. Am. J. Ophthalmol. 4, 238–250.

Marr, D. (1969) A theory for cerebellar cortex. J. Physiol. (London) 202, 437–470.

Marr, D. (1982) Vision. A Computational Investigation into the Human Representation and Processing of Visual Information. W.H. Freeman, San Francisco.

Matsnev, E.I., Yakovleva, I.Y., Tarasov, I.K., Alekseev, V.N., Kornilova, L.N., Mateev, A.D. & Gorgiladze, G.I. (1983) Space Motion Sickness: Phenomenology, Countermeasures, and Mechanisms. Aviat. Space Environ. Med. 54, 312–317.

Matsuo, V., Cohen, B., Raphan, T., deJong, V. & Henn, V. (1979) Asymmetric velocity storage for upward and downward nystagmus. Brain Res. 176, 159–164.

Matsuo, V., Büttner-Ennever, J., Cohen, B., Fradin, J. & Blumenfeld, H. (1983) Effects of pretectal lesions on components of the horizontal optokinetic response. Soc. Neurosci. Abstr. 9, 749.

Matsuoka, I., Domino, E.F. & Morimoto, M. (1973) Adrenergic and cholinergic mechanisms of single vestibular neurons in the cat. Adv. Oto-Rhino-Laryngol. 19, 163–178.

Maxwell, S.S. (1923) Labyrinth and Equilibrium, Lippincott, Philadelphia.

Mays, L. & Sparks, D. (1980) Saccades are spatially, not retinocentrically, coded. Science 208, 1163–1165.

Meienberg, O., Zangemeister, W.H., Rosenberg, M., Hoyt, W.F. & Stark, L. (1981) Saccadic eye movement strategies in patients with homonymous hemianopsia. Ann. Neurol. 9, 537–544.

Meiry, J.L. (1971) Vestibular and proprioceptive stabilization of eye movements. In: P. Bach-y-Rita, C.C. Collins & J. Hyde (Eds.) Control of Eye Movements. Academic Press, New York, pp. 483–496.

Melvill Jones, G. (1964) Predominance of anticompensatory oculomotor response during rapid head rotation. Aerosp. Med. 35, 965–968.

Melvill Jones, G. (1966) Interactions between optokinetic and vestibulo-ocular responses during head rotation in various planes. Aerosp. Med. 37, 172–177.

Melvill Jones, G. (1974a) The functional significance of size in the semicircular canals. In: H.H. Kornhuber (Ed) Handbook of Sensory Physiology, Vol. VI. Springer Verlag, Berlin, pp. 171–184.

Melvill Jones, G. (1974b) Adaptive neurobiology in space flight. Proc. Skylab Life Sciences Symp. Vol. 2, NASA TM X–58154, pp. 847–859.

Melvill Jones, G. (1977) Plasticity in the adult vestibulo-ocular reflex arc. Phil. Trans. R. Soc. London Ser. B 278, 319–334.

Melvill Jones, G. (1983a) Adaptive "tuning": The key to perceptual "truth"? Proc. Int. Union Physiol. Sciences, Vol. XV, XXIX Cong. Sydney, Australia, p. 385.

Melvill Jones, G. (1983b) Auto-adaptive control of central plasticity. Observations and speculations. In: H. Basar, H. Flohr, H. Haken & A.J. Mandell (Eds.) Synergetics of the brain. Springer Verlag, Berlin, Heidelberg, New York, Tokyo, pp. 122–138.

Melvill Jones, G. & Berthoz, A. (1981) Vestibulo-ocular compensation during transient head rotation: is it adaptively reversed by long term vision reversal? Soc. Neurosci. Abstr. 7, 298.

Melvill Jones, G. & Davies, P.R.T. (1976) Adaptation of cat vestibulo-ocular reflex to 200 days of optically reversed vision. Brain Res. 103, 551–554.

Melvill Jones, G. & Drazin, D.H. (1961) Oscillatory motion in flight. Flying Personnel Research Committee Report No. FPRC 1168, Air Ministry, London. Also In: A.B. Barbour & H.E. Whittingham (Eds) (1962) Human Problems of Supersonic and Hypersonic Flight. Pergamon Press, London, pp. 134–151.

Melvill Jones, G. & Gonshor, A. (1975) Goal-directed flexibility in the vestibulo-ocular reflex arc. In: G. Lennerstrand & P. Bach-y-Rita (Eds) Basic Mechanisms of Ocular Motility and Their Clinical Implications. Pergamon Press, New York, pp. 227–245.

Melvill Jones, G. & Gonshor, A. (1982) Oculomotor response to rapid head oscillation (0.5 − 5.0Hz) after prolonged adaptation to vision-reversal. Exp. Brain Res. 45, 45–58.

Melvill Jones, G. & Mandl, G. (1979) Effects of strobe light on adaptation of vestibulo-ocular reflex (VOR) to vision reversal. Brain Res. 164, 300–303.

Melvill Jones, G. & Mandl, G. (1981) Motion sickness due to vision reversal: its absence in stroboscopic light. In: B. Cohen (Ed.) Vestibular and Oculomotor Physiology. Ann. N.Y. Acad. Sci. 374, 303–313.

Melvill Jones, G. & Mandl, G. (1983) Neurobionomics of adaptive plasticity: Integrating sensory-motor function with environmental demands. In: J.E. Desmedt (Ed.) Motor Control Mechanisms in Health and Disease. Raven Press, pp. 1047–1071.

Melvill Jones, G. & Milsum, J.H. (1971) Frequency response analysis of central vestibular unit activity resulting from rotational stimulation of the semicircular canals. J. Physiol. (London)219, 191–215.

Melvill Jones, G. & Sugie, N. (1972) Vestibulo-ocular responses in man during sleep. EEG Clin. Neurophysiol. 32, 43–53.

Melvill Jones, G. & Young, L.R. (1978) "Subjective detection of vertical acceleration: A velocity dependent response?" Acta Oto-Laryngol. 85.45–53.

Melvill Jones, G., Mandl, G. & Cynader, M. (1980) Modification of optokinetic tracking by maintained vision reversal in normal and strobe-reared cats. Soc. Neurosci. Abstr. 6, 473.

Melvill Jones, G., Mandl, G., Cynader, M & Outerbridge, J.S. (1981) Eye oscillations in strobe-reared cats. Brain Res. 209, 47–60.

Melvill Jones, G., Guitton, D., Berthoz, A. & Volle, M. (1983) Rapid effects of vision reversal on head-eye coordination. Soc. Neurosci. Abstr. 9, 867.

Melvill Jones, G., Berthoz, A. & Segal, B. (1984) Adaptive modification of the vestibulo-ocular reflex by mental effort in darkness. Exp. Brain Res. 56, 149–153.

Menzio, P. (1949) Rapporti fra la corteccia cerebrale e di fenomeni di emislabirintazione. Arch. Fisiol. 49, 97–104.

Mertens, R.A. & Collins, W.E. (1967) Unilateral caloric habituation of nystagmus in the cat. Effects on rotational and bilateral caloric responses. Acta Oto-Laryngol. 64, 281–297.

Messenger, J.B. (1970) Optomotor responses and nystagmus in intact, blinded and statocystless cuttlefish (Sepia officinalis L.). J. Exp. Biol. 53, 789–796.

Meyer zum Gottesberge, A. & Maurer, W. (1949) Über den Funktionsmechanismus des vertikalen Bogengangsystems bei der Entstehung des rotatorischen und vertikalen Nystagmus. Archiv Ohren Nasen Kehlkopfheilk. Hals Nasen Ohrenheilk. 155, 705–725.

Milder, D.G. & Reinecke, R.D. (1983) Phoria adaptation to prisms: a cerebellar dependent response. Arch. Neurol. 49, 339–342.

Miledi, R. (1980) Intracellular calcium and desensitization of acetylcholine receptors. Proc. R. Soc. London Ser. B, 209, 447–452.

Miles, F.A. (1974) Single unit firing patterns in the vestibular nuclei related to voluntary eye movements and passive body rotation in conscious monkeys. Brain Res. 71, 215–224.

Miles, F.A. (1982) Information processing at the cellular and systems levels in complex organisms. In: H.M. Pinsker & W.D. Willis, Jr. (Eds.) Information Processing in the Nervous System. Raven Press, New York, pp. 313–329.

Miles, F.A. & Braitman, D.J. (1980) Long-term adaptive changes in primate vestibuloocular reflex. II. Electrophysiological observations on semicircular canal primary afferents. J. Neurophysiol. 43, 1426–1436.

Miles, F.A. & Eighmy, B.B. (1980) Long-term adaptive changes in primate vestibuloocular reflex. I. Behavioral observations. J. Neurophysiol. 43, 1406–1425.

Miles, F.A. & Fuller, J.H. (1974) Adaptive plasticity in the vestibulo-ocular responses of the rhesus monkey. Brain Res. 80, 512–516.

Miles, F.A. & Fuller, J.H. (1975) Visual tracking and the primate flocculus. Science 189, 1000–1002.

Miles, F.A. & Judge, S.J. (1982) Optically-induced changes in the neural coupling between vergence eye movements and accommodation in human subjects. In: G. Lennerstrand, D.S. Zee & E.L. Keller (Eds.) Functional Basis of Ocular Motility Disorders. Pergamon, New York. pp. 93–96.

Miles, F.A. & Lisberger, S.G. (1981a) The "error" signals subserving adaptive gain control in the primate vestibulo-ocular reflex. In : B. Cohen (Ed.) Vestibular and Oculomotor Physiology. Ann. N.Y. Acad. Sci. 374, 513–525.

Miles, F.A. & Lisberger, S.G. (1981b) Plasticity in the vestibulo-ocular reflex: a new hypothesis. Annu. Rev. Neurosci. 4, 273–299.

Miles, F.A., Braitman, D.J. & Dow, B.M. (1980a) Long-term adaptive changes in primate vestibulo-ocular reflex. IV. Electrophysiological observations in flocculus of normal monkeys. J. Neurophysiol. 43, 1437–1476.

Miles, F.A., Fuller, J.H., Braitman, D.J. & Dow, B.M. (1980b) Long term adaptive changes in primate vestibulo-ocular reflexes. III. Electrophysiological observations in flocculus of adapted monkeys. J. Neurophysiol. 43, 1477–1495.

Miller, A.D. & Wilson, V.J. (1983). "Vomitting center" reanalyzed: An electrical stimulation study. Brain Res. 270, 154–158.

Miller, E.F. (1962) Counterrolling of the human eyes produced by tilt with respect to gravity. Acta Oto-Laryngol. 54,479–501.

Miller, E.F. & Graybiel, A. (1965) Otolith function as measured by ocular counterrolling in: the Role of the Vestibular Organs in Space Exploration NASA SP–77, pp. 121–132.

Miller, E.F. & Graybiel, A. (1973) Experimental M–131 — Human vestibular function. Aerosp. Med. 44, 593–608.

Millodot, M. (1972) Variation of visual acuity in the central region on the retina. Br. J. Physiol. Optics 27, 24–29.

Miyashita, Y. (1984) Eye velocity responsiveness and its proprioceptive component in the floccular Purkinje cells of the alert pigmented rabbit. Exp. Brain Res. 55, 81–90.

Miyoshi, T. & Pfaltz, C.R. (1972) Studies on optokinetic habituation. ORL 34, 308–319.

Miyoshi, T., Pfaltz, C.R. & Piffko, P. (1973) Effect of repetitive optokinetic stimulation upon optokinetic and vestibular responses. Acta Oto-Laryngol. 75, 259–265.

Mohindra, I., Held, R. Gwiazda, J. & Brill, S. (1978) Astigmatism in infants. Science 202, 329–331.

Money, K.E. (1970) Motion sickness. Physiol. Rev. 50, 1–39.

Money, K.E. & Oman, C.M. (1983) Medical monitoring and therapy of space motion sickness. In : L.G. Napolitano (Ed.) Space 2000. Am. Inst. Aero Astronautics. pp. 311–326.

Money, K.E. & Scott, J.W. (1962) Functions of separate sensory receptors of non-auditory labyrinth of the cat. Am. J. Physiol. 202 (6), 1211–1220.

Money, K.E., Myles, W.S. & Hoffert, B.M. (1974) The mechanism of positional alcohol nystagmus. Can. J. Otolaryngol. 3, 302–313.

Montarolo, P.G., Raschi, F. & Stratta, P. (1981) Are the climbing fibres essential for the Purkinje cell inhibitory action? Exp. Brain Res. 42, 215–218.

Montigny, C. de & Lamarre, Y. (1973). Rhythmic activity induced by harmaline in the olivo-cerebellar-bulbar system of the cat. Brain Res. 53, 81–95.

Moran, W.B. (1974) The changes in phase lag during sinusoidal angular rotation following labyrinthectomy in the cat. Laryngoscope 84, 1707–1728.

Morasso, P., Bizzi, E. and Dichgans, J. (1973) Adjustments of saccade characteristics during head movements. Exp. Brain Res. 16, 492–500.

Morgan, M.W. (1944a) The nervous control of accommodation. Am. J. Optom. Arch. Am. Acad. Optom. 21, 87–93.

Morgan, M.W. (1944b) Accommodation and its relationship to convergence. Am. J. Optom. Arch. Am. Acad. Optom. 21, 183–195.

Morgan, M.W. (1947) The direction of visual lines when fusion is broken as in duction tests. Am. J. Optom. Arch. Am. Acad. Optom. 24, 8–12.

Morgan, M.W. (1954) The ciliary body in accommodation and accommodation-convergence. Am. J. Optom. Arch. Am. Acad. Optom. 31, 219–229.

Morgan, M.W. (1968) Accommodation and vergence. Am. J. Optom. Arch. Am. Acad. Optom. 45, 417–454.

Morris, E.J. & Lisberger, S.G. (1983) Signals used to maintain smooth pursuit eye movements in monkeys: Effects of small retinal position and velocity errors. Soc. Neurosci. Abstr. 9, 866.

Moses, R.E., (Ed.) (1970) Adler's Physiology of the Eye. Fifth Ed. Mosby, St. Louis, Mo.

Mowrer, O.H. (1935) The electrical response of the vestibular nerve during adequate stimulation. Science 81, 180–181.

Mowrer, O.H. (1936) Maturation vs. learning in the development of vestibular and optokinetic nystagmus. J. Genet. Psychol. 48, 383–404.

Mowrer, O.H. (1937) The influence of vision during bodily rotation upon the duration of post-rotational vestibular nystagmus. Acta Oto-Laryngol. 25, 351–364.

Mueller, J. (1826) In: Elements of Physiology (Translated from German by W. Baly (1843)) Vol. 2, Taylor & Walton, London. pp. 1147–1148.

Muratore, R. & Zee, D.S. (1979) Pursuit after-nystagmus. Vision Res. 19, 1057–1059.

Murphy, B.J. (1978) Pattern thresholds for moving and stationary gratings during smooth eye movement. Vision Res. 18, 521–530.

Nakao, S. (1983) Effects of vestibulo-cerebellar lesions upon dynamic characteristics and adaptation of vestibulo-ocular and optokinetic responses in pigmented rabbits. Exp. Brain Res. 53, 36–46.

Nakao, S., Sasaki, S., Schor, R.H., & Shimazu, H. (1982) Functional organization of premotor neurons in the cat medial vestibular nucleus related to slow and fast phases of nystagmus. Exp. Brain Res. 45. 371–385.

Nakayama, K. (1974) Photographic determination of the rotational state of the eye using matrices. Am. J. Optom. Physiol. Optics 51, 736–742.

Nashner, L. & Berthoz, A. (1978) Visual contribution to rapid motor responses during postural control. Brain Res. 150, 403–407.

Nashner, L.M., Owen Black, F. & Wall, C., III (1982). Adaptation to altered support and visual conditions during stance: Patients with vestibular deficits. J. Neurosci. 2, 536–544.

Nasiell, V. (1924) Zur Frage des Dunkelnystagmus und über postrotatorischen Nystagmus und Deviation der Augen bei Lageveränderungen des Kopfes und des Körpers gegen den Kopf beim Dunkelkaninchen. Acta Oto-Laryngol. 6, 175–177.

Noda, H. (1981) Visual mossy fiber inputs to the flocculus of the monkey. In: B. Cohen (Ed.) Vestibular and Oculomotor Physiology. Ann.N.Y. Acad. Sci. 374, 465–475

Noda H. & Suzuki, D.A. (1978) The role of the flocculus of the monkey in saccadic eye movements. J. Physiol. (London) 294, 317–334.

Norman, J.R. (1934) A systematic monograph of the flatfishes (Heterosomata), Vol. 1. Psettotidae, Botheidae, Pleuronectidae. British Museum, London.

North, R. & Henson, D.B. (1981) Adaptation to prism-induced heterophoria in subjects with abnormal binocular vision or asthenopia. Am. J. Optom. Physiol. Optics 58, 746–752.

Northington, P. & Barrera, S.E. (1934) Effects of unilateral and bilateral labyrinthectomy and intracranial section of eighth nerve. AMA Arch Neurol. Psychiatr. 32, 51–71.

Obata, K. (1965) Pharmacological study on postsynaptic inhibition of Deiters' neurons. Proc. XXIII Int. Congr. Physiol. Sci., Tokyo, 958, 406.

Obata, K. & Highstein, S.M. (1970) Blocking by picrotoxin of both vestibular inhibition and GABA action on rabbit oculomotor neurons. Brain Res. 18, 538–541.

Obata, K., Ito, M., Ochi, R. & Sato, N. (1967) Pharmacological properties of the postsynaptic inhibition by Purkinje cell axons and the action of γ-aminobutyric acid on Deiters' neurons. Exp. Brain Res. 4, 43–57.

Ogle, K.N. (1966) The accommodative convergence-accommodation ratio and its relation to the correction of refractive error. Trans. Am. Acad. Opthalmol. Otolaryngol. 70, 322–330.

Ogle, K.N. & Prangen, A.H. (1953) Observations on vertical divergences and hyperphorias. Arch. Ophthalmol. 49, 313–334.

Ohm, J. (1919) Über die Beziehungen der Augenmuskeln zu den Ampullen der Bogengänge beim Menschen und Kaninchen. Klin. Monatsbl. Augenheilk. 62, 289–315.

Olla, B.L., Samet, C.E. & Studholme, A.L. (1972) Activity and feeding behavior of the summer flounder (*Paralichthys dentatus*) under controlled laboratory conditions. Fish. Bull. U.S. Fish Wildlife Service 70, 1127–1136.

Olson, C.R. & Pettigrew, J.D. (1974) Single units in visual cortex of kittens reared in stroboscopic illumination. Brain Res. 70, 189–204.

Olson, J.F., Wolfe, J.W. & Engelken, M.S. (1981) Responses to low-frequency harmonic acceleration in patients with acoustic neuromas. Laryngoscope 91, 1270–1277

Oman, C.M. (1982a) A heuristic mathematical model for the dynamics of sensory conflict and motion sickness. Acta Oto-Laryngol. Suppl., 392, 1–44.

Oman C.M. (1982b) Space motion sickness and vestibular experiments in Spacelab. SAE Tech. paper series, No. 820833 XII Int. Soc. Conf. Environ. Syst. San Diego, Ca. July 19–21, pp. 1–21.

Oman, C.M., Bock, O.L. & Huang, J.-K. (1980) Visually induced self-motion sensation adapts rapidly to left-right visual reversal. Science 209, 706–708.

Optican, L.M. (1982) Saccadic dysmetria. In: G. Lennerstrand, D.S. Zee & E. Keller (Eds.) Functional Basis of Ocular Motility Disorders. Pergamon, Oxford, pp. 441–451.

Optican, L.M. & Miles, F.A. (1979) Visually induced adaptive changes in oculomotor control signals. Soc. Neurosci. Abstr. 5, 380.

Optican, L.M. & Robinson, D.A. (1980) Cerebellar dependent adaptive control of primate saccadic system. J. Neurophysiol. 44, 1058–1075.

Optican, L.M., Zee, D.S., Miles F.A. and Lisberger, S.G. (1980) Oculomotor deficits in monkeys with floccular lesion. Soc. Neurosci. Abstr. 6, 474.

Optican, L.M., Chu, F.C., Hays, A.V., Reingold, D.B. & Zee, D.S. (1982) Adaptive changes of oculomotor performance in abducens nerve palsy. Soc. Neurosci. Abstr. 8, 418.

Ostriker, G., Pellionisz, A. & Llinás, R. (1985) Tensorial computer model of gaze. I. Oculomotor activity expressed in non-orthogonal natural coordinates. Neuroscience (in press).

Ott, J.F. (1982) Evoked field potentials measured in the vestibular nuclei before and after unilateral partial labyrinthectomy. Soc. Neurosci. Abstr. 8, 42.

Outerbridge, J.S. & Melvill Jones, G. (1971) Reflex vestibular control of head movements in man. Aerosp. Med. 42, 935–940.

Outerbridge J.S., Mandl, G. & Gorayeb, M. (1977) How do visual cells synthesize responses to moving light stimuli? Soc. Neurosci. Abstr. 3. 572.

Oyster, C.W., Takahashi, E. & Collewijn, H. (1972) Directions selective retinal ganglion cells and control of optokinetic nystagmus in the rabbit. Vision Res. 12, 183–193.

Ozawa, S., Precht, W. & Shimazu, H. (1974) Crossed effects on central vestibular neurons in the horizontal canal system of the frog. Exp. Brain Res. 19, 394–405.

Packard, A. (1972) Cephalopods and fish: The limits of convergence. Biol. Rev. 47, 241–307.

Paige, G.D. (1980) The vestibulo-ocular reflex and its interactions with visual following mechanisms in the squirrel monkey. PhD Thesis, University of Chicago, Chicago, U.S.A.

Paige, G.D. (1983a) Vestibulo-ocular reflex and its interactions with visual following mechanisms in the squirrel monkey. I. Response characteristics in normal animals. J. Neurophysiol. 49, 134–151.

Paige, G.D. (1983b) Vestibulo ocular reflex and its interactions with visual following mechanisms in the squirrel monkey. II. Response characteristics and plasticity following unilateral inactivation of horizontal canal. J. Neurophysiol. 49, 152–168.

Palay, S.L. & Chan-Palay, V. (Eds) (1982) The Cerebellum: New Vistas. Springer, New York.

Parker, D.E., Covell, W.P. & Von Gierke, H.E. (1968) Exploration of vestibular damage in guinea pigs following mechanical stimulation. Acta Oto-Laryngol. 239, 1–59.

Pasternak, T., Movshon, J.A. & Merigan, W.H. (1981) Creation of direction selectivity in adult strobe-reared cats. Nature, 292, 834–837.

Pearson, H.E. & Murphy, E.H. (1983) Effects of stroboscopic rearing on the response properties and laminar distribution of single units in the rabbit superior colliculus. Dev. Brain Res. 9, 241–250.

Pearson, H.E., Berman, N. & Murphy, E.H. (1983) Critical periods in development for susceptibility to the effects of stroboscopic rearing in rabbit visual cortex. Exp. Brain Res. 50, 367–372.

Pellionisz, A. (1983a) Sensorimotor transformation of natural coordinates via neuronal networks: conceptual and formal unification of cerebellar and tectal models. In: R. Lara & M. Arbib (Eds.) COINS Technical Report 83–19, U. Mass, Amherst, MA on II. Workshop on visuomotor coordination in frog and toad. Models and experiments.

Pellionisz, A. (1983b) Brain theory: connecting neurobiology to robotics. Tensor analysis: natural coordinates to describe, understand and engineer functional geometries of intelligent organisms. J. Theoret. Neurobiol. 2, 185–211.

Pellionisz, A. (1984a) Coordination: A vector-matrix description of transformations of overcomplete CNS coordinates and a tensorial solution using the Moore-Penrose generalized inverse. J. Theoret. Biol. 110, 353–375.

Pellionisz, A. (1984b) Tensorial brain theory in cerebellar modelling. In : J. Bloedel, J. Dichgans & W. Precht (Eds.) Cerebellar Functions. Springer, Berlin, pp. 201–229.

Pellionisz, A. (1984c) Tensorial computer movie of the genesis and modification of cerebellar networks as dyadic expansions of the Eigenvectors stored in the inferor olive. Soc. Neurosci. Abstr. 10, 540.

Pellionisz, A. & Llinás, R. (1979a) Cerebellar coordination: Covariant analysis and contravariant synthesis via metric tensor. A tensorial approach to the geometry of brain function. Soc. Neurosci. Abstr. 5, 105.

367

Pellionisz, A. & Llinás, R. (1979b) Brain modeling by tensor network theory and computer simulation. The cerebellum: distributed processor for predictive coordination. Neuroscience 4, 323–348.

Pellionisz, A. & Llinás, R. (1980) Tensorial approach to the geometry of brain function. Cerebellar coordination via a metric tensor. Neuroscience 5, 1125–1136.

Pellionisz, A. & Llinás, R. (1982a) Space-time representation in the brain. The cerebellum as a predictive space-time metric tensor. Neuroscience 7, 2949–2970.

Pellionisz, A. & Llinás, R. (1982b) Tensor theory of brain function. The cerebellum as a space-time metric. Chapter 23. In: S. Amari & M.A. Arbib (Eds.) Competition and Cooperation in Neural Nets. Springer-Verlag Berlin, Heidelberg, New York, pp. 394–417.

Pellionisz, A., Llinás, R. & Perkel, D. (1977). A computer model of the cerebellar cortex of the frog. Neuroscience 2, 19–35.

Peterson, B.W. & Goldberg, J. (1982) Role of vestibular and neck reflexes in controlling eye and head position. In: A. Roucoux & M. Crommelinck (Eds) Physiological and Pathological Aspects of Eye Movements. Dr. W. Junk, The Hague, 351–364.

Petrofrezzo, A.J. (1966) Matrices and Transformations. Dover, New York.

Petrosini, L. & Troiani, D.C. (1979) Vestibular compensation after hemilabyrinthectomy; effects of trigeminal neurotomy. Physiol. Behav. 22, 133–137.

Pfaltz, E.R. (Ed.) (1983) Advances in Oto-Rhino-Laryngology. Neurophysiological and Clinical Aspects of Vestibular Disorders. Karger, Basel.

Phillips, S.R. (1974) Ocular neurological control systems: accommodation and the near response triad. Ph.D. Dissertation, Univ. California, Berkeley.

Phillips, S. & Stark, L. (1977) Blur: a sufficient accommodative stimulus. Doc. Opthalmol. 43, 65–89.

Platt, C. (1973a) Central control of postural orientation in flatfish. I. Postural change dependence on central neural changes. J. Exp. Biol. 59, 491–521.

Platt, C. (1973b) Central control of postural orientation in flatfish. II. Optic-vestibular efferent modification of gravistatic input. J. Exp. Biol. 59, 523–541.

Platt, C. (1976) Asymmetry of semicircular canal-extraocular muscle function in flatfish. Soc. Neurosci. Abstr. 2, 1532.

Poggio, G.F. & Fischer, B. (1977) Binocular interaction and depth sensitivity in striate and prestriate cortex of behaving rhesus monkey. J. Neurophysiol. 40, 1392–1405.

Pola, J. & Robinson, D.A. (1978) Oculomotor signals in the medial longitudinal fasciculus of the monkey. J. Neurophysiol. 41, 245–259.

Pola, J. & Wyatt, H.J. (1980) Target position and velocity: The stimuli for smooth pursuit eye movements. Vision Res. 20, 523–534.

Policanski, D. (1982) The asymmetry of flounders. Sci. Am. 246, 116–122.

Pompeiano, O. (1972) Reticular control of the vestibular nuclei: physiology and pharmacology. In: A. Brodal & O. Pompeiano (Eds.) Basic Aspects of Central Vestibular Mechanisms. Progress in Brain Research 37, Elsevier, Amsterdam, pp. 601–618.

Pompeiano, O. (1975) Vestibulo-spinal relationships. In: R.F. Noughton (Ed.) The Vestibular System. Academic Press, New York, San Francisco, London, pp. 147–180.

Pompeiano, O. & Hoshino, K. (1977) Responses to static tilts of lateral reticular neurons mediated by contralateral labyrinthine receptors. Arch. Ital. Biol. 115, 211–236.

Precht, W. (1974) Characteristics of vestibular neurons after acute and chronic destruction. In H.H. Kornhuber (Ed.) Handbook of Sensory Physiology, Vol. VI/2, Psychophysics, Applied Aspects and General Interpretation. Springer Verlag, Berlin, pp. 451–462.

Precht, W. (1978) Neuronal operations in the vestibular system. In: H.B. Barlow, E. Florey, O.J. Grüsser & H. von der Loos (Eds.) Studies of Brain Function. Springer Verlag, Berlin, Heidelberg, New York, pp. 1–226.

Precht, W. (1979) Labyrinthine influences on the vestibular nuclei. In: R. Granit, & O. Pompeiano (Eds) Reflex Control of Posture and Locomotion, Progress in Brain Research Vol. 50. Elsevier, Amsterdam, pp.369–381.

Precht, W. (1981) Visual-vestibular interaction in vestibular neurons. Functional pathway organization. In : B. Cohen (Ed.) Vestibular and Oculomotor Physiology. Ann. N.Y. Acad. Sci. 374, 230–248.

Precht, W. (1982) Anatomical and functional organisation of optokinetic pathways. In: G. Lennerstrand, D.S. Zee & E.L. Keller (Eds.) Functional Basis of Ocular Motility Disorders. Pergamon Press, Oxford, pp. 291–302.

Precht, W. & Cazin, L. (1979) Functional deficits in the optokinetic system of albino rats. Exp. Brain Res. 37, 183–186.

Precht, W., Shimazu, H. & Markham, C. H. (1966) A mechanism of central compensation of vestibular function following hemilabyrinthectomy. J. Neurophysiol. 29, 996–1010.

Precht, W., Grippo, J. & Wagner, A. (1967) Contribution of different types of central vestibular neurons to the vestibulospinal system. Brain Res. 4, 119–123.

Precht, W., Llinás, R. & Clarke, M. (1971) Physiological responses of frog vestibular fibers to horizontal angular acceleration. Exp. Brain Res. 13, 378–407.

Precht, W., Baker, R. & Okada, Y. (1973a) Evidence for GABA as the synaptic transmitter of the inhibitory vestibuloocular pathway. Exp. Brain Res. 18, 415–428.

Precht, W., Schwindt, P.C. & Baker, R. (1973b) Removal of vestibular commissural inhibition by antagonists of GABA and glycine. Brain Res. 62, 222–226.

Precht, W., Maioli, C., Dieringer, N. & Cochran, S. (1981) Mechanisms of compensation of the vestibuloocular reflex after vestibular neurotomy. In: H. Flohr & W. Precht (Eds) Lesion-induced Neuronal Plasticity in Sensorimotor systems. Springer Verlag, Berlin, Heidelberg, pp. 222–230.

Precht, W., Cazin, L., Blanks, R. & Lannou, J. (1982) Anatomy and physiology of the optokinetic pathways to the vestibular nuclei in the rat. In: A. Roucoux & M. Crommelinck (Eds). Physiological and Pathological Aspects of Eye Movements. D.W. Junk, The Hague, pp. 153–172.

Prince, J.H. (1956) Comparative Anatomy of the Eye. C.C. Thomas, Springfield, U.S.A.

Pulaski, P.D., Zee, D.S., & Robinson, D.A. (1981) The behavior of the vestibulo-ocular reflex at high velocities of head rotation. Brain Res. 222, 159–165.

Purkinje, J. (1820) Beyträge zur näheren Kenntniss des Schwindels aus heautognostischen Daten. Med. Jahrb. Österr. Staates 6, 79–125.

Putkonen, P.T., Courjon, J.H. & Jeannerod, M. (1977) Compensation of postural effects of hemilabyrinthectomy in the cat. A sensory substitution process? Exp. Brain Res. 28, 249–257.

Rall, W. (1974) Dendritic spines, synaptic potency and neuronal plasticity. In: C.D. Woody, K.A. Brown, T.J. Crow & J.D. Knispel (Eds.) Cellular Mechanisms subserving changes activity. Brain Inf. Serv. Res. Rep. 3, 13–21.

Ramón y Cajal, S. (1911) Histologie du Système Nerveux de l'Homme et des Vertébrés, Vol. 1–2, Maloine, Paris.

Raphan, T. & Cohen, B. (1981) The role of integration in oculomotor control. In: B. Zuber (Ed.) Models of oculomotor behavior and control. CRC Press, West Palm Beach, Fl, pp. 91–109.

Raphan, T., Cohen, B, & Matsuo, V. (1977) A velocity storage mechanism responsible for optokinetic nystagmus (OKN), optokinetic afternystagmus (OKAN) and vestibular nystagmus. In: R. Baker & A. Berthoz (Eds.) Control of Gaze by Brain Stem Neurons. Elsevier, Amsterdam, pp. 37–47.

Raphan, T., Matsuo, V. & Cohen, B. (1979) Velocity storage in the vestibulo-ocular reflex arc (VOR). Exp. Brain Res. 35, 229–248.

Raphan, T., Cohen B. & Henn, V. (1981) Effects of gravity rotatory nystagmus in monkeys. In: B. Cohen (Ed.) Vestibular and Oculomotor Physiology. Ann. N. Y. Acad. Sci. 374, 337–346.

Raphan, T., Cohen, B., Suzuki, J.I. & Henn V. (1983a) Nystagmus generated by pitch while rotating. Brain Res. 276, 165–172.

Raphan, T., Waespe, W. & Cohen, B. (1983b) Labyrinthine activation during rotation about axes tilted from the vertical. Proc. Barany Soc. ORL 30, 50–53.

Rashbass, C. & Westheimer, G. (1961) Disjunctive eye movements. J. Physiol. (London) 159, 339–360.

Ratliff, F. & Riggs, L. (1950) Involuntary motions of the eye during monocular fixation. J. Exp. Psychol. 40, 687–701.

Rauschecker, J & Harris, L.R. (1983) Auditory compensation of the effects of visual deprivation in the cat superior colliculus Exp. Brain. Res. 50, 69–83.

Reason J.T. (1978) Motion sickness adaptation: A neural mismatch model. J. R. Soc. Med. 71, 819–829.

Reason, J.T. & Brand, J.J. (1975) Motion Sickness Academic Press, London.

Reber, J. & Goldsmith, W. (1979) Analysis of large head-neck motions. J. Biomech. 12, 211–222.

Renaud, L.P., Blume, H.W., Pittman, Q.J., Lamour, Y. & Tan, A.T. (1979) Thyrotropin-releasing hormone selectively depressed glutamate excitation of cerebral cortical neurons. Science 205, 1275–1277.

Retzius, G. (1881) Das Gehörorgan der Wirbeltiere: morphologisch-histologische Studien. I. Das Gehörorgan der Fische und Amphibien. Samson & Wallin, Stockholm.

Retzius, G. (1884) Das Gehörorgan der Wirbeltiere. II. Das Gehörorgan der Reptilien, der Vogel und der Säugetiere. Samson & Wallin, Stockholm.

Richter, A. (1974) Antworten der Vestibulariskernneurone des Frosches bei natürlicher Labyrinthreizung. Doct. Thesis, Univ. Frankfurt.

Ried, S., Maioli, C. & Precht, W. (1984) Vestibular nuclear neuron activity in chronically hemilabyrinthectomized cats. Acta Oto-Laryngol. 98, 1–13.

Riggs, L.A. & Niehl, E.W. (1960) Eye movements recorded during convergence and divergence. J. Optom.Soc. Am. 50, 913–920.

Riggs, L. Ratliff, R., Cornsweet, J.C. & Cornsweet, T.N. (1953) The disappearance of steadily fixated visual test objects. J. Optom. Soc. Am. 43, 495–501.

Ripps, H., Chin, N.B., Siegel, I.M. & Breinin, G.M. (1962) Effect of pupil size on accommodation convergence and the AC/A ratio. Invest. Ophthalmol. 1, 127–135.

Ritchie, L. (1976) Effects of cerebellar lesions on saccadic eye movements. J. Neurophysiol. 39, 1246–1256.

Robinson, D.A. (1963) A method of measuring eye movement using a scleral search-coil in magnetic field. IEEE Trans. Biomed. Eng. 10, 137–145.

Robinson, D.A. (1964) The mechanics of human saccadic eye movement. J. Physiol. (London) 174, 245–264.

Robinson, D.A. (1968) The oculomotor control system: A review. Proc. IEEE 56, 1032–1049.

Robinson, D.A. (1970) Oculomotor unit behavior in the monkey. J. Neurophysiol. 38, 393–404.

Robinson, D.A. (1973) Models of the saccadic eye movement control system. Kybernetik 14, 71–83.

Robinson, D.A. (1974) The effect of cerebellectomy on the cat's vestibulo-ocular integrator. Brain Res 71, 195–207.

Robinson, D.A. (1975a) Oculomotor control signals. In: G. Lennerstrand & P. Bach-y-Rita (Eds.) Basic Mechanisms of Ocular Motility and their Clinical Implications. Pergamon Press, Oxford, pp. 337–374.

Robinson, D.A. (1975b) A quantitative analysis of extraocular muscle cooperation and squint. Invest. Ophthalmol. 14, 801–825.

Robinson, D.A. (1975c) How the oculomotor system repairs itself. Invest. Ophthalmol. 14, 413–415.

Robinson, D.A. (1976) Adaptive gain control of vestibulo-ocular reflex by the cerebellum. J. Neurophysiol. 39, 954–969.

Robinson, D.A. (1977a) Vestibular and optokinetic symbiosis: an example of explaining by modelling. In: R. Baker & A. Berthoz (Eds.) Control of Gaze by Brain Stem Neurons. Elsevier, Amsterdam, pp. 49–58.

Robinson, D.A. (1977b) Linear addition of optokinetic and vestibular signals in the vestibular nucleus. Exp. Brain Res. 30, 447–450.

Robinson, D.A. (1980) Visual-vestibular interaction in motion perception and the generation of nystagmus. Neurosci. Res. Prog. Bull. 18, 457–661.

Robinson, D.A. (1981a) The use of control systems analysis in the neurophysiology of eye movements. Annu. Rev. Neurosci. 4, 463–503.

Robinson, D.A. (1981b) Control of eye movements. In: V.B.

Brooks, American Physiological Society (Ed.) The Nervous System, Handbook of Physiology, Vol. II, Part 2. Williams & Wilkins, Baltimore, pp. 1275–1320.

Robinson, D.A. (1982) The use of matrices in analyzing the three-dimensional behavior of the vestibulo-ocular reflex. Biol. Cybern. 46, 53–66.

Robles, S.S. & Anderson, J.H. (1978) Compensation of vestibular deficits in the cat. Brain Res. 147, 183–187.

Rönne, H. (1923) Mouvements apparents, produits à la vision par verres de lunettes et la correction de ces mouvements par les canaux semicirculaires. Acta Oto-Laryngol. 5, 108–110.

Rothfeld, J. (1913) Die Physiologie des Bogengangapparates. Verh. Ges. Dtsch. Naturforsch. Ärzte, (85, Versammlung) Vol. 1, 269–322.

Rothfeld, J. (1914) Das "Oto-ophthalmotrop," ein Apparat zur Demonstration der vom Ohrlabyrinthe ausgelösten kompensatorischen Augenbewegungen. Berl. Klin. Wochenschr. 51, 256–258.

Roucoux, A. & Crommelinck, M. (Eds.) (1982) Physiological and pathological aspects of eye movements. Dr. W. Junk, The Hague, 448 pp.

Roucoux, A., Guitton, D. & Crommelinck, M. (1980) Stimulation of the superior colliculus in the alert cat. II. Eye and head movements evoked when the head is unrestrained. Exp. Brain Res. 39, 75–85.

Roucoux, A., Crommelinck, M., Guerit, J.M. & Meulders, M. (1981) Two modes of eye head coordination and the role of the vestibulo-ocular reflex in these two strategies. In: A. Fuchs & W. Becker (Eds.) Functional basis of ocular motility disorders. Amsterdam, Elsevier, 309–315.

Roucoux, A., Culee, C. & Roucoux, M. (1982a) Gaze fixation and pursuit in head free human infants. In: A. Roucoux and M. Crommelinck (Eds.) Physiological and Pathological Aspects of Eye Movements. Dr. W. Junk, The Hague, 23–31.

Roucoux, A., Vidal, P.P., Veraart, C., Crommelinck, M. & Berthoz, A. (1982b) The relation of neck muscles activity to horizontal eye position in the alert cat. I Head free. In: A. Roucoux & M. Crommelinck (Eds.) Physiological and Pathological Aspects of Eye Movements. Dr. W. Junk, The Hague, pp. 371–378.

Roucoux, A., Culee, C. & Roucoux, M. (1983) Development of fixation and pursuit eye movements in human infants. Behav. Brain Res. 10, 133–139.

Routh, E.J. (1960) Dynamics of a System of Rigid Bodies. Dover Press, New York.

Rovainen, C.M. (1976) Vestibulo-ocular reflex in adult sea lampreys. J. Comp. Physiol. 112, 159–164.

Rubia, F.J. & Kolb, F.P. (1979) Responses of cerebellar units to a passive movement in the decerebrate cat. Exp. Brain Res. 31, 387–401.

Rudge, R. & Chambers, B.R. (1982) Physiological basis for enduring vestibular symptoms. J. Neurol. Neurosurg. Psychiatry 45, 126–130.

Sandeman, D.C. (1983) The balance and visual systems of the swimming crab — their morphology and interaction. In: E. Horn (Ed.) Fortschr. Zool. Vol 28, Ch. 14. Fischer Verlag, Stuttgart.

Sandeman, D.C. & Okajima, A. (1972) Statocyst induced eye movements in the crab Scylla serrata. I. The sensory input from the statocyst. J. Exp. Biol. 57, 187–204.

Sandeman, D.C. & Okajima, A. (1973a) Statocyst induced eye movements in the crab Scylla serrata. II. The responses of the eye muscles. J. Exp. Biol. 58, 197–212.

Sandeman, D.C. & Okajima, A. (1973b) Statocyst induced eye movements in the crab Scylla serrata. III. The anatomical projections of sensory and motor neurons and the responses of the motor neurons. J. Exp. Biol. 59, 17–38.

Sandoval, M.E. & Cotman, C.W. (1978) Evaluation of glutamate as a neurotransmitter of cerebellar parallel fibers. Neuroscience. 3, 199–206.

Sasaki, K. & Gemba, H. (1982) Development and change of cortical field potentials during learning processes of visually initiated hand movements in the monkey. Exp. Brain Res. 48, 429–437.

Sato, Y., Kawasaki, T. & Ikarashi, K. (1982a) Zonal organization of the floccular Purkinje cells projecting to the vestibular nucleus in cats. Brain Res. 232, 1–15.

Sato, Y., Kawasaki, T. & Ikarashi, K. (1982b) Zonal organization of the floccular Purkinje cells projecting to the group y of the vestibular nuclear complex and the lateral cerebellar nucleus in the cats. Brain Res. 234, 430–434.

Schaefer, K.-P. & Meyer, D.L. (1973) Compensatory mechanisms following labyrinthine lesions in the guinea pig. A simple model of learning. In: H.P. Zippel (Ed.) Memory and Transfer of Information. Plenum Press, New York, London, pp. 203–232.

Schaefer, K.P., Meyer, D.L. (1974) Compensation of vestibular lesions. In: H.H. Kornhuber (Ed.) Handbook of Sensory Physiology, Vol. VI/2. Springer Verlag, Berlin, Heidelberg, New York, pp. 463–490.

Schaefer, K.-P. & Meyer, D.L. (1981) Aspects of vestibular compensation in guinea pigs. In: H. Flohr & W. Precht (Eds.) Lesion-induced Neuronal Plasticity in Sensorimotor Systems. Springer-Verlag, Berlin, Heidelberg, New York, pp. 197–207.

Schaefer, K.P., Schott, D. & Meyer, D.L. (1975) On the organization of neuronal circuits involved in the generation of the orienting response (visual grasp reflex). Fortschr. Zool. Vol. 23, pp. 199–212, Fischer Verlag, Stuttgart.

Schaefer, K.-P., Wilhelms, G. & Meyer, D.L. (1978) Der Einflurss von Alkohol auf die zentralnervösen Ausgleichsvorgänge nach Labyrinthausschaltung. Z. Rechtsmed. 81, 249–260.

Schairer, J.O. & Bennett, M.V. (1978) VOR gain changes produced by target rotation without head movement in goldfish. Soc. Neurosci. Abstr. 4, 167.

Schairer, J.O. & Bennett, M.V. (1981) Cerebellectomy in goldfish prevents adaptive gain control of the VOR without affecting the optokinetic system. In: T. Gualtierrotti (Ed.) Vestibular Function and Morphology. Springer Verlag, Berlin, Heidelberg, New York, pp. 463–477.

Scheich, H. & Bullock, T.H. (1974) The role of electroreceptors in the animal's life. The detection of the electric fields. In: A. Fessard (Ed.) Handbook of Sensory Physiology, Vol. III/3. Springer Verlag, New York, pp. 201–256.

Schmid, R. & Jeannerod, M. (1979) Organization and control of the vestibulo-ocular reflex. In: R. Granit & O. Pompeiano

370

(Eds.) Reflex Control of Posture and Movements. Progress in Brain Research, Vol. 50. Elsevier, Amsterdam, pp. 477–489.

Schmid, R., Jeannerod, M. & Zambarbieri, D. (1980) A multilevel model of vestibular habituation. In: G. Kaphan (Ed.) Proc. 2nd Mediterranean Conf. Med. Biol. Eng., SEE Publications, pp. 189–190.

Schmidt, D., Dell'Osso, L.F., Abel, L.A. & Daroff, R.B. (1980) Myasthenia gravis: dynamic changes in saccadic waveform gain and velocity. Exp. Neurol. 68, 365–377.

Schöne, H. (1954) Statozystenfunktion und statische Lageorientierung bei dekapoden Krebsen. Z. Vergl. Physiol. 36, 241–260.

Schöne, H. (1964) Über die Arbeitsweise der Statolithenapparate bei Plattfischen. Biol. Jahresh. 4, 135–156.

Schor, C.M. (1979a) The influence of rapid prism adaptation upon fixation disparity. Vision Res. 19, 757–765.

Schor, C.M. (1979b) The relationship between fusional vergence eye movements and fixation disparity. Vision Res. 19, 1359–1367.

Schor, C.M. (1980) Fixation disparity: a steady state error of disparity-induced vergence. Am. J. Optom. Physiol. Optics 57, 618–630.

Schor, C.M. (1982) Vergence eye movements: basic aspects. In: G. Lennerstrand, D.S. Zee, & E.L. Keller (Eds.) Functional Basis of Ocular Motility Disorders. Pergamon, New York, pp. 83–91.

Schor, C.M. (1983) Analysis of tonic and accommodative vergence disorders of binocular vision. Am. J. Optom. Physiol. Optics 60, 1–14.

Schor, R.H. (1974) Responses of cat vestibular neurons to sinusoïdal roll tilt. Exp. Brain Res. 20, 347–362.

Schor, R.H. & Miller, A. (1981) Vestibular reflexes in neck and forelimb muscles evoked by roll tilt. J. Neurophysiol. 46, 167–178.

Schor, R.H. & Miller, A.D. (1982) Relationship of cat vestibular neurons to otolith-spinal reflexes. Exp. Brain Res. 47, 137–144.

Schubert, G. (1943) Grundlagen der beidaugigen motorischen Koordination. Pfluegers Arch. Gesamte Physiol. Menschen Tieren 247, 279–291.

Schultheis, L.W. & Robinson, D.A. (1981) Directional plasticity of the vestibulo-ocular reflex in the cat. In: B. Cohen (Ed.) Vestibular and Oculomotor Physiology. Ann. N.Y. Acad. Sci. 374, 504–512.

Segal, B.N. (1985) Post-suppression vestibulo-ocular reflex in man: Pursuit and non-pursuit mechanisms. Exp. Brain Res., Submitted.

Selhorst, J.B., Stark, L., Ochs, A.L. & Hoyt, W.F. (1976) Disorders in cerebellar ocular motor control. II. Macrosaccadic oscillations: an oculographic control system and clinico-anatomical analysis. Brain 99, 509–522.

Semmlow, J.L. & Hung, G. (1979) Accommodative and fusional components of fixation disparity. Invest. Ophthalmol. 18, 1082–1086.

Semmlow, J.L. & Tinor, T. (1978) Accommodative convergence response to off-foveal retinal images. J. Opt. Soc. Am. 68, 1497–1501.

Semmlow, J.L. & Venkiteswaran, N. (1976) Dynamic accommodative vergence components in binocular vision. Vision Res. 16, 403–410.

Semmlow, J.L. & Wetzel, P. (1979) Dynamic contributions of binocular vergence components. J. Opt. Soc. Am. 69, 639–645.

Sharpe, J.A., Goldberg, H.J., Lo, A.W. & Herishanu, Y.O. (1981) Visual-vestibular interaction in multiple sclerosis. Neurology 31, 427–433.

Sherrington, C. (1906) The integrative action of the nervous system. Scribner, New York.

Shimazu, H. & Precht, W. (1965) Tonic and kinetic responses of cat's vestibular neurons to horizontal angular acceleration. J. Neurophysiol. 28, 991–1013.

Shimazu, H. & Precht, W. (1966) Inhibition of central vestibular neurons from the contralateral labyrinth and its mediating pathway. J. Neurophysiol. 29, 467–492.

Shimazu, H. & Smith, C.M. (1971) Cerebellar and labyrinthine influences on single vestibular neurons identified by natural stimuli. J. Neurophysiol. 34, 493–508.

Shirachi, D., Monk, D. & Black, J. (1978) Head rotational spectral characteristics during two dimensional smooth pursuit tasks. IEEE Trans. Syst. Man. Cybern. 8, 715–722.

Simpson, J.I. (1979) Erroneous zones of the cerebellar flocculus. Soc. Neurosci. Abstr. 5, 107.

Simpson, J.I. (1983) Transformation of coordinates intrinsic to the vestibuloocular reflex. Soc. Neurosci. Abstr. 9, 315.

Simpson, J. & Alley, K.E. (1974). Visual climbing fiber input to rabbit vestibulocerebellum: A source of direction-specific information. Brain Res. 82, 302–308.

Simpson, J.I. & Graf, W. (1981) Eye muscle geometry and compensatory eye movements in lateral-eyed and frontal-eyed animals. In: B. Cohen (Ed.) Vestibular and Oculomotor Physiology. Ann. N.Y. Acad. Sci. 374, 20–30.

Simpson, J.I., Soodak, R.E. & Hess, R. (1979) The accessory optic system and its relation to the vestibulo-cerebellum. In: R. Granit & O. Pompeiano (Eds.) Reflex Control of Posture and Movements, Progress in Brain Research, Vol. 50. Elsevier, Amsterdam, pp. 715–724.

Simpson, J.I., Graf, W. & Leonard, C.S. (1981a) The coordinate system of visual climbing fibers to the flocculus. In: A.F. Fuchs & W. Becker (Eds.) Progress in Oculomotor Research. Elsevier, New York, pp. 475–484.

Simpson, J.I. Graf, W. & Leonard, C.S. (1981b) Spatial coordinates of visual messages in the flocculus. Soc. Neurosci. Abstr. 7, 133.

Sirkin & Precht (1984) Brain Res. 302, 245 – 256.

Skavenski, A.A. & Robinson, D.A. (1973) Role of abducens neurons in vestibuloocular reflex. J. Neurophysiol. 36, 724–738.

Skavenski, A.A., Hansen, R.M., Steinman, R.M. & Winterson, B.J. (1979) Quality of retinal image stabilization during small retinal and artificial body rotations in man. Vision Res. 19, 675–683.

Skavenski, A.A., Blair, S.M. & Westheimer, G. (1981) The effect of habituating vestibular and optokinetic nystagmus on each other. J. Neurosci. 1, 351–357.

Smiles, K.A., Hite, D., Hams, V.J. & Junker, A.M. (1975) Effects of labyrinthectomy on the dynamic vestibuloocular counterroll reflex in the Rhesus monkey. Aviat. Space Environ. Med. 46, 1017–1022.

Smithline, L.M. (1974) Accommodative response to blur. J. Opt. Soc. Am. 64, 1512–1516.

Snow, R. & Vilis, T. (1983) Selective gain control of the vestibulo-ocular reflex. Proc. Can. Fed. Biol. Soc., 26, 167, Abstr. PO–25.

Spiegel, E.A. & Demètriades, T.D. (1925) Die zentrale Kompensation des Labyrinthverlustes. Pfluegers Arch. Gesamte Physiol. Meuschen Tiere 201, 215–222.

Stahle, J. (1958) Electronystagmography in the caloric and rotating test. Acta Oto-Laryngol. Suppl. 137, 1–83.

Stark, L. (1968) Neurological Control Systems. Plenum, New York.

Stark, L. (1982) The cerebellum as a calibrator organ. In: G. Lennerstrand, D. Zee & E. Keller (Eds.) Functional Basis of Ocular Motility Disorders. Pergamon Press, Oxford, pp. 467–470.

Stark, L. & Takahashi, Y. (1965) Absence of an odd-error signal mechanism in human accommodation. IEEE Trans. Biomed. Eng. BME–12, 138–146.

Stark, L., Vossius, G. & Young, L. (1962) Predictive control of eye tracking movements. IRE Trans. Hum. Factors Electron. HFE–3, 52–57.

Steer, R.W. (1970) Progress in vestibular modeling. Part I. Response of semicircular canals to constant rotation in a linear acceleration field. In: Fourth Symposium on the Role of the Vestibular Organs in Space Exploration. NASA SP–187, 353–360.

Steiner, F.A. & Weber, G. (1964) Die Beeinflussung vestibulär erregbarer Neurone des Hirnstamms durch elektrophoretisch appliziertes Acetylcholin. Helv. Physiol. Pharmacol. Acta. 22, C44–C46.

Steinhausen, W. (1933) Über die Beobachtung der Cupula in den Bogengansampullen des Labyrinths des lebenden Hechts. Arch. Ges. Physiol. 232, 500–512.

Steinman, R.M. & Collewijn, H. (1980) Binocular retinal image motion during active head rotation. Vision Res. 20, 415–429.

Steinman, R.M., Cushman, W.B. & Martins, A.J. (1982) The precision of gaze. Human Neurobiol. 1, 97–109.

Stensiö, E.A. (1927) The Downtonian and Devonian Vertebrates of Spitsbergen, Part 1. Family Cephalaspidae. Skr. om Svalbard og Nordischavet Nr. 12. Norske Vidensk. Akad., Oslo.

Stephens, P.R. & Young, J.Z. (1978) Semicircular canals in squids. Nature 271, 444–445.

Stephens, P.R. & Young, J.Z. (1982) The statocyst of the squid Loligo. J. Zool. London 197, 241–266.

Stone, J. (1978) The number and distribution of ganglion cells in the cat's retina. J. Comp. Neurol. 180, 753–772.

Stratton, G.M. (1897). Vision without inversion of the retinal image. Psychol. Rev. 4, 341–360.

Streeter, G.L. (1906/1907) On the development of the membranous labyrinth and the acoustic and facial nerves in the human embryo. Am. J. Anat. 6, 139–166.

Strong, N.P., Malach, R., Lee, P. & Van Sluyters, R.C. (1984) Horizontal optokinetic nystagmus in the cat. Recovery from cortical lesions. Der. Brain Res. 13, 179–192.

Stryker, M.P. & Sherk, H. (1975) Modification of cortical orientation selectivity in the cat by restricted visual experience. A reexamination. Science 190, 904–905.

Suzuki, J.-I., Cohen, B. & Bender, M.B. (1964) Compensatory eye movements induced by vertical semicircular canal stimulation. Exp. Neurol. 9, 137–160.

Szentágothai, J. (1943) Die zentrale Innervation der Augenbewegungen. Arch. Psychiatr. Nervenkr. 116, 721–760.

Szentágothai, J. (1950) The elementary vestibulo-ocular reflex arc. J. Neurophysiol. 13, 395–407.

Szentágothai, J. (1963) Ujabb adatok a synapsis functionalis anatómiájához. Magy. Tud. Akad. Biol. Orv. Oszt. Közl. 6, 217–227.

Tait, J. & McNally, W.J. (1934) Some features of the action of the utricular maculae (and of the associated action of the semicircular canals) of the frog. Phil. Trans. R. Soc. London, Ser. B 224, 241–268.

Takahashi, M., Igarashi, M. & Wright, W.K. (1977a) Damped pendular rotation nystagmus after unilateral labyrinthectomy or unilateral lateral semicircular canal block in squirrel monkeys. J. Otolaryngol. 6, 157–165.

Takahashi, M., Igarashi, M. & Homick, J.L. (1977b) Effect of otolith end organ ablation on horizontal optokinetic nystagmus and optokinetic after-nystagmus in the squirrel monkey. ORL 39, 74–81.

Takahashi, M., Uemura, T. & Fujishiro, T. (1980) Studies of the vestibulo-ocular reflex and visual-vestibular interactions during active head movements. Acta Oto-Laryngol. 90, 115–124.

Takahashi, M., Uemura, T. & Fufishiro, T. (1981) Compensatory eye movements and gaze fixation during active head rotation in patients with labyrinthine disorders. Ann. Oto-Laryngol. 90, 241–245.

Takeda, T. & Maekawa, K. (1976) The origin of the pretectoolivary tract. A study using the horseradish peroxi-dase method. Brain Res. 117, 319–325.

Takemori, S. & Cohen, B. (1974) Loss of visual suppression of vestibular nystagmus after flocculus lesions. Brain Res. 72, 213–224.

Tauber, E.S. & Atkin, A. (1968) Optomotor responses to monocular stimulation: relation to visual system organization. Science 160, 1365–1367.

Taylor, J.G. (1962) The behavioural basis of perception. Yale Univ. Press, New Haven and London.

Ten Bruggencate, G. & Engberg, I. (1971) Iontophoretic studies in Deiters' nucleus of the inhibitory actions of GABA and related amino acids and the interactions of strychnine and picrotoxin. Brain Res. 25, 431–448.

Ter Braak, J.W. (1936) Untersuchungen über optokinetischen Nystagmus. Arch. Neerl. Physiol. 21, 309–376.

Thach, W.T. (1968) Discharge of Purkinje and cerebellar nuclear neurons during rapidly alternating arm movements in the monkey. J. Neurophysiol., 31, 785–797.

Toates, F.M. (1972) Accommodation function of the human eye. Physiol. Rev. 52, 828–863.

Tolu, E., Mameli, O., Azzena, M.T. & Azzena, G.B. (1980) Dynamic responses of vestibular cells during spinal decompensation. Physiol. Behav. 25, 637–640.

Tomlinson, R.D., Saunders, G.E. & Schwarz, D.W. (1980) Analysis of human vestibulo-ocular reflex during active head movements. Acta Oto-Laryngol. 90, 184–190.

Tomlinson, R.D. & Robinson, D.A. (1981) Is the vestibulo-ocular reflex cancelled by smooth pursuit? In: A.F. Fuchs and W. Becker (Eds.) Progress in Oculomotor Research. Elsevier, Amsterdam, New York, pp. 533–539.

Tompsett, D.H. (1939) Sepia. L.M.B.C. Mem. Typ. Br. mar. Plant Anim. Liverpool 32.

Toupet, M. & Pialoux, P. (1981) Le nystagmus perverti. Ann. Oto-Laryngol. (Paris) 98, 319–338.

Trabal, I., Macadar, O., Cibilis, D. & Pereda, A. (1980) Dynamic analysis of the rightening reflex in the toad; the effects of hemilabyrinthectomy. Neurosci. Lett. Suppl. 5, 282.

Trendelenburg, W. & Kühn, A. (1908) Vergleichende Untersuchungen zur Physiologie des Ohrlabyrinthes der Reptilien. Arch. Anat. Suppl. 160–188.

Tretter, F., Singer, W. & Cynader, M. (1975) Modification of direction selectivity of neurons in the visual cortex of kittens. Brain Res. 84, 143–149.

Troelstra, A., Zuber, B.L., Miller, D. & Stark, L. (1964) Accommodative tracking: a trial-and-error function. Vision Res. 4, 585–594.

Tsukahara, N. (1981) Synaptic plasticity in the mammalian central nervous system. Ann. Rev. Neurosci. 4, 351–381.

Tsukahara, N. & Fujito, Y. (1976) Physiological evidence of formation of new synapses from cerebellum in the red nucleus neurons following cross-union of forelimb nerves. Brain Res. 106, 184–188.

Uchino, Y., Hirai, N. & Watanabe, S. (1978) Vestibulo-ocular reflex from the posterior canal nerve to extraocular motoneurons in the cat. Exp. Brain Res. 32, 337–388.

Uchino, Y., Hirai, N., Suzuki, S. & Watanabe, S. (1980a) Axonal branching in the trochlear and oculomotor nuclei of single vestibular neurons activated from the posterior semicircular nerve in the cat. Neurosci. Lett. 18, 283–288.

Uchino, Y., Suzuki, S. & Watanabe, S. (1980b) Vertical semicircular canal inputs to cat extraocular motoneurons. Exp. Brain Res. 41, 45–53.

Uchino, Y., Hirai, N. & Suzuki, S. (1982) Branching pattern and properties of vertical- and horizontal-canal related excitatory vestibulo-ocular neurons in the cat. J. Neurophysiol. 48, 891–903.

Uchino, Y. & Suzuki, S. (1983) Axon collaterals to extraocular motoneuron pools of inhibitory vestibuloocular neurons activated from the anterior, posterior, and horizontal semicircular canals in the cat. Neurosci. Lett. 37, 129–135.

Uemura, T. & Cohen, B. (1973) Effects of vestibular nuclei lesions on vestibulo-ocular reflexes and posture in monkeys. Acta Oto-Laryngol Suppl. 315, 1–71.

Uemura, T., Arai, Y. & Shimazaki, C. (1980) Eye-head coordination during lateral gaze in normal subjects. Acta Oto-Laryngol. 90, 191–198.

Valentinuzzi, M. (1967) An analysis of the mechanical forces in each semicircular canal of the cat under single and combined rotation. Bull. Math. Biophysics 29, 267–289.

Van der Steen, J. & Collewijn, H. (1984) Ocular stability in the horizontal, frontal and sagittal planes in the rabbit. Exp. Brain Res. 56, 263–274.

Versteegh, C. (1927) Ergebnisse Partieller Labyrinth Extirpation bei Kaninchen. Acta Oto-Laryngol. 9, 393–408.

Vidal, P.P., Roucoux, A. & Berthoz, A. (1982) Horizontal eye position related activity in neck muscles of the alert cat. Exp. Brain Res. 46, 448–453.

Vidal, P.P., Corvisier, J. & Berthoz, A. (1983a) Eye and neck motor signals in periabducens reticular neurons of the alert cat. Exp. Brain Res. 53, 16–28.

Vidal, P.P., Roucoux, A., Berthoz, A. & Crommelinck, M. (1983b) Eye position-related activity in deep neck muscles of the alert cat. In: E.R. Pfaltz (Ed.) Advances in Oto-Rhino-Laryngology, Neurophysiological and Clinical Aspects of Vestibular Disorders. Karger, Basel, Paris, London, New York, pp. 27–29.

Vidic, T.R., Barlow, J.S., Oman, C.M., Tole, J.R., Weiss. A.D. & Young, L.R. (1976) Human eye tracking during vertical and horizontal motion Soc. Neurosci. Abstr. II, 1062.

Vilis, T. & Hore, J. (1981) Characteristics of saccadic dysmetria in monkeys during reversible lesions of medial cerebellar nuclei. J. Neurophysiol. 46, 828–838.

Vilis, T., Snow, R. & Hore, J. (1982) Is cerebellar saccadic dysmetria equal in both eyes? Soc. Neurosci. Abstr. 12, 418.

Vilstrup, T. (1950) Studies on the Structure and Function of the Semicircular Canals. E. Munksgaard, Copenhagen.

Vital-Durand, F. & Jeannerod, M. (1974a) Maturation of the optokinetic response. Genetic and environmental factors. Brain Res. 71, 249–257.

Vital-Durand, F. & Jeannerod, M. (1974b) Role of visual experience in the development of optokinetic response in kittens. Exp. Brain Res. 20, 297–302.

Viviani, P. & Berthoz, A. (1975) Dynamics of the head neck system in response to small perturbations: analysis and modeling in the frequency domain. Biol. Cybern. 19, 19–37.

Volkmann, A.W. (1869) Zur Mechanik der Augenmuskeln. Ber. Sachs. Gesamte Akad. Wiss. 21, 28–69.

Voogd, J. & Bigaré, F. (1980) Topographical distribution of olivary and cortico nuclear fibers in the cerebellum: A review. In: J. Courville et al. (Eds.) The Inferior Olivary Nucleus. Raven Press, New York, pp. 207–234.

Vossius, G. (1972) Adaptive control of saccadic eye movements. Bibl. Ophthalmol. 82, 244–250.

Waespe, W. & Cohen, B. (1983) Flocculectomy and unit activity in the vestibular nuclei during visual-vestibular interactions. Exp. Brain Res. 51, 23–35.

Waespe, W. & Henn, V. (1977a) Neuronal activity in the vestibular nuclei of the alert monkey during vestibular and optokinetic stimulation. Exp. Brain Res. 27, 523–538.

Waespe, W. & Henn, V. (1977b) Vestibular nuclei activity during optokinetic afternystagmus (OKAN) in the alert monkey. Exp. Brain Res. 30, 323–330.

Waespe, W. & Henn, V. (1978a) Conflicting visual-vestibular stimulation and vestibular nucleus activity in alert monkeys. Exp. Brain Res. 33, 203–211.

Waespe, W. & Henn, V. (1978b) Reciprocal changes in primary and secondary optokinetic after-nystagmus (OKAN) produced by repetitive optokinetic stimulation in the monkey.

Arch. Psychiatr. Nervenkr. 225, 23–30.

Waespe, W. & Henn, V. (1979a) The velocity response of vestibular nucleus neurons during vestibular, visual, and combined angular acceleration. Exp. Brain Res. 37, 337–347.

Waespe, W. & Henn, V. (1979b) Motion information in the vestibular nuclei of alert monkeys: visual and vestibular input vs. optomotor output. In: R. Granit & O. Pompeiano (Eds.) Reflex Control of Posture and Movement. Progress in Brain Research Vol. 50. Elsevier, Amsterdam, pp. 683–693.

Waespe, W. & Henn, V. (1981) Visual-vestibular interaction in the flocculus of the alert monkey. II. Purkinje cell activity. Exp. Brain Res. 43, 349–360.

Waespe, W. & Henn, V. (1985) The primate flocculus in visualvestibular interactions: conceptual, neurophysiological and anatomical problems. In: J.R. Bloedel, J. Dichgans & W. Precht (Eds.) – Cerebellar Functions. Springer Verlag, Berlin, New York, pp. 109–125.

Waespe, W., Henn, V. & Miles, T.S. (1977) Activity in the vestibular nuclei of the alert monkey during spontaneous eye movements and vestibular and optokinetic stimulation. In: R. Baker & A. Berthoz (Eds.) Control of Gaze by Brain Stem Neurons. Elsevier, Amsterdam, pp. 269–278.

Waespe, W., Henn, V. & Isoviita, V. (1980) Nystagmus slow-phase velocity during vestibular, optokinetic, and combined stimulation in the monkey. Arch. Psychiatr. Nervenkr. 228, 275–286.

Waespe, W., Buettner, U. & Henn, V. (1981) Visual-vestibular interaction in the flocculus of the alert monkey. I. Input activity. Exp. Brain Res. 43, 337–348.

Waespe, W., Cohen, B. & Raphan, T. (1983) Role of the flocculus and paraflocculus in optokinetic nystagmus and visual-vestibular interactions: effects of lesions. Exp. Brain Res. 50, 9–33.

Waespe, W., Cohen, B. & Raphan, T. (1985) Dynamic modifications of the vestibulo-ocular reflex by the nodulus and uvula. Science, in press.

Wall, C., O'Leary, D.P. & Black, F.O. (1978) Systems analysis of vestibulo-ocular system response using white noise rotational stimuli. In: J.D. Hood (Ed.) Vestibular Mechanisms in Health and Disease. Academic Press, London, pp. 157 164.

Wallach, H., Frey, K.J. & Romney, G. (1969) Adaptation to field displacement during head movement unrelated to the constancy of visual direction. Percept. Psychophys. 5, 253–256.

Wallman, J., Velez, J., Weinstein, B. & Green, A.E. (1982) Avian vestibuloocular reflex: adaptive plasticity and developmental changes. J. Neurophysiol. 48, 952–967.

Watanabe, E. (1984) Neuronal events correlated with long-term adaptation of horizontal vestibuloocular reflex in the primate flocculus. Brain Res. 297, 169–174.

Watanabe, E. & Balaban, C.D. (1983) Functional representation of eye movements in the flocculus of monkeys (*Macaca fuscata*). Neurosci. Lett. Suppl. 13, S26.

Watt, D.G. & Tomi, L.M. (1983) Further studies of otolith-spinal reflex adaptation to altered gravity. Neurosci. Abstr. Vol. 9, p. 523, Abstr. 152.3.

Weaver, R.S. (1965) Theoretical aspects of the role of angular acceleration in vestibular stimulation. Acta Oto-Laryngol.

Suppl. 205, 5–37.

Weiland, C. (1898) Are our present ideas about the mechanism of the eye-movements correct? Arch. Ophthal., 27, 46–64.

Weiss, L. (1875) Zur Bestimmung des Drehpunktes im Auge. Albrecht von Graefes Arch. Ophthalmol. 21/2, 132–180.

Werner, C. F. (1930) Das Ohrlabyrinth der Elasmobranchier. Z. Wiss. Zool. 136, 485–579.

Werner, C. F. (1933) Das Ohrlabyrinth der Tiere. Ein Versuch seine Formverschiedenheit zu erklären. Passow-Schäfer's Beitr. Hals. Nas. Ohrenheilk. 30, 390–408.

Werner, C. F. (1960) Das Gehörorgan der Wirbeltiere und des Menschen. VEB Georg Thieme, Leipzig.

Wessely, K. (1916) Über den Einfluss der Augenbewegungen auf den Augendruck. Arch. Augenheilk. 81, 102–119.

Westheimer, G. (1955a) The relationship between accommodation and accommodative convergence. Am. J. Optom. Arch. Am. Acad. Optom. 32, 206–212.

Westheimer, G. (1955b) The inconstancy of the AC/A ratio. Am. J. Optom. Arch. Am. Acad. Optom. 32, 435–436.

Westheimer, G. (1957) Kinematics of the eye. J. Opt. Soc. Am. 67, 967–974.

Westheimer, G. (1963) Amphetamine, barbiturates, and accommodation-convergence. Arch. Ophthalmol. 70, 830–836.

Westheimer, G. (1982) Pathological physiology of binocular parallelism. In: G. Lennerstrand, D.S. Zee & E.L. Keller (Eds.) Functional Basis of Ocular Motility Disorders. Pergamon, Oxford, pp. 195–197.

Westheimer, G. & Blair, S.M. (1972) Mapping the visual sensory onto the visual motor system. Invest. Ophthalmol. 11, 490–496.

Westheimer, G. & Blair, S.M. (1973) Oculomotor defects in cerebellectomized monkeys. Invest. Ophthalmol. 12, 618–621.

Westheimer, G. & McKee, S.P. (1975) Visual acuity in the presence of retinal-image motion. J. Opt. Soc. Am. 65, 847–850.

Westheimer, G. & Mitchell, D. (1969) The sensory stimulus for disjunctive eye movements. Vision Res. 9, 749–755.

Whiteside, T.C. (1957) The Problems of Vision in Flight at High Altitude. Butterworths, London.

Whittaker, S.G. & Eaholtz, G. (1982) Learning patterns of eye motion for foveal pursuit. Invest. Ophthalmol. 23, 393–397.

Whittington, D., Lestienne, F. & Bizzi, E. (1984) Behaviour of preoculomotor brain stem neurons during eye-head coordination. Exp. Brain Res. 55, 215–222.

Wicklegren, B.G. & Sterling, P. (1969) Influence of visual cortex on receptive fields in the superior colliculus of the cat. J. Neurophysiol. 32, 16–23.

Wied, de, D. & Gispen, W.H. (1977) Behavioral effects of peptides. In: H. Gainer (Ed.) Peptides in Neurobiology. Plenum Press, New York, London, pp. 397–448.

Wiesel, T.N. & Hubel, D.H. (1965) Comparison of the effects of unilateral and bilateral eye closure on cortical unit responses in kittens. J. Neurophysiol. 28, 1029–1040.

Williams, P.L. & Warwick, R. (1975) Functional Neuroanatomy of Man. Saunders, Philadelphia.

Williams, S.R. (1902) Changes accompanying the migration of the eye and observations on the tractus opticus and tectum opticum in *Pseudopleuronectes americanus*. Bull. Mus. Comp. Zool. Harv. Univ. 40, 1–57.

Wilson, V.J. & Felpel, L.P. (1972) Specificity of semicircular canal input to neurons in the pigeon vestibular nuclei. J. Neurophysiol. 35, 253–264.

Wilson, V.J. & Melvill Jones, G. (1979) Mammalian Vestibular Physiology. Plenum, New York. 365 pp.

Wilson, V.J., Precht, W. & Dieringer, N. (1983) Responses of different compartments of cat's Splenius muscle to optokinetic stimulation. Exp. Brain Res. 50, 153–156.

Winterson, B.J. & Steinman, R.M. (1978) The effect of luminance on human smooth pursuit of perifoveal and foveal targets. Vision Res. 18, 1165–1172.

Wist, E.R., Brandt, T.H. & Krafczyks, S. (1983) Oscillopsia and retinal slip. Evidence supporting a clinical test. Brain 106, 153–168.

Witmack, K. (1909) Über die Veränderungen im Innen-Ohr nach Rotationen. Verh. Dtsch. Otol. Ges. 18, 105–156.

Woellner, R.C. & Graybiel, A. (1959) Counterrolling of the eyes and its dependence on the magnitude of gravitational or inertial force acting laterally on the body. J. Appl. Physiol. 14, 632–634.

Woellner, R.C. & Graybiel, A. (1960) The loss of counterrolling of the eyes in three persons presumably without functional otolith organs. Ann. Oto. Rhino. Laryngol. 69, 1–7.

Wolfe, J.W. & Kos, C.M. (1977) Nystagmic responses of the rhesus monkey to rotational stimulation following unilateral labyrinthectomy: final report. Trans. Am. Acad. Ophthalmol. Otolaryngol. 84, 38–45.

Wolpaw, J.R., Braitman, D.J. & Seegal. R.F. (1983a) Adaptive plasticity in primate spinal stretch reflex: Initial development. J. Neurophysiol. 50, 1296–1311.

Wolpaw, J.R., Seegal, R.F. & O'Keefe, J.A. (1983b) Adaptive plasticity in spinal stretch reflex: Behaviour of synergist and antagonistic muscles. J. Neurophysiol. 50, 1312–1329.

Wood, C.C., Spear, P.D. & Braun, J.J. (1973) Direction-specific deficits in horizontal optokinetic nystagmus following removal of visual cortex in the cat. Brain Res. 60, 231–237.

Wurtz, R.H. (1969). Response of striate cortex neurons to stimuli during rapid eye movements in the monkey. J. Neurophysiol. 32, 975–986.

Xerri, C. & Lacour, M. (1980) Compensation des déficits posturaux et cinétiques après neurectomie vestibulaire unilatérale chez le chat. Rôle de l'activité sensori-motrice. Acta Oto-Laryngol. 90, 414–424.

Xerri, C., Manzoni, D. & Pompeiano, O. (1981a) Response characteristics of lateral reticular neurons to sinusoidal tilt after unilateral labyrinthectomy. Arch. Ital. Biol. 119, 226–254.

Xerri, C., Manzoni, D. & Pompeiano, O. (1981b) Effects of cerebellectomy on responses of lateral reticular neurons to sinusoidal tilt after ipsilateral labyrinthectomy. Arch. Ital. Biol. 119, 255–277.

Xerri, C., Gianni, S., Manzoni, D. & Pompeiano, O. (1983) Response characteristics of lateral vestibular nucleus neurons to sinusoidal tilt after acute or chronic vestibular deafferentations. Acta Oto-Laryngol. 30,  – .

Yagi, T., Shimizu, M., Sekine, S. & Kamio, T. (1981) New neurootological test for detecting cerebellar dysfunction. Ves-

tibulo-ocular reflex changes with horizontal vision-reversal prisms. Ann. Otol. 90, 276–280.

Yamamoto, C. (1967) Pharmacologic studies of norepinephrine, acetylcholine and related compounds on neurons in Deiters' nucleus and the cerebellum. J. Pharmacol. Exp. Ther. 156, 39–47.

Yamamoto, M. (1978) Localization of rabbit's flocculus Purkinje cells projecting to the cerebellar lateral nucleus and the nucleus prepositus hypoglossi, investigated by means of the horseradish peroxidase retrograde axonal transport. Neurosci. Lett. 12, 29–34.

Yamazaki, A. & Zee, D.S. (1979) Rebound nystagmus: EOG analysis of a case with a floccular tumor. Br. J. Ophthalmol. 63, 782–786.

Yee, R.D., Baloh, R.W., Honrubia, V., Lau, C.G.Y. & Jenkins, H.A. (1979) Slow build-up of optokinetic nystagmus associated with downbeat nystagmus. Invest. Ophthalmol. 18, 622–629.

Yingcharoen, K. & Rinvik, E. (1983) Ultrastructural degeneration of a projection from the flocculus to the nucleus prepositus hypoglossi in the cat. Exp. Brain Res. 51, 192–198.

Yoshida, K., McCrea, R., Berthoz, A. & Vidal, P.-P. (1982) Morphological and physiological characteristics of inhibitory burst neurons controlling horizontal rapid eye movements in the alert cat. J. Neurophysiol. 48, 761, 784.

Young, J.Z. (1960) The statocysts of *Octopus vulgaris*. Proc. R. Soc. London Ser. B 152, 3–29.

Young, L. R. (1969) Biocybernetics of the vestibular system. In: L.D. Proctor (Ed) Biocybernetics of the central nervous system. Little, Brown and & Co. Boston, pp. 79–117.

Young, L.R. (1962) A sampled data model for eye tracking movements. Sc. D. Thesis, Dept. Aeronautics and Astronautics, MIT, Cambridge, Ma.

Young, L.R., (1982) Human orientation in space. AIAA Dryden Lecture in Research. AIAA–82–0422, 20th Aerospace Sciences Meeting, Orlando, FL.

Young, L.R. (1984) Perception of the body in space. In: I. Darian-Smith (Ed.) Handbook of Physiology — The Nervous System III, American Physiological Association. Waverly Press, Baltimore, MD, pp. 1023–1066.

Young, L.R., & Henn, V.S. (1974) Selective habituation of vestibular nystagmus by visual stimulation. Acta Oto-Laryngol. 77, 159–166.

Young, L.R. & Henn, V. (1975) Nystagmus induced by pitch and yaw rotation in monkeys. Fortschr. Zool. 23, 235–246.

Young, L.R. & Henn, V.S. (1976) Selective habituation of vestibular nystagmus by visual stimulation in the monkey. Acta Oto-L aryngol. 82, 165–171.

Young, L.R. & Graybiel, A. (1985) Linear acceleration detection by labyrinthine defective subjects. (in prep.)

Young, L.R. & Meiry, J.L. (1968) A revised dynamic otolith model. Aerosp. Med. 39, 606–608.

Young, L.R., Lichtenberg, B.K., Arrott, A.P., Crites, T.A., Oman, C.M. & Edelman, E.R. (1981) Ocular torsion on earth and in weightlessness. In: B. Cohen (Ed.) Vestibular and Oculomotor Physiology. Ann. N.Y. Acad. Sci. 374, 80–92.

Young, L.R., Watt, D.G., Money, K.E. & Lichtenberg, B.K. (1984) Spatial orientation in weightlessness and readaptation to earth's gravity. Science 225, 205–208.

Yules, R.B., Krebs, C.Q. & Gault, F.P. (1966) The physiology of the lateral vestibular nucleus. Exp. Neurol. 16, 172–180.

Zadeh, L. & Desoer, C. (1964) Linear System Theory: A State Approach. McGraw Hill, New York.

Zangemeister, W.H. & Stark, L. (1981) Active head rotation and eye-head coordination. In: B. Cohen (Ed.) Vestibular and Oculomotor Physiology. Ann. N.Y. Acad. Sci. 374, 540–559.

Zangemeister, W.H. & Stark, L. (1982) Gaze latency: variable interactions of head and eye latency. Exp. Neurol. 75, 389–406.

Zangemeister, W.H., Jones, A. & Stark, L. (1981a) Dynamics of head movement trajectories: main sequence relationship. Exp. Neurol. 71, 76–91.

Zangemeister, W.H., Lehman, S.L. & Stark, L. (1981b) Simulation of head movement trajectories: model and fit to main sequence. Biol. Cybern. 41, 19–32.

Zangemeister, W.H., Meinberg, O., Stark, L. & Hoyt, W.F. (1982) Eye-head coordination in homonymous hemianopsia. J. Neurol 226, 243–254.

Zasorin, N.L., Baloh, R.W., Yee, R.D. & Honrubia, V. (1983) Influence of vestibulo-ocular reflex gain on human optokinetic responses. Exp. Brain Res. 51, 271–274.

Zee, D.S. (1977) Disorders of eye-head coordination. In: B. Brooks & E.J. Bajandas (Eds.) Eye Movements. Plenum press, New York, pp. 9–40.

Zee, D.S. (1982) Ocular motor abnormalities related to lesions in the vestibulocerebellum in primate. In: G. Lennerstrand, D.S. Zee & E.L. Keller (Eds.) Functional Basis of Ocular Motility Disorders. Pergamon, Oxford, pp. 423–430.

Zee, D.S. & Robinson, D.A. (1979) Clinical applications of oculomotor models. In: H.S. Thompson, R. Daroff, L. Frisén, J.S. Glaser & M.D. Sanders (Eds.) Topics in Neuro-Ophthalmology. Williams & Wilkens, Baltimore, pp. 266–285.

Zee, D.S., Friendlich, A.R. & Robinson, D.A. (1974) The mechanism of downbeat nystagmus. Arch. Neurol. 30, 227–237.

Zee, D.S., Yee, R.D., Cogan, D.G., Robinson, D.A. & Engel, W.K. (1976a) Ocular motor abnormalities in hereditary cerebellar ataxia. Brain 99, 207–234.

Zee, D.S., Yee, R.D. & Robinson, D.A. (1976b) Optokinetic responses in labyrinthine-defective human beings. Brain Res. 113, 423–428.

Zee, D.S., Optican, L.M., Cook, J.D., Robinson, D.A., & Engel, W.K. (1976c) Slow saccades in spinocerebellar degeneration. Arch. Neurol. 33, 243–251.

Zee, D.S., Yamazaki, A., Butler, P.H. & Güger, G. (1981) Effects of ablation of flocculus and paraflocculus on eye movements in primate. J. Neurophysiol. 46, 878–899.

Zee, D.S., Preziosi, T.J. & Proctor, L.R. (1982a) Bechterew's phenomenon in a human patient. Ann. Neurol. 12, 495–496.

Zee, D.S., Butler, P.H., Optican, L.M., Tusa, R.J.& Gucer, G. (1982b) Effects of bilateral occipital lobectomies on eye movements in monkeys: preliminary observations. In: A. Roucoux & M. Grommelinck (Eds.) Physiological and Pathological Aspects of Eye movements. Dr. W. Junk, The Hague, pp. 225–232.

Zuckerman, H. (1967) The physiological adaptation to unilateral semicircular canal inactivation. McGill Med. J. 36, 8–13.

# Subject Index